Immunoassays
for the
80s

Immunoassays for the 80s

Edited by

**A. VOLLER, A. BARTLETT
and D. BIDWELL**

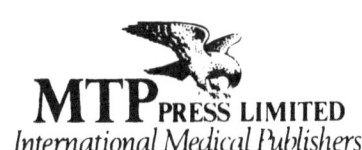

MTP PRESS LIMITED
International Medical Publishers

Published by
MTP Press Limited
Falcon House
Lancaster, England

Copyright © 1981 MTP Press Limited
Softcover reprint of the hardcover 1st edition 1981
First published 1981

ISBN-13: 978-94-009-8056-3   e-ISBN-13: 978-94-009-8056-3
DOI: 10.1007/978-94-009-8056-3
Phototypeset in 'Monophoto' Times New Roman by
Servis Filmsetting Limited, Manchester
Printed in Great Britain by
Robert MacLehose & Co. Limited, Renfrew

Contents

v

List of Contributors

E. M. E. ABU ELZEIN
Animal Virus Research Institute,
Woking, UK

S. AVRAMEAS
Unité d'Immunocytochimie,
Department de Biologie Moléculaire,
Institut Pasteur,
Paris, France

R. R. A. BACON
Immunoassay Section,
Department of Clinical Chemistry,
Edinburgh University,
Edinburgh, UK

IRENE BATTY
Consultant Immunologist,
Wellcome Foundation Executive Director,
European Committee for Clinical
  Laboratory Standards,
London, UK

A. E. BOLTON
Division of Biochemistry,
North East London Polytechnic,
London E15 4LZ, UK

C. L. CAMBIASO
Unit of Experimental Medicine,
ICP – Université Catholique de Louvain,
Brussels, Belgium

D. CATTY
Department of Immunology,
University of Birmingham,
Birmingham, UK

G. S. CHALLAND
ARES Applied Research Systems Ltd,
Welwyn Garden City, UK

SHIREEN CHANTLER
Wellcome Research Laboratories,
Beckenham, UK

M. D. CHAPMAN
Division of Immunological Medicine,
Clinical Research Centre,
Harrow, UK

M. F. CLARK
Department of Plant Pathology,
East Malling Research Station,
Maidstone, UK

D. COLLET-CASSART
Unit of Experimental Medicine,
ICP – Université Catholique de Louvain,
Brussels, Belgium

R. R. A. COOMBS
Department of Pathology,
University of Cambridge,
Addenbrooke's Hospital,
Hills Road,
Cambridge CB2 2QQ, UK

J. R. CROWTHER
Experimental Pathology (Immunology
  Section),
Animal Virus Research Institute,
Woking, UK

J. A. DIMENT
Wellcome Research Laboratories,
Beckenham, UK

C. C. DRAPER
Ross Institute of Tropical Hygiene,
London School of Hygiene and Tropical
  Medicine,
London, UK

R. EKINS
Sub-Department of Molecular Biophysics,
Institute of Nuclear Medicine,
The Middlesex Hospital Medical School,
London W1N 8AA, UK

C. C. ENTWISTLE
UK Transplant Service,
South West Regional Transfusion Centre,
Bristol, UK

P. S. GARDNER
Division of Microbiological Reagents and
    Quality Control,
Central Public Health Laboratory,
London, UK

P. G. H. GELL
Department of Pathology,
University of Cambridge,
Tennis Court Road,
Cambridge, UK

A. A. GLYNN
Department of Bacteriology,
Wright-Fleming Institute,
St. Mary's Hospital Medical School,
London, UK

K. GRIFFITHS
Tenovus Institute for Cancer Research,
Welsh National School of Medicine,
Heath Park,
Cardiff CF4 4XX, UK

M. HJELM
Department of Chemical Pathology,
The Hospital for Sick Children,
Great Ormond Street,
London WC1N 3JH, UK

E. J. HOLBOROW
Bone & Joint Research Unit,
University of London,
London, UK

W. M. HUNTER
MRC Immunoassay Team,
Edinburgh, UK

C. ISON
Bacteriology Department,
Wright-Fleming Institute,
St. Mary's Hospital Medical School,
London WA 1PG, UK

G. D. JOHNSON
Bone and Joint Research Unit,
University of London,
London, UK

B. G. JOYCE
Tenovus Institute for Cancer Research,
Welsh National School of Medicine,

Heath Park,
Cardiff CF4 4XX, UK

R. S. KAMEL
Department of Chemical Pathology,
St. Bartholomew's Hospital,
London, UK

HEATHER A. KEMP
Department of Medical Biochemistry,
Welsh National School of Medicine,
Heath Park,
Cardiff, UK

K. W. KEMP
Department of Mathematical Statistics and
    Operations Research,
University College,
Cardiff, UK

J. LANDON
Department of Chemical Pathology,
St. Bartholomew's Hospital,
London, UK

N. R. LING
Department of Immunology,
University of Birmingham,
Birmingham, UK

J. A. LOWE
Department of Immunology,
University of Birmingham,
Birmingham, UK

D. W. R. MACKENZIE
Mycological Reference Laboratory,
London School of Hygiene and Tropical
    Medicine,
London, UK

I. McKENZIE
MRC Immunoassay Team,
Edinburgh, UK

M. L. McLAREN
Ross Institute of Tropical Hygiene,
London School of Hygiene and Tropical
    Medicine,
London, UK

C. G. MAGNUSSON
Unit of Experimental Medicine,
ICP – Université Catholique de Louvain,
Brussels, Belgium

RUTH MARCH
Bone and Joint Research Unit,

University of London,
London, UK

V. MARKS
Department of Biochemistry,
University of Surrey,
Guildford GU2 5XH, UK

P. L. MASSON
Unit of Experimental Medicine,
ICP – Université Catholique de Louvain,
Brussels, Belgium

L. R. MATHIESEN
Enterovirus Department,
State Serum Institute,
Copenhagen, Denmark

L-A. NILSSON
Departments of Bacteriology and Clinical
    Immunology,
Institute of Medical Microbiology,
Göteborg, Sweden

A. B. J. NIX
Department of Mathematical Statistics and
    Operations Research,
University College,
Cardiff, UK

T. OLSSON
Department of Clinical Chemistry,
Huddinge University Hospital,
S-141 42 Huddinge, Sweden

M. B. PEPYS
Department of Immunological Medicine,
Royal Postgraduate Medical School,
London, UK

T. A. E. PLATTS-MILLS
Division of Immunological Medicine,
Clinical Research Centre,
Harrow, UK

C. RAYKUNDALIA
Department of Immunology,
University of Birmingham,
Birmingham, UK

G. F. READ
Tenovus Institute for Cancer Research,
Welsh National School of Medicine,
Heath Park,
Cardiff CF4 4XX, UK

JANE REEBACK
Bone and Joint Research Unit,

University of London,
London, UK

DIANA RIAD-FAHMY
Tenovus Institute for Cancer Research,
Welsh National School of Medicine,
Heath park,
Cardiff CF4 4XX, UK

R. J. ROWLANDS
Department of Mathematical Statistics and
    Operations Research,
University College,
Cardiff, UK

K. E. RUBENSTEIN
Project Administration,
Syva Company,
Palo Alto,
California, USA

C. J. M. SINDIC
Unit of Experimental Medicine,
ICP – Université Catholique de Louvain,
Brussels, Belgium

A. THORE
Department of Clinical Chemistry,
Huddinge University Hospital,
S-141 42 Huddinge, Sweden

E. TOVEY
Division of Immunological Medicine,
Clinical Research Centre,
Harrow, UK

M. VEJTORP
Rubella Department,
State Serum Institute,
Copenhagen, Denmark

N. J. WALD
ICRF Cancer Epidemiology and Clinical
    Trials Unit,
Radcliffe Infirmary,
Oxford, UK

R. F. WALKER
Tenovus Institute for Cancer Research,
Welsh National School of Medicine,
Heath Park,
Cardiff CF4 4XX, UK

D. W. WILSON
Tenovus Institute for Cancer Research,
Welsh National School of Medicine,
Heath Park,
Cardiff CF4 4XX, UK

J. S. WOODHEAD
Department of Medical Biochemistry,
Welsh National School of Medicine,
Heath Park,
Cardiff, UK

A. J. ZUCKERMAN
Department of Medical Microbiology,
London School of Hygiene and Tropical
  Medicine,
London, UK

Preface

Analyses for naturally occurring biological substances or administered materials have been with us for many years. These were usually based on the physical or chemical characteristics of the substances to be measured. However in recent years there has been an explosion of interest in analytical methods which made use of the high specificity and sensitivity of immunological reactions. These methods can be very simple in terms of technical procedures and can usually be performed on minute samples of biological fluids – factors which have ensured their ready acceptance in most laboratories.

Recently there have been numerous meetings on technical aspects of particular immunoassays and on their application in specific diseases. We felt however that the time was ripe for an 'overview' of the whole field. To this end a conference on 'Immunoassays for the 80s' was held at the Zoological Society of London in 1980, and this book is largely based on that meeting. Both the immunoassay techniques and their numerous applications were discussed and are dealt with at length in this volume.

The editors wish to thank all the contributors for their chapters and to acknowledge the debt they owe to Jean Ryan (NLCM) without whose organization and assistance this volume would not have been completed.

A.V., D.B., A.B.

Part I
Immunoassay
Techniques

1
Historical Perspectives

P. G. H. GELL

Immunological methods have been used for analysis ever since the demonstration of 'optimal proportions' in the early 1920s, at a time when playing with such things was still a 'hobby for gentlemen'. One may say nevertheless that quantitative immunology dated from this discovery, which led to a crucially important clinical advance, namely the definition of 'units' of toxins and antitoxins. This made possible rational immunotherapy and immunoprophylaxis in diphtheria and other diseases. Based on this understanding, *in vivo* tests using groups of animals allowed estimations down to the microgram level of either reagent; and the tests were good in that the activities measured (toxicity of toxin, protective power of antisera) were those relevant to clinical use. Developments in the 1930s gave a clearer picture of the nature of determinant groups of epitopes. The immunogenicity of chemically combined haptens was described and determinant groups were shown to have molecular sizes of around 200–1000 daltons. After the development of isotopic labelling the complete set-up was available for very precise immunoassays of high, medium or low molecular weight substances by competition methods. The very great advances of the 1950s in knowledge of antibody structure and cellular immunology were only marginally relevant to immunoassays. In view of the passage of 30 years it is disappointing that the assay of small molecules, such as drugs and neurotransmitters, has not developed more rapidly. However methods for estimating peptide and other hormones of intermediate molecular weight have proceeded in step with their discovery.

A real advance in convenience and sensitivity has been gained in recent years by the use of enzyme-labelled, instead of radio labelled, reagents. This allows one to use simple colorimeters rather than gamma-counters, which are not always reliable. It is possible that a current major advance is in the use of monoclonal antibodies in immunoassays. This means that we can obtain antibodies of uniform avidity and affinity directed at a single definable epitope. Although these properties may appear at first to be just a nuisance, compared to the blunderbuss activities of conventional antisera, there is little doubt that in spite of the formidable difficulties in defining the precise specificity of a monoclonal antibody derived from a hybridoma, and the influence upon experimental conditions entailed by the uniform and possibly not very high avidity, the improved precision of such antibodies cannot fail to contribute to improvement of test systems.

2
Merits and Disadvantages of Different Labels and Methods of Immunoassay

R. EKINS

INTRODUCTION

Antibodies comprise molecules of biological origin generally possessing a very high degree of structural specificity; this renders them especially suitable for use as 'specific reagents' in assays designed for the measurement of biological substances such as hormones, vitamins, viral and tumour antigens, etc. – particularly those of large molecular size and complex composition. Nevertheless antibodies constitute only one of several classes of biological compound endowed with a high capacity for molecular recognition, sharing this property with – for example – hormone 'receptors' located within or on the surface of target cells, specific 'transport' proteins, enzymes, etc. Each of these classes of 'binding substance' can be exploited, for assay purposes, in techniques virtually identical in concept and in experimental detail with 'immunoassay'. In short, from the standpoint of the assayist, antibodies are distinguished from other specific 'binding proteins' chiefly by virtue of their origin and mode of production; otherwise there is little to distinguish 'immunoassay' methods from a wide group of analogous techniques relying on essentially identical analytical principles.

Thus, in this presentation I propose to use the term 'immunoassay' as representing an analytical method relying on the use of an antibody as the 'specific reagent'* whilst recognizing that many of the concepts herein

* The term 'immunoassay' has also frequently been used to describe assays in which an antibody represents the analyte irrespective of whether or not an antibody is used as the 'specific reagent' in the procedure. Although hallowed by tradition, this use of the term departs from the general convention, whereby the prefix applied to the word 'assay' is descriptive of the nature of the assay system rather than that of the analyte, e.g. 'bioassay'.

5

discussed have a wider applicability than to those assays which are based on antibodies *per se*.

BASIC PRINCIPLES OF IMMUNOASSAY

All assays fundamentally rely on interaction between the analyte and a 'specific' analytical reagent. The term 'specific' as employed here is, of course, a relative one; virtually no reagent is absolutely specific in the sense that it will react solely with a single analyte of unique molecular composition or structure. Although the specificity of an assay system often relies heavily on the specificity of the 'analytical reagent' used in the basic analytical reaction, additional specificity may be imparted to a system relying on an analytical reagent of low specificity by extraction and purification of the analyte prior to its exposure to the 'reagent' (e.g. by chromatographic techniques).

The term 'analytical reagent' as used above is intended to embrace both physical reagents (e.g. ultraviolet light, electron beams) and chemical reagents (e.g. specific binding proteins). Moreover it is intended to refer essentially to the reagent which, by interaction with the analyte, enables the amount of the latter to be quantified (i.e. it is not intended to refer to substances such as solvents, or to other reagents which are used, for example, in connection with preliminary extraction or purification procedures).

Immunoassay systems (i.e. those relying on antibody as the specific analytical reagent) may be subdivided into two main classes distinguished by their respective reliance on (a) observation of the reagent (antibody) and (b) observation of the analyte, following interaction between the two, as the basis of the analytical measurement. For reasons discussed below, it is usual (though not obligatory) that the design of assays of Type I is based on the use of an *excess* (usually large) of antibody over analyte; conversely assays of Type II rely on the use of an amount of antibody *less than* the amount of analyte in the system (i.e. a 'saturable' amount of antibody). Expressed in their simplest form, the concepts underlying the two forms of assay may be expressed thus:

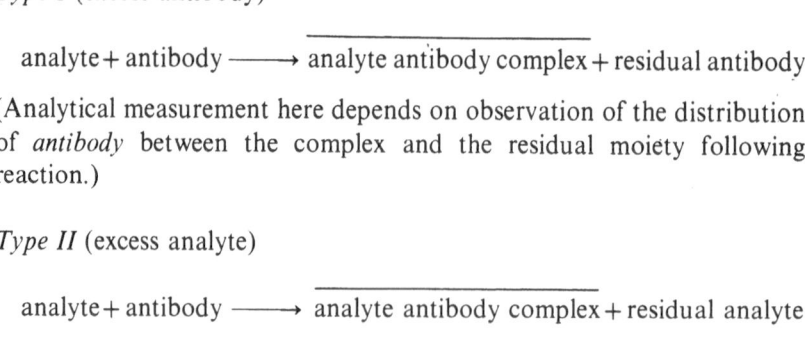

Type I (excess antibody)

analyte + antibody ⟶ analyte antibody complex + residual antibody

(Analytical measurement here depends on observation of the distribution of *antibody* between the complex and the residual moiety following reaction.)

Type II (excess analyte)

analyte + antibody ⟶ analyte antibody complex + residual analyte

(Analytical measurement here depends on observation of the distribution of *analyte* between the complex and the residual fraction following reaction.)

These two forms of assay inevitably share many methodological features; nevertheless the fundamental difference in the concepts on which they rely manifests itself, *inter alia*, in the manner in which assays of each type should be 'designed' and in their relative sensitivity and specificity characteristics. This difference arises essentially from the differing impact of the Law of Mass Action on systems of each type.

With regard to the ultimate sensitivities attainable by the two approaches, it is evident that, considering an assay of Type I, however little analyte may be present in a test sample, an amount of antibody may be introduced into the assay system sufficient to ensure that *some* of the antibody will combine with analyte to form the complex in a given time-interval, however short this may be. This follows from consideration of the rate of formation of complex which is given by:

$$\text{rate of complex formation} = k_1[\text{An}][\text{Ab}]$$

where k_1 = associative rate constant
and [An] and [Ab] are the analyte and antibody concentrations respectively.

Indeed, the existence of even a single molecule of analyte can, in principle, be revealed by introducing a sufficiency of antibody into the system to ensure that the analyte molecule will react to form the antibody–analyte complex. These considerations reveal that

(1) the ultimate sensitivity of an assay system of Type I is one molecule of the analyte; and
(2) that maximal sensitivity in such a system is attained using an amount of Ab approaching infinity.

In contrast, systems of Type II essentially depend on the notion of 'saturation' of antibody-binding sites by analyte. Although this notion represents something of an over-simplification, it may readily be shown that maximal sensitivity of an assay system in this category is achieved when the antibody concentration approaches zero[1].

However, it also follows that the measurement of very small concentrations of analyte necessarily demands the use of very low concentrations of antibody; this in turn implies exceedingly low rates of analyte–antibody complex formation, and a correspondingly low concentration of complex in the mixture following attainment of thermodynamic equilibrium.

The upshot of these considerations is that it may be shown that the ultimate sensitivity of a 'Type II' or 'saturation assay' system is governed by the equilibrium constant (K) of the reaction between analyte and antibody, and is given by ε/K where ε is the relative error in the experimental estimate of the amount (or fraction) of analyte in the complex[2]. In practice, since the equilibrium constants characterizing even the most avid antigen–antibody reactions seldom surpasses 10^{12} l/mol, and since the experimental errors incurred in assay systems of this type never, in practice, fall below 1% the maximal sensitivity theoretically attainable in a Type II system using conventionally prepared antibodies is of the order of 1×10^{-14} mol/l, i.e. approximately 10^7 molecules/ml. In practice assays of this type have never achieved sensitivities significantly superior to this.

SPECIFICITY

Non-specificity of an immunoassay system can arise as a result of two prime effects:

(1) 'cross-reaction' of substances structurally resembling the analyte;
(2) effects of ions and other substances on the kinetics of the analyte–antibody reaction.

(Other causes of assay non-specificity also exist: they are of less fundamental importance and will not be considered in the present discussion.)

The effects of each of these two sources of non-specificity are different in assays of either type and are best considered separately.

'Cross-reaction'

Type I assays

The notion of 'cross-reaction' rests on the proposition that an antibody is capable of reaction with two molecules sharing a common, or closely similar, antigenic determinant. Assuming that a single 'monoclonal' antibody population is present in large excess *vis-à-vis* two cross-reacting antigens, it is evident that the number of antibodies forming complexes with each of the two antigens will be broadly proportional to the respective numbers of antigen molecules present, irrespective of the respective energies of reaction between the two antigens and the antibody. In short, the two antigens will appear 'equipotent' in this type of system.

In addition to true 'cross-reactivity', the question of antibody heterogeneity must also be considered. Assuming an antiserum to comprise a mixed population of antibodies endowed with differing 'structural specificities', and assuming that any antibody purification procedures have not succeeded in isolating a single 'species' of antibody, then it is plausible that certain antibodies in the mixture will react with antigens other than the antigen of interest. Such substances will likewise appear equipotent in the assay system.

Type II assays

In this type of assay system – as a result of the reliance on amounts of antibody less than, or comparable to, the amount of analyte present – the effect of cross-reacting antigens is considerably more complex. In essence, the potency of a cross-reactant is a complex function of the 'occupancy' of antibody by the analyte or – alternatively stated – of the fractional binding by antibody of the analyte. In the simplest circumstances, in which a single species of antibody is present, the effect on the assay system of a cross-reactant may be expressed thus[3]:

$$\text{Relative potency (of cross-reactant)} = b + \left(f \frac{K_c}{K*} \right)$$

where b = fraction of analyte bound to antibody

f = fraction of analyte 'free'

$K*, K_c$ = equilibrium constants of analyte v. cross-reactant respectively.

The implication of this equation is that, in circumstances in which the analyte is entirely antibody-bound following reaction, the cross-reactant will be equipotent; conversely, in circumstances in which the analyte is entirely free, then the cross-reactant will display a relative potency given by the ratio of the two equilibrium constants. (These represent extremes which, of course, are never normally attained in a practical assay system.)

The situation is naturally greatly complicated by the presence in antisera of heterogeneous antibody-binding sites possessing differing 'cross-reactivities' characterized by varying 'avidity ratios' ($K_c/K*$) and by the relative concentrations of antibodies falling within each class, etc. A particular point of dissimilarity from assays falling into Type I is that the existence of antibodies in the mixture reacting with antigens other than the analyte, and entirely non-reactive with the analyte, have no influence on the system, i.e. such antigens have a zero relative potency in Type II assays as compared with a relative potency of unity in Type I assays.

The outcome of these general considerations is that, in a Type I system, much greater reliance is implicitly placed on the 'purity' of the specific antibody employed. Moreover all cross-reactants tend to display equal potencies in such a system. In contrast, in Type II assays, homogeneity of antibody is less important; indeed it is conventional to set up such assays using antiserum *per se* rather than an isolated and purified antibody. Because the majority of 'cross-reactants' are likely to be less avidly bound than the analyte by the principal specific antibody present, a Type II system is inherently more specific than one of Type I, albeit the additional measures of antibody purification which are frequently adopted in the development of Type I systems usually preclude a straightforward comparison.

Effects on kinetics of antibody–analyte reactions

Type I assays

Because, in assays of this type, the antibody is normally introduced in considerable excess (thus 'driving' the analyte towards complex formation), such systems are relatively invulnerable to any environmental influences which alter the equilibrium constant of the reaction. In this sense Type I assays are highly specific, i.e. influenced by substances (such as salt, urea) which influence the kinetics of antibody–antigen reactions.

Type II assays

In contrast, the design constraints placed upon Type II assays render them especially vulnerable to influences which alter the equilibrium constant of the basic reactions; they are, in short, more responsive to substances in biological fluids which, whilst not explicitly competing with the analyte in its reaction with the specific antibody, disturb its distribution between bound and free moieties, and thereby bias the assay result.

Thus, in summary, it is evident that the differing assay designs (arising from the quest for high assay sensitivity) which are imposed in the two forms of assay system have contrasting implications with respect to assay specificity. In general the 'saturation assay' systems (Type II) are more susceptible to disturbances arising from the presence of substances which influence the kinetics of antibody–antigen reactions, whilst being less influenced by cross-reacting antigens. Converse effects are seen in Type II assays, albeit direct comparison is made difficult by the practice of antibody 'purification' which is normally performed in the course of the setting up of Type I assays.

'SANDWICH' OR 'TWO-SITE' IMMUNOASSAYS

This type of assay essentially comprises a Type I system which is preceded by 'immuno-extraction' of the analyte. Typically an antibody is coupled to a solid support such as cellulose or Sephadex particles, a plastic surface, or glass micro-beads and exposed to the analyte-containing biological fluid. This results in removal of the analyte in the form of a primary antibody–analyte complex which is subsequently exposed to a second specific antibody, generally directed towards a second antigenic site on the analyte molecule. Assuming the analyte to be of sufficient molecular size, and the antigenic sites on its surface to be situated in such a manner that no steric hindrance between the two antibodies occurs, an antibody 'sandwich' will be formed in which the analyte constitutes the 'filling'. The analytical measurement ultimately depends on observation of the final distribution of the second antibody between analyte-bound and free moieties in the way characteristic of Type I assays. Clearly the particular advantage of this approach is that the analyte must be characterized by two geometrically separated and (usually) molecularly distinct binding sites. This imparts a much higher degree of specificity to the overall system.

USE OF 'LABELS'

In the foregoing discussion, two basic principles of measurement using antibodies as specific assay reagents have been identified. 'Labelling' agents, such as radioisotopes, enzymes, red cells, may be employed in assay techniques of either category primarily to assist in the observation of the distribution of antibody (Type I) or analyte (Type II) respectively. Clearly an assay of Type I relies upon labelling of the reagent (i.e. antibody); an assay of Type II on the labelling of analyte. Hence alternative descriptions of these two forms of technique are 'labelled antibody' and 'labelled analyte' methods respectively. For the purposes of the present discussion, we can assume that the presence of the label does not alter the reaction behaviour of the antibody or analyte in each case, and the effects on sensitivity and/or specificity of using a 'labelled analyte' chemically different, and displaying altered reactivity, from the unlabelled analyte will not be pursued here.

It is convenient to distinguish the two forms of analytical approach by distinctive nomenclature: for example, radioimmunoassay (RIA) represents a Type II form of technique in which the analyte is labelled with a radioisotope. Conversely, immunoradiometric assay (IRMA) represents a radiolabelled antibody, or Type I assay. Likewise enzyme immunoassay (EIA) and immunoenzymometric assay (IEMA) are terms which can be applied to analogous techniques using enzyme labels. Unfortunately the clarity and logical advantages of such a nomenclature have not prevailed, and terms such as 'RIA', for example, are often applied indiscrimately to techniques falling into both Type I and Type II categories. This is particularly unfortunate in so far as the misuse of nomenclature has tended to confuse discussion regarding, for example, the relative merits of different labels, as when the sensitivity of enzyme-labelled antibody techniques is compared with that of radioimmunoassay[4]. Such comparisons are clearly misleading in that, whilst purporting to illustrate the relative advantages of different forms of label, they implicitly reflect the relative merits of two underlying analytical principles.

EFFECTS OF LABEL ON ASSAY SENSITIVITY

In an earlier section, we have seen that the theoretical sensitivity of the labelled antibody (Type I) techniques is one molecule of analyte; that of the labelled analyte (Type II) techniques is ε/K. These ultimate sensitivity limits are a direct consequence of Mass Action effects; however, another constraint is imposed, in assays of each type, by the characteristics of the 'signal detection' system which is used to perceive the labelled antibody or analyte as the case may be.

In assays of Type I, the practical sensitivity (or detection limit) of the system is governed by the minimum number of antibody molecules bound to analyte which can be distinguished from any 'noise' or background level that may exist. There are, in short, two prime factors which govern the detection limit of these systems:

(1) the background or noise level and its statistical variation;
(2) the 'specific activity' of the labelled antibody, i.e. the number of observable events/unit time for each antibody molecule.

Thus the theoretical sensitivity limit of a labelled antibody assay system (one molecule of analyte) will only be attained in practice if there exists a negligible 'background' signal, and the labelled antibody binding to the analyte molecule emits a perceptible signal during the period of observation.

Clearly different labels will possess different characteristics in relation to each of the above parameters. For example, if we assume that, using a sandwich-type IRMA technique, we entirely remove 'free' labelled antibody from the solid-linked antibody–analyte-labelled antibody complex, we will nevertheless be faced with a typical radioactive background of 30 c/min. Meanwhile assuming the use of monoiodinated ^{125}I-labelled antibody, and a counter efficiency of 50%, the 'signalling rate' yielded by the labelled antibody will be approximately 1 ct/min per 250 000 molecules. A simple calculation will demonstrate that, given counting times of a minute or two, a minimum of the order of 10^6 labelled molecules will be required to yield a signal which is statistically distinguishable from the background count.

Radioactive labels are, in short, of relatively low specific activity when this parameter is expressed in terms of the proportion of labelled antibody molecules that generate a detectable event within a given time-interval and implicitly restrict the sensitivity attainable using labelled antibody techniques.

Other labels – for example enzymes – are capable of signal amplification in so far as a single molecule of enzyme may catalyse the conversion of many molecules of substrate to form an observable product. Nevertheless little benefit will stem from amplification of this kind if the detection system employed to measure the product of this reaction is itself relatively insensitive.

Meanwhile yet other labels, whilst they may be capable of yielding high 'specific activities', may be associated with high noise, or background, levels generated by components of the assay system other than the labelled antibody *per se*. Typical of such labels are fluorophores such as fluorescein, whose fluorescence must generally be viewed against a background of fluorescence generated by biological materials such as proteins, antibody supports such as plastics, etc.

A general disadvantage of the majority of non-isotopic labels in the present context is their vulnerability to environmental effects which modulate the activity of the label *per se*. Clearly, the radioactive labels, whose disintegration is quite unaffected by chemical or physical factors, are exceedingly 'rugged' in this sense.

In assays of the labelled analyte variety (Type II systems), assay sensitivity is fundamentally constrained by ε (the relative error in the measurement of bound analyte – assuming that observation is made of the bound moiety) and the equilibrium constant (K) of the reaction.

The error in the measurement of the bound moiety is, in turn, made up of two components: the error in the measurement of the signal *per se*, and the error introduced by the various manipulations – pipetting of antibody and labelled analyte; separation of antibody–analyte complex from free analyte, etc. Thus, the sensitivity attainable in Type II systems may be expressed as:

$$\frac{1}{K} \sqrt{\varepsilon_s^2 + \varepsilon_e^2}$$

where ε_s and ε_e are the signal detection and manipulation components of the error respectively.

The effect of the use of labels of different specific activities in such systems is somewhat complex: in particular the introduction of a relatively large amount of labelled analyte of low specific activity into such a system, whilst minimizing the signal detection error, may enlarge the 'manipulation error' as a result of statistical variations in the pipetting of the labelled analyte. Nevertheless it may readily be shown that increase in the specific activity of the label beyond a certain point has little or no effect on assay sensitivity since this is ultimately constrained by the many other factors which determine the magnitude of ε_e.

This phenomenon has been long recognized in the field of RIA, and the fact that increased sensitivity cannot be achieved by increasing the specific activity of the radioactively labelled analyte used in these procedures is now generally accepted.

A fundamental implication of this observation is that the sensitivity of conventional RIA cannot, in general, be improved upon by the use of alternative labels in assays of Type II. Indeed, since the error in the signal measurement *per se* in the radioisotopic techniques can normally be readily reduced to 1% or less, and since the precision of measurement of many other labels is generally rather less than this in practice, it is not surprising that other labels rarely, if ever, yield assay systems possessing the sensitivities attainable by RIA.

PRACTICAL IMPLICATIONS

In the foregoing sections we have been generally concerned, in the broadest sense, with the characteristics of the two fundamental principles of analytical measurement based on the use of antibodies as specific reagents. Amongst the general conclusions that can be drawn are:

(1) that 'labelled antibody' methods are intrinsically capable of sensitivities many orders of magnitude greater than 'labelled analyte' methods;
(2) that radiolabelled antibody methods (IRMA) – because of specific activity considerations – are unlikely to prove of significantly greater sensitivity than radiolabelled analyte (RIA) methods;
(3) that – because of Mass Action effects – the speed of labelled antibody methods can be made much greater than the labelled analyte methods, i.e. significantly shorter incubation times are demanded;
(4) that assay specificity is enhanced by the use of sandwich or two-site antibody recognition systems;
(5) that the sensitivity of RIA methods cannot in general be enhanced by the use of non-isotopic labels; conversely the sensitivity of IRMA techniques can be significantly increased by the use of non-isotopic labels (possibly involving signal amplification) and which display higher 'specific activities' than those characterizing radioisotopes.

These general predictions find total support in the experimental experience gained during the past two decades. Despite very large investments by academic and industrial institutions, non-isotopic assays of Type II (i.e. those relying on the use of labelled analytes) have only rarely approached, and have never surpassed, the sensitivities attainable by RIA. Likewise IRMA techniques have generally been of the same order of sensitivity as RIA (i.e of the order of 10^{-15} to 10^{-14} mol/l). However a recently described labelled antibody assay system[5], relying on the enzyme alkaline phosphatase as label, and its catalysis of the conversion of a radioisotopically labelled substrate ([^{3}H]AMP) to a labelled product ([^{3}H]adenosine), has demonstrated the validity of the proposition that labelled antibody methods are capable of sensitivities orders of magnitude greater than labelled analyte techniques by attaining a sensitivity of 10^{-21} moles (i.e. 600 molecules).

These considerations point to the replacement of RIA techniques as the principle and most ubiquitous immunoassay method in the last decade, by labelled antibody techniques in the next. One of the principal impediments to this development is the ready availability of relatively large quantities of pure antibody for the particular analyte of interest; this limitation is ultimately likely to be circumvented by the development of the hybridoma techniques pioneered by Milstein and Köhler[6] during the past two or three years and which are to be discussed in later chapters.

Meanwhile to exploit the full sensitivity potential implicit in labelled antibody methods, it is necessary to develop labels capable of yielding very high effective specific activities. One possible line of attack lies in the use of chemiluminescent molecules as described by Simpson et al[7]. Another is the use of fluorescent markers – accompanied by noise-reduction techniques – particularly the chelated rare-earth fluorophores[8]. These fluorescent materials possess the particular merit of a delayed fluorescence arising from the time-lapse involved in the transfer of energy from the chelating molecule to the chelated metal ion. The effect of this is to prolong the pulse of fluorescent light (generated by a pulse of incident light from a pulsed laser or xenon source) as compared with the fluorescence yielded by the majority of fluorescent materials found in biological fluids, plastics, etc. By appropriate electronic gating, and the use of very fast circuitry, it is possible to delay observation of the fluorescent light pulse until virtually all background fluorescence has decayed away, thus greatly enhancing the signal/noise ratio. Moreover, because incident light pulses can be of exceedingly short duration, very high energy inputs, amounting to many kilowatts of light energy, can be directed upon fluorescently labelled molecules without danger of overheating or bleaching and consequent destruction of the marker.

Such a technique offers, in short, the possibility of extremely high specific activities – far higher than those characterizing radioisotopes – whilst keeping the background down to low and entirely acceptable levels, and enabling individual sample measurements to be made in a second or less.

Such studies are in a comparatively early stage, but it is clear that techniques of this kind open up the possibility of immunoassay techniques far superior to current immunoassay methodology in terms of sensitivity, performance time, convenience and overall reliability. These benefits will stem as a result of the combination of the use of labelled antibody methods (with the associated advantages they offer in regard to reaction speed, specificity, etc.) and of the use of 'stable' labels of exceedingly high specific activity, deriving the energy input they require to yield a signal, not as a result of past neutron activation in an atomic reactor, but from powerful physical or chemical energy sources present at the time of measurement.

Although it might be argued that increased sensitivity and/or reaction speed is unnecessary for the measurement of many analytes, it is nevertheless the case that there are many substances, including many hormones, which currently are beyond the sensitivity range of all but the radioisotopic methods, either RIA or IRMA. Indeed some hormones lie beyond the sensitivity range of RIA other than when present in body fluids at abnormally elevated levels. Moreover, we are entering an era when the measurement of 'free' rather than total, or 'protein-bound' hormones may – because of their physiological importance – emerge as the preferred diagnostic measurement. Simple general methods for measurement of 'free' hormones have now been evolved[9], albeit they necessitate significantly higher sensitivities than are required for the assay of 'total' hormone concentrations.

The emergence of immunoassay methods which – whilst obviating the environmental and instability problems which characterize the use of radioisotopes – are of sufficient sensitivity to encompass the concentration ranges which are currently the preserve of the radioassays, will be of enormous benefit. Clearly there is little point in developing labels which are restricted in their use to analytes falling within limited concentration ranges as is the case with the present generation of non-isotopic labels. However, in some of the newer fluorescence techniques, it is possible that we have found labels which are capable of covering the entire range of biological measurement.

References

1. Ekins, R. P. (1978). Quality control and assay design. In *Radioimmoassay and Related Procedures in Medicine 1977*, Vol. II, p. 39. (Vienna: IAEA)
2. Ekins, R. P. and Newman, G. B. (1970). Theoretical aspects of saturation analysis. In *Proceedings of the Second Karolinska Symposium on Research Methods in Reproductive Endocrinology, Stockholm, 1970*, p. 11
3. Ekins, R. P. (1974). Basic principles and theory (radioimmunoassay and saturation analysis). *Br. Med. Bull., 30*, 3
4. Ekins, R. P. (1976). ELISA: A replacement for radioimmunoassays? *Lancet, 2*, 569
5. Harris, C. C., Yolken, R. H., Krokan, H. and Chang Hsu, I. (1979). *Proc. Natl. Acad. Sci. USA, 76*, 5336
6. Milstein, C. and Köhler, G. (1977). Cell fusion and the derivation of cell lines producing specific antibody. In *Antibodies in Human Diagnosis and Therapy*, p. 271. (New York: Raven Press)
7. Simpson, J. S. A., Campbell, A. K., Ryall, M. E. T. and Woodhead, J. S. (1979). A stable chemiluminescent-labelled antibody for immunological assays. *Nature (London), 279*, 646
8. Soini, E. and Hemmilä, I. (1979). Fluoroimmunoassay: present status and key problems. *Clin. Chem., 25/3*, 353
9. Ekins, R. P., Filetti, S., Kurtz, A. B. and Dwyer, K. (1980). A simple general method for the assay of free hormones (and drugs): its application to the measurement of serum-free thyroxine levels and the bearing of assay results on the 'free thyroxine' concept. *Endocrinology, 85*, 29–30P

3
Assays Utilizing Red Cells as Markers

R. R. A. COOMBS

INTRODUCTION

I will attempt to present very briefly the ways in which red cells have been used:

(1) By virtue of their lysability, in reactions to investigate the structure of complement and to study antigen–antibody interactions by means of complement absorption.
(2) By virtue of their agglutinability in agglutination tests. Many elaborations have been developed from simple haemagglutination, but in all, the red cell acts as carrier for antigen. These reactions are fairly well known.
(3) Thirdly, I shall spend more time on the recent and very important developments, where red cells are used as carrier, marker or label for antibody.

These recent developments, where the red cell is used as the *label* for antibody, bring red cell assays, in my view, to the very forefront of immunoassay procedures. While focusing on these newer developments, I hope to stress in proper perspective their antecedents. More and more today a supposedly new finding is, in fact, a rediscovery. This was brought home to my colleagues and myself in 1945 when we first reported the antiglobulin reaction[1].

ASSAYS INVOLVING COMPLEMENT

Immune haemolysis

Ever since Bordet's discovery of alexin and haemolysin in 1898 and of the so-called Bordet–Gengou phenomenon of complement fixation in 1901, the red cell has been an invaluable and unsurpassable asset for the study and assay of complement. It is on the red cell that the complement system has been dissected, analysed and extensively characterized. In recent years the study of polymorphic forms of various complement components have been greatly promoted by the so-called overlay techniques used by Lachmann and Hobart[2]. Following biophysical separation of complement sera with, say, electrofocusing, antibody-sensitized red cells and R reagents (that is complement deficient in the one component being tested) are added as an overlay to the gels.

Complement-fixation tests

In diagnostic serology the traditional complement-fixation test for either antigen or antibody is possible only by virtue of antibody-sensitized red cells being an extremely sensitive indicator for free complement. This is still an excellent reaction where the antigen is ill-defined, in a crude tissue extract and possibly of lipoid nature. It is extensively used in epidemiological studies.

Another type of complement-mediated reaction involving red cells is the conglutination reaction[3] in which non-haemolytic complements – together with conglutinin – produce, not haemolysis, but intense flocculation of red cells. The special advantages of the conglutinating complement absorption test stem from the fact that complement from most animal species can be used and that some of these are better absorbed or fixed than is the haemolytic complement of the guinea-pig. Also, only with conglutination tests can conglutinin itself or immunoconglutinin be measured.

Haemolysis of red cells in gels

I have already mentioned overlay techniques[2] in investigations into the polymorphic forms of complement components. Jerne[4] was, I think, the first to show plaques (haemolysed red cells in gels) around antibody-producing lymphoid cells. The antibody-secreting lymphoid cell secretes red cell antibody which diffuses into a gel containing red cells and complement giving an area of lysis or a plaque.

This principle has been adapted by Russell and his colleagues[5,6] in the single radial haemolysis technique for measuring influenza and rubella antibodies. The gel contains virus-coupled red cells. Sera to be tested are diffused from wells and complement is then added. It is an excellent assay procedure for IgG antibody.

Adherence reactions

Red cells are important in complement-mediated reactions not only as a consequence of their property of undergoing lysis, but also by virtue of surface receptors they possess. Human red cells[7] with receptors for fixed C3b give immune adherence, while guinea-pig red cells[8] have receptors for fixed C4.

Both red cells can be used in discriminatory rosetting reactions which I shall mention later.

VIRUS HAEMAGGLUTINATION

Before discussing antibody-mediated haemagglutination, I would like to mention the singular contribution of the red cell in viral haemagglutination (that is aggregation of red cells by virus haemagglutinin). This is an extremely sensitive and convenient method for measuring virus haemagglutinin. As the virus haemagglutinin, in a standard dose, can be inhibited by specific antibody to the haemagglutinin, an *important* assay procedure is also afforded for antibody to the virus using an inhibition test. It is the stability of red cell suspensions and the ease with which they can be haemagglutinated (and the ease with which this can be read) that makes haemagglutination such a valuable diagnostic procedure.

ANTIBODY-INDUCED HAEMAGGLUTINATION

Direct haemagglutination and the antiglobulin reaction

Not only has haemagglutination been used to define blood groups and to investigate blood group antigens and antibodies, but because of the ideal properties of red cells as such, haemagglutination has been used as a model to investigate the agglutination reaction itself. Why, for instance, is the human red cell so agglutinable and the ox red cell[9] so inagglutinable? The effect of the density of antigen sites and the distance of these sites from the sheer plane of the cell surface can be investigated.

It was the human red cell carrying, but unagglutinated by, IgG Rh antibody that allowed the rediscovery of the antiglobulin reaction in 1945. In this reaction the adsorbed Rh antibody is detected in a second stage with the application of an antiglobulin reagent. The principle of this antiglobulin stage is now incorporated in many of the immunoassay reactions in general use. Other labels for the antiglobulin antibody include radioisotopes (radioimmunoassay or RIA), enzymes (as in the enzyme linked immunosorbent assay or ELISA reaction) or fluorescent chemicals (as in the indirect immunofluorescence reaction). In this chapter I shall be commending the use of the red cell itself as a label for the antiglobulin.

Passive haemagglutination

Besides the innate antigens on the red cell membrane, other extraneous antigens can be adsorbed or coupled to red cells, whose role then becomes that

of passive carrier of the antigen in question – so-called passive haemagglutination (Figure 3.1). Passive haemagglutination tests have been very successful

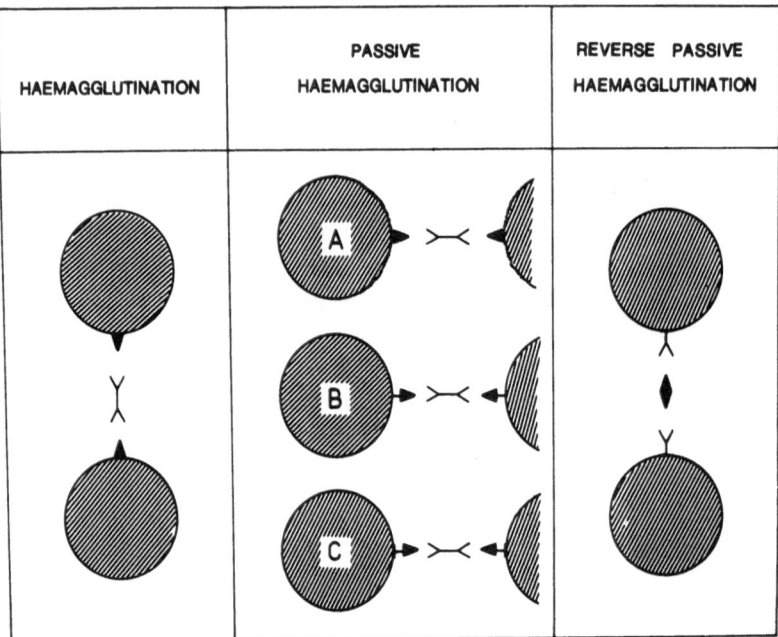

Figure 3.1   Haemagglutination, passive haemagglutination and reverse passive haemagglutination. Haemagglutination: antibody reacting with innate antigen on red cell membrane. Passive
haemagglutination: antigen adsorbed passively on to the red cell membrane, (A) protein antigen
adsorbed on tanned red cells (method of Boyden), (B) antigen covalently coupled to the red cell
membrane, (C) lipopolysaccharide antigen binding by natural affinity to the red cell membrane.
Reverse passive haemagglutination: antibody coupled to the red cell, leaving antigen-specific
receptors free to react with antigen

With polysaccharide and lipopolysaccharide antigens extracted from the cell
walls of Gram-negative bacteria. The extracted lipopolysaccharides bind
naturally to the red cell membrane[10]. The coated red cells are agglutinated by
antibody and an antiglobulin stage is possible to enhance the titre of IgG
antibodies. The polysaccharide of *Haemophilus influenzae*, for example, may
be detected in cerebrospinal fluid by a specific inhibition assay.

With most protein antigens special coupling procedures have to be used.
Boyden[11] first described adsorption of protein antigens following mild
tanning of the red cells. This has proved a very trustworthy procedure but
often far from optimal. It certainly excludes a second amplification stage with
an antiglobulin reagent. A series of covalent linking procedures have been
reported[12]. A coupling procedure which we use with great success was
originally described by Gold and Fudenberg[13] and involves cross-linking by
chromic chloride.

At one time we developed, after a great expenditure of effort, a red cell linked antigen–antibody reaction (RCLAAR)[14]. This was specially designed to make it possible to use a final antiglobulin stage to augment the sensitivity and to allow discrimination of the different classes of reacting antibody. It was possible to detect IgE antibody by this test[15], but as its debut coincided with that of the RAST (radio allergosorbent test) it aroused little interest as it did not have the sensitivity of the latter reaction.

Reverse passive haemagglutination

The next development I wish to refer to, is reverse passive haemagglutination (RPH), in which the antibody immunoglobulin itself is adsorbed onto or coupled to the red cell. These antibody-coupled red cells may then be agglutinated by antigen (Figure 3.1).

Many investigators have recently used reverse passive agglutination of latex particles in tests for microbial antigens[16] and in the identification of species proteins[17] in forensic investigations. Many people will be aware of the RPH tests for HBsAg put out by various companies in which preserved red cells are coated with antibody to hepatitis B surface antigen.

In RPH, a great deal depends on the physical state of the carrier red cell and the finesse in coupling the antibody. This holds especially for those reactions described later, in which RPH forms the final stage of more complex reactions. Before discussing these, we must first discuss mixed agglutination and rosetting reactions.

MIXED AGGLUTINATION AND ROSETTING REACTIONS

Mixed agglutination

Mixed agglutination is the direct and mixed agglutination of two distinct cell types. In a pure agglutinating system, mixed aggregates of two distinct cell types, say red cell and tissue cell, can only occur if both cell types possess a common antigen. So a control red cell with the antigen in question (say blood group A antigen) is used to test for the presence of this antigen on tissue cells[18]. This reaction (Figure 3.2) has been successfully used to demonstrate blood group antigens on tissue cells[19], to group blood stains[20] and to check the species identity of tissue cells growing *in vitro* in cell culture[21]. These reactions are qualitative only.

Mixed antiglobulin (rosetting) reaction (MARR)

Where it is not possible to select an indicator (red) cell with the antigen in question, then attached antibody Ig can be detected by the mixed antiglobulin reaction – a hybrid of mixed agglutination and the antiglobulin reaction. The indicator red cell has attached Ig and this is used to detect Ig (i.e. the same

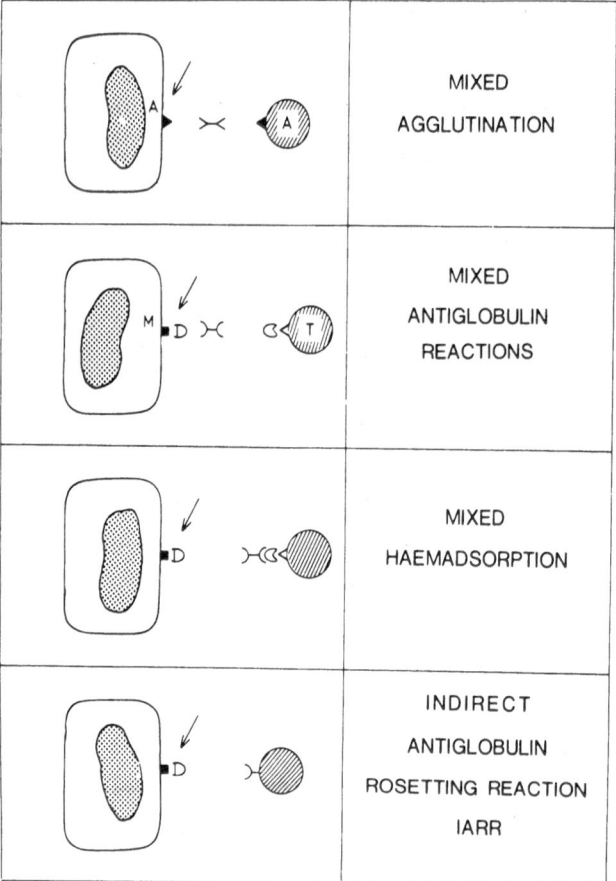

Figure 3.2 Mixed agglutination, mixed antiglobulin reaction, mixed haemadsorption and indirect antiglobulin rosetting reaction, showing evolution of reaction mechanisms. In mixed agglutination – identical antigen on the two distinct cell types – say epidermal cell and red cell. Object of test to reveal the A antigen on the epidermal cell. In mixed antiglobulin reaction the M antigen – or anti-M antibody (Ig) reacting with it is revealed by mixed agglutination using antiglobulin and indicator red cells carrying (Ig) antibody. In mixed haemadsorption (a development of the mixed antiglobulin reaction) the antiglobulin is first reacted with the Ig-carrying indicator red cell – and then the antiglobulin-carrying red cells are added to the test cells being examined for antibody adsorption. In the indirect antiglobulin rosetting reaction, the antiglobulin is coupled direct to the indicator red cells

antigen) on the test cell using an antiglobulin reagent[18].

An operational development was made by Fagraeus and Espmark[22], who reacted the antiglobulin with the Ig-carrying indicator red cells before adding to the washed antiserum-treated test cells (Figure 3.2). This variant was called 'mixed haemadsorption'. It could be performed as a mixed cell or rosetting reaction in suspension or as a plate test. It has been used to measure antibodies to tissue cells[23], to virus at cell surfaces and to protein antigens adsorbed on glass[24].

The MARR[25, 26] found an important application in differentiating B lymphocytes which have surface membrane immunoglobulin (SmIg) on their surface from T lymphocytes, which do not possess detectable SmIg. Rosetted B lymphocytes can be counted and expressed as a percentage of the total lymphocyte population. This reaction also has now been streamlined. It has been made more elegant and easier to perform by first coupling chemically the antiglobulin antibody directly to the indicator red cells (Figure 3.3). We call this the direct antiglobulin rosetting reaction (or DARR).

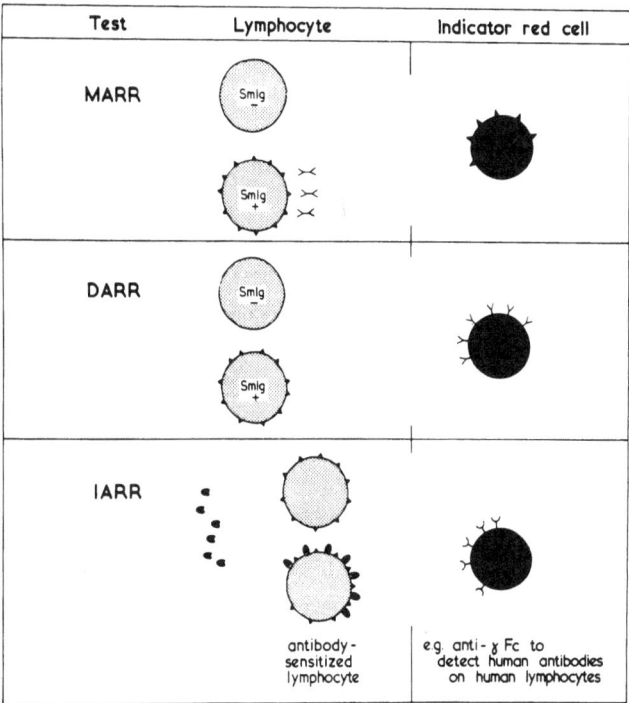

Figure 3.3   Diagrammatic representation of the mixed antiglobulin rosetting reaction (MARR), direct antiglobulin rosetting reaction (DARR) and indirect antiglobulin rosetting reaction (IARR). In the latter reaction on human lymphocytes the indicator red cells may be coupled with anti-human γFc as only 1% or 2% of human lymphocytes have γ chain determinants

Direct antiglobulin rosetting reaction (DARR)

The first reports were by Giuliano *et al.*[27], Molinaro and Dray[28], Parish and Hayward[29] and Haegert and Coombs[30]. As presently performed in our laboratory[31], the carrier red cells are pre-treated with trypsin which increases the sensitivity of the reaction. It can be used as a very sensitive rosetting reaction for enumerating and investigating B lymphocytes. Its much greater sensitivity over direct immunofluorescence[32,33] has suggested to us the concept of B major and B minor subpopulations of lymphocytes[34].

Antiglobulin reagents of all specificities may be coupled for investigational purposes. Besides antiglobulin reagents, antibodies to a host of specificities may be coupled, for instance anticomplement components, anti-C reactive protein, anti-α_2 macroglobulin or antinucleotidase. With these coupled red cells various tissue cells may be examined for the corresponding antigens on their cell membranes.

On the technical side, many aspects which cannot be dealt with here are nevertheless exceedingly important. I would mention that there is no problem related to IgGFc receptors on the cells being tested, because using chromic chloride as we do, the Fc reactive sites on the coupled IgG are no longer reactive. Rosetted lymphocytes or other cells under investigation may be not only enumerated, but separated from non-reactive cells on gradients. Besides depletion[29], suspensions can be enriched[35] for reactive cells.

Indirect antiglobulin rosetting reaction (IARR)

An *indirect* antiglobulin rosetting reaction (IARR) to measure antibody reacting with cells such as lymphocytes has also been developed[36,37] (Figures 3.2 and 3.3). On the human lymphocyte there is no great problem as SmIg is mainly IgM and IgD with only about 1% of peripheral blood lymphocytes having γ heavy chains on their membrane. Therefore suspensions of mixed B and T lymphocytes can be exposed to a human serum to be tested for IgG lymphocyte alloantibodies, either anti-HLA A, B or C or anti-HLA Dr, the latter supposedly reacting with B lymphocytes only. Mixed rosetting, with an unstained red cell carrying anti-γFc and fluorescein-stained sheep red cells as an indicator for human T lymphocytes, can indicate which antibodies are being measured (see Figure 3.4). Both complement-mediated cytolysis and this rosetting reaction have their advantages and disadvantages.

The IARR has also been used successfully to measure antibodies reacting with granulocytes[38] or to measure adsorbed antigen–antibody complexes on granulocytes.

Other rosetting reactions

There are, of course, many other rosetting reactions appropriately using red cells as the indicator satellite cells forming a corolla around the test or disc cell under investigation. The applications and methodology of rosetting have recently been reviewed[39]. There are basically four categories of rosetting reactions:

(1) *Rosetting for antigen-specific receptors:* used to reveal antigen-specific receptors on lymphoid cells or passively acquired cytophilic antibody on

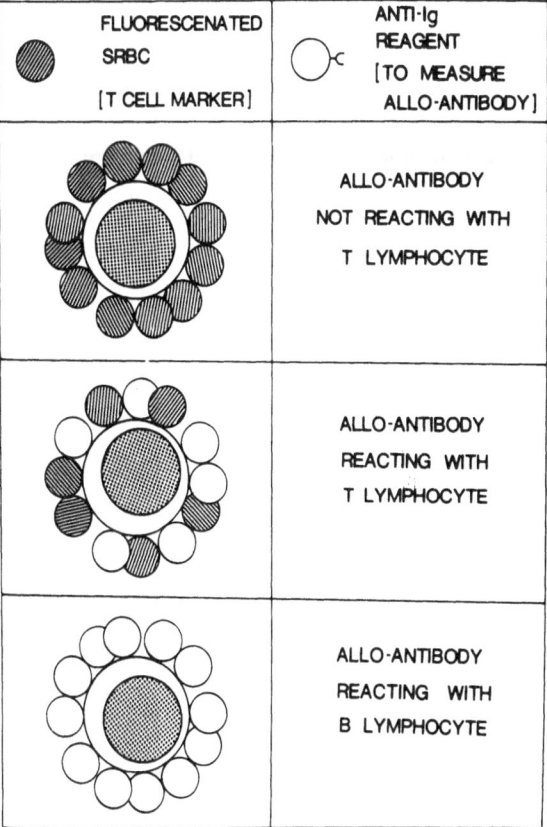

Figure 3.4 Rosetting reaction with mixed indicator red cells, fluorescenated sheep red cells are markers for human T lymphocytes and unstained ox red cells coupled with anti-human γFc are indicator red cells for adsorbed IgG allo-antibody (see reference 37)

other cells, such as macrophages or basophils.

(2) *Rosetting for cell surface determinants:* using some adaptation of either mixed agglutination or mixed antiglobulin reaction. Some of these have already been discussed.

(3) *Rosetting reactions involving receptors for IgG Fc and complement.*

(4) *Special affinity rosetting reactions:* where particular red cells (or bacteria and viruses) have a natural affinity for, adhere to and form rosettes around other cells.

These rosetting reactions, because of their excellence as probes and their great sensitivity, are playing an ever-increasing part in analytical immunological investigations. However, automated procedures for enumerating rosetted cells need to be developed if rosetting reactions are to become an accepted part of routine clinical laboratory practice.

MIXED REVERSE PASSIVE ANTIGLOBULIN HAEMAGGLUTINATION (MrPAH)

While working on the IARR the idea struck me that the same principle might be developed and adapted in a fairly simple procedure for measuring not only the titre of bacterial antibodies, but also the full spectrum of their Ig classes or even subclasses. Portions of a bacterial suspension are exposed to the dilutions of a serum titration. After incubation the bacteria are washed and aliquots of each washed suspension (carrying adsorbed specific antibodies) added to a series of red cells coupled with class-specific anti-Ig reagents – say anti-γFc, anti-μFc and anti-αFc. Adsorbed antibody Ig of the appropriate class gives a RPH (actually MrPAH), and this is read visually by simple haemagglutination in microtitre plates (Figure 3.5).

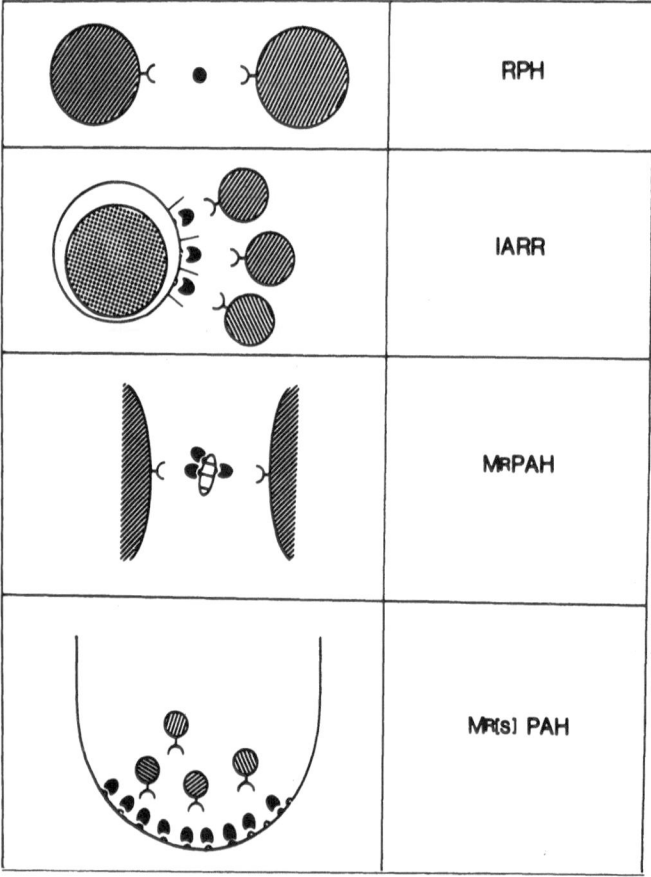

Figure 3.5 Evolution of MrsPAH (mixed reverse (solid phase) passive antiglobulin haemagglutination) from reverse passive haemagglutination (RPH) and indirect antiglobulin rosetting reaction (IARR). ● = immunoglobulin or antibody

The first investigations[40, 41] were performed on *Brucella abortus*, *Salmonella enteritidis* and *Streptococcus mutans*. The special advantages of this MrPAH reaction are:

(1) It is extremely sensitive if the carrier red cell is specially prepared (equivalent to ELISA).
(2) In the one test the titre of each class of reacting antibody may be measured without the need to fractionate.
(3) The test is set out and read on microtitre plates using either a serum dilution[40] or a bacterial dilution[41] procedure; the latter giving a greater economy of labour.

Protein A

Before any bacterium (especially streptococci and those with ubiquitous antibodies) can be used in any immunoassay for antibody using antiglobulin, whether it be a radiolabelled, ELISA or MrPAH test, it is essential to ensure that the bacterium is free of protein A or protein A-like substances. This can

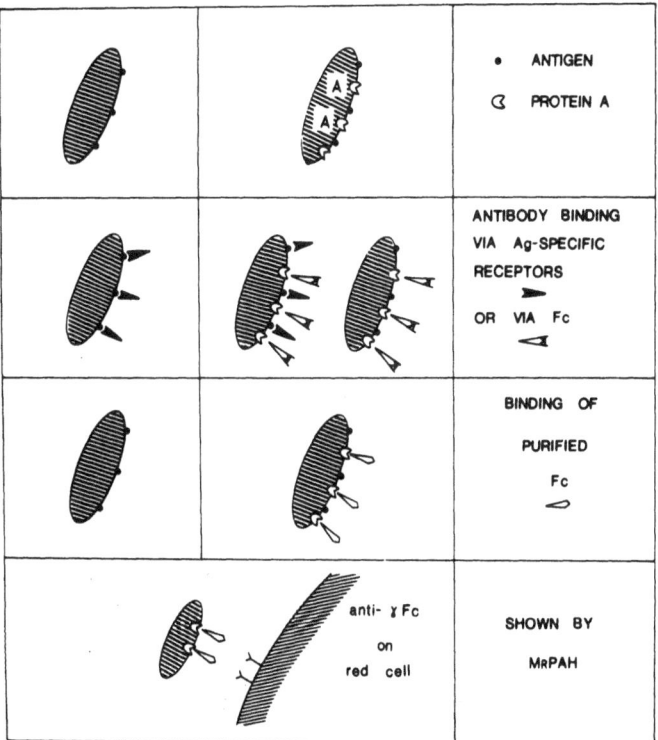

Figure 3.6 Adsorption on to a bacterium of antibody Ig via antigen-specific receptors and of IgG or IgG Fc via interaction with protein A-like substances on the bacterial surface (non antigen-specific). Absorption in both cases shown by MrPAH

be done elegantly by the MRPAH reaction itself using a test sample of purified γFc[42] (Figure 3.6). If the bacterium is found not to take up the purified γFc, then its surface membrane can be considered to be free of protein A-like substance and the organisms used in MRPAH tests to measure specific reactive antibodies.

Antigen-coated microtitre plates (MRsPAH)

MRPAH has been brought more into line with other immunoassay procedures such as RIA and ELISA by using antigen-coated microtitre plates (Figure 3.5). The 's' in the name MRsPAH refers to the reaction being performed on a solid phase. In our original study[43] with Dr Thornley, plates coated with gonococcal antigen extracts were used to test sera and urethral washings for gonococcal antibody. As in all such tests Tween 20 was added to the washing fluid. The procedure had the same sensitivity as was obtained using radiolabelled antiglobulin.

It is an easy step to the examination of sera for viral antibodies. With Drs Cranage and Stott we are investigating the detection of antibodies to rubella and respiratory syncytial virus. The important measure of IgM antibodies, indicative of recent infection, presents no difficulty in principle.

Again, it is a short step to harnessing MRsPAH for the assay of antibodies of all immunoglobulin classes to inhalant, food and other allergens[47]. The only special consideration is finding the optimal conditions for adsorbing and fixing the various allergens to the plastic microtitre plates so that:

(1) the allergen and adsorbed antibodies are not washed off with the washing diluent containing Tween 20; and
(2) immunoglobulin does not bind to the plate in the absence of fixed allergen.

IgE antibodies can be measured and comparisons with RAST are in progress, with especial regard to sensitivity[48].

Coupled red cells as label for antibody

At this point I wish to digress and without going into technical details stress the importance of the fullest consideration being given to the preparation of the coupled red cells. With sheep, human (and of course ox) red cells, pretreatment with trypsin before linking with IgG antibody greatly increases the sensitivity of these indicator red cells in the DARR, MRPAH and RPH – most noticeably however in the simple RPH. In many cases with monomeric antigens one may achieve no RPH unless the carrier red cells are first treated with trypsin.

With Drs Bradburne and Stott we have good experience using RPH with antirotavirus and antirespiratory syncytial virus systems. With Professor Lachmann we are examining the assay of complement components. Also, because of the great sensitivity of RPH, Drs Scott, Thornley and myself are comparing it with RIST (a solid-phase radioimmunoassay for IgE) for the assay of IgE in serum[49].

SOLID-PHASE AGGREGATION OF COUPLED ERYTHROCYTES (SPACE)

SPACE is a simple extension of RPH, where antibody is not only coupled to indicator red cells, but also to the wall (solid phase) of a microtitre plate well, which first captures the antigen to present it to antibody-coupled red cells subsequently added (Figure 3.7). It is totally comparable to the double-antibody ELISA plate test. Dr Bradburne[44], colleagues and ourselves have

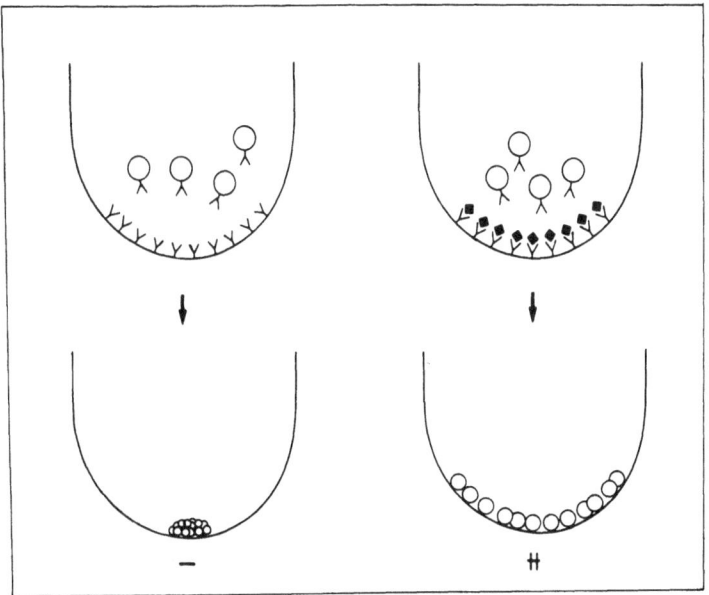

Figure 3.7 SPACE, or solid phase aggregation of coupled erythrocytes, to measure antigen (say a virus) in a system where simple RPH is not possible

applied this very successfully to detection of rotavirus in faeces; i.e. detection of antigen in a 'dirty' medium (faeces) that could easily lyse or aggregate red cells for other reasons. Again the test is read by the simple haemagglutination pattern.

DISCUSSION

In these reactions involving the principle of reverse passive haemagglutination, whether it is the DARR, IARR or M_R (and M_{RS}) PAH, the red cell is the label, tag or marker for antibody. The red cell replaces radioisotope, enzyme, fluorescein or other molecular label. These reactions (DARR, IARR and M_RPAH) have no special problems not shared with all other reactions using an antiglobulin stage in the test. For example, uptake of non-specific IgG through IgG Fc binding is a complication in all antiglobulin procedures, but this can be controlled for and avoided.

I shall list what I consider to be the particular advantages of M_R (and M_{RS}) PAH especially:

(1) The method has great sensitivity, probably equivalent to that of ELISA but possibly a little less sensitive than radioimmunoassay, although even this differential may be removed (i) with further improvement of the carrier indicator red cell, and (ii) with the greater use of affinity purified or monoclonal antibodies to couple to the red cells.
(2) Its simplicity of concept and execution; it is unsophisticated and easy to read.
(3) No expensive equipment is required. This means that a laboratory can take it up and put it down again without commitment as a consequence of heavy investment in apparatus.
(4) There are no health hazards due to handling radioisotopes or possibly carcinogenic chemicals.
(5) Results can be obtained very speedily. It is likely to be one stage shorter than other tests involving an antiglobulin stage and counting or colorimetric estimation is also eliminated. This augurs well for rapid diagnosis. Rapid diagnosis gets high priority these days.
(6) Another great advantage is its great adaptability for either diagnostic or research purposes. This I consider to be very important. Some systems are straight-jacketed by their machinery.

On the debit side:

(1) Haemagglutination reading is to some extent subjective and end-point determinations do not allow the fuller quantitative analyses derived from comparison of slopes of reactivity. It may be impossible to derive a background value to subtract from more intense positive results.
(2) At the moment, radiolabelled and enzyme-linked reagents have a longer 'shelf life' than antibody-coupled red cells. At present red cells labelled with antibody will keep at $+4°C$ for 2–3 weeks or even longer with special attention to the medium.

Experiments presently in progress by Dr Pegg, Mr Diaper, Miss Yeo and myself[45] indicate that it will probably be possible to cryopreserve standard antibody-coupled indicator red cells frozen in protective media over liquid nitrogen, allowing reconstitution when required.

It is also not impossible that the carrier red cell could be fixed or preserved by some chemical treatment to give a reagent with a prolonged shelf life at room temperature. It is my guess, however, that it may be some time before a preserved cell is achieved which has the sensitivity and other excellent properties of the fresh cell. Ling and his colleagues[46], however, have already made an incursion into this problem with a trial of red cells fixed with dimethyl suberimidate.

Although automation is an area in which I have no experience, I believe haemagglutination and its recording have been accomplished in the Auto-Analyser system. So I expect that that system or similar systems could be harnessed to reverse passive haemagglutination.

In conclusion, my brief was to survey the contributions of the red cell in immunoassay procedures. Up until the present, these have mainly derived from:

(1) the lysability of the cells and the use of this as an indicator of complement activity; and
(2) the superb agglutinability of the cells exploited in passive haemagglutination tests where the cells are used as carriers for antigen.

For the future, I have emphasized the potential significance of the red cell as carrier for antibody in developments involving the principle of RPH. I am confident that reactions such as DARR, IARR and MrPAH, especially with the indicator red cells linked with affinity-purified or monoclonal antibodies, will become everyday reactions both in diagnostic and research laboratories of the 1980s.

References

1. Coombs, R. R. A., Mourant, A. E. and Race, R. R. (1945). A new test for the detection of weak and incomplete Rh agglutinins. *Br. J. Exp. Pathol.*, **26**, 255
2. Lachmann, P. J. and Hobart, M. J. (1978). Complement technology. In Weir, D. M. (ed.) *Handbook of Experimental Immunology*, pp. 5A1–5A23. (Oxford: Blackwell Scientific Publications)
3. Coombs, R. R. A., Coombs, A. M. and Ingram, D. G. (1960). *The Serology of Conglutination and its Relation to Disease.* (Oxford: Blackwell Scientific Publications)
4. Jerne, N. K., Nordin, A. A. and Henry, C. (1963). The agar plaque technique for recognizing antibody producing cells. In Amos, B. and Koprowski, B. (eds.) *Cell-bound Antibodies.* (Philadelphia: Wistar Institute Press)
5. Russell, S. M., McCahon, D. and Beare, A. S. (1975). A single radial haemolysis technique for the measurement of influenza antibody. *J. Gen. Virol.*, **27**, 1
6. Russell, S. M., Benjamin, S. R., Briggs, M., Jenkins, M., Mortimer, P. P. and Payne, S. B. (1978). Evaluation of the single radial haemolysis (SRH) technique for rubella antibody measurement. *J. Clin. Pathol.* **31**, 521

7. Nelson, D. S. (1963). Immune adherence. *Adv. Immunol.*, **3**, 131

8. Wilson, A. B., Prichard-Thomas, S., Lachmann, P. J. and Coombs, R. R. A. (1980). Receptors on guinea pig erythrocytes specific for cell-bound fourth component of human complement (C4). *Immunology*, **39**, 195

9. Uhlenbruck, G., Seaman, G. V. F. and Coombs, R. R. A. (1967). Factors influencing the agglutinability of red cells. III. Physico-chemical studies on ox red cells of different classes of agglutinability. *Vox Sang.*, **12**, 420

10. Neter, E. (1956). Bacterial haemagglutination and haemolysis. *Bact. Rev.*, **20**, 166

11. Boyden, S. V. (1951). Adsorption of proteins on erythrocytes treated with tannic acid and subsequent haemagglutination by anti-protein sera. *J. Exp. Med.*, **93**, 107

12. Gell, P. G. H. and Coombs, R. R. A. (1975). Basic immunological methods. In Gell, P. G. H. Coombs, R. R. A. and Lachmann, P. J. (eds.) *Clinical Aspects of Immunology*, pp. 14–15. (Oxford: Blackwell Scientific Publications)

13. Gold, E. R. and Fudenberg, H. H. (1967). Chromic chloride: a coupling reagent for passive haemagglutination reactions. *J. Immunol.*, **99**, 859

14. Coombs, R. R. A. and Fiset, M. L. (1954). Detection of complete and incomplete antibodies to egg albumin by means of a sheep red cell egg albumin antigen unit. *Br. J. Exp. Pathol.*, **35**, 472

15. Coombs, R. R. A., Hunter, A., Jonas, W. E., Bennich, H., Johanssen, S. G. O. and Panzani, R. (1968). Detection of IgE (Ig ND) specific antibody (probably reagin) to castor bean allergen by the red cell linked antigen–antiglobulin reaction. *Lancet*, **1**, 1115

16. Bloomfield, N., Gordon, M. A. and Elmendorf, D. F. Jr (1963). Detection of cryptococcus neoformans antigen in body fluids by latex particle agglutination. *Proc. Soc. Exp. Biol. Med.*, **114**, 64

17. Cayzer, I. and Whitehead, P. H. (1973). The use of sensitized latex in the identification of human blood stains. *J. Forensic Sci. Soc.*, **13**, 179

18. Coombs, R. R. A. and Franks, D. (1969). Immunological reactions involving two cell types. *Prog. Allergy*, **13**, 174

19. Coombs, R. R. A., Bedford, D. and Rouillard, L. M. (1956). A and B blood group antigens on human epidermal cells demonstrated by mixed agglutination. *Lancet*, **1**, 461

20. Coombs, R. R. A. and Dodd, B. (1961). Possible application of the principle of mixed agglutination in the identification of blood stains. *Med. Sci. Law*, **1**, 359

21. Coombs, R. R. A., Daniel, M. R., Gurner, B. W. and Kelus, A. (1961). Recognition of the species of origin of cells in culture by mixed agglutination. 1. Use of antisera to red cells. *Immunology*, **4**, 55

22. Fagraeus, A. and Espmark, A. (1961). Use of a mixed haemadsorption method in virus infected tissue cultures. *Nature (London)*, **190**, 370

23. Fagraeus, A., Espmark, J. A. and Jonsson, J. (1965). Mixed haemadsorption: a mixed antiglobulin reaction applied to antigens on a glass surface. *Immunology*, **9**, 161

24. Jonsson, J. (1969). Application of mixed haemadsorption – a mixed antiglobulin reaction – to soluble antigens fixed on glass slides. *Acta Path Microbiol. Scand.*, Suppl. 202

25. Coombs, R. R. A., Gurner, B. W., Janeway, A., Wilson, A. B., Gell, P. G. H. and Kelus, A. S. (1970). Immunoglobulin determinants on the lymphocytes of normal rabbits. 1. Demonstration by the mixed antiglobulin reaction of determinants recognised by anti-γ, anti-μ, anti-Fab and anti-allotype sera anti-AS4 and anti-AS6. *Immunology*, **18**, 417

26. Haegart, D. G. (1978). Technical improvements in the mixed antiglobulin rosetting reaction with consequent demonstration of high numbers of immunoglobulin-bearing lymphocytes in viable preparations of human peripheral blood. *J. Immunol. Methods*, **22**, 73

27. Giuliano, V. J., Jasin, B. H. E., Herd, E. R. and Ziff, M. (1974). Enumeration of B lymphocytes in human peripheral blood by a rosette method for the detection of surface-bound immunoglobulin. *J. Immunol.*, **112**, 1494

28. Molinaro, G. A. and Dray, S. (1974). Antibody coated erythrocytes as a manifold probe for antigens. *Nature (London)*, **248**, 515

29. Parish, C. R. and Hayward, J. A. (1974). The lymphocyte surface. I. Relation between Fc receptors, C′3 receptors and surface immunoglobulin. *Proc. R. Soc. Lond.*, **187**, 47. II. Separation of Fc receptors C′3 receptor and surface immunoglobulin-bearing lymphocytes. *Proc. R. Soc. Lond.*, **187**, 65

30. Haegert, D. G. and Coombs, R. R. A. (1976). Immunoglobulin-positive mononuclear cells in human peripheral blood: detection by mixed antiglobulin and direct antiglobulin rosetting reactions. *J. Immunol.*, **116**, 1426

31. Coombs, R. R. A., Wilson, A. B., Eremin, O., Gurner, B. W., Haegert, D. G., Lawson, Y. A., Bright, S. and Munro, A. J. (1977). Comparison of the direct antiglobulin rosetting reaction with the mixed antiglobulin rosetting reaction for the detection of immunoglobulin on lymphocytes. *J. Immunol. Methods*, **18**, 45

32. Haegert, D. G., Hurd, C. and Coombs, R. R. A. (1978). Comparison of the direct antiglobulin rosetting reaction with direct immunofluorescence in the detection of surface membrane immunoglobulin on human peripheral blood lymphocytes. *Immunology*, **34**, 533

33. Binns, R. M., Licence, S. T., Symons, D. B. A., Gurner, B. W. and Coombs, R. R. A. (1979). Comparison of the direct antiglobulin rosetting reaction (DARR) and direct immunofluorescence (DIF) for demonstration of SIg-bearing lymphocytes in pigs, sheep and cattle. *Immunology*, **36**, 549

34. Haegert, D. G. and Coombs, R. R. A. (1979). Do human B and Null lymphocytes form a single immunoglobulin-bearing population? *Lancet*, **2**, 1051

35. Eremin, O., Kraft, D., Coombs, R. R. A., Franks, D., Ashby, J. and Plumb, D. (1977). Surface characteristics of the human K (killer) lymphocyte. *Int. Arch. Allergy Appl. Immunol.*, **55**, 112

36. Bright, S., Munro, A. J., Lawson, Y. A., Joysey, V. C. and Coombs, R. R. A. (1977). An indirect anti-immunoglobulin rosetting reaction to detect alloantibodies to human lymphocytes. *J. Immunol. Methods*, **18**, 55

37. Bright, S., Munro, A. J., Lawson, Y. A. and Coombs, R. R. A. (1978). The detection of alloantibodies to subpopulations of human lymphocytes: an adaptation of the indirect anti-immunoglobulin rosetting reaction (IARR). *J. Immunol. Methods*, **24**, 175

38. Wilson, A. B., Prichard-Thomas, S. and Coombs, R. R. A. (1980). (In preparation)

39. Coombs, R. R. A. and Wilson, A. B. (1981). Rosette forming reactions. In Lachmann, P. J. and Peters (eds.) *Clinical Aspects of Immunology*, 4th Edn. (Oxford: Blackwell Scientific Publications; in press)

40. Coombs, R. R. A., Edebo, L., Feinstein, A. and Gurner, B. W. (1978). The class of antibodies sensitizing bacteria measured by mixed reverse passive antiglobulin haemagglutination (MʀPAH). *Immunology*, **34**, 1037

41. Eggert, F. M., Edebo, L. B., Gurner, B. W. and Coombs, R. R. A. (1979). A simplified procedure for measuring the class of anti-bacterial antibodies by mixed reverse passive antiglobulin haemagglutination (MʀPAH). *J. Immunol. Methods*, **26**, 125

42. Freimer, E. H., Raeder, R., Feinstein, A., Herbert, J., Gurner, B. W. and Coombs, R. R. A. (1979). Detection of protein A-like substances on haemolytic streptococci prior to use in mixed reverse passive antiglobulin haemagglutination (MʀPAH). *J. Immunol. Methods*, **31**, 219

43. Thornley, M. J. and Coombs, R. R. A. (1979). The measurement of gonococcal antibodies in serum and secretions by mixed reverse passive antiglobulin haemagglutination (MʀPAH). *J. Med. Microbiol.*, **12**, v

44. Bradburne, A. F., Almeida, J. D., Gardner, P. S., Moosai, R. B., Nash, A. A. and Coombs, R. R. A. (1979). A solid phase system (SPACE) for the detection and quantitation of rotavirus in faeces. *J. Gen. Virol.*, **44**, 615

45. Pegg, D., Diaper, M., Yeo, S. and Coombs, R. R. A. (1980). (In preparation)

46. Ling, N. R., Stephens, G., Bratt, P. and Dhaliwal, H. S. (1979). Attachment of antigens and antibodies to fixed red cells; their use in rosette and haemagglutination tests; a comparison with fresh red cells. *Mol. Immunol.*, **16**, 637

47. Kieffer, Marianne, Frazier, P. J., Daniels, N. W. R., Ciclitira, P. J. and Coombs, R. R. A. (1981). Serum antibodies (measured by MRSPAH) to alcohol-soluble gliadins in adult coeliac patients. *J. Immunol. Methods* (In press)

48. Scott, M. L., Thornley, Margaret J. and Coombs, R. R. A. (1981). Comparison of red-cell linked anti-IgE and ^{125}I-labelled anti-IgE in a solid-phase system for the measurement of IgE specific for castor bean allergen. *Int. Arch. Allergy Appl. Immunol.* (In press)

49. Scott, M. L., Thornley, Margaret J., Coombs, R. R. A. and Bradwell, A. R. (1981). Measurement of human serum IgE and IgA by reverse passive antiglobulin haemagglutination. *Int. Arch. Allergy Appl. Immunol.* (In press)

4
Particle Counting Immunoassay (PACIA): An Automated Non-Radioisotopic Immunoassay Method, suitable for Antigens, Haptens, Antibodies and Immune Complexes

P. L. MASSON, D. COLLET-CASSART, C. G. MAGNUSSON, C. J. M. SINDIC AND C. L. CAMBIASO

INTRODUCTION

The principle of PACIA (particle counting immunoassay) is based on the agglutination of polystyrene particles 0.8 μm diameter, usually called 'latex'. The novelty of the method consists in the measurement of agglutination by determination of the number of residual non-agglutinated particles by means of a Technicon AutoCounter, an instrument designed for the counting of blood cells[1]. The advantages of the method are:

(1) radioisotopes are not used;
(2) reagent stability;
(3) analysis rate of 60/h;
(4) no separation step is required – that is, the assay is completely homogeneous;

(5) all assays are completed within 30 min;

(6) the sensitivity of the technique equals or exceeds that of RIA;

(7) probably all determinations possible with RIA are equally possible with PACIA.

The aim of this chapter is to describe the many applications of this technique which we have used not only for the determination of antigens and haptens but also for the titration of antibodies and the determination of circulating immune complexes. We will show the high sensitivity, simple operation and, in the first applications, the accuracy and precision of this technique.

The instrumental system consists of four basic units:

(1) A new sampler/reaction module called DIAS in which the reagents are added to automatically aliquoted samples and agglutination occurs under precise conditions of mixing, incubation and time.

(2) A Pump III and continuous-flow manifold providing a second dilution of the latex and connecting the DIAS to the AutoCounter.

(3) The AutoCounter with an upper and lower size threshold, so that only 0.8 μm particles are counted.

(4) The recorder which traces peaks whose heights correspond to the number of non-agglutinated particles.

As the system has been described in detail in a recent Monograph[2], we will not describe the instrument but concentrate on its performance. Four variations of the PACIA technique have been developed to date, corresponding to the determination of the four main categories of substances to be assayed. These techniques are:

for antigens	direct agglutination
for haptens	mixed agglutination inhibition
for antibodies	latex agglutination with IgM rheumatoid factor
for immune complexes	agglutination inhibition of selected agglutinators

DETERMINATION OF ANTIGENS

Up to now we have used the PACIA system for the determination of 18 antigens – from serum proteins to peptide hormones and including various infectious antigens (Table 4.1). For these tests, the latex particles are coated by antibodies and the antigen is determined by the concentration of latex agglutinated. The advantage of this method over others to be described lies in its simplicity, there being no need for purified antigen as a competitor, or for a second antibody as a detector.

Table 4.1 Antigens which can be determined by the PACIA system

Hormones		Immunoglobulins	
Insulin		IgG	$(r=0.95; n=100)$ †
Growth hormone		IgA	$(r=0.97; n=49)$ †
HPL	$(r=0.99; n=32)*$	IgM	$(r=0.94; n=98)$ †
		IgE	$(r=0.96; n=25)*$
Various		*Infectious antigens*	
Ferritin	$(r=0.98; n=92)*$	Measles	
Lactoferrin	$(r=0.97; n=20)*$	Herpes	
α_1-Fetoprotein	$(r=0.98; n=127)*$	Streptococcus C and D	
β_2-Microglobulin	$(r=0.93; n=24)*$	Trypanosomes	
C_3			
TBG			
Myoglobin			

* Correlation with RIA
† Correlation with AIP

Sensitivity is in the order of 0.1–1 μg/l, for most of the proteins in Table 4.1. In the case of insulin determination, a meaningful agglutination has been observed down to 1 ng/l. This measurement demonstrates the extraordinary sensitivity of the PACIA method which, in this case, is about 20 femtomolar $(20 \times 10^{-15}$ mol/l). That such a sensitivity is possible with insulin is doubly surprising in view of its small size (6000 Daltons) and few binding sites.

In spite of its short incubation time, the sensitivity of PACIA equals and, in certain cases improves on, that of radioimmunoassay (RIA). A single antigen molecule is sufficient to agglutinate two particles and only 3000 particles are necessary for counting. These two factors account for the very high sensitivity of the method. Further, the volume of reagents required is low; 1 ml of antiserum is sufficient to prepare 2.7 ml of latex suspension (100 g/l) which is sufficient to carry out 18 000 determinations.

At present, detailed studies have been carried out for seven protein determinations including HPL[3], ferritin, α_1-fetoprotein, IgE, IgG, IgA and IgM. These methods can be considered as ready for use. They conform to the performance criteria usually expected in clinical chemistry. The sigmoidal standard curves extend from 1 to 50 μg/l. Serum predilution is usually required, but this step is not yet automated.

Information on the accuracy of PACIA is based on recovery studies (Table 4.2) and correlations with RIA results (Table 4.1). As to reproducibility (Table 4.3), for ferritin the day-to-day coefficient of variation is not more than 7%. Values of 12.7% and 13.2% were obtained for long-term precision of two concentrations of α_1-fetoprotein.

High-sensitivity latex agglutination tests have until now not been possible in serum owing to the agglutinating factors, the most common being IgM rheumatoid factor. This antibody reacts with the Fc region of homologous and heterologous IgG and can, therefore, agglutinate particles covered with

Table 4.2 Recovery in the PACIA method

	No. of sera	Initial concentration (μg/l)	Added concentration (μg/l)	Recovery (%) ($\pm$ CV)
α_1-Fetoprotein	30	0–94	18.6	98.4$\pm$11.6
	10	0–43	4.6	93.5$\pm$ 9.5
	10	0–43	13.3	97.4$\pm$ 5.2
Ferritin	25	10–239	20.0	99.5$\pm$ 5.6
	30	16–158	8.0	96.7$\pm$ 9.0

Table 4.3 Precision of the PACIA method

Proteins	Concentration (μg/l)	Precision (%CV) 10 times a day	Precision (%CV) 8 days/once a day
α_1-Fetoprotein	8.2	2.8	7.5
	16.2	4.0	13.2
	18.3	4.8	8.2
	18.7	4.9	8.1
	35.7	8.1	12.7
Ferritin	2.2	0.9	3.1
	4.8	1.5	5.1
	12.2	3.3	2.2
	15.3	1.3	4.4
	25.2	1.4	6.7

rabbit or goat IgG. For use in the PACIA system we therefore coat latex with $F(ab')_2$ fragments rather than with whole IgG. The fragments are bound to the particles by simple adsorption or by covalent binding to carboxyl or amino groups[4]. To eliminate all non-specific reactions with various serum proteins, we further use high ionic strength solutions which prevent protein–protein interactions of feeble affinity.

As a result of the interference study we realized that in many cases the possible error due to rheumatoid factor has not been considered in techniques as commonly used as RIA and immunonephelometry. With M. Lievens of this laboratory, we have shown that recovery by immunonephelometry of horse ferritin added to a serum rich in rheumatoid factor can be as high as 150% at a dilution of 1:50. By combining with antibody–antigen complexes, rheumatoid factor increases their size and hence their nephelometric effect. In RIA the use of solid-phase antibodies, which act as a target for rheumatoid factor, can cause considerable errors. A recent paper draws attention to the fact that, in enzyme-linked sandwich immunoassay, it is also necessary to use $F(ab')_2$ fragments rather than whole antibodies[5].

PACIA is only rarely affected by turbidity in the samples; blank determinations are only necessary for frozen samples and here centrifugation and freon treatment can clarify the sample sufficiently. A problem for all agglutination methods, including PACIA, is the prozone effect, i.e. a reduction in agglutination in presence of excess agglutinating agent. For ferritin and α_1-fetoprotein, however, where normal values are respectively 125–200 μg/l and 0–25 μg/l, no decrease of agglutination has been observed up to concentrations of 10 mg/l. This resistance to the prozone effect is probably due to the large excess of antibodies bound to the latex particles.

DETERMINATION OF HAPTENS

The application of PACIA to haptens is still under development. Haptens are determined by agglutination inhibition. For the determination of T_4 we use particles coated with antibodies, the agglutinating agent being dextran (molecular weight 150 000) carrying 15 T_4 residues per molecule. T_4 is conjugated to dextran by cyanogen bromide. The determination of this hormone has not yet been carried out using the system with DIAS, but preliminary results obtained with incubation in a continuously vibrating coil show that sensitivity is largely sufficient (1 μg/1)*. The correlation coefficient for a first correlation with RIA on 18 samples was 0.96.

Preliminary results have been obtained with three other hapten determinations (T_3, digoxin and progesterone) using a slightly different method. In this case, the 0.8 μm latex particles were coated by the hapten, while the agglutinating agent was a synthetic macromolecule, i.e. a 0.2 μm latex particle coated by the antibody. These particles have a high agglutinating power but due to their small size they are not detected by the AutoCounter. In order to bind the hapten to latex, we first coupled the hapten residues to a protein using carbodi-imide or diazotization, the conjugate being then adsorbed on polystyrene particles.

This mixed agglutination system, in which the hapten is determined by its inhibiting power, is about 10 times more sensitive than the procedure used for T_4. A sensitivity of about 100 ng/l was achieved for the three haptens tested. To date, correlation results with RIA are available only for digoxin ($r = 0.97$ for 18 samples, a concentration range 0.1–2.5 μg/l).

DETERMINATION OF ANTIBODIES

IgM antibodies are titrated using their agglutinating activity on particles coated with antigen. At present our experience is limited to rheumatoid factor which we have studied in man and mouse. In certain mouse strains such as 129/Sv, rheumatoid factor is essentially IgA in nature. Due to its spontaneous polymerization, this antibody has high agglutinating activity. Using the

---

* Since this paper was written, T_4 has been determined by the current PACIA system including DIAS using as agglutinator dextran–T_4 conjugate.

inverse of the serum volume capable of reducing the number of particles by 50% as the unit of agglutination. J. van Snick established a correlation with an RIA determination; the coefficient of correlation for 20 samples was 0.97[6].

As IgG antibodies are not good agglutinators, a second reagent is necessary to titrate them. The reagent we used was IgM rheumatoid factor which agglutinates latex according to its IgG loading and hence according to the quantity of IgG antibodies bound to the antigen coupled with the particles. Interference of endogenous rheumatoid factor is avoided by systematically treating all samples with dithiothreitol which inactivates IgM antibodies by reducing sulphide bridges. Up to now we have applied this method to the determination of antibodies to rabbit basic myelin protein and to anti-herpes antibodies. A study of the level of anti-herpes antibodies in the cerebrospinal fluid of a patient suffering from herpes encephalitis showed that PACIA is clearly more sensitive than complement fixation. Whereas the latter test becomes negative after 5 weeks evolution of the disease, PACIA remained positive up to the 37th week.

DETERMINATION OF CIRCULATING IMMUNE COMPLEXES

The level of immune complexes is determined by their affinity for rheumatoid factor[7] or for another latex agglutinating agent present in mouse serum which we have called MAG[8]. By reacting with these agents, the complexes inhibit their agglutinating activity on IgG coated latex. Amongst the many methods available for the detection of circulating immune complexes, we believe that PACIA is one of the best for the following reasons. Due to the complete automation of the method and to the stability of the agglutinators used (i.e. serum rich in rheumatoid factor and mouse serum) the reproducibility is satisfactory, contrary to techniques based on the use of reagents such as Clq or Raji cells. The use of two reagents with different specificities widens the spectrum of complexes which can be detected by PACIA. Rheumatoid factor detects complexes consisting of IgG1, IgG2 and IgG4, whereas MAG reacts with IgM and IgG1 complexes. By treating all samples with dithiothreitol, interference by rheumatoid factor in certain samples is avoided. Unlike tests in which endogenous serum Clq interferes, there is no interference from complement with PACIA, as the pH 9.2 and high ionic strength used effectively avoid this source of interference.

At present, the determination of immune complexes is required essentially to monitor so-called immune diseases such as disseminated lupus erythematosus, vasculitis, nephritis, arthritis, etc. Cancer specialists are interested in the tests as they believe that it may provide prognostic information. Two other applications which seem promising are the selection of blood donors and the early detection of postnatal infections by analysis of cord serum.

CONCLUSION

PACIA appears to be a flexible method which will probably be suitable for all the applications previously carried out by radioimmunoassay. In addition to the fact that no radioisotopes are required, the main advantages of PACIA are: simple reagent preparation and reagent stability; complete automation including the short incubation time; strict control of interference. As a result of our experience with the routine determination of five proteins and circulating immune complexes, we can strongly recommend the technique.

References

1. Cambiaso, C. L., Leek, A. E., De Steenwinkel, F., Billen, J. and Masson, P. L. (1977). Particle counting immunoassay (PACIA). I: A general method for the determination of antibodies, antigens and haptens. *J. Immunol. Methods*, **18**, 33

2. Technicon PACIA System, Monograph 1: *Instrumentation* (Geneva: Technicon International Division SA)

3. •Leek, A. E., De Steenwinkel, F., Cambiaso, C. L. and Masson, P. L. (1980). Particle counting immunoassay (PACIA). V: Its application to the determination of human placental lactogen. *J. Autom. Chem.*, **2**, 149

4. Limet, J. N., Moussebois, C. H., Cambiaso, C. L., Vaerman, J. P. and Masson, P. L. (1979). Particle counting immunoassay. IV: The use of F(ab')$_2$ fragments and N$^\varepsilon$-chloroacetyl lysine N-carboxyanhydride for their coupling to polystyrene latex particles. *J. Immunol. Methods*, **28**, 25

5. Kato, K., Umeda, U., Suzuki, F., Hayashi, D. and Kosaka, A. (1979). Use of antibody Fab' fragments to remove interference by rheumatoid factors with the enzyme-linked sandwich immunoassay. *FEBS Lett.*, **102**, 253

6 Van Snick, J. L. and Masson, P. L. (1979). Age-dependent production of IgA and IgM autoantibodies against IgG2a in a colony of 129/Sv mice. *J. Exp. Med.*, **149**, 1519

7. Cambiaso, C. L., Riccomi, H., Sindic, C. and Masson, P. L. (1978). Particle counting immunoassay (PACIA). II: Automated determination of circulating immune complexes by inhibition of the agglutinating activity of rheumatoid sera. *J. Immunol. Methods*, **23**, 29

8. Cambiaso, C. L., Sindic, C. and Masson, P. L. (1979). Particle counting immunoassay (PACIA). III: Automated determination of circulating immune complexes by inhibition of an agglutinating factor of mouse serum. *J. Immunol. Methods*, **28**, 13

5
Precipitation and Related Immunoassay Techniques

L.-Å. NILSSON

INTRODUCTION

Immunoprecipitation, the formation of visible antigen–antibody complexes when a soluble macromolecular antigen and an antiserum containing the corresponding antibodies are mixed, dates back to the beginning of modern immunology. As early as 1897 Kraus[1] gave a description of this phenomenon, obtained after mixing a bacterial culture supernatant and the serum from immunized animals. This finding was the basis for the extensive immunochemical work performed by Heidelberger and Kendall[2] in the 1920s and 1930s. Only a few years after Kraus' publication, Bechhold[3], in 1905, reported on the performance of precipitin reactions in a gel milieu rather than in a fluid medium. The immunological implications of the latter findings were, however, not fully realized until about 40 years later with the rediscovery and further development of modern immunodiffusion techniques by Oudin[4], Ouchterlony[5], Elek[6], Grabar and Williams[7], Laurell[8] and others.

The antigen–antibody reaction leading to precipitate formation may be regarded as a two-step reaction: the first stage – combination of antigenic determinants and corresponding antibodies, being extremely rapid, whereas the second stage – formation of a visible precipitate, sometimes occurs very slowly. The reaction is accompanied by a change in energy, which seems to take place mainly during the first stage. Several hypotheses have been advanced in order to explain the nature of the precipitin reaction (for a review see, e.g. Boyd[9]). The most popular of these is still the lattice theory, originally formulated by Marrack[10], implying the formation of a network of multivalent antigenic particles and bivalent antibodies. Lattice formation seems to be initiated by the development of differently sized and composed soluble antigen–antibody complexes which successively display a hydrophobic character, leading to

43

the formation of an insoluble precipitate[11,12]. Factors which influence the amount of precipitate are the relative proportions between antigen and antibody (see below), the possible presence of complement, pH, salt concentration, temperature, reaction time, and volume of reaction mixture[9].

Recent evidence indicates not only that the immunospecific interaction between the antigenic determinants and the antigen-binding site on the Fab portion of the immunoglobulin molecule is of importance for the development of the lattice but that the Fc portion of the molecule contributes substantially to precipitate formation[11,13,14]. This 'non-specific' effect, called Fc-mediated immune precipitation, is most pronounced in the low antigen-excess and in the equivalence zones. It has been postulated that this enhancing effect on precipitation is due to an Fc–Fc interaction between individual immunoglobulin molecules, operating mainly during the second, insolubilization stage of precipitation[15]. Evidence was also obtained, indicating that the Fc-mediated precipitation is due to the interaction between antigen-rich soluble immune complexes and antibody-rich insoluble immune complexes.

The basis for the use of precipitation methods as an accurate quantitative immunochemical tool was elaborated in the classical works by Heidelberger and Kendall[16]. Their original precipitation technique made precise immunochemical analysis on a molecular basis possible. The theoretical considerations of this technique have been extensively treated by, for example, Kabat[17] and Day[18]. A representative precipitation curve obtained after mixing increasing amounts of antigen with a constant amount of antibody (the so-called α-procedure) is schematically outlined in Figure 5.1. A characteristic feature of this curve is the initial continuous increment of the precipitate as increasing amounts of antigen are added. In this region of the

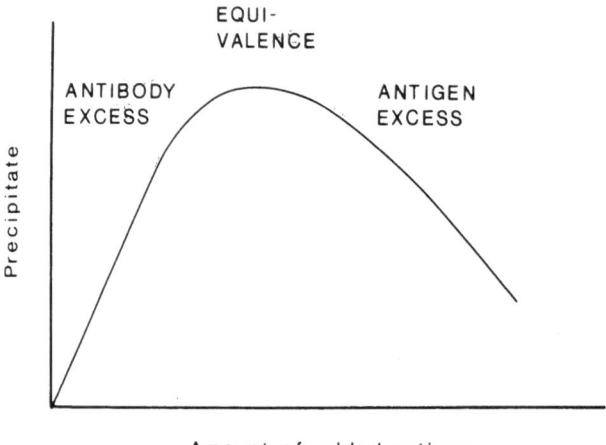

Figure 5.1 Schematic course of precipitation curve obtained by addition of increasing amounts of antigen to a constant amount of antibodies. For explanation, see text

curve (antibody excess) there is no free antigen in the soluble phase. When a certain relationship between the amounts of antigen and antibody is reached (optimal ratio – OR) a maximal amount of precipitated material is registered. For some, but not all, precipitating systems the OR coincides with the so-called equivalence zone, being recognized by the absence in the supernatant of both free antigen and free antibody. As still more antigen is added the antigen–antibody complexes formed will become more soluble, leading to a decrease of the amount of precipitate (region of antigen excess). The solubility of complexes formed in antigen or antibody excess will to some extent depend on the type of immune serum employed; for example horse antisera to protein antigens often give complexes which are more soluble in antigen excess than those formed by rabbit immune sera.

The quantitative immunoprecipitation technique, as originally described, implies rather laborious chemical analysis of precipitates. The substitution of such analysis by recording of the turbidity of solutions containing mixtures of antigen and antisera was a prerequisite for the further development of nephelometric techniques with possible automation in quantitative immunochemical work. The development of immunoprecipitation methods for analytical work advanced rapidly after the substitution of fluid media with stabilized gels for performance of the precipitin reaction, mainly due to the impressive resolution power attained.

This chapter gives brief presentations of a series of immunoprecipitation methods in current use. Some practical aspects of their performance are emphasized, such as simplicity, cost and technical skill involved. Other factors influencing the range of their application are also discussed, for example precision, sensitivity and resolving power.

The milieu in which the precipitation reaction takes place is of prime importance for the analytical possibilities offered by the various techniques, and distinction will therefore be made between assays performed in a solution as opposed to those taking place in conjunction with diffusion or electrophoretical separation of serological reactants in a gel. Some of the novelties in the field will be emphasized. A recently described solid-phase serological technique – thin layer immunoassay (TIA) – may in certain situations improve the analytical possibilities of immunodiffusion assays. The prime advantage of TIA is, however, not the combination of the two techniques. TIA has seroanalytical potentialities as a method *per se* and a description of this technique will be included.

ASSAYS BASED ON IMMUNOPRECIPITATION IN SOLUTION

The addition of antigen in solution to the corresponding antibodies results in the formation of immune complexes. The amount of immune complexes formed in antibody excess (cf. Figure 5.1), being proportional to the amount of added antigen, may be measured by registration of the turbidity (turbidimetry) or the light-scattering (nephelometry) of the mixture. By comparison with reference samples with known concentration, the unknown samples can be expressed in quantitative terms. Since both turbidity and light-scattering properties vary in different patients' sera, the subtraction of an individual serum blank value is required for each separate analysis. A review of automated immunoanalysis has recently been published[19].

Turbidimetry

The development by Libby of the photron reflectometer made possible simple measurement of immune complexes by registration of the turbidity[20]. A linear relationship was observed between galvanometer readings and amount of precipitate obtained by mixing varying amounts of antigen and antiserum at constant proportions[21]. The validity of the principles for the use of turbidimetric techniques for registration of precipitation reactions was later confirmed and extended by Boyden et al.[22]. Subsequently, systems for quantitation of various antigens on a larger scale were developed by Ritchie[23] and Schultze and Schwick[24]. The procedure is simple and rapid, and the suitability for automation implies a large capacity and accuracy of the assay. By spectrophotometric registration of the turbidity, the sensitivity of this assay is about 0.5–1 μg/ml. Shortened reaction time and increased sensitivity may be attained after enhancement of immune complex formation by the addition of polyethylene glycol[25].

A possible source of error which may occur in assays based on immunoprecipitation in solution is the antigen excess which may occur in, for example, paraproteinaemia. Taking the course of the classical precipitin curve into consideration it may be noted that most readings of the amount of precipitate correspond to two different antigen concentrations. Accurate quantitation is only yielded in the region of antibody excess (ascending portion of the Heidelberger curve). This source of error may be excluded by further addition of antiserum to the reaction cuvette followed by another turbidimetric or nephelometric reading. In the region of antibody excess no increase of the turbidity or the light-scattering will be registered. This procedure will, however, increase the consumption of antiserum as well as the time required for analysis. The above-mentioned problems of turbidity or light-scattering caused by factors other than the antigen–antibody complexes, as well as the disclosure of antigen excess, may be circumvented by the use of kinetic turbidimetry employing an automatic centrifugal analyzer[26,27]. In this modification the change in absorbance between readings obtained at a certain time interval (e.g. 10 and 255 s) is registered. Another approach, difference turbidimetry, was used by Jacobsen and Stensgaard[28]. The technique, involving the use of tandem cuvettes, provides the opportunity of using the separate antigen and antibody solutions as blanks. A twofold increase of sensitivity was obtained by measuring turbidity at low wavelengths (280 nm) rather than at 340–360 nm.

Nephelometry

Determination of the light-scattering properties of antigen–antibody mixtures was used as a measure of precipitate formation by, for example, Killingsworth and Savory[29, 30]. The instruments initially employed measured the scattering of light at an angle of 90°. An extension of this development was the introduction of a new generation of instruments, introduced in the mid-1970s, the methodological principle of which was the measurement of forward light-scattering rather than light-scatter measurement at an angle of 90°[31-33]. In some instruments a laser, emitting light at 632.8 nm, is used as radiation source. Such systems are available as specially designed nephelometers[33, 35] or they may be incorporated into regular centrifugal analysers[31, 36]. This methodology is, like turbidimetry, characterized by simplicity, rapid processing of sample results, a high degree of sensitivity and precision as well as a range of measurement which seems to be adequate for the quantitation of many proteins. Like turbidimetry, nephelometry can be automated, thus reducing labour cost. A disadvantage of the technique may be the high purchase price of the instrument.

Nephelometry has been applied to the quantitative determination of immunoglobulins[29, 31, 33, 35, 41, 42, 44], complement factors[33, 35, 44], rheumatoid factor[37, 38] and immune complexes[39, 40]. Method comparison between nephelometric assays and immunoprecipitation-in-gel techniques, such as single radial immunodiffusion (SRID) or electroimmunoassay (EIA) (see below) generally showed good correlation, at least for samples from normal individuals[33, 35, 41-44, 46].

Immunochemical quantitation of M-components and IgA by precipitation-in-gel procedures imposes a special problem[45], one reason being the possibly different physicochemical properties of the molecules assayed with regard to molecular size and charge as compared to those of the reference sample. Another reason is the possible antigenic deficiency of an M-component as compared to normal serum immunoglobulins. Such factors may lead to too high or too low values for the components assayed. Since the methodological errors connected with diffusion or electrophoretic migration in a gel are not present in nephelometry, immunoglobulin determination by this technique should not be affected by differences in physicochemical characteristics. This assumption is substantiated by the comparison study of Virella and Fudenberg[46] including pathological sera. The quantitation of M-components – often being antigenically deficient as compared to the reference antigen may, however, be subject to errors similar to those encountered in any immunochemical assay, including those performed in gel. Erroneous results may also be obtained in nephelometric assays of physicochemically labile proteins such as ceruloplasmin and C3. This is probably due to *in vitro* degradation of the native protein leading to changes both of physicochemical properties and antigenic mosaic[47]. One disadvantage of nephelometry, as compared to SRID or EIA, is the need to clear lipaemic sera by centrifugation[48].

It should be mentioned that a competitive nephelometric immunoassay has been described for determination of anti-epileptic drugs[49]. In this assay the inhibition of immunoprecipitation by hapten (the drug) is employed.

Immunoassays based on turbidimetry or nephelometry are generally rapid, precise, sensitive and technically simple to perform. It may be anticipated that the use of these techniques will increase. Their main advantage compared to immunoprecipitation assays performed in gel is their suitability for automation. In order to be able to compete economically with the last-mentioned techniques, however, a rather large bulk of analyses is required because of the high cost of procuring the necessary instrumentation. Another disadvantage of these techniques is that results are only obtained as plain figures whereas gel precipitation techniques also give qualitative information which may give hints of possibly erroneous results as well as diagnostically valuable information.

ASSAYS BASED ON IMMUNOPRECIPITATION-IN-GEL

The performance of precipitation reactions in gel media offers certain advantages. By means of diffusion or electrophoresis a concentration gradient of one or both of the serological reactants involved is established in the stabilized medium. Precipitation will occur where antigen and antibody are present in an optimal ratio (OR). When complex mixtures of antigens are analysed by means of antisera containing the corresponding antibodies, the location in the gel of the OR for the separate systems will most often vary depending on different properties of the antigens in the mixture. This will lead to the formation of one precipitation line for each separate antigen–antibody system.

A characteristic property of immunoassays employing precipitation in gel is therefore the high resolution obtained. Depending on the character of the gel employed, mixtures of antigenic substances may be separated and analysed with regard to differences in concentration, diffusion coefficient, molecular weight or electrical charge. For more extensive accounts of the various techniques the reader is referred to the handbooks listed in references 50–54.

Immunodiffusion assays

Immunodiffusion assays may be subdivided into techniques by which one (simple diffusion) or both (double diffusion) of the serological reactants (antigen and antibody) diffuse into the gel (see Figure 5.2).

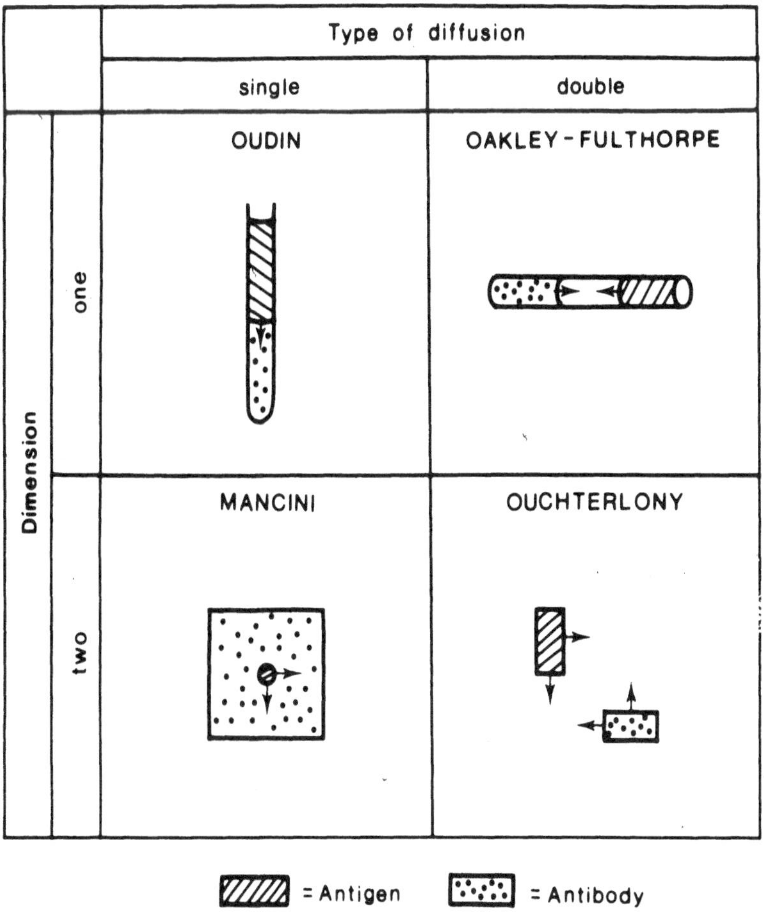

Figure 5.2 Schematic representation of the four main principles of assays based on diffusion-in-gel techniques

Simple diffusion in one dimension

This principle was originally described by Oudin[4]. In this technique, performed in tubes, antigen diffuses into an agar gel containing antibody. The resulting precipitate is gradually displaced and 'migrates' through the gel at a rate which is dependent on the original antigen concentration, the diffusion coefficient of the antigen and the concentration of the antiserum incorporated in the gel. This technique has been of great importance for the analysis of various antigens – for example, rabbit immunoglobulin allotypes – as well as for the development of more sophisticated immunodiffusion techniques.

c

Simple diffusion in two dimensions, also called single radial immunodiffusion (SRID)

This principle was originally described by Ouchterlony[55]. In this technique antigen radially diffuses from a circular well into a gel layer containing homogeneously distributed monospecific antiserum. A successively growing, circular precipitation zone will appear around the well. The growth of this zone will continue until equilibrium between the diffusing antigen and the reacting antibodies in the antiserum incorporated in the gel is attained. The implications of this technique for quantitative purposes were first described by Mancini *et al.*[56]. A rectilinear relationship exists between antigen concentration and area (D^2) of the zone enclosed by the precipitate. In some modifications of SRID the size of the precipitation zone is registered before equilibrium is reached[57]. In this instance a rectilinear dose–response curve may be obtained when log antigen concentration is plotted against the diameter (D) of the precipitation ring. For greatest accuracy, however, SRID tests should be measured at equivalence, *i.e.* after completed diffusion[58]. The sensitivity level of SRID, 0.5–1 $\mu g/ml$, is about the same as for nephelometric or turbidimetric techniques.

Since quantitation by SRID implies diffusion-in-gel, a requirement for the use of this technique for quantitative purposes is that the diffusion coefficient of the substance to be quantitated is the same in the various test samples as in the reference sample. This is a possible source of error in the quantitation of, for example, IgA which may be present both as monomers and polymers in varying proportions in serum, and as secretory IgA in secretions. In order to obtain acceptable accuracy it is essential that the proportion of various antigenic determinants reacting serologically is similar in the test and the reference samples. Pronounced deviation from this ideal condition may be found when sera containing M-components are subject to quantitation. Variation in the antibody content and specificity of various antisera may also be a source of error of results obtained by SRID. Recommendation of test procedures for antisera to be used in SRID have recently been advanced by the MRC working party on the clinical use of immunological reagents[59]. The importance of standardization of reagents and techniques cannot be over-emphasized[60]. An extensive evaluation of various technique modifications has been made by Berne[58].

Summing up, SRID is a simple and inexpensive quantitative technique with high precision and without requirement for any equipment except that which is usually available in any laboratory. In contrast to nephelometric techniques SRID may be used for quantitation of lipaemic sera without pretreatment of sera. The technique has the disadvantage as compared to EIA or nephelometry that test results are not available for 3–4 days instead of 1–2 days. Because of its simplicity, however, SRID has become widely used and it is presently one of the established, standard techniques with which new methods for quantitative determination of various antigenic substances are often compared. The test may hold its position as a standard technique if more sophisticated automation possibilities are developed. One system, permitting semi-automated evaluation of quantitative SRID plates, has been described[61].

Double diffusion in one dimension

This technique, as described by, for example, Oakley and Fulthorpe[62] employs the diffusion in a tube of antigen and antibody into an interjacent inert gel. By the use of this principle of diffusion in combination with large reactant volumes a slightly higher sensitivity and resolution power is attained as compared to the Oudin technique.

Double diffusion in two dimensions (Ouchterlony technique, DD)[63,64]

This method employs diffusion of antigen and antibody in two dimensions from separate sources into a gel. A distinctive characteristic of the double diffusion-in-gel technique is the high resolving power with regard to the analysis of complex mixtures of antigens and antibodies, each separate antigen–antibody system giving rise to an individual precipitation line. The information yielded by this technique is mainly qualitative. The possibility of using different basin arrangements makes the DD technique particularly suited for the comparison of serologically related materials of different origin. The type patterns which may be obtained at comparative analysis have been described and interpreted by Ouchterlony[64]. The technical performance, the principles for evaluation and interpretation of results and possible pitfalls in the evaluation and interpretation of results have been extensively dealt with in several reviews to which the reader is referred[50-52,63-65].

Immunoelectrophoretic techniques

Immunoelectrophoresis (IE)

Originally described by Grabar and Williams[7], this technique combines the principles of electrophoretic separation of the antigenic material and immunoprecipitation in a gel. The development of the technique was of great importance for immunochemical protein research. By this procedure the analytical resolving power was further increased as compared to the double diffusion-in-gel technique. The information yielded is at most semiquantitative, but IE forms the basis for the modern quantitative immunoelectrophoretic techniques (see below). By using suitable basin arrangements it is possible to use IE for qualitative comparative purposes. Further information concerning the performance of the regular IE technique, as well as modifications suitable for qualitative comparative analysis, may be found in references 52, 66 and 67. Results are essentially interpreted according to the principles given by Ouchterlony, referred to above[64].

Counter-current immunoelectrophoresis[68]

Antigen and antibody are forced towards each other in an agar gel under the influence of an electrical field. Usually the antigen is applied to the cathodic well and the antibody to the anodic. By selection of suitable pH the negatively charged antigen moves towards the anode whereas the antibodies migrate towards the cathode under the influence of the electroendosmotic flow. Due to the selectively directed migration of serological reactants, counter-current electrophoresis is more sensitive than the previously mentioned precipitation-in-gel techniques. For example, it was possible to detect as low a concentration as $0.05\,\mu g/ml$ of pneumococcal polysaccharide in cerebrospinal fluid[69]. Other advantages of the technique are simplicity and rapidity, results often being obtained within a few hours. The analytical resolution power is, however, not as good as for the previously mentioned gel techniques. A major field of application is in the rapid diagnosis of infectious diseases characterized by the presence of free microbial antigen in body fluids[69, 70].

Electroimmunoassay (EIA)

In EIA, originally described by Laurell[71], an antigen, which may be present in a mixture of proteins, is propagated by electrophoresis into an antibody-containing gel. The resulting precipitate resembles a rocket[72] (hence the name rocket immunoelectrophoresis) the height of which is proportional to the original antigen concentration in the sample. The principal difference between SRID and EIA is that the migration of the antigen in the latter technique is caused by electrophoresis rather than diffusion. By this procedure equilibrium between antigen and antibody is attained faster than in the SRID assay, implying that a quantitative result may be available in a couple of hours rather than days.

The sensitivity of EIA is in the same range as SRID, i.e. about $0.5-1\ \mu g/ml$ for protein antigens. By the use of a special device for application of large sample volumes it has, however, been possible to achieve a sensitivity level comparable to that of tracer techniques $(1-5\,ng/ml)$[73]. Another modification of EIA, having a very high sensitivity, was recently described[74]. This technique is based on photography of a plate with otherwise invisible precipitates which had been enhanced by ethidium bromide staining followed by ultraviolet illumination. By this procedure DNA concentrations of $0.1-20\,\mu g$ DNA/ml corresponding to a minimum quantifiable amount of DNA of 0.4 ng were demonstrated.

The precision of EIA is about the same as for SRID. Practical considerations regarding the performance of the assay have been extensively dealt with by Laurell[75] and Weeke[76]. It should be noted that a possible disadvantage of EIA is the electrophoretic separation; antigens with an electrical charge similar to that of antibodies may preferentially be quantitated by SRID rather than by EIA. Quantitation of immunoglobulins is, however, possible after changing the molecular charge by e.g. carbamylation of the samples.

The quantitative analysis of immunoglobulins is of particular interest. The increasing use of nephelometric techniques for quantitation of immunoglobulins has tended to supersede immunodiffusion techniques mainly due to the automation possibilities of the former technique. It has, however, been claimed that quantitative analysis of immunoglobulins cannot replace analysis of the electrophoretic pattern[77-79]. Both qualitative and quantitative information of the antigen assayed may be obtained by means of EIA[75,77,79].

As mentioned, the main advantage of EIA over SRID is its speed. The capacity of EIA for screening analysis is, however, limited in comparison to that of SRID and the choice of technique will therefore depend on the number of samples analysed daily and the possible clinical need for a rapid answer.

Crossed immunoelectrophoresis (CIE)

CIE, first described by Ressler[80], later developed by Laurell[8], employs electrophoretic separation of a sample as a two-step procedure. In the first step the sample is subjected to electrophoresis, usually in an agarose gel. In a second step, electrophoresis of the separated components is performed into an antibody-containing gel at a direction perpendicular to that of the first step.

In the original procedure described by Laurell, the electrophoresis strip of the first step is cut out and transferred to a second plate with the antibody-containing gel. A modification, permitting more accurate quantitative evaluation of the precipitation pattern obtained in CIE, was later described by Clarke and Freeman[81]. Various procedures for the application of antiserum have been used[82,83].

As mentioned above, CIE is usually performed in agarose. In order to take advantage of different properties of the gel matrix for the separation of complex mixtures of antigens, several attempts have been made to use different gel matrices in the two electrophoresis steps. Agarose is commonly used for the second dimension and polyacrylamide, starch gel or cellulose acetate have been used as substitutes for agarose during the first dimension separation. One problem encountered in the combination of different gels is the different endosmotic properties of the media. This may lead to accumulation of buffer fluid at the interface resulting in mechanical interruption of the continuity. Various solutions of this problem have been presented[84,85].

CIE possesses higher resolving power and simpler identification possibilities than regular IE, the patterns obtained making it suitable for the qualitative analysis of protein heterogeneity and complex mixtures of proteins

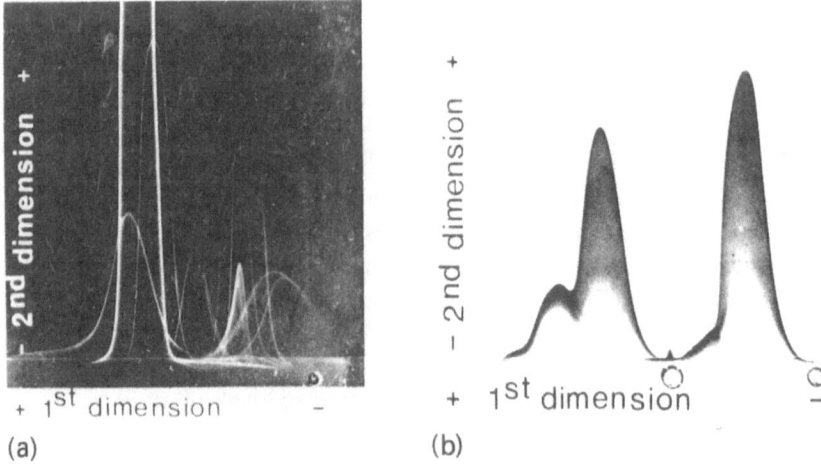

Figure 5.3 Photographs of crossed immunoelectrophoresis plates: (a) analysis of human serum by means of anti-human serum, incorporated in the gel during the second step; (b) analysis of native serum (right) and serum treated with bacterial lipopolysaccharide (LPS) (left) by means of anti-human C3 serum incorporated in the gel during the second step

(cf. Figures 5. 3a and 5. 3b). In the analysis of serum proteins, for example, the patterns obtained are often too complex to allow the general application of CIE in routine work.

The technical performance requires some experience, as does the interpretation of results. An extensive literature survey giving more than 500 references on quantitative immunoelectrophoretic methods has been published[86].

Modifications of quantitative immunoelectrophoresis

A large number of technique variations based on combinations of EIA, CIE and other precipitation-in-gel techniques have been elaborated for various analytical purposes. One of these may be mentioned in particular, since it employs a non-serological reactant. In the immunoaffino-electrophoresis technique[87] an intermediate gel containing ConA was employed in order to selectively trap *Candida albicans* cell wall antigens during electrophoresis. By this procedure it was possible to analyse cytoplasmic antibodies exclusively, thus increasing the diagnostic specificity of the assay. A detailed account of other quantitative IE techniques is beyond the scope of the present review but the interested reader is referred to references 53 and 54 for technical performance, as well as for numerous examples of applications.

Immunofixation

Immunofixation is a very simple technique which combines the principles of electrophoretic separation in a gel and subsequent precipitation *in situ* of antigen by means of suitable monospecific antiserum[88]. The antiserum is applied as an even layer over the surface of the gel immediately after completion of the electrophoresis. After washing the gel in order to remove unreacted material, the precipitated antigen is visualized by protein staining. Since diffusion of the separated material is minimal, excellent resolution is attained. The technique is therefore suitable for the study of microheterogeneity of protein antigens. In order to obtain optimal results it is important to adjust the concentration of the antiserum to the expected antigen concentration in the separated sample since a large antigen excess may lead to the formation of soluble immune complexes which are not trapped in the gel and thus will not show up after staining.

Immunofixation has been used for demonstration of Gc-globulin types, genetic polymorphism of ceruloplasmin and α_1-antitrypsin, C3 conversion products[88, 89], and analysis of M-components[90, 91]. Figure 5.4 shows the

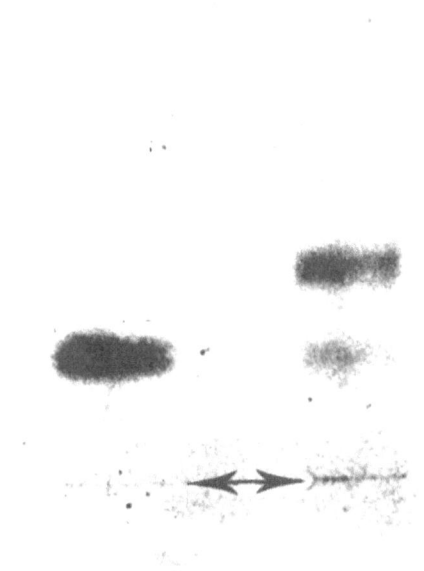

Figure 5.4 Photograph of immunofixation plate, showing analysis of native serum (left) and serum treated with immune complexes in order to induce C3 conversion (right). Application basins indicated by arrows. Anode to the top. After electrophoresis the agar surface was covered with a filter paper soaked in anti-C3, followed by washing and protein staining

demonstration of C3 conversion products by means of immunofixation. The immunofixation technique is much more sensitive than regular electrophoresis, the level of sensitivity being about 1 μg/ml[90].

The immunofixation technique seems to be very suitable for analysis of discrete M-components, especially of IgA or IgM types. These are often difficult to reveal by conventional immunoprecipitation techniques, such as IE, due to the effect of the high concentration of normal IgG, making identification of M-components of other immunoglobulin classes difficult or sometimes even impossible. A possible source of error connected with analysis of monoclonal bands by use of anti-Ig sera is the possible concomitant presence of rheumatoid factor which may react indiscriminately with various anti-Ig sera forming band-like precipitates.

A technique developed for the electrophoretic characterization of specific antibodies, imprint electroimmunofixation, was recently described[92]. An electrophoresis plate with separated serum samples is placed in close contact with an agar plate containing homogeneously distributed antigen. Specific antibodies are trapped, after diffusion, in the antigen-containing gel and after fixation the antibodies may be visualized by means of treatment of the plate with isotope-labelled anti-immunoglobulin followed by autoradiography.

Another immunofixation technique which, however, does not employ electrophoretic separation of the sample was elaborated for quantitative purposes by Wadsworth[93]. In this technique, called the specific immunoprecipitate spot (SIS) assay, antigen applied on the surface of a gel reacts with antibodies in the corresponding antiserum incorporated in the gel. This technique seems to be useful for quantitation of proteins, for example, various immunoglobulins, for which differing results may be obtained by SRID or EIA due to the previously mentioned heterogeneity of the assayed material with regard to molecular size or electrophoretic mobility.

In another modification of the spot assay, spot immunoprecipitate assay (SIA)[94,95], precipitation occurs after spot-wise application of both antigen and antiserum to an inert gel. In this technique a substantial saving of antibody may be obtained as compared to the previously mentioned techniques.

THIN LAYER IMMUNOASSAY (TIA)

General considerations

Thin layer immunoassay (TIA) is a recently developed solid phase technique which has certain principal features in common with the enzyme-labelled immunosorbent assay, ELISA. In solid-phase techniques one of the serological reactants, either antigen or antibody, is firmly attached to a solid phase, usually a plastic tube (ELISA) or a plastic plate (TIA), which can be used for demonstration of the corresponding reactant.

In TIA the principles of performing the antigen–antibody reaction on a flat polystyrene surface, and the visualization of the reaction by condensation of water vapour, have been combined[99]. The main steps in the performance of TIA for demonstration of antibodies are schematically outlined in Figure 5.5.

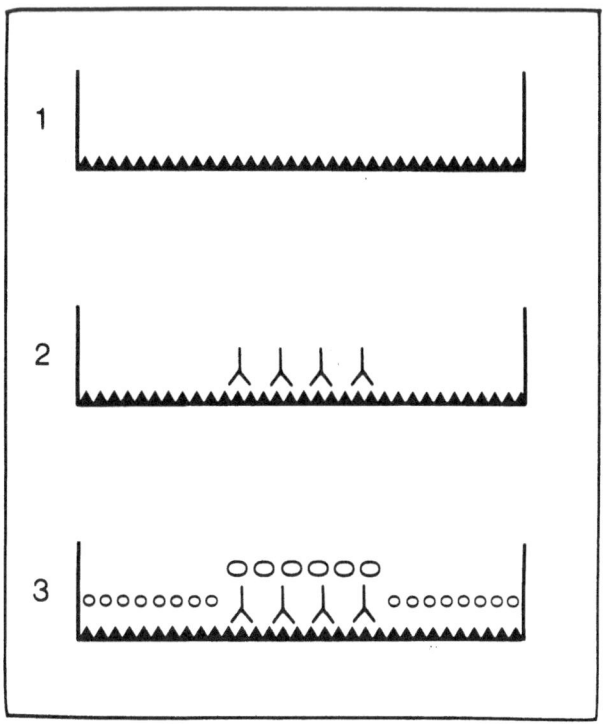

Figure 5.5   Schematic representation of the principle of TIA; (1) coating of plastic surface with antigen; (2) application of antiserum containing specific antibodies; (3) visualization of the antigen–antibody reaction by exposure of the surface to water vapour

A plastic surface is coated by incubation with an antigen-containing solution. After washing the antiserum is applied to the coated surface. After removal of unbound material by further careful washing of the surface, the antigen–antibody reaction is visualized by exposure of the plate to water vapour, either by breathing on the plate or by exposure of the surface to water vapour at about 60° for 60 s (vapour condensation on surface – VCS – technique). The latter procedure, although somewhat less sensitive than the former, gives a comparatively stable condensation pattern, which may be documented photographically. Provided that the primary coating does not increase the wettability of the surface extensively, antigen–antibody reactions may be seen as relatively hydrophilic areas with large condensation drops (increased wettability) against the background of antigen-coated polystyrene surface which is more hydrophobic (smaller condensation drops). The changed condensation pattern is generally easily recognizable by the naked eye (see Figure 5.6). In this connection it should be mentioned that visualization is not restricted to the VCS technique, but may be accomplished by a procedure analogous to that used in ELISA[100].

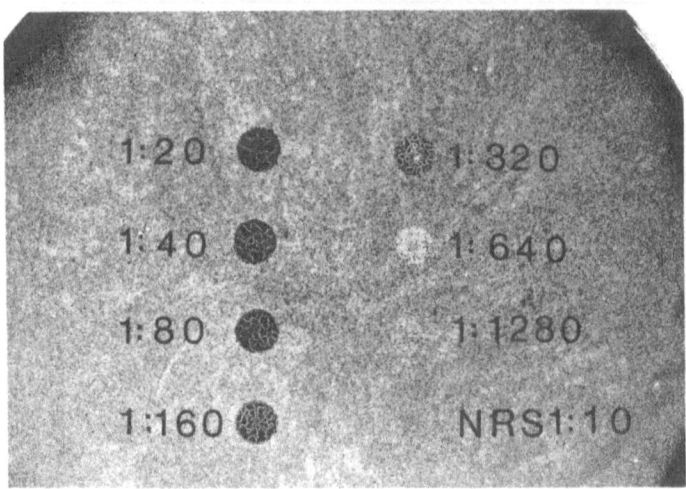

Figure 5.6 Photograph of spot-TIA plate which has been coated with bovine serum albumin (BSA) (100 μg/ml). Indicated dilutions of rabbit anti-BSA were applied spot-wise. After rinsing, visualization of antigen–antibody reactions by condensation of water vapour was performed

Quantitative determination of antibodies by TIA may be done either by spot-wise application of serial dilutions of the antiserum on the coated plate (spot-TIA)[101] or by letting the undiluted antiserum diffuse radially in a gel layer which has been applied on top of the antigen-coated surface (DIG-TIA)[99,102]. In the former modification of TIA the quantity of antibody is shown as the highest dilution of the antiserum giving a positive reaction (end-point titration). The change from a positive to a negative reaction occurs within a rather limited concentration interval corresponding to less than $\pm 50\%$ (one titre step in a 1/2 dilution series). The precision of spot-TIA is comparable to that of other end-point titration assays such as haemagglutination assays.

In DIG-TIA the size of the circular positive reaction zone is related to the antibody concentration of the applied serum, the areas or, under certain conditions, the diameters of the TIA zones being proportional to the logarithmic expression of the antibody concentration. In contrast to reversed SRID[103], diffusion of antibodies does not reach equilibrium in DIG-TIA as performed but is interrupted by rinsing off the supporting gel after a suitable time interval. The sensitivity of DIG-TIA as regularly performed for demonstration of antibodies is 1–3 μg Ab/ml.

It is possible to increase the sensitivity of TIA about ten times by treating the plates with an anti-immunoglobulin serum (reinforcement) before the visualization of antigen–antibody reactions. By using heavy chain specific antisera it is also possible to obtain information on the immunoglobulin class of the antibodies bound to the surface. It should be noted, however, that TIA in this respect is subject to the same limitations as other solid-phase techniques because of the possible competition for available antigenic sites between antibodies of different avidity and Ig class in the serum tested.

One factor which is of importance for the sensitivity of TIA is the concentration of the serological reactant used for coating. For most of the serological systems involving purified antigens which have been studied so far, a maximal plateau sensitivity of the assay is noted when the antigen solution used for coating reaches a certain concentration[101,102]. A decrease of the sensitivity is noted when lower coating concentrations are used. This has been explained as being due to an increased distance between the adsorbed molecules (spacing effect) resulting in failure to attain the sensitivity level of the visualization technique. For the serological systems studied so far, the coating concentration giving the above-mentioned plateau sensitivity was about 5–10 mg/l. From a practical point of view it may be worth mentioning that when purified antigen is available in sufficient amounts, we have used coating concentrations which are about ten times higher than those giving the plateau sensitivity. It should also be noted that one and the same antigen solution may be used for coating of several plates in succession. For instance a solution of IgG (100 mg/l) could be used for coating at least 50 plates without impairment of the serological reactivity. Elwing and Glantz, using a BSA–anti-BSA model system, recently showed that the amount of antigen adsorbed to the plastic surface is about $0.1–1.0 \mu g/cm^2$ depending on the coating concentration employed[104].

The spacing described above, leading to a decreased sensitivity, may be encountered in another situation; namely when the antigen used for coating is present in a mixture of different antigenic components. Due to possible competition between separate molecular species with regard to absorption, the surface concentration of the relevant antigen may become too low to allow subsequent visualization of bound antibodies by the VCS technique. This problem may be overcome by using purified antigen for coating as exemplified below with the studies on herpes simplex virus antigen. When TIA is used for determination of antibodies against various micro-organisms it is important to consider that an increased level of sensitivity of the assay implies an increase in cost and labour for purification of the coating antigen. It may be useful to compare different antigen preparations with various degrees of purity in preliminary trials under 'field conditions'.

Demonstration of antigen by TIA may be done either directly on plates which have been coated with specific antibodies, or by an inhibition technique (see Figure 5.7). The former technique has been used for demonstration of hepatitis B surface antigen (HBsAg) on plates coated with the γ-globulin

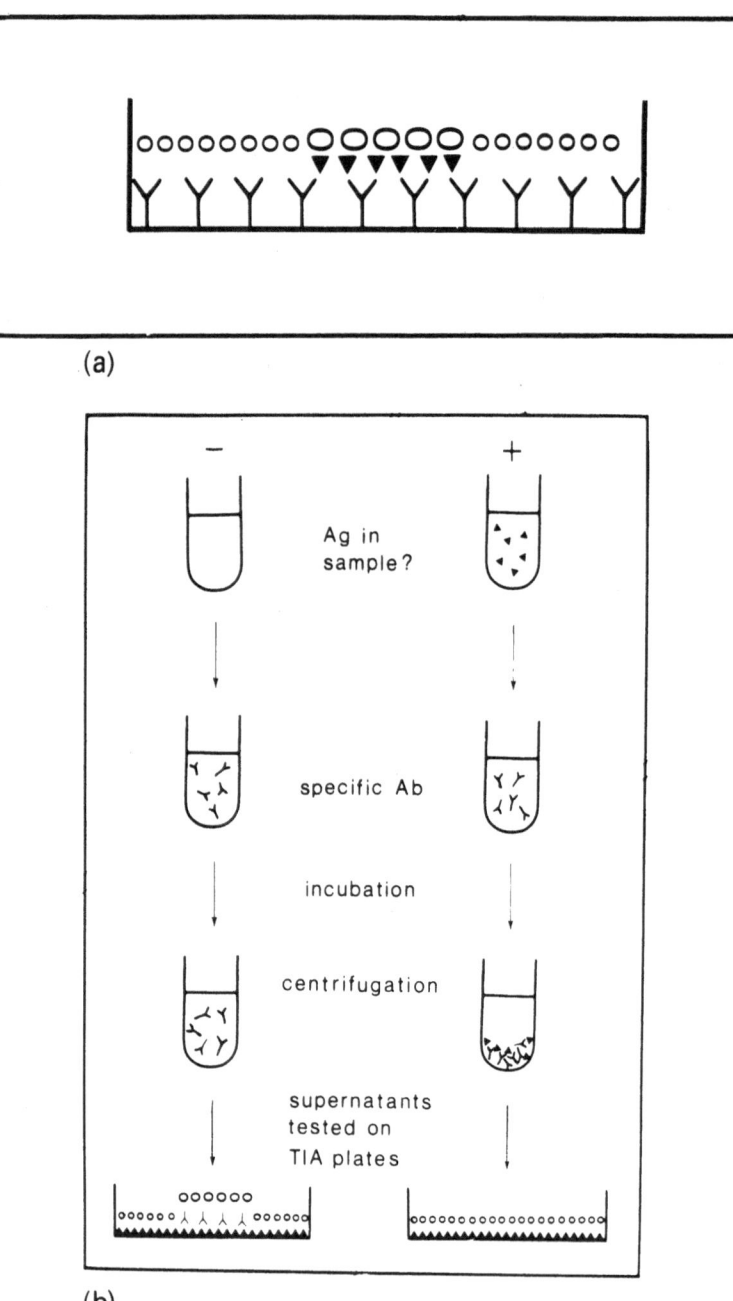

(a)

(b)

Figure 5.7   Schematic representation of procedures for demonstration of antigen by TIA: (a) direct demonstration of antigen by means of TIA plate coated with specific antibodies; (b) indirect technique for demonstration of antigen, employing an inhibition procedure

fraction of a specific goat hyperimmune serum against HBsAg[105]. Similarily carcinoembryonic antigen (CEA) and albumin were demonstrated on plates coated with specific CEA and albumin antibodies respectively, purified from hyperimmune sera by affinity chromatography[106]. The inhibition assay is performed by the addition of the antigen-containing sample to an antibody solution. After a suitable incubation period the presence or absence of antibody in the supernatant is determined on antigen-coated plates. When spot TIA was adapted for demonstration of antigen by means of the inhibition procedure the sensitivity attained ranged from 0.2 to 0.8 μg/ml depending upon the antigen–antibody system analysed[101].

Differences of sensitivity level relating to the previously mentioned spacing effect should also be considered when specific antibodies are used for coating in assays for demonstration of antigen. For practical reasons three different levels of sensitivity may be considered. When an unfractionated hyperimmune serum is used for coating, the spacing of the individual specific antibodies will be rather large due to the simultaneous adsorption of serologically irrelevant material in the immune serum, resulting in low sensitivity of the assay. The second possibility is coating of plates with the IgG fraction of the hyperimmune serum. Because of a less pronounced spacing of specific antibody molecules this procedure leads to an intermediate sensitivity. The highest level of sensitivity is obtained using plates coated with purified specific antibodies. In this connection it should be mentioned that when serum is assayed for antigen, the presence of rheumatoid factor (RF) is a possible source of error which may give falsely positive results in TIA as well as in other solid-phase immunoassays in which labelled anti-immunoglobulin is used to indicate the antigen–antibody reaction. Any RF may be detected by parallel testing of the sera on a set of plates coated with a solution of purified, normal IgG without specific antibodies (see applications).

Combination of the principles of immunoprecipitation-in-gel and TIA resulted in a new technique (PAS-TIA)[107], giving extended analytical possibilities as compared to the two basic techniques. Briefly, a regular double diffusion-in-gel analysis is performed in an agar gel prepared on top of a plastic surface which has been coated with a suitable antigen. After establishment of the precipitation pattern the gel is removed from the surface. Antigen–antibody complexes form a precipitation line containing the same serological specificity as the coating antigen are adsorbed to the surface. Visualization of the adsorbed complexes is performed by the VCS technique. The technique has been used in conjunction with comparative immunodiffusion analysis in order to identify a single precipitate formed by a purified antigen with its counterpart in a complex precipitation pattern. This technique should also be useful for the identification of which particular antigen in a complex mixture used for coating adsorbs to a plastic surface in TIA.

Applications

Virology

Antibodies to herpes simplex virus (HSV) were quantitated by DIG-TIA using plates coated with purified HSV antigen[108]. Since preliminary experiments had shown that crude HSV antigen, as contained in culture fluid, was not suitable for coating of plates, a procedure for purification of antigen implying a series of salt precipitation steps followed by wheat germ lectin chromatography was elaborated. When DIG-TIA, carried out on plates coated with the purified antigen, was compared with a HSV neutralization test, complete agreement with regard to positive or negative results was obtained. It was also possible to demonstrate a significant increase in antibody concentration by TIA in paired acute – and convalescent – phase sera from patients with HSV-1 infections showing a titre rise in neutralization and complement fixation tests.

HBsAg in serum was demonstrated in preliminary experiments by testing reference sera with known amounts of HBsAg on TIA plates which had been coated with the purified IgG fraction of a goat hyperimmune serum against HBsAg[105]. The sensitivity of the assay was similar to that of countercurrent immunoelectrophoresis. Attempts to increase the sensitivity by using purified specific antibodies for coating will be made.

Parasitology

Antibodies to *Schistosoma mansoni* were demonstrated in most sera from patients with schistosomiasis, using TIA plates coated with a crude extract from adult *S. mansoni*[109]. The diagnostic specificity of the assay was ascertained by the negative results obtained when sera from patients with schistosomiasis, as well as other parasitic diseases (filariasis, fascioliasis, echinococcosis, toxoplasmosis), were cross-tested on TIA plates which had been coated with crude extracts from the corresponding parasites. When TIA and ELISA were compared with regard to their ability to detect antibodies in known cases of infections with *S. mansoni* the performances of the two tests were almost identical, about 95% of the investigated sera being positive[110]. There was also an excellent correlation between the tests when antibodies against *S. haematobium*, both in human cases and in experimentally infected baboons, were determined. Extensive cross-reactions were noted when *S. mansoni* sera were tested on plates coated with *S. haematobium* and vice-versa. Work is in progress to overcome this possible disadvantage by preparation of species-specific antigen.

TIA has also been used for demonstration of antibodies against *Entamoeba histolytica* in sera from patients with entamoebiasis, and in blood donors[111]. The results with regard to positive or negative reactions agreed well with those obtained by the passive haemagglutination and immunodiffusion techniques.

Rheumatoid factor (RF)

RF could be determined quantitatively using DIG-TIA plates which had been coated with human IgG[112]. A reasonably good agreement between the results obtained by DIG-TIA and the Waaler-Rose test (AAF) was obtained when the two tests were compared. All AAF-positive sera were positive in DIG-TIA. Positive DIG-TIA reactions were also noted for some of the AAF-negative patient sera, but the possible clinical significance of this finding has yet to be established. When the TIA plates were reinforced with anti-IgA or anti-IgM an increase in size of the hydrophilic zones was noted for both antisera in most RF-positive sera analysed, indicating the simultaneous presence of RF of IgM and IgA type. Reinforcement with anti-IgG was not possible in these experiments since this resulted in an increased wettability of the whole surface. Reinforcement with anti-human IgG should be possible using DIG-TIA plates coated with rabbit IgG; such studies are in progress.

Ligand–receptor interactions

The use of TIA is not restricted to the study of antigen–antibody interactions; the technique has also been adapted for demonstration of ligand–receptor interactions of various other types. For instance, it was possible to demonstrate by TIA the binding of cholera toxin to a plastic surface coated with GM1, a ganglioside which has been postulated to constitute the natural cell membrane receptor for this toxin.

Indications for the probable structure of the receptors for tetanus toxin and Sendai virus respectively were obtained by applying the toxin or the virus preparation to surfaces which had been coated with different well-characterized gangliosides. It was shown that tetanus toxin adsorbed most strongly to the G1b series of gangliosides (GT1b, GQ1b and GD1b), whereas Sendai virus attached best to the ganglioside GQ1b[113]. Another similar type of interaction which has been studied by this technique is the binding of C-reactive protein to pneumococcal C-polysaccharide. It seems probable that TIA may be useful for the demonstration of other types of interactions as well, notably between cell receptors and toxins, viruses and hormones.

Acknowledgments

Part of the studies referred to, carried out at the author's laboratory, were supported by grants from WHO Special Programme for Tropical Diseases and the Swedish Agency for Research Cooperation with developing countries. I am grateful to Professor Örjan Ouchterlony for critical reading of the manuscript and to Ms Sally Bodin and Ms Diana Bruning for skilful typing.

References

1. Kraus, R. (1897). Über spezifische Reaktionen in keimfreien Filtraten aus Cholera-, Thyphus- und Pestbouillonkulturen, erzeugt durch homologes Serum. *Wien. Klin.Wochenschr.*, **10**, 736

2. Heidelberger, M. and Kendall, F. E. (1935). The precipitin reaction between type III pneumococcus polysaccharide and homologous antibody. III. A quantitative study and a theory of the reaction mechanism. *J. Exp. Med.*, **61**, 563

3. Bechhold, H. (1905). Strukturbildung in Gallerten. *Z. Phys. Chem.*, **52**, 185

4. Oudin, J. (1946). Méthode d'analyse immunochimique par précipitation spécifique en milieu gélifié. *C. R. Acad. Sci.*, **222**, 115

5. Ouchterlony, Ö. (1948). Antigen–antibody reactions in gels. *Arkiv för Kemi, Mineralogi och Geologi*, **Bd 26B**, No. 14, 1

6. Elek, S. D. (1948). The recognition of toxicogenic bacterial strains *in vitro. Br. Med. J.*, **1**, 493

7. Grabar, P. and Williams, C. A. (1953). Méthode permettant l'étude conjuguée des propriétés électrophorétiques et immunochimiques d'un mélange de protéines. Application au sérum sanguin. *Biochim. Biophys. Acta*, **10**, 193

8. Laurell, C.-B. (1965). Antigen–antibody crossed electrophoresis. *Analyt. Biochem.*, **10**, 358

9. Boyd, W. C. (1966). *Fundamentals of Immunology*, 4th Edn., p. 349. (New York, London, Sydney: Interscience Publishers)

10. Marrack, J. R. (1938). The chemistry of antigens and antibodies. Medical Research Council (Britain), Spec. Rep. Ser. No. 230

11. Marrack, J. R. and Richards, C. B. (1971). Light-scattering studies of the formation of aggregates in mixtures of antigen and antibody. *Immunology*, **20**, 1019

12. Steensgaard, J. and Frich, J. R. (1979). A theoretical approach to precipitin reactions. Insight from computer simulation. *Immunology*, **36**, 279

13. Møller, N. P. H. (1979). The precipitin reaction: the importance of the Fc-portion of IgG. *Protides Biol. Fluids*, **26**, 83

14. Møller, N. P. H. (1979). Fc-mediated immune precipitation. I. A new role of the Fc-portion of IgG. *Immunology*, **38**, 631

15. Møller, N. P. H. and Steensgaard, J. (1979). Fc-mediated immune precipitation. II. Analysis of precipitating immune complexes by rate-zonal ultra-centrifugation. *Immunology*, **38**, 641

16. Heidelberger, M. (1939). Quantitative absolute methods in the study of antigen–antibody reactions. *Bacteriol. Rev.*, **3**, 49

17. Kabat, I. (1976). *Structural Concepts in Immunology and Immunochemistry.* (New York: Holt, Rinehart & Winston)

18. Day, E. D. (1966). *Foundations of Immunochemistry*, p. 209. (Baltimore: The Williams & Wilkins Company)

19. Ritchie, R. (ed.) (1978). *Automated Immunoanalysis.* (New York and Basel: Marcel Dekker, Inc.)

20. Libby, R. L. (1938). The photonreflectometer – an instrument for the measurement of turbid systems. *J. Immunol.*, **34**, 71

21. Libby, R. L. (1938). A new and rapid quantitative technic for the determination of the potency of types I and II antipneumococcal serum. *J. Immunol.*, **34**, 269

22. Boyden, A., Bolton, E. and Gemeroy, D. (1947). Precipitin testing with special reference to the photoelectric measurement of turbidity. *J. Immunol.*, **57**, 211

23. Ritchie, R. F. (1967). A simple, direct, and sensitive technique for measurement of specific protein in dilute solution. *J. Lab. Clin. Med.*, **70**, 512

24. Schultze, H. E. and Schwick, G. (1959). Quantitative immunologische Bestimmung von Plasmaproteinen. *Clin. Chim. Acta*, **4**, 15

25. Lizana, J. and Hellsing, K. (1974). Manual immunonephelometric assay of proteins with the use of polymer enhancement. *Clin. Chem.*, **20**, 1181

26. Finley, P. R., Williams, R. J., Lichti, D. A., Griffith, F. and Thies, A. C. (1979).

Immunochemical determination of human immunoglobulins; use of kinetic turbidimetry and a 36-place centrifugal analyzer. *Clin. Chem.*, **25**, 526

27. Dito, W. R. (1979). Rapid immunonephelometric quantitation of eleven serum proteins by centrifugal fast analyzer. *Am. J. Clin. Pathol.*, **71**, 301

28. Jacobsen, C. and Steensgaard, J. (1979). Measurements of precipitin reactions by difference turbidimetry: a new method. *Immunology*, **36**, 293

29. Killingsworth, L. M. and Savory, J. (1972). Manual nephelometric methods for immunochemical determination of immunoglobulins IgG, IgA, and IgM in human serum. *Clin. Chem.*, **18**, 335

30. Killingsworth, L. M. and Savory, J. (1973). Nephelometric studies of the precipitin reaction: a model system for specific protein measurements. *Clin. Chem.*, **19**, 403

31. Buffone, G. J., Savory, J., Cross, R. E. and Hammond, J. E. (1975). Evaluation of kinetic light scattering as an approach to the measurement of specific proteins with the centrifugal analyzer. I. Methodology. *Clin. Chem.*, **21**, 1731

32. Buffone, G. J., Savory, J. and Hermans, J. (1975). Evaluation of kinetic light scattering as an approach to the measurement of specific proteins with the centrifugal analyzer. II. Theoretical considerations. *Clin. Chem.*, **21**, 1735

33. Deaton, C. D., Maxwell, K. W., Smith, R. S. and Creveling, R. L. (1976). Use of laser nephelometry in the measurement of serum proteins. *Clin. Chem.*, **22**, 1465

34. Smith, R. S., Deaton, C. D., Creveling, R. L. and Maxwell, K. W. (1976). Manual laser nephelometry. An improved concept to quantitate serum proteins. *Am. J. Clin. Pathol.*, **66**, 464

35. Sieber, A. and Gross, J. (1977). Protein determination by laser nephelometry. *Med. Lab.*, **2**, 17

36. Buffone, G. J., Savory, J. and Cross, R. E. (1974). Use of a laser-equipped centrifugal analyzer for kinetic measurement of serum IgG. *Clin. Chem.*, **20**, 1320

37. Virella, G., Waller, M. and Fudenberg, H. H. (1978). Nephelometric method for determination of rheumatoid factor. *J. Immunol. Methods*, **22**, 247

38. Finley, P. R., Hicks, M. J., Williams, R. J., Hinlicky, J. and Lichti, D. A. (1979). Rate nephelometric measurement of rheumatoid factor in serum. *Clin. Chem.*, **25**, 1909

39. Roberts-Thomson, P. J. and Bradley, J. (1979). A nephelometric study of the reaction of monoclonal rheumatoid factor with heat aggregated gamma globulin and sera from patients with immune complex diseases. *Clin. Exp. Immunol.*, **37**, 408

40. Höffken, K., Bestek, U., Sperber, U. and Schmidt, C. G. (1979). Quantitation of immune complexes by nephelometry. *J. Immunol. Methods*, **29**, 237

41. Daigneault, R. and Lemieux, D. (1978). Evaluation of a Behring laser-nephelometer prototype in the measurement of IgG, IgA and IgM. *Clin. Biochem.*, **11**, 28

42. Whicher, J. T., Perry, D. E. and Hobbs, J. R. (1978). An evaluation of the Hyland laser nephelometer PDQ system for the measurement of immunoglobulins. *Ann. Clin. Biochem.*, **15**, 77

43. Heuck, C. C. and Schlierf, G. (1979). Nephelometry of apolipoprotein B in human serum. *Clin. Chem.*, **25**, 221

44. Alexander, R. L., Jr. (1980). Comparison of radial immunodiffusion and laser nephelometry for quantitating some serum proteins. *Clin. Chem.*, **26**, 314

45. Roberts, N. B. and Nance, L. A. (1979). Hyland laser nephelometer compared with radial-immunodiffusion assay for quantitation of individual immunoglobulins, and an assessment of the excess-antigen effect. *Clin. Chem.*, **25**, 1509

46. Virella, G. and Fudenberg, H. H. (1977). Comparison of immunoglobulin determinations in pathological sera by radial immunodiffusion and laser nephelometry. *Clin. Chem.*, **23**, 1925

47. Buffone, G. J., Brett, E. M., Lewis, S. A., Iosefsohn, M. and Hicks, J. M. (1979). Limitations of immunochemical measurement of ceruloplasmin. *Clin. Chem.*, **25**, 749

48. Keren, D. F., Frye, R. M., Datiles, T. B. and Grindon, A. J. (1978). A modification of the automated immune precipitin method for quantitation of human serum immunoglobulins.

Am. J. Clin. Pathol., **70**, 41

49. Nishikawa, T., Kubo, H. and Saito, M. (1979). Competitive nephelometric immunoassay method for antiepileptic drugs in patient blood. *J. Immunol. Methods*, **29**, 85

50. Crowle, A. J. (1961). *Immunodiffusion*, p. 333. (New York and London: Academic Press)

51. Backhausz, R. (1967). *Immunodiffusion und Immunoelectrophorese*, p. 516. (Jena: Gustav Fischer Verlag)

52. Ouchterlony, Ö. and Nilsson, L.-Å. (1978). Immunodiffusion and immunoelectrophoresis. In Weir, D. M. (ed.). *Handbook of Experimental Immunology*, Chap. 19. (Oxford: Blackwell Scientific Publications)

53. Axelsen, N. H., Kröll, J. and Weeke, B. (eds.) (1973). A manual of quantitative immunoelectrophoresis. Methods and applications. *Scand. J. Immunol.*, **2** (Suppl), 1

54. Axelsen, N. H. (ed.) (1980). *Techniques of Immunoprecipitation-in-gel.* In press (Oxford: Blackwell Scientific Publications)

55. Ouchterlony, Ö. (1949). Antigen–antibody reactions in gels. *Acta Pathol. Microbiol. Scand.*, **26**. 507

56. Mancini, G., Carbonara, A. O. and Heremans, J. F. (1965). Immunochemical quantitation of antigens by single radial immunodiffusion. *Immunochemistry*, **2**, 235

57. Fahey, J. L. and McKelvey, E. M. (1965). Quantitative determination of serum immunoglobulins in antibody-agar plates. *J. Immunol.*, **94**, 84

58. Berne, B. H. (1974). Differing methodology and equations used in quantitating immunoglobulins by radial immunodiffusion – a comparative evaluation of reported and commercial techniques. *Clin. Chem.*, **20**, 61

59. MRC Working Party. (1971). Characterization of antisera as reagents. Recommendations made by the MRC Working Party on the clinical use of immunological reagents. *Immunology*, **20**, 3

60. Reimer, C. B., Smith, S. J., Hannon, W. H., Ritchie, R. F., van Es, L., Becker, W., Markowitz, H., Gauldie, J. and Anderson, S. G. (1978). Progress towards international reference standards for human serum proteins. *J. Biol. Stand.*, **6**, 133

61. Johnson, J. D., Butts, G. and Dahlgren, D. A. (1973). Instrumentation for quantitation of radial immunodiffusion (RID) patterns. *Clin. Chem.*, **19**, 683

62. Oakley, C. L. and Fulthorpe, A. J. (1953). Antigenic analysis by diffusion. *J. Pathol. Bacteriol.*, **65**, 49

63. Ouchterlony, Ö. (1958). Diffusion-in-gel methods for immunological analysis. In Kallós, P. (ed.) *Progress in Allergy*, Vol. 5, p. 1. (Basel: Karger)

64. Ouchterlony, Ö. (1962). Diffusion-in-gel methods for immunological analysis. II. In Kallós, P. and Waksman, B. H. (eds.) *Progress in Allergy*, Vol. 6, p. 30. (Basel: Karger)

65. Nilsson L.-Å. (1980). Double diffusion-in-gel. In Axelsen, N. (ed.) *Techniques of Immunoprecipitation-in-gel.* In press. (Oxford: Blackwell Scientific Publications)

66. Grabar, P. and Burtin, P. (1964). *Immunoelectrophoretic Analysis.* (Amsterdam: Elsevier Publishing Company)

67. Nilsson, L.-Å. (1980). Immunoelectrophoresis. In Axelsen, N. (ed.). *Techniques of Immunoprecipitation-in-gel.* In press. (Oxford: Blackwell Scientific Publications)

68. Bussard, A. (1959). Description d'une technique combinant simultanement l'électrophorèse et la précipitation immunologique dans un gel: l'électrosynérèse. *Biochim. Biophys. Acta*, **31**, 258

69. Myhre, E. B. (1974). Rapid diagnosis of bacterial meningitis. Demonstration of bacterial antigen by counterimmunoelectrophoresis. *Scand. J. Infect. Dis.*, **6**, 237

70. Tosswill, J., Ridley, D. S. and Warhurst, D. C. (1980). Counter current immunoelectrophoresis as a rapid screening test for amoebic liver abscess. *J. Clin. Pathol.*, **33**, 33

71. Laurell, C.-B. (1966). Quantitative estimation of proteins by electrophoresis in agarose gel containing antibodies. *Anal. Biochem.*, **15**, 45

72. Cann, J. R. (1975). A phenomenological theory of rocket and crossed immunoelectrophoresis. *Immunochemistry*, **12**, 473

73. Krøll, J. (1976). Immunoelectrophoretic quantitation of trace proteins. *J. Immunol. Methods*, **13**, 333

74. Steinman, C. R. (1979). Quantitation of submicrogram concentrations of DNA by a modified Laurell electrophoresis method. *J. Immunol. Methods*, **31**, 373

75. Laurell, C. -B. (1972). Electroimmuno assay. *Scand. J. Clin. Lab. Invest.*, **29** (Suppl. 124), 21

76. Weeke, B. (1973). Rocket immunoelectrophoresis. In Axelsen, N., Krøll, J. and Weeke, B. (eds.) A manual of quantitative immunoelectrophoresis: methods and applications. *Scand. J. Immunol.*, **2** (Suppl. 1)

77. Laurell, C.-B. (1973). Electrophoresis, specific protein assays, or both in measurement of plasma proteins? *Clin. Chem.*, **19**, 99

78. Gilliland, B. C. (1977). Immunologic quantitation of serum immunoglobulins. *Am. J. Clin. Pathol.*, **68**, 664

79. Oxelius, V. -A. (1978). Crossed immunoelectrophoresis and electroimmunoassay of human IgG subclasses. *Acta Pathol. Microbiol. Scand. (C)*, **86**, 109

80. Ressler, N. (1960). Two-dimensional electrophoresis of protein antigens with an antibody containing buffer. *Clin. Chim. Acta*, **5**, 795

81. Clarke. H. G. M. and Freeman, T. (1968). Quantitative immunoelectrophoresis of human serum proteins. *Clin. Sci.*, **35**, 403

82. Crowle, A. J. (1977). Templates for antiserum application in immunoelectrophoresis and two-dimensional electroimmunodiffusion. *J. Immunol. Methods*, **14**, 197

83. Kuusi, N. (1979). A technical improvement for crossed immunoelectrophoresis. *J. Immunol. Methods*, **31**, 361

84. Ekwall, K., Söderholm, J. and Wadström, T. (1976). Disc-crossed immuno- electrophoresis. A simple 'laying-on' technique permitting the use of commercially available agarose. *J. Immunol. Methods*, **12**, 103

85. Groc, W., Harms, A. and Lahn, W. (1975). Electrophoretic separation of serum proteins on cellulose acetate followed by electrophoresis in antibody-containing agarose gel. *Clin. Chim. Acta*, **60**, 371

86. Verbruggen, R. (1975). Quantitative immunoelectrophoretic methods: a literature survey. *Clin. Chem.*, **21**, 5

87. Syverson, R. E., Buckley, H. R. and Gibian, J. R. (1978). Increasing the predictive value positive of the precipitin test for the diagnosis of deep-seated candidiasis. *Am. J. Clin. Pathol.*, **70**, 826

88. Alper, C. A. and Johnson, A. M. (1969). Immunofixation electrophoresis: A technique for the study of protein polymorphism. *Vox Sang.*, **17**, 445

89. Whicher, J. T., Higginson, J., Riches, P. G. and Radford, S. (1980). Clinical applications of immunofixation. I. The detection and quantitation of complement activation. *J. Clin. Pathol.* (In press)

90. Whicher, J. T., Hawkins, L. and Higginson, J. (1980). Clinical applications of immunofixation. II. A more sensitive technique for the detection of Bence-Jones protein. *J. Clin. Pathol.* (In press)

91. Ritchie, R. F. and Smith, R. (1976). Immunofixation. III. Application to the study of monoclonal proteins. *Clin. Chem.*, **22**, 1982

92. Nordal, H. J., Vandvik, B. and Norrby, E. (1978). Demonstration of electrophoretically restricted virus-specific antibodies in serum and cerebrospinal fluid by imprint electroimmunofixation. *Scand. J. Immunol.*, **7**, 381

93. Wadsworth, C. (1977). A new specific quantitation-in-gel method differentiating commercial human serum standards intended for RID analyses. *Scand. J. Immunol.*, **6**, 97

94. Wadsworth, C. (1977). A rapid spot immunoprecipitate assay method applied · to quantitating C-reactive protein in pediatric sera. *Scand. J. Immunol.*, **6**, 1263

95. Wadsworth, C. (1980). Spot immunoprecipitate assay and stained protein assay. In Axelsen, N. (ed.). *Techniques of Immunoprecipitation-in-gel*. In press. (Oxford: Blackwell Scientific Publications)

96. Langmuir, I. and Schaefer, V. (1937). Optical measurement of the thickness of a film adsorbed from a solution. *J. Am. Chem. Soc.*, **59**, 2400

97. Vroman, L. and Adams, A. (1969). Identification of rapid changes at plasma–solid interfaces. *J. Biomed. Mater. Res.*, **3**, 43

98. Adams, A. L., Klings, M., Fischer, G. C. and Vroman, L. (1973). Three simple ways to detect antibody–antigen complex on flat surfaces. *J. Immunol. Methods*, **3**, 227

99. Elwing, H., Nilsson, L.-Å. and Ouchterlony, Ö. (1976). Visualization principles in thin-layer immunoassays (TIA) on plastic surfaces. *Int. Arch. Allergy Appl. Immunol.*, **51**, 757

100. Elwing, H. and Nygren, H. (1979). Diffusion in gel-enzyme linked immunosorbent assay (DIG-ELISA): A simple method for quantitation of class-specific antibodies. *J. Immunol. Methods*, **31**, 101

101. Elwing, H., Nilsson, L.-Å. and Ouchterlony, Ö. (1977). A simple spot technique for thin layer immunoassays (TIA) on plastic surfaces. *J. Immunol. Methods*, **17**, 131

102. Elwing, H. and Nilsson, L.-Å. (1980). Diffusion-in-gel thin layer immunoassay (DIG-TIA). Optimal conditions for quantitation of antibodies. *J. Immunol Methods* (In press)

103. Vaerman, J.-P., Lebacq-Verheyden, A.-M., Scolari, L. and Heremans, J. F. (1969). Further studies on single radial immunodiffusion. II. The reversed system: diffusion of antibodies in antigen-containing gels. *Immunochemistry*, **6**, 287

104. Elwing, H. and Glantz, P.-O. (1980). Water wettability of antigen and antigen–antibody adsorbed on solid surfaces. (In preparation)

105. WHO. (1979). Detection of antigens and IgM antibodies for rapid diagnosis of viral infections: a WHO memorandum. *Bull. WHO*, **57**, 925

106. Elwing, H. and Nilsson, L.-Å. Unpublished observations.

107. Elwing, H., Nilsson, L.-Å. and Ouchterlony, Ö. (1977). A precipitate adsorption on surface technique: a combination of immunodiffusion and thin-layer immunoassay. *Int. Arch. Allergy Appl. Immunol.*, **55**, 82

108. Jeansson, S., Elwing, H. and Nilsson, L.-Å. (1979). Thin-layer immunoassay for determination of antibodies to herpes simplex virus. *J. Clin. Microbiol.*, **9**, 317

109. Nilsson, L.-Å., Björck, L., Capron, A., Elwing, H. and Ouchterlony, Ö. (1980). Application of thin layer immunoassay (TIA) as a serodiagnostic tool in schistosomiasis. A preliminary report. *Trans. R. Soc. Trop. Med. Hyg.*, **74**, 201

110. Ismail, M., Draper, C., Ouchterlony, Ö., Nilsson, L.-Å. and Terry, R. (1979). A comparison between a new serological method, thin layer immunoassay (TIA), and the enzyme-linked immunosorbent assay (ELISA) for the detection of antibodies in schistosomiasis. *Parasite Immunol.*, **1**, 251

111. Nilsson, L.-Å., Petchclai, B. and Elwing, H. (1980). Application of thin layer immunoassay (TIA) for demonstration of antibodies against *Entamoeba histolytica*. *Am. J. Trop. Med. Hyg.*, **29**, 524

112. Nilsson, L.-Å., Björck, L., Elwing. H. and Ouchterlony, Ö. (1980). Determination of rheumatoid factor by means of thin layer immunoassay (TIA). *Int. Arch. Allergy Appl. Immunol.*, **63**, 294

113. Holmgren, J., Elwing, H., Fredman, P., Strannegård, Ö. and Svennerholm, L. (1980). Gangliosides as receptors for bacterial toxins and Sendai virus. In Svennerholm, L., Mandel, P., Dreyfus. H. and Urban, P. F. (eds.). *Structure and Function of Gangliosides*. (New York: Plenum Press).

6
Radioimmunoassay

A. E. BOLTON

INTRODUCTION

Radioimmunoassay (RIA) is currently one of the most widely applied of all immunoassay procedures. The increasing application of this technique in many routine clinical diagnostic tests has resulted in requirements for improved reliability and reproducibility, greater rapidity and larger sample throughput. The more demanding performance requirements for RIAs has been reflected in an evolution of the technology associated with these methods, particularly in the area of automation and experimental procedures relating to the use of automated equipment.

RIA is one example of a limited reagent or saturation assay type of method[1], three component parts of which are labelled tracer ligand, specific binding reagent (antibody) and a means whereby that fraction of labelled ligand bound to antibody can be measured. In the specific case of RIA the tracer ligand is labelled with a radioisotope, and consequently measurement of that proportion bound to antibody can only be accomplished after physical separation of bound from free fractions.

TRACER LIGAND

Many of the problems encountered in RIA procedures are caused by difficulties associated with the radioligand. The advantages of using radioactively labelled tracer ligands are the ease, reliability, rapidity, sensitivity and precision of their quantitation. There are two types of labelled ligand preparation. In the first, the radioactive nuclide replaces a non-radioactive isotope of the same element which is present in the native molecule. This is generally confined to ^{14}C or ^{3}H labelling of small molecules (haptens), for example drugs and steroids, although radioactive iodine can be substituted for non-radioactive iodine in the thyroid hormones thyroxine and tri-iodothyronine. Most labelled ligand preparations for RIA are of the second type in which a foreign radioactive atom is used, i.e. an atom which is not part of the structure of the native material.

The most widely used element for foreign labelling is iodine as this can be readily substituted by simple chemical methods into proteins and other molecules. Suitable radioactive nuclides of iodine are available (Table 6.1),

Table 6.1 Some properties of ^{125}I and ^{131}I

	^{131}I	^{125}I
Half life	8 days	60 days
Specific radioactivity (theoretical, at 100% isotopic abundance)	16 000 Ci/matom	2200 Ci/matom
Isotopic abundance normally available	20%	95%
Counting efficiency (average)	30%	70%
Approximate count rate for 1 atom/mol of iodine and peptide of MW 20 000 (ct min^{-1} μg^{-1})		
Fresh iodine	105.6×10^6	160.9×10^6
Iodine 1 week old	59.4×10^6	151.6×10^6

particularly ^{125}I. This combines the advantages of high isotopic abundance, high specific radioactivity and high counting efficiency with the fact that, as a γ-emitting radionuclide, no special preparation of samples is required before counting. Such are the advantages of γ-emitting labelled ligands that even in cases where tritiated tracers are available, e.g. many steroids, radioiodine-labelled derivatives have been prepared for use in radioimmunoassays[2]. These overcome the need for the tedious and expensive liquid scintillation counting systems required for β-emitting radionuclides. In addition to ease of counting ^{125}I has a much higher count rate than ^3H – 1 gram atom of ^{125}I gives approximately 75 times the count rate produced by 1 gram atom of ^3H.

Radioiodination of proteins

As radioiodination of proteins is foreign labelling, it follows that the labelled product is chemically different from the immunogen. There may, therefore, be differences in binding by antiserum of labelled ligand and unlabelled material. It is important that any loss in affinity of binding of tracer ligand to antibody should be minimal, and radioiodination techniques have been developed and optimized to minimize such differences.

Reduction in affinity can be caused by structural alterations consequent upon the substitution of iodine into the protein, chemical alteration of the protein caused by the iodination reagents used and possible impurities present in the radioiodide solution, and alterations resulting from manipulation of the protein in dilute, carrier-free solution before and during labelling.

The effect of iodine substitution on the affinity of binding of protein to antibody can best be demonstrated with small peptides of known amino acid sequence where antibodies with specificities to different parts of the amino acid sequence are available, e.g. ACTH[3].

Chemical alteration of amino acids by iodination reagents, particularly by oxidizing agents used in radioiodination reactions, has been demonstrated. Thus tryptophan is oxidized to the oxindole[4], cysteine to cystine[5] and methionine is oxidized to the sulphoxide[5]. Parallel experiments have demonstrated marked differences in tracer affinity for antibody when labelled ligands have been prepared using radioiodide from more than one source[6,7], suggesting that impurities in the radioiodide solution may be responsible for some alterations in labelled protein preparations.

Protein iodination methods can be divided into two groups: direct methods in which radioiodine is directly substituted into amino acid residues of the protein (often tyrosine), and conjugation methods in which a radioiodine-containing moiety is conjugated to a specific amino acid residue (often lysine). All the former (direct) methods suffer from the potential problem of exposure of the protein to possible noxious impurities in the radioiodide solution – a problem avoided by the conjugation methods.

Direct iodination methods

The most widely used method for protein radioiodination utilizes chloramine-T (N-chloro-p-toluenesulphonamide) as oxidizing agent[8,9]. Radioiodide ($^{125}I^-$) is oxidized in the presence of the protein to yield an active form of iodine, thought to be cationic (I^+)[10], which substitutes into the phenolic groups of tyrosine[11] or the imidazole ring of histidine[12] depending on the experimental conditions used. The reaction is then quenched and any remaining active species of radioiodine reduced to $^{125}I^-$ by the addition of excess reducing agent. As first described, a relatively large amount of oxidizing agent (88 μg chloramine-T) was employed, and sodium metabisulphite (240 μg) was used for quenching[8]. Such high levels of iodination reagents may in part account for the sporadic occurrence of reduced binding to antibody of protein ligands prepared by this method[13]. Reduction in the amount of oxidizing and reducing agents used has been described, e.g. 10 μg chloramine-T and 24 μg metabisulphite[14], 5 μg each of chloramine-T and metabisulphite[15], and 1 μg of chloramine-T[16]. The use of alternative and less damaging reducing agents to terminate the reaction, or quenching the reaction by the addition of an excess of protein, e.g. albumin[16], should minimize reductive alteration of the protein during the labelling reaction.

In order to minimize the oxidative alteration of proteins during labelling, alternative oxidizing agents to chloramine-T have been investigated. Sodium hypochlorite[17] and chlorine[18] have been used and claimed to be milder in their effects on proteins. However, neither method has apparently gained wide acceptance.

As an alternative to soluble oxidizing agents, Fraker and Speck[19] proposed the use of a sparingly soluble chloramide for protein radioiodination.

A film of the chloramide, 1,3.4.6-tetrachloro-3α,6α-diphenylglycoluril (commercially available under the name Iodogen from Pierce & Warriner UK Ltd) is deposited in the iodination tube by evaporation of a solution in methylene chloride. Such reaction tubes may be stored for up to 6 months when desiccated at room temperature[20]. Protein and radioiodide solutions are then added to the tube and the reaction allowed to proceed for 5 min at 0 °C in an ice bath. The iodination can be terminated by removal of the reaction mixture from the tube[19]. However, active iodide may still be present in solution, and this is sometimes capable of iodinating carrier proteins etc. after removal from the reaction vessel (Table 6.2). To obviate such effects, either a

Table 6.2 Radioiodination of fibrinogen using Iodogen as oxidizing agent

Reactants added to tube with Iodogen	Reactants added after removal from Iodogen tube	Incorporation of ^{125}I into protein
Protein	Na^{125}I	0%
Na^{125}I	Protein	9.2%
Protein Na^{+125}I	—	29.8%

Protein (5 μg in 10 μl phosphate buffer, pH 7.5) and Na^{125}I (10 μl, 1 mCi) were added as indicated above to tubes containing 2 μg of Iodogen.

reducing agent may be added, or the reaction mixture diluted and allowed to stand for 15 min for the active iodine to decay[21]. Alternatively, the reaction conditions can be adjusted such that all the radioiodide is incorporated into the tracer – in such cases the radiolabelled ligand can apparently be used directly in the radioimmunoassay without any further purification[22].

Use of 1,3,4,6-tetrachloro-3α,6α-diphenylglycoluril as oxidizing agent for the preparation of radioiodinated proteins has been shown to yield radioligands with small improvements in affinity of binding to antibody in the case of IgG to anti-IgG[19], and improvements both in binding to antibody and stability in the case of some hormones[21,22], particularly small peptides[21]. However, this method has been shown to yield tracers with a markedly lowered affinity for antibody and high instability compared with other methods in the case of human spleen ferritin[23].

Enzymatic methods of oxidative iodination, first developed for trace-labelling immunoglobulins[24], has been applied to the preparation of high specific-radioactivity tracers for use in RIAs[25]. Lactoperoxidase is mixed with protein solution, radioiodide solution and hydrogen peroxide, and the reaction allowed to continue for 2–10 s[25]. Alternatively, lower concentrations of hydrogen peroxide added sequentially to minimize protein oxidation[26], and a longer reaction time, may be used. The reaction can be terminated by dilution[25] or by the addition of cysteine[24]. The use of a glucose oxidase–glucose system to generate hydrogen peroxide[27] should further reduce the likely damaging effects of this added oxidizing agent. The reaction conditions need careful optimization[28], and lactoperoxidase-catalysed iodinations have a clearly defined pH optimum around 5.0[29]. Tyrosine is the major amino acid iodinated, although histidine is also substituted to a lesser extent[30]. Proteins labelled by the enzyme-catalysed iodination method have been found to maintain their structural integrity[31]. To minimize contamination of the radioligand preparation with labelled enzyme protein, which inevitably forms during the reaction, the enzyme can be coupled to an insoluble support medium and used in this form. The labelling reaction can then be terminated simply by removal of the reactants from the solid-coupled enzyme after centrifugation. Insoluble copolymers of glucose oxidase and lactoperodidase have been described[32], and insoluble forms of these enzymes are available along with radioiodide commercially as an iodination kit (New England Nuclear, Boston, USA).

Conjugation labelling methods

Such methods in which a radioactive moiety is conjugated to a protein obviate direct exposure of the protein being labelled to oxidizing and reducing agents, and to radioiodide solutions (Figure 6.1). Three conjugation-labelling methods have been described, using radioiodinated N-succinimidyl 3-(4-hydroxyphenyl) propionate[33], using radioiodinated methyl-p-hydroxybenzimidate hydrochloride[34], and using [^{125}I]di-iodofluorescein isothiocyanate[35]. The first of these is probably the most widely used in radioligand preparation for RIA, and is available commercially in a ready-iodinated form (Bolton–Hunter Reagent, New England Nuclear, Boston, USA and the Radiochemical Centre, Amersham, UK). For certain proteins, for example ferritin[23,36] conjugation, labelling has been found to yield more stable tracers with higher affinity of binding to antibody than other methods. There is also some evidence that this method gives tracers of more reliable performance in a routine RIA laboratory than those prepared by the oxidative chloramine-T method[37].

Labelling of proteins with the Bolton–Hunter reagent results in a predominance of labelled lysine residues, with a small degree of labelling of tyrosine and histidine[38].

Conjugation labelling methods tend to result in low yields of radioligand. This problem can be minimized by increasing the concentration of reactants[37], and is less important in those cases where radiolabelled can be

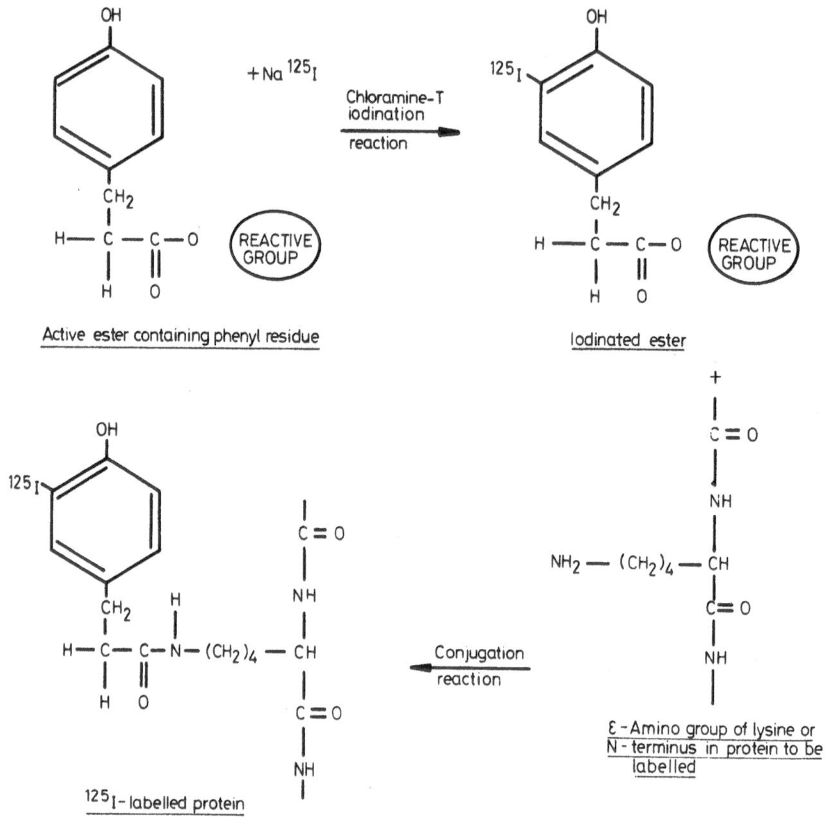

Figure 6.1 The conjugation labelling reaction

separated from unlabelled protein, since in such cases, tracers of high specific radioactivity can still be obtained[16].

In general, the use of a simple, high-yield direct iodination procedure is to be recommended for first attempts at preparing radioligands of proteins, and if problems are encountered, the lower yield but probably more reliable conjugation method should be tried.

Radioiodination of haptens

The convenience and high count rate of ^{125}I have led to the development and widespread application of methods of labelling haptens with this radionuclide. Such methods also allow the development of assays for compounds for which no tritiated or other radioactive tracer is readily available. The incorporation of a γ-emitting radionuclide into hapten tracers for radioimmunoassay also more readily permits the application of automated systems to such assays.

Radioiodine can be directly substituted into certain haptens, e.g. into the phenolic ring of oestrogens, by a simple oxidative iodination reaction. However, such radioligand derivatives of oestradiol-17β remain almost completely unbound by antisera to oestradiol-17β[2]. Direct incorporation of radioiodine into testosterone has also been described[39] by melting the steroid with Na[125]I. Such a radioligand yielded a RIA for testosterone with very similar characteristics to one using a tritiated testosterone tracer[39]. The precise chemical identity of this iodinated derivative is not understood.

Most radioiodinated ligands for use in RIA systems have been prepared using derivatives of the hapten containing a phenolic or imidazole group. Such derivatives can either be radioiodinated directly after conjugation of the hapten to the group into which the label can be substituted[40], or the hapten can be conjugated to an already labelled group[41]. This latter technique can be applied where the hapten itself would become labelled if the whole conjugate were to be exposed to the iodination reaction, e.g. oestrogens. Conjugates of some non-polar steroids have also been found to be difficult to iodinate directly[42]. Histamine derivatives may give fewer products after conjugation to hapten than tyrosine derivatives, and are thus preferred[2].

Although ^{125}I-labelled radioligands for hapten radioimmunoassay have great advantages of convenience of counting, there are certain disadvantages in their use. Haptens are rendered immunogenic by chemical linkage to a protein, and antisera are raised by immunizing such protein–hapten conjugates. The position of linkage in the hapten molecule, and the type of chemical linkage employed, can affect the specificity of the antiserum obtained[43]. Often the same hapten derivatives are used both to link the protein to form the immunogen and to prepare the derivatives for radiolabelling. Antisera to conjugates of proteins with haptens have specificities to the hapten, to the protein, and to the link between the two. As this linkage region is also present in the tracer, and the antibodies directed towards it often have very high affinities[44], it follows that the radioligand used in the assay often has a greater affinity for the antibody than the unmodified hapten being measured. This results in a reduction in the sensitivity of the assay system[45], although this can be overcome to some extent by employing a different chemical linkage in the hapten–protein conjugate and in the radioligand[46]. Another potential problem is that metabolites may be present in the sample being assayed which resemble the tracer more closely than the hapten being investigated. This can result in an amplification of interference by such metabolites in an assay[47]. Some examples of linkages which can be used in the preparation of radioiodinated ligands or immunogens for haptens are listed in Table 6.3.

ANTIBODY

The antibodies selected for use in radioimmunoassay procedures, like those for other saturation assay type methods, should exhibit high structural specificity and energy of reaction to yield assays of maximum specificity and

Table 6.3 Chemical groups utilized in the preparation of immunogens and tracer ligands for hapten radioimmunoassay

Linkage	Reference
Carboxymethyl-oxime	67
Hemisuccinate	67
Chlorocarbonate	67
Thioether alkanoic acid	68
Glucuronide	69

Table 6.4 An immunization schedule for raising antisera

Day	Immunogen (ml)	Bleed (ml)
0	1	–
14	1	–
21	–	20
28	1	–
35	–	20
42	1	–
49	–	20

Immunogen in physiological saline is emulsified with an equal volume of Freund's complete adjuvant before injecting. 100–500 μg of immunogen per animal for each dose is effective. Each 1 ml dose is given at four sites subcutaneously (two over shoulder blades, two inside the thighs)

potential sensitivity. The immunization schedule and route of immunization vary considerably among different workers in the field. One schedule, involving multiple intradermal injections of low doses of immunogen, has been described and claimed to give highly specific antisera in a few weeks with minimal doses of immunogen[48]. A schedule that has proved successful in the author's laboratory is shown in Table 6.4.

Polypeptides and proteins of molecular weight above about 4000 are immunogenic. Materials of lower molecular weight, including steroids, drugs and thyroid hormones, can be rendered immunogenic by coupling to a carrier protein – often bovine serum albumin or keyhole limpet haemocyanin.

The specificity of an antiserum obtained depends in part on the response of the individual animal immunized. However, in the case of immunogenic polypeptides and proteins the purity of the immunogen can play an important part. Thus, for example, in the case of the pituitary glycoprotein hormones, which share a common α-subunit and a hormone specific β-subunit, antisera raised against the whole molecule will have a high chance of containing specificities towards both subunits. Hence such antisera will cross-react with other glycoprotein hormones. Antisera raised against the hormone-specific β-subunit should be more specific.

The specificity of antisera to low molecular weight haptens depends to a great extent on the site of attachment of the molecule to the carrier protein used in the immunogen[43]. In principle a site in the hapten molecule should be selected for linking to the protein such that the structurally specific sites of the molecule remain exposed. Thus, for example, antiserum to oestradiol-17β linked via the 6 position[49] and progesterone linked via the 11 position[50] are highly specific.

SEPARATION SYSTEM

In the case of assays using a radioactive ligand, a physical separation of the antibody-bound and free tracer has to be effected before that fraction of labelled ligand bound to antibody can be measured. Such separation is generally carried out by precipitation or insolubilization of the antibody-bound or free fraction, and separating the phases by centrifugation or filtration. Antibody-bound ligand can be precipitated chemically, using ethanol or ammonium sulphate for example, or unbound ligand can be adsorbed for example onto dextran-coated charcoal. Such methods, while inexpensive, require careful optimization and can only be applied to a limited number of assays. More general separation systems utilize the immunological precipitation of the bound fraction (double-antibody methods), the use of the first or second antibodies in an insoluble form (solid-phase methods), or various preparations of staphylococcal protein-A.

Double-antibody separation systems

Optimized double-antibody systems[10] provide a reproducible and non-disruptive method for the separation of antibody-bound from free radioligand in RIA procedures. However, with increasing pressure for rapid production of results, the relatively long incubation time (generally overnight) required for this method mitigates against its use. Although the rate of reaction between first and second antibody is rapid, the formation of the precipitate which is the basis of the separation system is a more protracted process. This can be speeded up by increasing the concentration of second antibody used; however, this increases the use of an already expensive reagent. Alternatively the rate of precipitation can be increased by the addition of some form of accelerator, for example ammonium sulphate or dextran[51]. In our laboratory we have found that polyethylene glycol 6000 is an effective accelerator of precipitation, provided that a concentration is used that does not cause non-specific precipitation of the ligand being measured.

Solid-phase methods

Insoluble forms of both first and second antibodies have been used. Whole antisera, or the IgG fraction, can either be covalently coupled to a solid support medium such as Sephadex or cellulose[52], rendered insoluble by polymerization[53], or physically adsorbed to a solid support, for example the surface of assay tubes[54]. The latter system allows the simplest possible manual approach to RIA. Tracer and sample are added to the coated tube and separated after the incubation period by aspirating or pouring the contents from the tube. The preparation of suitably coated tubes with acceptable batch-to-batch reproducibility may pose technical problems, and different tube types may have different properties. However, commercially produced assay kits based on such separation systems are available.

Solid-phase separation systems have advantages of simplicity – no additional manipulations are required to effect separation other than the removal of the unbound ligand (in the liquid phase) after centrifugation or filtration. The separation is efficient, and precision is high. Problems associated with low recovery of antibody activity and reduced assay sensitivity have been described[55], and particulate solid preparations need to be kept in suspension to minimize incubation times. This can be tedious if mechanical rotators or shakers are used; however, increasing the viscosity of the incubation medium[56], or the use of magnetized particles[57] and a magnetic field can overcome these problems.

Solid-phase second antibody systems[58] retain the advantages of solid-phase first antibody systems, and overcome many of their problems such as low recovery of antibody and reduced assay sensitivity. Using agarose-coupled second antibody, Hunter has described a system in which the antibody-bound fraction separates by sedimentation through a layer of sucrose, eliminating the need for centrifugation and washing of the solid residue[59].

Staphylococcal protein-A

Protein-A is a cell wall-associated protein of *Staphylococcus aureus*[60]. It binds specifically to the Fc region of immunoglobulins from humans and other animal species[61]. The use of a suspension of formaldehyde-treated heat-killed staphylococci for separating antibody-bound from free ligand in radio-immunoassays has been described[62], and provided sufficient excess of this reagent is added to bind all the IgG present in samples[63], the separation system is apparently unaffected by patient's sera.

AUTOMATION

Although many automated systems exist for sample dilution and reagent addition these result in only semi-automated RIA procedures. The necessity of physically separating antibody-bound from free ligand in radioimmunoassays imposes considerable technical difficulties in the development of fully automated systems. The length of incubation times often involved in RIA procedures may also require samples to come 'off-line' during this period. Equipment can be based either on continuous-flow principles, or the automated handling of samples in individual reaction tubes.

The first approach, continuous flow, is exemplified by the Technicon system. This utilizes antibodies coupled to solid magnetized particles[57] as the separation system – these are retained in a magnetic field while the unbound ligand is washed away. The particles are then released into the counting head. One drawback to continuous-flow systems is that only assays with short incubation times can be handled satisfactorily. A second disadvantage to the Technicon system (as with many other commercially available systems) is that one is dependent on specialized materials (in this case magnetized solid-coupled antibodies) obtained from the manufacturer – such reagents may be expensive.

The second approach – automated handling of samples in individual reaction tubes, is exemplified by the system developed by Bagshawe for human chorionic gonadotrophin[64] and now updated and available commercially (Kemteck). Samples are diluted into tubes in cassettes and reagents added. The cassettes can then be incubated 'off-line'. Separation is effected by a double-antibody system, the precipitate being removed by filtration onto discs set in plastic tape. The tape then moves on to the detector. Because the samples come 'off-line' protracted incubation times can be utilized if required.

Solid-phase double antibody separated by sedimentation through a sucrose solution[59] has also been used as the basis for a proposed system of automation[65, 66].

These latter two systems would appear to be somewhat more flexible in their requirements for reagents and less dependent on commercial materials. New developments in the automation of RIA techniques can be expected in the future.

CONCLUSIONS

Radionuclides do not occur in normal clinical or biological samples in readily measurable amounts. Furthermore, γ-emitting nuclides can be quantitated reliably and this quantitation is not affected or quenched by organic materials. Thus it follows that, in RIAs utilizing radioligands labelled with ^{125}I, there can be no non-specific intrusion at the counting stage unless the patient's samples contain radionuclides used for therapy or *in vivo* diagnostic procedures. Quantitation of immunoassays using other forms of detection systems, e.g. enzymes or fluorimetry, or RIAs using tritiated tracers, are all prone, to a greater or lesser extent, to non-specific effects produced by biological materials. Because of this inherent robustness in the assay systems, it is likely that the RIA will be a favoured method for the measurement of low concentrations of clinically important substances in the future. New areas of application can be anticipated; e.g. increasing applications of this technique in haematology seem likely. One area of technology specific to RIA that may become more widely exploited – the use of two radionuclides with non-overlapping emission spectra to measure two compounds simultaneously in the same tube – has already been validated in combined assays for vitamin B_{12} and folate (Simultrac, commercial kit from Shwarz/Mann) using ^{51}Co and ^{125}I as radionuclides.

References

1. Ekins, R. P. (1976). General principles of hormone assay. In Loraine, J. A. and Bell, E. T. (eds.). *Hormone Assays and their Clinical Application*, 4th Edn., pp. 1–72. (Edinburgh: Churchill Livingstone)

2. Hunter, W. M., Nars, P. -W. and Rutherford, F. J. (1975). Preparation and behaviour of ^{125}I-labelled radioligands for phenolic and neutral steroids. In Cameron, E. H. D., Hillier, S. G. and Griffiths, K. (eds.). *Steroid Immunoassay: Proceedings of the Fifth Tenovus Workshop*, pp. 141–52 (Cardiff: Alpha Omega Publishing)

3. Landon, J., Livanou, T. and Greenwood, F. C. (1967). The preparation and immunological properties of ^{131}I-labelled adrenocorticotrophin. *Biochem. J.*, **105**, 1075

4. Alexander, N. M. (1974). Oxidative cleavage of tryptophanyl peptide bonds during chemical, and peroxidase, catalysed iodinations. *J. Biol. Chem.*, **249**, 1946–52

5. Schechter, Y., Burstein, Y. and Patchornik, A. (1975). Selective oxidation of methionine residues in proteins. *Biochemistry (USA)*, **14**, 4497

6. Buckle, R. M. (1971). Radioimmunoassay of parathyroid hormone: studies on iodination and purification of labelled hormone. In Kirkham, K. E. and Hunter, W. M. (eds.). *Radioimmunoassay Methods: European Workshop*, pp. 42–54. (Edinburgh: Churchill Livingstone)

7. Chesworth, J. M. (1977). Radioimmunoassays of ovine LH and ovine prolactin using polymerized second antisera. *Anal. Biochem.*, **80**, 31

8. Hunter, W. M. and Greenwood, F. C. (1962). Preparation of iodine-131-labelled human growth hormone of high specific activity. *Nature (London)*, **194**, 495

9. Greenwood, F. C., Hunter, W. M. and Glover, J. S. (1963). The preparation of ^{131}I-labelled human growth hormone of high specific radioactivity. *Biochem. J.*, **89**, 114

10. Hunter, W. M. (1973). Radioimmunoassay. In Weir, D. M. (ed.). *Handbook of Experimental Immunology*, pp. 17.1–17.36. (Oxford: Blackwell Scientific Publications)

11. Krohn, K. A., Knight, L. C., Haring, J. F. and Welch, M. J. (1977). Differences in the sites of iodination of proteins following four methods of radioiodination. *Biochim. Biophys. Acta*, **490**, 497

12. Chrisholm, D. J., Young, J. D. and Lazarus, L. (1969). The gastrointestinal stimulus to insulin release. 1. Secretin. *J. Clin. Invest.*, **48**, 1453

13. Hunter, W. M. (1971). The preparation and assessment of iodinated antigens. In Kirkham, K. E. and Hunter, W. M. (eds.) *Radioimmunoassay Methods. European Workshop*, pp. 3-23 (Edinburgh: Churchill Livingstone)

14. Wide, L., Nillius, S. J., Gemzell, C. and Roos, P. (1973). Radioimmunosorbent assay of follicle-stimulating hormone and luteinizing hormone in serum and urine from men and women. *Acta Endocrinol.*, **73** (Suppl. 174), 7

15. Stadil, F. and Rehfeld, J. F. (1972). Preparation of ^{125}I-labelled synthetic human gastrin 1 for

radioimmunoanalysis. *Scand. J. Clin. Lab. Invest.*, **30**, 361

16. Heber, D., Odell, W. D., Schedewie, H. and Wolfsen, A. R. (1978). Improved iodination of peptides for radioimmunoassay and membrane radioreceptor assay. *Clin. Chem.*, **24**, 796

17. Redshaw, M. R. and Lynch, S. S. (1974). An improved method for the preparation of iodinated antigens for radioimmunoassay. *J. Endocrinol.*, **60**, 527

18. Butt, W. R. (1972). The iodination of follicle-stimulating and other hormones for radioimmunoassay. *J. Endocrinol.*, **55**, 453

19. Fraker, P. J. and Speck, J. C. (1978). Protein and cell membrane iodinations with a sparingly soluble chloroamide, 1,3,4,6-tetrachloro-3α,6α-diphenylglycoluril. *Biochem. Biophys. Res. Commun.*, **80**, 849

20. Markwell, M. A. K. and Fox, C. F. (1978). Surface-specific iodination of membrane proteins of viruses and eucaryotic cells using 1,3,4,6-tetrachloro-3α,6α-diphenylglycoluril. *Biochemistry (USA)*, **17**, 4807

21. Salacinski, P. R. P., McLean, C., Sykes, J. E. C., Clement-Jones, V. V. and Lowry, P. J. (In preparation)

22. Salacinski, P., Hope, J., McLean, C., Clement-Jones, V., Sykes, J., Price, J. and Lowry, P. J. (1979). A new simple method which allows theoretical incorporation of radioiodine into proteins and peptides without damage. *J. Endocrinol.*, **81**, 131

23. Bolton, A. E., Lee-Own, V., McLean, R. K. and Challand, G. S. (1979). Three different radioiodination methods for human spleen ferritin compared. *Clin. Chem.*, **25**, 1826

24. Marchalonis, J. J. (1969). An enzymic method for the trace iodination of immunoglobulins and other proteins. *Biochem. J.*, **113**, 299

25. Thorell, J. I. and Johansson, B. G. (1971). Enzymic iodination of polypeptides with iodine-125 to high specific activity. *Biochim. Biophys. Acta*, **251**, 363

26. Phillips, D. R. and Morrison, M. (1971). Exposed protein on the intact human erythrocyte. *Biochemistry (USA)*, **10**, 1766

27. Hubbard, A. L. and Cohn, Z. A. (1972). The enzymatic iodination of the red cell membrane. *J. Cell Biol.*, **55**, 390

28. Miyachi, Y., Vaitukaitis, J. L., Nieschlag, E. and Lipset, M. B. (1972). Enzymatic radioiodination of gonadotrophins. *J. Clin. Endocrinol. Metab.*, **34**, 23

29. Morrison, M. and Bayse, G. S. (1970). Catalysis of iodination by lactoperoxidase. *Biochemistry (USA)*, **9**, 2995

30. Krohn, K. A. and Welch, M. J. (1974). Studies of radioiodinated fibrinogen. II. Lactoperoxidase iodination of fibrinogen and model compounds. *Int. J. Appl. Radiat. Isot.*, **25**, 315

31. Miyachy, Y. and Chrambach, A. (1972). Structural integrity of gonadotrophins after enzymatic iodination. *Biochem. Biophys. Res. Commun.*, **48**, 464

32. Karonen, S. L., Mersky, P., Siren, M. and Seuderling, V. (1975). An enzymatic solid-phase method for trace iodination of proteins and peptides with ^{125}iodide. *Anal. Biochem.*, **67**, 1

33. Bolton, A. E. and Hunter, W. M. (1973). The labelling of proteins to high specific radioactivities by conjugation to a ^{125}I-containing acylating agent. *Biochem. J.*, **133**, 529

34. Wood, F. T., Wu, W. M. and Gerhart, J. C. (1975). The radioactive labelling of protein with an iodinated amidination reagent. *Anal. Biochem.*, **69**, 339

35. Gabel, C. A. and Shapiro, B. M. (1978). ^{125}I-diiodofluoroscein isothyocyanate: its synthesis and use as a reagent for labelling protein and cells to high specific radioactivity. *Anal. Biochem.*, **86**, 396

36. Goldie, D. J. and Thomas, M. J. (1978). Measurement of serum ferritin by radioimmunoassay. *Ann. Clin. Biochem.*, **15**, 102

37. Bolton, A. E. Bennie, J. G. and Hunter, W. M. (1977). Innovations in labelling techniques. In Peeters, H. (ed.) *Protides of the Biological Fluids, 24th Colloquium*, pp. 687–93. (Oxford: Pergamon Press)

38. Knight, L. C., and Welch, M. J. (1978). Sites of direct and indirect halogenation of albumin. *Biochim. Biophys. Acta*, **534**, 185

39. Hampl, R., Dvorak, P., Lukesova, S., Kozak, I., Chrpova, M. and Starka, L. (1978). The use

D

of iodinated steroid as radioligand for testosterone radioimmunoassay. *J. Steroid Biochem.*, **9**, 771

40. Oliver, G. C., Parker, B. M., Brasfield, D. L. and Parker, C. W. (1968). The measurement of digitoxin in human serum by radioimmunoassay. *J. Clin. Invest.*, **47**, 1035

41. Nars, P. -W. and Hunter, W. M. (1973). A method for labelling oestradiol-17β with radioiodine for radioimmunoassay. *J. Endocrinol.*, **57**, xlvii

42. Scarisbrick, J. J. and Cameron, E. H. D. (1975). Radioimmunoassay of progesterone: comparison of (1,2,6,7-^{3}H4)-progesterone and progesterone-(^{125}I)-iodohistamine radioligand. *J. Steroid Biochem.*, **6**, 51

43. Niswender, G. D., Nett, T. N., Meyer, D. L. and Hagerman, D. D. (1975). Factors influencing the specificity of antibodies to steroid hormones. In Cameron, E. H. D., Hillier, S. G. and Griffiths, K. (eds.) *Steroid Immunoassay: Proceedings of the Fifth Tenovus Workshop*, pp. 61–6. (Cardiff: Alpha Omega Publishing)

44. Jeffcoat, S. L., Edwards, R., Gilby, E. D. and White, N. (1975). The use of ^{3}H-labelled ligands in steroid radioimmunoassays. In Cameron, E. H. D., Hillier, S. G. and Griffiths, K. (eds.) *Steroid Immunoassay: Proceedings of the Fifth Tenovus Workshop*, pp. 133–40. (Cardiff: Alpha Omega Publishing)

45. Ekins, R. P. (1975). In Cameron, E. H. D., Hillier, S. G. and Griffiths, K. (eds.) *Steroid Immunoassay: Proceedings of the Fifth Tenovus Workshop*, pp. 172–4. (Cardiff: Alpha Omega Publishing)

46. Gomez-Sanchez, C., Milwich, L. and Holland, O. B. (1977). Radioiodinated derivatives for steroid radioimmunoassay. Application to the radioimmunoassay of cortisol. *J. Lab. Clin. Med.*, **89**, 902

47. Bolton, A. E. and Rutherford, F. J. (1976). Evidence for the presence of 6-keto-oestradiol-17β in human plasma – implications for oestradiol-17β radioimmunoassays. *J. Steroid Biochem.*, **7**, 71

48. Vaitukaitis, J., Robbins, J. B., Nieschlag, E. and Ross, G. T. (1971). A method for producing specific antisera with small doses of immunogen. *J. Clin. Endocrinol. Metab.*, **33**, 988

49. Lindner, H. R., Perel, E. and Friedlander, A. (1970). In Finkelstein, M., Conti, C., Klopper, A. and Cassano, C. (eds.) *Research in Steroids*, Vol. 4, p. 197. (Oxford: Pergamon Press)

50. Dighe, K. K. and Hunter, W. M. (1974). A solid-phase radioimmunoassay for plasma progesterone. *Biochem. J.*, **143**, 219

51. Martin, M. J. and Landon, J. (1975). In Pasternak, C. A. (ed.) *Radioimmunoassay in Clinical Biochemistry*, pp. 269–81. (London: Heyden)

52. Wide, L. (1969). Radioimmunoassays employing immunoadsorbents. *Acta Endocrinol.*, **63**, (Suppl. 142), 207

53. Donini, S. and Donini, P. (1969). Radioimmunoassay employing polymerized antisera. *Acta Endocrinol.*, **63** (Suppl. 142), 257

54. Catt, K. J. (1969). Radioimmunoassay with antibody-coated discs and tubes. *Acta Endocrinol.*, **63** (Suppl. 142), 222

55. Bolton, A. E. and Hunter, W. M. (1973). The use of antisera covalently coupled to agarose, cellulose and Sephadex in radioimmunoassay systems for proteins and haptens. *Biochim. Biophys. Acta*, **329**, 318

56. Bolton, A. E., Dighe, K. K. and Hunter, W. M. (1975). Steroid antibody immunoadsorbents. In Cameron, E. H. D., Hillier, S. G. and Griffiths, K. (eds.) *Steroid Immunoassay: Proceedings of the Fifth Tenovus Workshop*, pp. 257–66. (Cardiff: Alpha Omega Publishing)

57. Nye, L., Forrest, G. C., Greenwood, H., Gardner, J. S., Jay, R., Roberts, J. R. and Landon, J. (1976). Solid-phase, magnetic particle radioimmunoassay. *Clin. Chim. Acta*, **69**, 387

58. den Hollander, F. C. and Schuurs, A. H. W. M. (1971). In Kirkham, K. E. and Hunter, W. M. (eds.) *Radioimmunoassay Methods: European Workshop*, pp. 419–22. (Edinburgh: Churchill Livingstone)

59. Hunter, W. M. (1977). Simplified solid-phase radioimmunoassay without centrifugation. *Acta Endocrinol.* (Suppl. 212), 260

60. Verwey, E. F. (1940). A type-specific protein derived from the *Staphylococcus. J. Exp. Med.*, **71**, 635

61. Forsgreen, A. and Sjoquist, J. (1966). Protein A from *S. aureus.* 1. Pseudo-immune reaction with human γ-globulin. *J. Immunol.*, **97**, 822

62. Jonsson, S. (1978). Protein-A-containing *Staphylococcus aureus* as an immunoglobulin-binding reagent in radioimmunoassay and in non-radioactive surface immunoassay. In *Radioimmunoassay and Related Procedures in Medicine 1977*, Vol. 1, pp. 161–75. (Vienna: IAEA)

63. Jonsson, S. and Kronvall, G. (1974). The use of protein A-containing *Staphylococcus aureus* as a solid-phase anti-IgG reagent in immunoassays as exemplified in the quantitation of α-fetoprotein in normal human adult serum. *Eur. J. Immunol.*, **4**, 29

64. Butler, H. A., Bagshawe, K. D., Marchant, D. and Verdin, A. (1971). In Kirkham, K. E. and Hunter, W. M. (eds.) *Radioimmunoassay Methods: European Workshop*, pp. 635–8. (Edinburgh: Churchill Livingstone)

65. Hunter, W. M. (1975). UK P.A. 47078/75

66. Hunter, W. M. (1976). UK P.A. 50517/76

67. Erlanger, B. F., Borek, F., Beiser, S. M. and Lieberman, S. (1957). Steroid–protein conjugates. 1. Preparation and characterization of conjugates of bovine serum albumin with testosterone and with cortisone. *J. Biol. Chem.*, **228**, 713

68. Kohen, F., Bauminger, S. and Lindner, H. R. (1976). Preparation of antigenic steroid–protein conjugates. In Cameron, E. H. D., Hillier, S. G. and Griffiths, K. (eds.) *Steroid Immunoassay: Fifth Tenovus Workshop*, pp. 11–22. (Cardiff: Alpha Omega Publishing)

69. Kellie, A. E., Lichman, K. V. and Samarajeewa, P. (1976). Chemistry of steroid–protein conjugate formation. In Cameron, E. H. D., Hillier, S. G. and Griffiths, K. (eds.) *Steroid Immunoassay: Proceedings of the Fifth Tenovus Workshop*, pp. 33–46. (Cardiff: Alpha Omega Publishing)

7
Heterogeneous Enzyme Immunoassays

S. AVRAMEAS

INTRODUCTION

Enzyme immunoassays can be defined as quantitative immunological procedures in which the extent of an antigen–antibody reaction is evaluated by enzyme measurement. Such procedures are based on the use of enzymes as labels[1,2] for antigens or antibodies and on the fact that the quantity of an enzyme can be accurately determined by appropriate enzymatic techniques. Humoral[3-5] as well as tissue[6] constituents can be measured using enzyme immunoassays. In all cases the basic principles of the procedures employed are the same as those developed for various quantitative radioimmunoassays (RIAs), but measurement of enzyme activity is substituted for radioactivity counting.

GENERAL CONSIDERATIONS

As for RIA, competitive[3-5, 7-9] and non-competitive procedures[9-14] have also been used in enzyme immunoassay. When dealing with the measurement of multivalent antigens, we have found that non-competitive assays are more sensitive than competitive assays and also more suitable for routine work. This procedure presents the additional advantage of requiring labelled antibody rather than labelled antigen. Enzyme-labelled antibody preparations are easier to standardize and are more universal tools than labelled antigens in enzyme immunoassays.

Regardless of whether competitive or non-competitive procedures are used, the sensitivity, specificity and reproducibility of the various enzyme im-

85

munoassays depend mainly upon the insoluble phase used to immobilize the antigen or the antibody, the enzyme used as the label and the effectiveness of the enzyme conjugate employed.

SOLID-PHASE ANTIGEN OR ANTIBODY

To immobilize antigens or antibody a number of solid phases have been employed. Like other investigators[10, 15, 16], we have found that the adsorption of antibodies to plastic surfaces, a procedure introduced by Catt and Tregear[17] for RIA, produced immobilized antibody preparations equally effective for enzyme immunoassays. The advantages of this kind of immobilization are its simplicity, its ease of handling, and the fact that it requires only small quantities of antibody. Although plastic solid phases have many advantages, one has to bear in mind that by this procedure only a small quantity of material is fixed, that due to hydrophobicity, denaturation of the adsorbed macromolecules may take place with time, and that sometimes desorption of the immobilized antibody can occur. However, the main disadvantage of the plastic surface is that the quantity of antibody adsorbed varies from one batch of plastic to another, and even the adsorption capacity of different wells of the same microplate may vary.

Covalent coupling of antibody to cellulose[18], agarose[19] or polyacrylamide beads[6, 14] produces stable immobilized antibody preparations which give more reproducible results in enzyme immunoassays. However, a serious drawback of covalent immobilization on beads is that all washing steps have to be carried out by successive centrifugations, thus making the overall procedures tedious and time-consuming. Therefore, this technique should be confined to situations in which a high degree of precision for quantitative evaluation is required. However, when a large number of samples has to be tested, and when the precision of the assay is not so fundamental, it is preferable to use plastic microplates.

In an effort to improve the use of covalently immobilized antibody in enzyme immunoassays we have recently developed magnetic polyacrylamide agarose beads[14]. These beads are prepared by adding iron oxide during the polymerization of the polyacrylamide.

Active aldehyde groups can be introduced onto these beads through the polyacrylamide moieties using glutaraldehyde[20] or, alternatively, active imine groups through the agarose by cyanogen bromide treatment[21]. Antigens and antibodies can then be covalently immobilized on these activated beads and used in enzyme immunoassays as follows: after each incubation or washing step, the tubes containing the beads are deposited on a rack supporting a series of small magnets. The beads are attracted by the magnets and are deposited on the wall of the tube which is in contact with the magnets. All the beads are deposited on the wall in 30–60 s. This technique avoids tedious and time-consuming successive centrifugations.

ENZYME AND SUBSTRATES

Chromogenic substrates

The enzymes most often used in enzyme immunoassays are horseradish peroxidase, *Aspergillus niger* glucose oxidase, *Escherichia coli* and veal intestinal alkaline phosphatase and *E coli* β-galactosidase. Using magnetic polyacrylamide agarose beads as the solid phase we have systematically compared[14] peroxidase, glucose oxidase, alkaline phosphatase, and β-galactosidase-labelled antibodies for their effectiveness in a non-competitive enzyme immunoassay for the measurement of human IgE. Although the four enzymes detected equally small quantities of IgE, the dose–response curves of alkaline phosphatase and β-galactosidase were superior to those of glucose oxidase and peroxidase. With alkaline phosphatase and β-galactosidase conjugates, a linear plot was obtained for quantities of human IgE ranging from 1 to 1000 iu. The sensitivities of the measurements in this case were equal to that achieved with RIA. Furthermore, best results in terms of reproducibility were also obtained when either alkaline phosphatase or β-galactosidase were used as the enzyme marker. The satisfactory results obtained with these two enzymes are probably due to their substrates (*p*-nitrophenylphosphate for alkaline phosphatase and *p*-nitrophenyl-β-*D*-galactopyranoside for β-galactosidase) which are more stable than those used to measure peroxidase and glucose oxidase (*o*-dianisidine, *o*-phenylenediamine, ABTS). The relative instability of the various substrates used to measure oxidoreductases like peroxidase and glucose oxidase can be a serious drawback in the use of oxidoreductases in enzyme immunoassays requiring a long incubation time.

Fluorogenic, radioactive and other non-chromogenic substrates

Using fluorescent radioactive and light-emission techniques, procedures have been developed which can measure extremely small quantities of enzyme. Such procedures, when applied to enzyme immunoassays, allow measurement of very ·small quantities of antigen or antibody. The use of radioactive substrates[22] has allowed the measurement of 10^{-17} g of cholera toxin. Using 4-methyl-umbelliferyl-β-*D*-galactopyranoside, a fluorogenic substrate for β-galactosidase, extremely small quantities of constituents have been measured[23,24]. In our hands, amounts of human IgE as low as 0.05 iu/ml have been measured using β-galactosidase as the enzyme marker and 4-methyl-umbelliferyl-β-*D*-galactopyranoside as its substrates[25].

Enzyme-labelled antibodies have been used to measure immunoglobulin antigenic determinants on the surface of lymphocytes. Using a peroxidase conjugate and chromogenic substrate (*o*-dianisidine and O_2H_2) at least 100 000 lymphocytes were needed in order to have a measurable amount of immunoglobulin[6]. With the same conjugate but using a light-emission technique capable of evaluating peroxidase at the femtogram level, 100–1000 lymphocytes were needed[26]. Finally, the use of a β-galactosidase conjugate in a fluorescent microtechnique made it possible to quantitate the immunoglobulins present on the surface of individual lymphocytes[27,28].

CONJUGATES

Enzyme conjugates are prepared by covalently coupling antigens or antibodies to enzymes. Various coupling procedures have been described (for a review see reference 29) but either glutaraldehyde[30,31] or sodium m-periodate[32] coupling procedures have been most commonly used. The periodate procedure is applied principally for the preparation of peroxidase conjugates while glutaraldehyde is used for the preparation of many other enzyme–protein conjugates employed in enzyme immunoassays.

In addition to the use of conjugates prepared by covalently coupling enzymes to antigens or antibodies, it is also possible to make use of non-covalent interactions[33-35]. More recently, we have developed two enzyme immunoassay procedures which are based on the non-covalent but exceptionally strong interaction of avidin with biotin[36].

In the first procedure, biotin-labelled antibody, biotin-labelled enzyme, and native unlabelled avidin were used. To quantitate an antigen, the antigen is allowed to react with the corresponding immobilized antibody. After washing, biotin-labelled antibody is added and allowed to incubate. After washing to eliminate the excess biotin-labelled antibody, avidin is added. After incubation and washing, a biotin-labelled enzyme is added. This step, after incubation and washing, is followed by measurement of the enzyme associated with the immobilized phase. The procedure is based on the principle that avidin possesses four active sites, not all of which are engaged in the interaction with the biotin-labelled antibody. The remaining free active sites can then operate as acceptors for the biotin-labelled enzyme, secondarily added to the system.

In the second procedure, biotin-labelled antibody and enzyme-labelled avidin are used. The labelled antibody is allowed to react with the antigen and, after washing, enzyme-labelled avidin is added. After further incubation and washing, the enzyme associated with the antigen is measured.

These procedures are of course more sophisticated and time-consuming than conventional ones where covalently prepared conjugates are used. However, they present the advantage of sequential addition of the reagents. Thus the antibody, the avidin and the enzyme label can be introduced independently at different concentrations chosen by the experimental design and in this way a substantial increase in sensitivity of enzyme immunoassays can be achieved.

CONCLUDING REMARKS

Compared to the other quantitative immunoassays, enzyme immunoassays present the following advantages:

(1) Enzyme-labelled antigens and antibodies stored under sterile conditions can be used for years without any appreciable loss of their enzymatic and immunological activities.

(2) Enzyme immunoassays are easy to manipulate and entail a minimal risk of contamination or pollution.

(3) There is no need for costly equipment and the assay can be performed in simply equipped laboratories, or even under field conditions.

(4) The possibility of using fluorogenic substrates makes enzyme immunoassays a tool of tremendous potential. In the years to come, substantial development in this direction can be expected.

References

1. Avrameas, S. and Uriel, J. (1966). Méthode de marquage d'antigènes et d'anticorps avec des enzymes et son application en immunodiffusion. *C. R. Acad. Sci. Paris*, **262**, 2543

2. Nakane, P. K. and Pierce, G. B. (1966). Enzyme-labelled antibodies. Preparation and application for the localization of antigens. *J. Histochem. Cytochem.*, **14**, 929

3. Avrameas, S. and Guilbert, B. (1971). Dosage enzymo-immunologique de protéines à l'aide d'immunoadsorbants et d'antigènes marqués aux enzymes. *C. R. Acad. Sci. Paris*, **273**, 2705

4. Engvall, E. and Perlmann, P. (1971). Enzyme-linked immunosorbent assay (ELISA). Quantitative assay of immunoglobulin G. *Immunochemistry*, **8**, 871

5. Van Weemen, B. K. and Schuurs, A.H.W.M. (1971). Immunoassay using antigen-enzyme conjugates. *FEBS Lett.*, **15**, 232

6. Avrameas, S. and Guilbert, B. (1971). A method for quantitative determination of cellular immunoglobulins by enzyme-labelled antibodies. *Eur. J. Immunol.*, **1**, 394

7. Avrameas, S. and Guilbert, B. (1972). Enzyme-immunoassay for the measurement of antigens using peroxidase conjugates. *Biochimie*, **54**, 837

8. Van Weemen, B. K. and Schuurs, A.H.W.M. (1972). Immunoassay using hapten-enzyme conjugates. *FEBS Lett.*, **24**, 77

9. Belanger, L., Sylvestre, C. and Dufour, D. (1973). Enzyme-linked immunoassay for alpha-fetoprotein by competitive and sandwich procedures. *Clin. Chim. Acta*, **48**, 15

10. Engvall, E. and Perlmann, P. (1972). Enzyme-linked immunosorbent by enzyme-labelled anti-immunoglobulin in antigen coated tubes. *J. Immunol.*, **109**, 129

11. Maiolini, R., Ferrua, B. and Masseyeff, R. (1975). Enzymoimmunoassay of human alpha-fetoprotein. *J. Immunol. Methods*, **6**, 355

12. Maiolini, P. and Masseyeff, R. A. (1975). A sandwich method for enzymoimmunoassay of human alpha-fetoprotein. *J. Immunol. Methods*, **6**, 355

13. Voller, A., Bartlett, A., Bidwell, D. E., Clark, M. G. and Adams, A. W. (1976). The detection of viruses by enzyme-linked immunosorbent assay (ELISA). *J. Gen. Virol.*, **33**, 165

14. Guesdon, J.-L. and Avrameas, S. (1977). Magnetic solid phase enzyme immunoassay. *Immunochemistry*, **14**, 443

15. Voller, A., Bidwell, D. E., Huldt, G. and Engvall, E. (1974). A microplate method of enzyme-linked immunosorbent assay and its application to malaria. *Bull. WHO*, **51**, 209

16. Pesce, A. J., Ford, D. J., Gaizutis, M. and Pollak, V. E. (1977). Binding of protein to polystyrene in solid-phase immunoassays. *Biochim. Biophys. Acta*, **492**, 399

17. Catt, K. and Tregear, G. W. (1967). Solid phase radioimmunoassay in antibody-coated tubes. *Science*, **158**, 1570

18. Ferrua, B., Maiolini, R. and Masseyeff, R. (1979). Coupling of gamma-globulin to microcrystalline cellulose by periodate oxidation, *J. Immunol. Methods*, **25**, 49

19. Streefkerk, J. G. and Deelder, A. M. (1975). Serodiagnostic application of immunohistoperoxidase reactions on antigen-coupled agarose beads. *J. Immunol. Methods*, **7**, 225

20. Ternynck, T. and Avrameas, S. (1976). Polymerization and immobilization of protein using ethylchloroformate and glutaraldehyde. *Scand. J. Immunol.*, Suppl. **3**, 29

21. Porath, J., Axen, R. and Ernback, S. (1967). Chemical coupling of proteins to agarose. *Nature (London)*, **215**, 1491

22. Harris, C. C., Yolken, R. H., Krokan, H. and Hsu, I. C. (1979). Ultra-sensitive enzymatic radioimmunoassay: application to detection of cholera toxin and rotavirus. *Proc. Natl. Acad. Sci. USA*, **76**, 5336

23. Kato, K., Hamaguchi, Y., Fukui, M. and Ishikawa, E. (1975). Enzyme-linked immunoassay. I. Novel method for synthesis of the insulin-β-D-galactosidase conjugate and its applicability for insulin assay. *J. Biochem.*, **78**, 235

24. Cameron, D. J. and Erlanger, B. F. (1976). An enzyme-linked procedure for the detection and estimation of surface receptors on cells. *J. Immunol.*, **116**, 1313

25. Labrousse, H., Guesdon, J.-L. and Avrameas, S. (1980). Chromogenic and fluorogenic substrates for the quantitation of human IgE by enzyme immunoassay using β-galactosidase conjugates. (In preparation)

26. Puget, K., Michelson, A. M. and Avrameas, S. (1977). Light emission techniques for the microestimation of femtogram levels of peroxidase. *Anal. Biochem.*, **79**, 447

27. Hösli, P., Avrameas, S., Ullmann, A., Vogt, E. and Rodrigot, M. (1978). Quantitative ultramicro-scale immunoenzymatic method for measuring Ig antigenic determinants in single cells. *Clin. Chem.*, **24**, 1325

28. Avrameas, S., Hösli, P., Stanislawski, M., Rodrigot, M. and Vogt, E. (1979). A quantitative study at the single cell level of immunoglobulin antigenic determinants present on the surface of murine B and T lymphocytes. *J. Immunol.*, **122**, 648

29. Avrameas, S., Ternynck, T. and Guesdon, J. -L. (1978). Coupling of enzymes to antibodies and antigens. *Scand. J. Immunol.*, **8**, 7

30. Avrameas, S. (1969). Coupling of enzymes to proteins with glutaraldehyde. Use of the conjugates for the detection of antigens and antibodies. *Immunochemistry*, **5**, 43

31. Avrameas, S. and Ternynck, T. (1971). Peroxidase-labelled antibody and Fab conjugates with enhanced intracellular penetration. *Immunochemistry*, **8**, 1175

32. Nakane, P. A. and Kawoi, A. (1974). Peroxidase-labelled antibody. A new method of conjugation. *J. Histochem. Cytochem.*, **22**, 1084

33. Avrameas, S. (1969). Indirect immunoenzyme techniques for the intracellular detection of antigens. *Immunochemistry*, **6**, 825

34. Mason, T. E., Phifer, R. F., Spicer, S. S., Swallow, R. A. and Dreskin, R. B. (1969). An immunoglobulin–enzyme bridge method for localizing tissue antigens. *J. Histochem. Cytochem.*, **17**, 563

35. Sternberger, L. A., Hardy, P. H., Jr., Cuculis, J. J. and Meyer, H. G. (1970). The unlabelled antibody–enzyme method of immunohistochemistry. Preparation and properties of soluble antigen–antibody complex (horseradish peroxidase–anti-horseradish peroxidase) and its use in identification of spirochetes. *J. Histochem. Cytochem.*, **18**, 315

36. Guesdon, J.-L., Ternynck, T. and Avrameas, S. (1979). The use of avidin–biotin interaction in immunoenzymatic techniques. *J. Histochem. Cytochem.*, **27**, 1131

8
Immunoassays Employing Reactants Labelled with a Fluorophore

J. LANDON AND R. S. KAMEL

INTRODUCTION

The immediate future of laboratory practice will continue to lie with immunoassay because of its specificity, potential sensitivity, practicality and, in particular, wide applicability. There has been considerable recent interest in the use of fluorescent molecules as a label for immunoassay purposes. This review attempts to explain simply the basis of immunoassay with particular reference to fluoroimmunoassay (FIA) and immunofluorimetric analysis (IFMA); to compare the advantages and disadvantages of fluorescent labels as compared with radioisotopes and other non-isotopic alternatives and to consider the many different analytical approaches made possible by use of a fluorescent tracer.

BASIS AND TYPES OF IMMUNOASSAY

As its name implies, an immunoassay is an analytical procedure based on the reaction between an antigen and a specific antibody, which obeys the Law of Mass Action:

$$\text{Ag} + \text{Ab} \underset{k_2}{\overset{k_1}{\rightleftharpoons}} \text{Ag:Ab}$$
$$\text{(free fraction)} \qquad \text{(bound fraction)}$$

where Ag represents the antigen, Ab the antibody and Ag:Ab the bound complex. At equilibrium, some of the free reactants will be combining, with a rate constant k_1, to form more of the complex, while some of the complex will be dissociating, with a rate constant k_2, to give free antigen and antibody.

Immunoassays are most commonly employed to quantitate antigens in biological fluids and it is with this role that the present review is primarily concerned. Nonetheless, it should be noted that immunoassays are also frequently used to detect the presence of circulating antibodies or immune complexes. Indeed, Berson and his colleagues' pioneer work in radioimmunoassay followed their use of ^{131}I-labelled insulin to demonstrate the presence of circulating antibodies in patients treated with insulin[1].

Immunoassays for the detection or quantitation of an antigen can be categorized into those in which no labelled reactant is required, those employing labelled antigen and others in which specific antibodies are labelled.

Non-labelled immunoassays

Several immunoassay techniques do not require use of a labelled reactant, as discussed in an earlier chapter by L.-A. Nilsson. Despite their extensive and rapidly increasing use, non-labelled techniques are limited to the assay of proteins and other large molecules present at relatively high concentrations, since only in such circumstances are the resultant antigen–antibody complexes sufficiently large to be detectable. Additional disadvantages include the need for relatively large amounts of monospecific antisera; problems with very turbid or haemolysed samples and the possibility of erroneous results in the presence of antigen excess – due to the prozone phenomenon.

Immunoassays employing labelled antigen

The use of antigen labelled with a radioisotope, by Yalow and Berson in a radioimmunoassay (RIA) for insulin[2], proved an important milestone. It made possible the assay of haptens (such as drugs and the thyroid and steroid hormones) as well as proteins; resulted in a million-fold increase in sensitivity; removed the need for monospecific antisera and markedly reduced the amounts of antisera required; avoided the problem of antigen excess and enabled the assay of haemolysed and turbid samples. In the same year Ekins had recognized the wider implications of this approach and developed techniques for both thyroxine (T_4) and vitamin B_{12} employing circulating carrier proteins as the binding protein[3,4]. His use of the general term 'limited reagent methods' was to indicate that the concentration of binding protein must be insufficient to bind all the ligand[5].

Immunoassays employing labelled antibodies

In 1968 Miles and Hales introduced an important new type of immunoassay which they termed immunoradiometric analysis (IRMA)[6], based on the use of isotopically labelled specific antibodies. IRMA differs markedly from RIA as an analytical technique. Excessive amounts of labelled antibody are added to ensure that all the antigen is bound, so that IRMA can be defined as a 'reagent excess' as distinct from a 'limited reagent' procedure – which shortens incubation times and potentially improves sensitivity[5]. It is necessary to separate the antibody (as opposed to the antigen) in the bound fraction from that in the free fraction and, finally, the counts in the bound fraction are related *directly* to the total amount of antigen present (as opposed to the *inverse* relationship of a RIA).

'Sandwich' techniques have also been developed for large molecules with more than one antigenic determinant – an approach pioneered by Wide and his colleagues[7]. Subsequently, this approach has been further modified by use of a common, isotopically labelled second antibody[8].

Non-isotopic immunoassays

The dominant reactant in all immunoassays for antigens is the antibody since it is this which, in large part, determines the specificity (which is a feature of the close 'fit' necessary for all antigen–antibody reactions) and ultimate sensitivity that can be attained – with the latter depending on the avidity with which the antibody binds the antigen[9]. The ability to raise antisera against an enormous range of molecules also explains the wide applicability of immunoassay. The labelled antigen or antibody in RIA or IRMA is employed only as a tracer and any label is suitable provided its determination is relatively simple and sufficiently sensitive for the purpose of the assay and means are available to covalently link the label to the antigen or antibody[10].

It is not surprising, therefore, that many different materials have been employed for labelling purposes. Thus, in addition to β-(^{3}H,^{14}C) and γ(^{125}I, ^{57}Co) emitting isotopes, these include enzymes; the coenzymes NAD and ATP; viruses; fluorescent, bioluminescent and chemiluminescent molecules; proteins; metals; free radicals; red blood cells and latex and other particles. While we have studied many of these alternative labels, recent work has been concentrated on the use of fluorescent molecules.

BASIS OF FLUORESCENCE AND FLUORIMETRY

A body which emits light because of its high temperature is said to exhibit incandescence, while all other forms of light emission are called luminescence. There are several different types of luminescence which differ only in the source of energy involved in exciting the molecule to a higher electronic state from which light may be emitted as it returns to the ground state. These include radioluminescence, with energy supplied by high energy particles;

electroluminescence, as in an electric light bulb; chemiluminescence, in which the energy is derived from a chemical reaction, with this being referred to as bioluminescence if the reaction involves, or takes place in, a biological system; and, finally, photoluminescence involving excitation by photons (units of electronic radiation) of infrared, visible or ultraviolet light.

Fluorescence

In photoluminescence, a photon of the appropriate energy (wavelength) excites the molecule from its ground state (S_0) to a higher electronic state $(S_1, S_2,$ etc), in which the outer atomic electrons remain paired but with one being promoted to a higher energy level. The luminescent properties of a molecule depend on the fate of the S_1 species (Figure 8.1). This may return to the ground

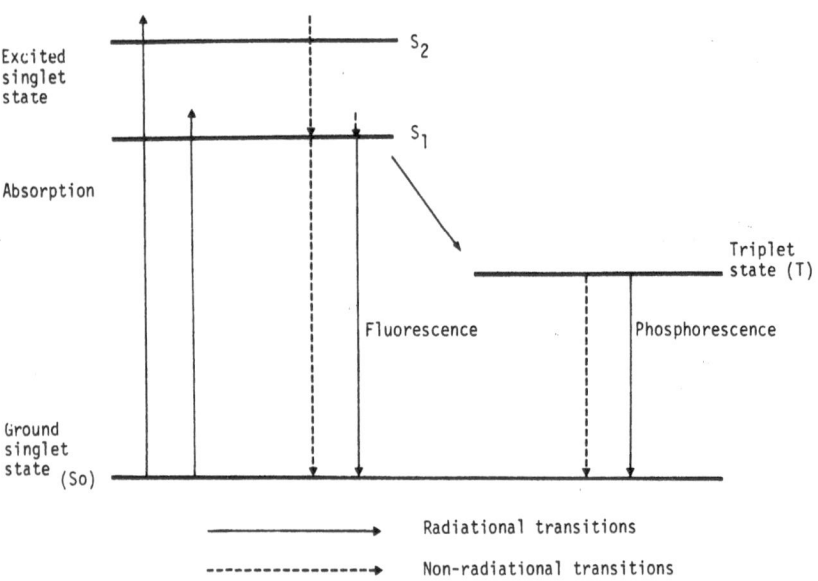

Figure 8.1 Simplified energy level diagram

state by non-radiative 'internal conversion' or by one of two light-emitting processes, namely:

(1) phosphorescence, in which the release of energy is delayed and occurs via the triplet state;
(2) fluorescence, in which the release of energy occurs in the form of a photon of longer wavelength. This term was applied by Sir G. Stokes, in 1852, to the blue-white light observed in the mineral fluospar and is derived from the Latin *fluo* – to flow.

The ultraviolet and visible regions of the spectrum are those of interest in fluorimetry and the energy associated with radiation of this frequency is quite high, being sufficient to cause breakdown of some absorbing molecules. The efficiency with which the excited molecules dissipate the energy by emission of light of a longer (and, therefore, less energetic) wavelength – the quantum efficiency, is defined as the number of quanta emitted/the number of quanta absorbed. This never exceeds unity.

Some problems in fluorescence

Various factors present in biological fluids can cause an apparent increase or decrease in the fluorescence exhibited by a fluorophore. Examples include:

Light-scattering

The incident beam of light can be scattered either from molecules (Rayleigh scattering) or from small particles in colloidal suspension (Tyndall scattering) and, thereby, summate with fluorescence – especially if the latter takes place at a wavelength close to that of the exciting light (as with a fluorophore having a small Stokes' shift). Some of the incident light can also be converted into vibrational and rotational energy and be scattered as light of low energy (long wavelength) characteristic for the solvent molecules – the Raman bands.

Endogenous fluorophores

A background signal can also be caused by compounds present in the sample which themselves fluoresce when excited by light of the same wavelengths as the fluorophore employed as the label.

Inner filter effects

These are due to the presence of compounds which absorb part of either the excitation or emission beam.

Quenching

Many changes in the environment of a fluorophore can give rise to changes in the quantum yield of its fluorescence. This is termed quenching when the fluorescence signal is decreased, and can be caused by such factors as a rise in temperature, a low pH, changes in polarity or the presence of trace oxidizing agents or dissolved oxygen. Specific or non-specific binding to antibodies and to albumin respectively can also impair fluorescence. Another mechanism, termed resonance energy transfer, is discussed in the chapter by K. E. Rubenstein as one approach to non-separation FIA and IFMA.

In assays on serum samples employing a fluorescein label the interfering factors, in order of importance, are the presence of endogenous fluorophores, in particular bilirubin; light-scattering by high concentrations of lipids and other large complexes; inner filter effects due to haemoglobin and bilirubin and quenching due to non-specific binding by albumin.

Choice of fluorophore

Among the fluorescent molecules most frequently used in immunochemistry are fluorescein, the rhodamines, some umbelliferones and, more recently, rare earth chelates.

Fluorescein is currently the label of choice in FIA and IFMA. Thus, in the dianion form which predominates in aqueous alkaline solution, it has a quantum yield approaching the maximum possible and a high extinction coefficient for the absorption of radiation; its fluorescence may be excited by a variety of common light sources and the green emission is well detected by conventional photomultipliers; it shows little photolability under normal fluorimetric conditions; its temperature coefficient is low; labelling techniques are relatively simple and the labelled product has a virtually indefinite shelf life and retains most of the quantum efficiency of the fluorescein molecule.

On the debit side, fluorescein has a small Stokes' shift with absorption and emission maxima of about 490 nm and 520 nm respectively. Thus light-scattering interference could be a problem were it not for the availability of dedicated and excellent filter systems. Of more importance, the absorption and emission bands occupy similar spectral regions to those of bilirubin; some fluorescein-labelled haptens bind non-specifically to albumin and, finally, the close proximity of several fluorescein groups on a molecule results in 'concentration quenching' of the fluorescence.

Fluorimetry

An important difference between colorimetry and fluorimetry is that while the fraction of a parallel beam of light absorbed by a sample is independent of its intensity and relates directly to the concentration of the absorbing species (the

Beer–Lambert law), the intensity of fluorescence emission is directly proportional to the intensity of the incident light. This explains why fluorimetry is a much more sensitive procedure.

In a fluorimeter, a solution of fluorescent molecules is excited with light of constant intensity and appropriate wavelength. Within a microsecond a steady state is reached with the rate at which the fluorophores are being excited to higher electronic states being balanced by the combined rates of radiative (fluorescent) and non-radiative deactivation. They can be divided into spectrophotofluorimeters and filter fluorimeters depending on the means employed to isolate light of a desired wavelength in the excitation and emission light beams. The large, relatively expensive fluorimeters are of the former type and employ a monochrometer to enable maximum versatility in wavelength selection. The latter employ optical filters of the absorbence or interference type, are less expensive, simpler to employ and, provided the filters used are well-matched and of good quality, are as sensitive as spectrofluorimeters.

Various light sources, including lasers, can be employed but it is important to avoid even small variations in light intensity, since any fluctuations are reflected as an instability of overall fluorimetric efficiency. In order to overcome this problem fluorimeters of the 'ratio-recording' type have been introduced in which the intensity of the light source is monitored independently and the fluorescence output presented as the ratio of the fluorescence of the sample solution to the reference signal. Such means of overcoming variations in light intensity are essential for the performance of reliable FIA and IFMA.

When fluorescein is employed as the label it is possible to introduce the assay tube directly, provided it is constructed of material that transmits both the exciting and emitted light and there is a suitable holder to ensure the accurate location of the tubes. A small flow-through cell, with a capacity of less than 100 μl, is also suitable.

COMPARISON OF FLUOROIMMUNOASSAY AND RADIOIMMUNOASSAY

The impact of fluorophores as a label will depend upon their advantages and disadvantages as compared with a γ-emitting isotope, such as ^{125}I. For convenience only assays employing labelled antigen (FIA and RIA) will be considered since most of the conclusions reached also relate to labelled antibody techniques.

Similarities

Since the only fundamental difference between a FIA and a RIA is the label employed, it follows that they have much in common. Both are dependent on the production of suitable antisera in animals and the same antisera can be employed for RIA and FIA. The same standards and quality control samples can also be used and identical separation techniques are applicable. Thus the only difference in the immunoassay kits for ligands is the labelled antigen.

Most of the steps involved in a RIA and a FIA are also the same. Thus, in a conventional assay, it is first necessary to accurately pipette the sample (or standard), labelled antigen and an appropriate dilution of the antiserum into the assay tube, usually in μl volumes. The reactants must then be incubated until equilibrium has been reached – which may take from a few minutes (for compounds in the μmol/l range) to many hours (for compounds in the low pmol/l range), depending on the concentration of the reactants. The means for data reduction and the calculation of results are also identical and the only steps that vary are the method of end-point detection and, in some instances, avoidance of the need to separate the antibody-bound and free fractions.

Finally many of the advantages of RIA are shared by FIA including specificity, practicality and wide applicability.

Differences

Avoidance of health hazard

Concern is sometimes expressed about the radiation hazards associated with RIA[11]. Care is essential in performing a radioiodination to produce the labelled antigen employed as the tracer, since several mCi of ^{125}I are commonly employed. However, performing a RIA involves the use of only about 0.1 μCi of radioactivity and there are no risks provided the most basic laboratory rules are followed. Nonetheless, some countries have so framed their legislation as to prohibit all but a few centres from performing RIA. Furthermore, there is an increasing emotive bias against the use of radioisotopes in most countries and, for example, few laboratory directors would let their female staff continue to perform such assays when pregnant. Use of a fluorophore as the label avoids these problems.

Preparation and stability of labelled reactant

Several excellent techniques have been developed to radioiodinate small and large antigens and antibodies both directly and by means of conjugation techniques. These have been referred to in the chapter by A. Bolton, who has made a number of important contributions in this area. Fluorescein labelling of proteins or of any molecules with a primary or secondary amino group is even easier, involving only their reaction with fluorescein isothiocyanate (FITC) at a slightly alkaline pH. When the species to be labelled has no amino group, other simple methods are often available. For example, coupling of an oestrogen by carbodi-imide condensation with fluorescein amine[12]. When no suitable reactive group is available it may be possible to label a structurally related molecule. Thus α, α-diphenylglycine labelled with FITC gave a labelled product suitable for the development of FIA for phenytoin[13].

The main disadvantage of antigens (or antibodies) labelled with ^{125}I or some other γ-emitting isotope is their short shelf-life – usually limited to some 6–24 weeks. This reflects the short half-life of the isotope (about 60 days in the case of ^{125}I), a progressive loss of immunoreactivity and of sensitivity of the assay and acute changes due to decay catastrophe. The short shelf-life necessitates frequent radioiodinations which, in turn, significantly increase the cost of kit production, quality assurance (which must be performed with each new label) and distribution. It also means that some of the contents of a kit may remain unused and, therefore, wasted at the time of its expiry date. In contrast, antigens or antibodies labelled with a fluorophore have a virtually indefinite shelf life (Figure 8.2). This is of inestimable value, especially from a commercial standpoint.

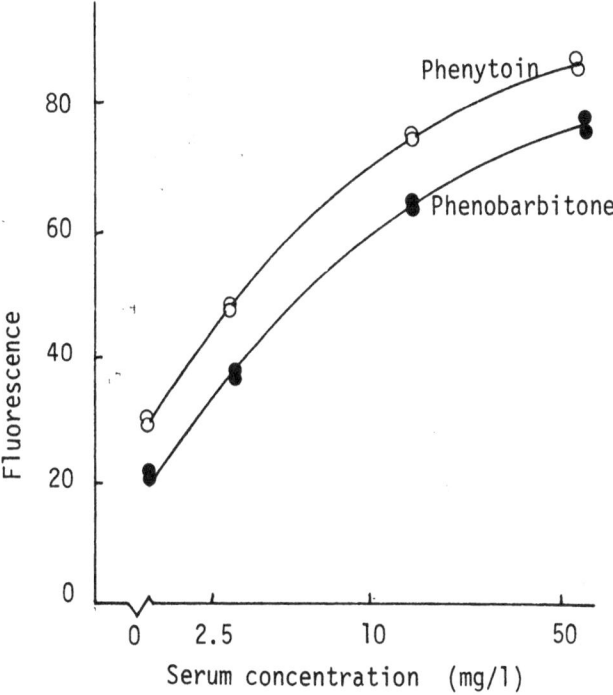

Figure 8.2 Simultaneous magnetizable solid-phase fluoroimmunoassay for phenytoin (measuring the free fraction) using 30 months' old (○) and freshly prepared tracer (●)

Variety of analytical approaches

RIA invariably requires a separation step prior to isotope counting because it is impossible to distinguish between the radioactivity in the antibody-bound and free fractions. This step is often technically demanding, time-consuming and one of the main sources of imprecision. Apart from the large number of different separation procedures available[14], there is little opportunity to adopt different analytical approaches in a RIA. Thus, apart from conventional assays in which the sample (or standard), labelled antigen and antiserum are added at the outset, the only common variant is to delay addition of the label – so-called 'late addition' assays.

This contrasts with the situation regarding immunoassays employing a fluorescent label where, as will be discussed in detail later, there are a plethora of different analytical approaches (Table 8.1) many of which do not require a separation step – usually because antibody binding either increases or decreases the signal. In FIA, virtually the entire range of separation techniques developed for RIA are applicable and such a step can serve a second important function, namely to remove endogenous fluorophores and other interfering constituents in the sample prior to end-point measurement.

Table 8.1   Types of immunoassay employing reactants labelled with a fluorophore

Employing labelled antigen (fluoroimmunoassay, FIA)	
With a separation step	simultaneous addition FIA
	sequential addition FIA
Without a separation step	signal from free fraction
	direct quenching FIA
	alternative binding FIA
	release FIA
	excitation transfer FIA
	signal from bound fraction
	enhancement FIA
	indirect quenching FIA
	polarization FIA
Employing labelled antibody (immunofluorimetric assays, IFMA)	
With a separation step	conventional IFMA
	two-site sandwich IFMA
Without a separation step	excitation transfer IFMA

Ease and speed of end-point detection

Relatively inexpensive and efficient (over 70% efficiency for [125I]) manual and automatic λ-counters are widely available, which are simple to use, involving only introduction of the tube into the well of the sodium iodide crystal. Counting precision is satisfactory and obeys known physical laws such that, for example, when 10 000 counts are collected, the coefficient of variation (CV) for repeated counts on the same sample is only 1%, and sufficient counts are usually generated in 60 s, or less. With the new multihead counters, it is possible to count several hundred tubes within 30 min and several fully automated RIA systems have been developed, both of the continuous-flow and discrete types.

Dedicated filter fluorimeters are inexpensive although not yet so widely available in immunoassay laboratories as γ-counters. They are as simple to use and provide a result more quickly (less than 5 s) than the time taken to obtain a significant number of counts when an isotope is employed as the label. Fluorimetry is also one of the few techniques more precise than isotope counting. Thus using a Perkin Elmer M1000 filter fluorimeter for repeated ($\times 21$) determinations of from 1.25 to 10 nmol/l of fluorescein, the CV ranged from 0.083 to 0.168%. When 5 pmol of human placental lactogen labelled with FITC was placed in 19 different cuvettes the CV was less than 0.3% and was only 1.7% when the end-point determinations were performed in different Sarstedt assay tubes – demonstrating that fluorimetry can be performed directly without transfer of the reactants into a cuvette.

Sensitivity

The main advantage of employing antigens labelled with a γ-emitting isotope is that they enable attainment of the maximum possible sensitivity, which often lies in the low pmol/l range. This is set by the avidity with which the antiserum employed in the particular immunoassay binds the ligand and the ability of RIA to achieve such sensitivity reflects three factors: the availability of methods to prepare labelled antigens of high specific activity; the efficiency of modern γ-counters; and, of special importance, freedom from interference by biological fluids with end-point detection. This high signal–noise ratio is virtually unique to isotopes because biological samples do not contain any radioactivity; nor do they influence the efficiency of detection of γ-emitting isotopes.

In contrast, as discussed earlier, biological samples contain many factors capable of interference with FIA and IFMA. It is this which explains why such assays have not, as yet, attained the sensitivity of RIA. However, FIA are now able to extend throughout the μmol/l and nmol/l into the pmol/l range and will inevitably attain the same sensitivity as RIA.

COMPARISON OF FLUOROIMMUNOASSAY AND OTHER NON-ISOTOPIC IMMUNOASSAYS

In several of the non-isotopic immunoassays (NIIA) summarized earlier, the complexity, time taken and/or the insensitivity of end-point detection is such as to virtually exclude their extensive use at their present stage of development. These include NIIA employing viruses, free radicals, metals, proteins and red blood cells as the label. Of the remainder, particles, enzymes and chemiluminescent molecules would appear the main contenders to fluorophores as the label of choice. Because of their present extensive use, brief attention will be given to enzyme immunoassay (EIA) and immunoenzymo-metric assays (IEMA).

Similarities

All types of NIIA share with FIA many similarities to RIA such as specificity and wide applicability; use of the same antisera, standards and quality assurance samples; and many of the analytical steps. Several also share many of the advantages of FIA including the stability of the labelled product; freedom from any health hazard or any emotive bias against their use; the potential for avoiding a separation step and a large number of possible analytical approaches. Unfortunately, most NIIA (like FIA but unlike RIA) experience problems with endogenous interfering factors in biological samples. For example, serum frequently contains enzymes with effects similar to those of the enzyme employed for labelling; other factors, such as the presence of enzyme inhibitors or haemolysis, may influence the label's activity.

Differences

There are some differences between EIA and FIA.

(1) The large size of enzymes (as compared with fluorescein) limits the method of separating the bound and free fractions to solid-phase and second-antibody techniques.

(2) It is necessary to actually separate the enzyme-labelled antigen in the bound from that in the free fraction because, even when precipitated, enzyme activity will persist. In FIA it is only necessary to clear one or other fraction from the light path.

(3) The single most important factor which differentiates the various types of NIIA and upon which future choice will be based is the means of end-point detection. Use of fluorescent molecules or particles shares with γ-emitting isotopes the advantage that immediate end-point measurement is possible after completion of the immunological reaction and the separation step (if required). In contrast, an additional chemical step is required when enzymes (and coenzymes) or chemiluminescent (and bioluminescent) molecules are employed. Thus, for example, the need to determine enzyme activity prolongs the assay, adds to its cost and complexity and increases imprecision. From the standpoint of end-point detection, instruments for determining enzyme activity are the most widely available. However, in addition to the extra step required, the amplification made possible by use of an enzyme to attain sensitivity will also magnify any error; values are difficult to check and changes in temperature influence enzymatic activity.

TYPES OF IMMUNOASSAY EMPLOYING FLUORESCENT LABELS

Labelled antigen techniques – with separation

One of the first separation FIA was for human γ-globulin[15]. We have developed such assays for determining serum gentamicin levels, using an ammonium sulphate separation step and measurement of the free fraction of the fluorescein-labelled antibiotic in the supernate[16] and serum phenytoin levels, using a sodium sulphate separation step, followed by measurement of either the free fraction (in the supernate) or the bound fraction (in the precipitate) after it had been redissolved in NaOH[17].

The separation step has two important functions. First, to separate the antibody-bound and free fractions and, second, to allow removal of any fluorophores or other interfering substances present in the sample prior to end-point detection. This second function enables the assay of larger serum volumes and markedly increases sensitivity provided there are adequate wash steps. In order to facilitate the latter and attain maximum precision, while keeping work to a minimum, there has been extensive use of solid-phase technology. Thus antibodies have been covalently bound to polyacrylamide beads and to magnetizable particles or adsorbed to the surface of a special paddle.

Use of magnetizable particles avoids the need for (and is much quicker than) centrifugation[18] since all that is required is the momentary application of a magnetic field. Furthermore, it is possible merely to sediment the particles at the bottom of the cuvette or assay tube and read the fluorescence directly in the supernate.

Simultaneous addition, separation fluoroimmunoassays

These are analogous to conventional RIA in that they involve addition of sample (or standard) and limited amounts of fluorescein-labelled antigen and antiserum. In one system, employed for the assay of thyroxine (T_4) and tri-iodothyronine (T_3), the antisera are covalently linked to small (2–5 μm) polyacrylamide beads. After incubation, the tubes are centrifuged and the supernate (containing the free fraction, endogenous fluorophores and other interfering factors) aspirated to waste. The beads are then resuspended and the fluorescence bound to them measured directly[19]. In one of our approaches (Figure 8.3), antisera are coupled to magnetizable particles and the bound fraction subsequently eluted. Such assays have been established for human albumin in serum, urine and cerebrospinal fluid[20], human IgG[21], cortisol[22], the bile acids[23], 17-hydroxyprogesterone and oestriol in pregnancy samples[24]. This type of FIA has also been applied to gentamicin, tobramicin, procainamide, N-acetyl-procainamide, propranolol, phenobarbitone and phenytoin[25] (Figure 8.3).

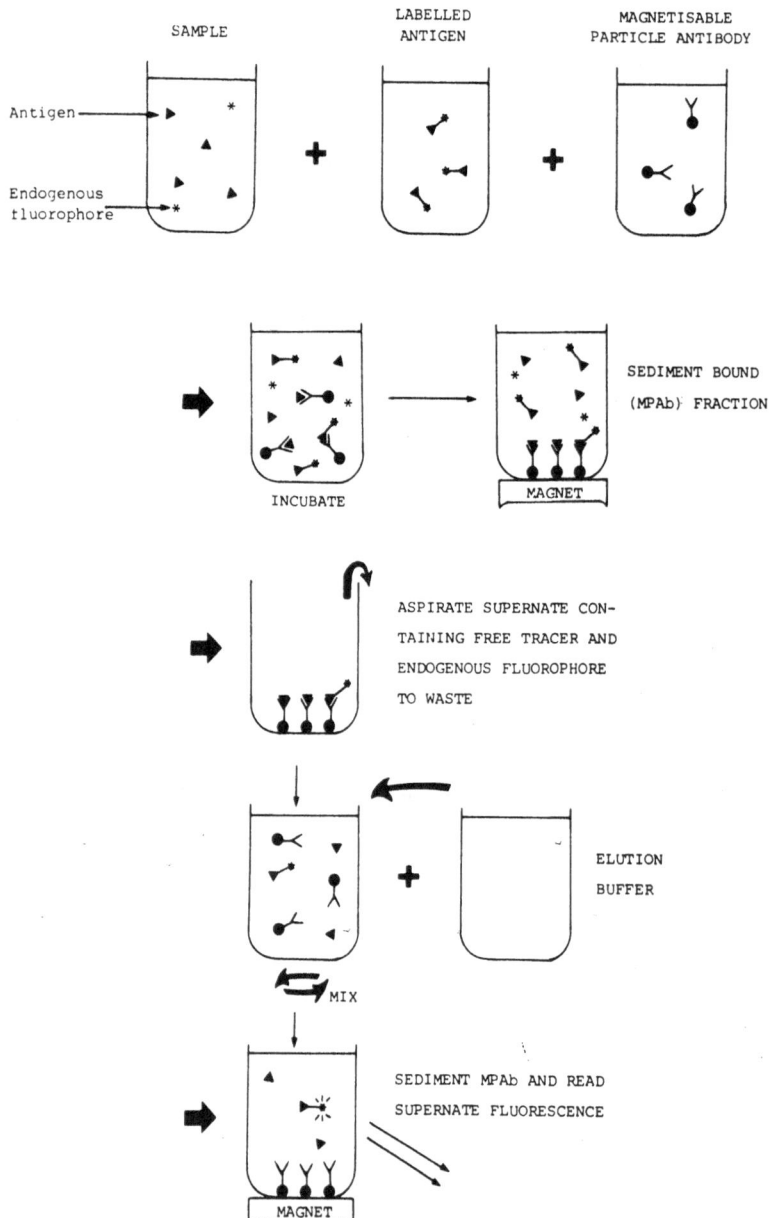

Figure 8.3   Simultaneous addition fluoroimmunoassay

As in an RIA, the level of the signal (fluorescence) is inversely related to the amount of antigen present in the sample (or standard). Others at this hospital have employed more conventional separation techniques for the FIA of human placental lactogen (HPL) in serum[26] and of α-fetoprotein in amniotic fluid[27] – but with poorer precision.

Sequential addition, separation fluoroimmunoassays

Another development has been the introduction of FIA in which reagents are added sequentially, analogous to the late addition of isotopically labelled antigen in RIA. This results in an improvement in sensitivity and facilitates the removal of interfering factors.

An excess of antiserum covalently linked to magnetizable particles (as opposed to the limited amount employed in a conventional FIA) is incubated with sample (or standard) until all the antigen has been bound – which is relatively quick because of the antiserum excess. The particles are then sedimented by momentary application of a magnetic field and the supernate, containing interfering compounds, aspirated to waste. An excess of fluorescein-labelled antigen is now added, of which some is bound to the remaining unoccupied antibody-binding sites while the remainder, left in the supernate, is read – with the reading being directly related to the antigen content of the initial sample.

One such FIA has been developed for thyroxine (T_4) with the standard curve covering the hypothyroid, euthyroid and hyperthyroid range. Results correlate closely with those of an RIA and precision is excellent[28]. Sequential addition, separation FIA have also been developed for human placental lactogen and, of particular note because of the sensitivity achieved (less than 0.5 μg/l), for digoxin.

Labelled antigen techniques – without separation

FIA not requiring a separation step can be divided into those in which the signal originates from the free fraction and others in which the signal is contributed by the antibody-bound labelled antigen. Some of these are discussed below.

Enhancement fluoroimmunoassays

FIA based on enhancement of the fluorescence of the labelled antigen upon antibody binding are possible, but unusual. In one study, fluorescein-labelled T_4 was found to give an abnormally low fluorescence yield, probably because of intramolecular quenching of the fluorophore by the iodine-containing thyroxine moiety. Antibody binding resulted in a four-fold increase in fluorescence (presumably by inhibiting the quenching effect), which served as the basis of an FIA[29].

Direct quenching fluoroimmunoassays

In direct contrast to the above are FIA which depend upon antibody binding leading to a reduction of fluorescence (Figure 8.4). If a limited amount of

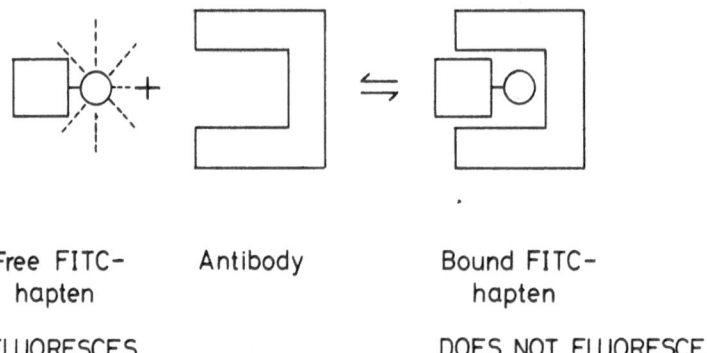

Free FITC-   Antibody   Bound FITC-
   hapten   hapten

FLUORESCES   DOES NOT FLUORESCE

Figure 8.4   Direct quenching fluoroimmunoassay

antiserum is incubated with labelled and unlabelled antigen, the amount of the labelled species which becomes antibody-bound (and, therefore, the extent of quenching) will be inversely related to the amount of unlabelled antigen present. Elimination of the need to separate greatly simplifies the method technically but account must be taken of the many factors in biological samples which may interfere.

Direct quenching FIA have been developed for determining serum levels of gentamicin[30] and for other aminoglycosides[31,32] (such as amikacin and netilimicin) which are amongst the simplest immunoassay methods yet devised. Such assays can also be fully automated employing standard Auto-Analyzer modules[33]. The high circulating concentrations of these antigens enable sufficient dilution of the sample to avoid interfering factors – unless the patient is icteric.

Indirect quenching fluoroimmunoassays

Direct quenching FIA are applicable only to the assay of haptens and, for example, antibody binding of a protein labelled with a fluorophore rarely results in any significant change in fluorescence intensity – probably because of the distance between the antigenic determinant and the site of label attachment. However, use can be made of the immunogenicity of fluorescein and the fact that binding of the fluorophore itself, and of fluorescein-labelled species by such antisera, causes virtually complete quenching. This approach, which we term indirect quenching FIA[34] and others have called fluorescence protection immunoassay[35], is discussed in the chapter by K. E. Rubenstein.

Indirect quenching FIA have been developed for human albumin in serum, urine and cerebrospinal fluid, and for human IgG and placental lactogen. This approach has also proved suitable for the detection of circulating antibodies.

Alternative binding fluoroimmunoassays

Only a minority of antisera raised against a hapten, such as gentamicin, are suitable for direct quenching FIA. Thus most antisera bind the fluorescein-labelled drug without influencing its fluorescence. Perhaps more surprisingly, the indirect quenching approach (despite a comment to the contrary[35]) is seldom applicable to haptens. The fluorescein-labelled hapten behaves as other small bifunctional antigens formed by the covalent linkage of two different antigens, which have been shown to cross-link mixtures of antibodies against the two[36]. The success of indirect quenching FIA for proteins (as opposed to haptens) probably reflects the multiplicity of their antigenic sites, with the several antibodies bound to those different sites effectively preventing binding of label by the anti-fluorescein serum added later.

However, we have developed a novel non-separation FIA approach for haptens using the same reagents as for an indirect quenching assay – with the important difference that the antibodies to the hapten and to fluorescein are incorporated into a complex. The principle of this 'alternative binding' FIA is that the labelled hapten can bind to only one antibody and if this is directed against fluorescein then fluorescence is decreased – whereas if it is directed against the hapten, fluorescence is unimpaired. Unlabelled hapten competes only for the anti-hapten binding sites so that its addition results in more of the tracer becoming bound to anti-fluorescein with a decrease in signal.

Release fluoroimmunoassay

Another type of non-separation FIA, introduced by Burd and his colleagues[37,38], involves the use of a non-fluorescent labelled antigen (for example, a derivative of umbelliferyl-β-galactoside) which releases a fluorophore when split by an appropriate hydrolytic enzyme. Steric hindrance by the antibody in the bound fraction inhibits the action of the enzyme so that only the free fraction contributes to the signal. A practical assay for determining serum levels of gentamicin has been described but such assays involve an extra step, namely addition of enzyme and measurement of rate of fluorescence increase, as compared with alternative non-separation FIA.

Fluorescent excitation transfer fluoroimmunoassay

This novel approach, introduced by the Syva Corporation, involves the use of one reactant labelled with fluorescein (F) as donor, and a second labelled with rhodamine (R) which acts as an acceptor – and is discussed in the chapter by K. E. Rubenstein.

Polarization fluoroimmunoassay

This technique was introduced independently by two groups for the assay of biological compounds[39, 40]. If a solution of fluorescent molecules is excited with polarized light, the polarization of the emitted light will depend on the extent of random Brownian rotation of the molecules which occurs during the lifetime of their excited state (4–5 ns in the case of fluorescein-labelled molecules). The smaller the labelled antigen the faster will be their random rotation, reflected by a low signal. Binding by the large antibody molecule is equivalent to an increase in effective size, and results in a greatly enhanced signal.

The principle of polarization FIA has been demonstrated in assay systems for human chorionic gonadotrophin (HCG), insulin and oestradiol-17β. However, its use for the assay of biological fluids and practical clinical applicability has been limited to the determination of urinary HCG[41] and serum levels of gentamicin[42], phenytoin[13] and angiotensin in an assay for plasma renin activity[43]. The technique has also been applied for the study of antibodies to insulin, conalbumin and penicillin by measurement of the increase in fluorescence polarization employing fluorophore-labelled antigens[44, 45].

Polarization FIA is simple, quick and precise, but has some major disadvantages. The first, and most important, obstacle to its wider use is the lack of availability of convenient, relatively inexpensive, specially constructed polarization fluorimeters capable of providing a direct readout. Second is the sensitivity, limited to the μmol/l and upper nmol/l range with respect to antigens in biological samples, and finally, is a lack of applicability to antigens with a molecular weight above about 20 000 – because it depends upon the detection of a marked increase in effective size following antibody binding.

Labelled antibody techniques – with separation

Early immunofluorometric assays (IFMA) were based on the precipitin reaction and separation of the bound complex from excess unreacted labelled antibody by centrifugation or filtration[46]. Techniques have also been developed in which the binding of labelled antibodies onto antigens attached to the surface of paper discs is assessed by a fluorimeter designed to measure surface fluorescence and in which agarose beads and microfluorimetry are employed. In the latter, it has proved possible to determine the fluorescence signal from individual beads and average the signal from several beads for quantitative purposes. However, the complexity of the microfluorimetric equipment poses a major limitation.

Most recent work relating to IFMA has involved use of the sandwich approach. Excess antibody attached to a solid phase is first used to bind all the antigen from the sample. After washing, fluorescent-labelled antibody is added in excess and that bound to the solid phase, via the antigen, gives a direct measurement of the amount of antigen. Quantitation can be achieved after elution of the labelled antibodies from the solid phase as in an assay for human IgG[47]. Alternatively, techniques have been developed that permit direct fluorimetry of bound fluorescent antibody on the solid phase.

The most extensively used is the commercial FIAX/StiQ system which comprises a fluorimeter especially designed to measure fluorescence on the surface of the StiQ sampler. The latter are designed to facilitate the several incubation and washing steps required in assays of this type and can be employed for both antigens and antibodies. Thus the system has been applied for the IFMA of IgG, IgA, IgM, C3, C4 and albumin, and for the detection of antibodies to rubella, toxoplasma, ANA and DNA. An IFMA has also recently been developed for oestradiol-17β[48].

Labelled antibody techniques – without separation

Spatially selective excitation of the fluorescence provides means of avoiding the separation step. Light undergoing total internal reflection at the quartz side of a quartz–water interface penetrates into the aqueous medium to a depth of only a few hundred nanometres. Thus if antigen is attached directly (or indirectly via an antibody) to the quartz surface and then fluorescent-labelled antibody is added to the aqueous medium, that bound to the antigen may be excited while unreacted labelled antibody will not encounter the exciting light and will not, therefore, fluoresce. A helium–cadmium laser has been employed to demonstrate the feasibility of this approach.

Syva have also developed a non-separation IFMA, as discussed in the chapter by K. E. Rubenstein.

CONCLUSIONS

It is likely that the 1980s will continue to witness a rapid increase in demand for immunoassays with their extension into many further medical and non-medical fields. This reflects the potential sensitivity, specificity, precision, practicality and, in particular, wide applicability of such assays.

The various types of immunoassay are, in general, complementary rather than exclusive with non-labelled techniques certain to continue to dominate for the quantitation of serum-specific proteins and radioimmunoassay for compounds present at low concentrations and for which precise results are required – such as for the assay of free hormones and tumour-specific products and for neonatal screening. Enzyme immunoassay will play a significant role, especially for qualitative and semi-quantitative assays (for example, to detect circulating antibodies) where a visual colour change offers the simplest end-point.

Nonetheless, it is probable that non-isotopic immunoassays will exhibit the most rapid rise and take over part of the roles both of radioimmunoassay and of non-labelled immunoassay. Thus they will dominate therapeutic drug monitoring and other new areas of expansion and take over progressively more of the high-volume assays. The speed, simplicity and precision of end-point detection indicates that fluoroimmunoassays will play an increasingly important role, especially as improvements in methodology (such as multilabelling) and in instrumentation (such as time-resolved fluorescence) result in a marked improvement in the sensitivity that can be achieved.

References

1. Berson, S. A., Yalow, R. S., Baumann, A., Rothschild, M. A. and Newerly, K. J. (1956). Insulin–^{131}I metabolism in human subjects: demonstration of insulin binding globulin in the . circulation of insulin treated subjects. *J. Clin. Invest.*, **35**, 170

2. Yalow, R. S. and Berson, S. A. (1960). Immunoassay of endogenous plasma insulin in man. *J. Clin. Invest.*, **39**, 1157

3. Ekins, R. P. (1960). The estimation of thyroxine in human plasma by an electrophoretic technique. *Clin. Chim. Acta*, **5**, 453

4. Barakat, R. M. and Ekins, R. P. (1961). Assay of vitamin B12 in blood. A simple method. *Lancet*, **2**, 25

5. Ekins, R. S. (1976). General principles of hormone assay. In Loraine, J. A. and Bell, E. T. (eds.) In *Hormone Assays and their Clinical Application*, p. 1. (Edinburgh: Churchill Livingstone)

6. Miles, L. E. M. and Hales, C. N. (1968). Labelled antibodies and immunological assay systems. *Nature (London)*, **219**, 186

7. Wide, L., Bennich, H. and Johansson, S. G. O. (1967). Diagnosis of allergy by an in-vitro test for allergen antibodies. *Lancet*, **2**, 1105

8. Beck, P. and Hales, C. N. (1975). Immunoassay of serum polypeptide hormone by using ^{RS}I-labelled anti (immunoglobulin G) antibodies. *Biochem. J.*, **145**, 607

9. Exley, D. (1979). Steroid immunoassay in clinical chemistry. *Pure Appl. Chem.*, **52**, 33

10. Landon, J. (1977) Enzymoimmunoassay: techniques and uses. *Nature (London)*, **268**, 483

11. Bogdanovic, E. M. and Strash, A. M. (1975). Radioiodine escape as an unexpected source of radioimmunoassay error and chronic low level environmental contamination. *Nature (London)*, **257**, 426

12. Dandliker, W. B., Hicks, A. N., Levison, S. A. and Brown, R. J. (1977). Fluorescein-labelled derivative of estradiol with binding affinity towards cellular receptors. *Biochem. Biophys. Res. Commun.*, **74**, 538

13. McGregor, A. R., Crookall-Greening, J. O., Landon, J. and Smith, D. S. (1978). Polarisation fluoroimmunoassay of phenytoin. *Clin. Chim. Acta*, **83**, 161

14. Ratcliffe, J. G. (1974). Separation techniques in saturation analysis. *Br. Med. Bull.*, **30**, 32

15. Tengerdy, R. P. (1965). Gamma globulin determination in human sera by the inhibition of the precipitation of fluorescein-labelled gamma globulin. *J. Lab. Clin. Med.*, **65**, 859

16. Shaw, E. J., Watson, R. A. and Smith, D. S. (1977). Fluoroimmunoassay of serum gentamicin. *Eur. J. Drug Metab. Pharmacokinet.*, **14**, 191

17. Kamel, R. S., McGregor, A. R., Landon, J. and Smith, D. S. (1978). Separation fluoroimmunoassay methods for phenytoin. *Clin. Chim. Acta*, **89**, 93

18. Nye, L., Forrest, G. C., Greenwood, H. A., Gardner, J. C., Jay, R., Roberts, J. R. and Landon, J. (1976). Solid-phase magnetic particle radioimmunoassay. *Clin. Chim. Acta*, **69**, 387

19. Curry, R. E., Heitzman, H., Riege, D. H., Sweet, R. V. and Simonsen, M. G. (1979). A systems approach to fluorescent immunoassay: general principles and representative applications. *Clin. Chem*, **25**, 1591

20. Nargessi, R. D., Landon, J., Pourfarzaneh, M. and Smith, D. S. (1978). Solid-phase fluoroimmunoassay of human albumin in biological fluids. *Clin. Chim. Acta*, **89**, 455

21. Nargessi, R. D., Pourfarzaneh, M., Smith, D. S. and Landon, J. (1980). Magnetisable solid-phase fluoroimmunoassay of immunoglobulin G in biological fluids. (Submitted to *Clin. Chim Acta*)

22. Pourfarzaneh, M., White, W., Landon, J. and Smith, D. S. (1980). Direct determination of cortisol in serum by fluoroimmunoassay with magnetisable solid-phase. *Clin. Chem.* (In press)

23. Shridi, F. A., Pourfarzaneh, M., Chitranukroh, A., Billing, B. H. and Ekeke, G. (1980). A direct fluoroimmunoassay for conjugated chenodeoxycholic acid using antiserum coupled to magnetisable particles. *Annals. Clin. Biochem.* (In press)

24. Ekeke, G., Landon, J., Edwards, C. R. W., White, G. W. and Shridi, F. (1980). Magnetisable solid-phase separation fluoroimmunoassay for total oestriol in pregnancy serum. *Clin. Chim. Acta*, (In press)

25. Kamel, R. S., Landon, J. and Smith, D. S. (1980). Magnetisable solid-phase fluoroimmunoassay of phenytoin in disposable test tubes. *Clin. Chem.*, **10** (In press)

26. Chard, T. and Sykes (1979). Fluoroimmunoassay for human choriomammotropin. *Clin. Chem.*, **25**, 973

27. Sinosich, M. J. and Chard, T. (1979). Fluoroimmunoassay of alphafetoprotein in amniotic fluid. *Ann. Clin. Biochem.*, **16**, 334

28. Nargessi, R. D., Ackland, J., Hassan, M., Forrest, G. C., Smith, D. S. and Landon, J. (1980). Magnetisable solid-phase fluoroimmunoassay of thyroxine by a sequential addition technique. *Clin. Chem.* (In press)

29. Smith, D. S. (1977). Enhancement fluoroimmunoassay of thyroxine. *FEBS Lett.*,**77**, 25

30. Shaw, E. J., Watson, R. A. A., Landon, J. and Smith, D. S. (1977). Estimation of serum gentamicin by quenching fluoroimmunoassay. *J. Clin. Pathol.*, **30**, 526

31. Shaw, E. J., Munro, A., Kamel, R. S. and Smith, D. S. (1978). *Development of Manual and Automated Fluoroimmunoassay for Drugs.* Laboratory Management and Automation, 8th Technicon International Congress Basingstoke: (Technicon Instruments Co, Ltd)

32. Broughton, A. and Frazier, M. (1978). A quenching fluoroimmunoassay for the aminoglycoside netilmicin. *Clin. Chem.*, **24**, 1033

33. Shaw, E. J., Watson, R. A. A. and Smith, D. S. (1979). Continuous-flow fluoroimmunoassay of serum gentamicin, with automatic sample blank correction. *Clin. Chem.*, **24**, 1033

34. Nargessi, R. D., Landon, J. and Smith, D. S. (1979). Use of antibodies against the label in non-separation non-isotopic immunoassay: 'indirect quenching' fluoroimmunoassay of proteins. *J. Immunol. Methods*, **26**, 307

35. Zuk, R. F., Rowley, G. L. and Ullman, E. F. (1979). Fluorescence protection immunoassay: a new homogeneous assay technique. *J. Immunol. Methods*, **26**, 307

36. Nitecki, D. E., Woods, V. and Goodman, J. W. (1977). Crosslinking of antibody molecules by bifunctional antigens. *Adv. Exp. Med. Biol.*, **86A**, 139

37. Burd, J. F., Carrico, R. J., Fetter, M. C., Buckler, R. T., Johnson, R. D., Boguslaski, R. C. and Christner, J. E. (1977). Specific protein-binding reaction monitored by enzymatic hydrolysis of ligand–fluorescent dye conjugate. *Anal. Biochem.*, **77**, 56

38. Burd, J. F., Wong, R. C., Feeney, J. E., Carrico, R. J. and Boguslaski, R. C. (1977). Homogenous reactant-labelled fluorescent immunoassay for therapeutic drugs exemplified by gentamicin determination in human serum. *Clin. Chem.*, **23**, 1402

39. Dandliker, W. B., Kelly, R. J., Dandliker, J., Farquhar, J. and Levin, J. (1973). Fluorescence polarization immunoassay theory and experimental method. *Immunochemistry*, **10**, 219

40. Spencer, R. D., Toledo, F. B., Williams, B. T. and Yoss, N. L. (1973). Design, construction and two applications for an automated flow-cell polarization fluorimeter with digital read

out: enzyme-inhibitor (antitrypsin) assay and antigen–antibody (insulin–insulin antiserum) assay. *Clin. Chem.*, **19**, 838

41. Urios, P., Cittanova, N. and Jayle, M. F. (1978). Immunoassay of the human chorionic gonadotrophin using fluorescence polarisation. *FEBS Lett.*, **94**, 54

42. Watson, R. A. A., Landon, J., Shaw, E. J. and Smith, D. S. (1976). Polarisation fluoroimmunoassay of gentamicin. *Clin. Chim. Acta*, **73**, 51

43. Maeda, H., Nakayama, M., Iwaoka, D., and Sato, T. (1978). *Assay of Angiotensin I by Fluorescence Polarisation Method.* Proceedings of International Symposium of Kinins, Angiotensin, Kini. (Plenum Publ. Co. Ltd)

44. Tengerdy, R. P. (1967). Quantitative determination of antibody by fluorescence polarisation. *J. Lab. Clin. Med.*, **70**, 707

45. Dandliker, W. B., Helbert, S. P., Florin, M. C., Alonso, R. and Schapiro, H. C. (1965). The synthesis of fluorescent penicilloyl haptens and their use in investigating 'penicillin' antibodies by fluorescence polarisation. *J. Exp. Med.*, **122**, 1029

46. Capel, P. J. A. (1974). A quantitative immunofluorescence method based on the covalent coupling of protein to sepharox beads. *J. Immunol. Methods*, **5**, 295

47. Aalberse, R. C. (1973). Quantitative fluoroimmunoassay. *Clin. Chim. Acta*, **48**, 109

48. Ekeke, G. I., Exley, D. and Abuknesha, R. (1979). Immunofluorimetric assay of estradiol-17β. *J. Steroid Biochem.*, **11**, 1597

9
Chemiluminescence and its Use in Immunoassay

T. OLSSON AND A. THORE

INTRODUCTION

Chemiluminescence is the basis of several new developments in analytical chemistry. Owing to the simplicity of luminometry and the extreme sensitivity by which chemiluminescent reactions can be measured, chemiluminescence analysis is becoming increasingly useful as a tool for research and routine in medicine, biology and biochemistry. Chemiluminescence analysis has been extensively discussed in several recent reviews[1-4].

The chemical basis for chemiluminescence analysis is the existence of chemical reactions, usually redox reactions involving oxygen or peroxide and an oxidizable organic substrate, in which energy is released as visible light. By measuring the rate of light emission in a luminometer or other suitable instrument for light detection the rate of the chemiluminescent reaction, and thereby the concentration of reactants, can be estimated. The sensitivity is often extremely high, detection limits of 10^{-15} mol or less are common.

During the last two decades more than 1000 research papers have appeared in which chemiluminescence has been used for various analytical purposes. Most assays are based on a limited group of chemiluminescent reactions, namely the enzyme catalysed bioluminescent reactions occuring in fireflies and certain bacteria, and two reactions based on oxidation of luminol (5-amino-1,2,3,4,-tetrahydrophtsalazine-1,4-dione) or pyrogallol by peroxide. The firefly reaction, catalysed by firefly luciferase, is used for analysis of adenosine triphosphate (ATP) and reactions which can be linked to ATP consumption or formation. The bacterial reaction catalysed by bacterial luciferase is used for analysis of reduced flavin mononucleotide ($FMNH_2$) or, by coupling to a NAD(P)H/FMN oxidoreductase for analysis of reduced nicotinamide adenine dinucleotides (NADH, NADPH) or redox reactions involving pyridine nucleotides. The luminol and pyrogallol reactions are used for analysis of peroxide, peroxidase or haemin, the latter two catalysing the reaction between peroxide and luminol. The reaction schemes are given below:

FIREFLY REACTION

$$ATP + luciferin + O_2 \xrightarrow{\text{luciferase}} AMP + PP + oxyluciferin + CO_2 + H_2O + light$$
$$(Eq.1)$$

BACTERIAL REACTIONS

$$FMNH_2 + CH_3(CH_2)_{8-12}CHO + O_2 \xrightarrow{\underset{Mg^{2+}}{\text{luciferase}}} FMN + CH_3(CH_2)_{8-12}COOH$$
$$+ H_2O + light \qquad (Eq.2)$$

$$NADH(NADPH) + FMN + H^+ \xrightarrow{\text{oxidoreductase}} NAD^+(NADP^+) + FMNH_2$$
$$(Eq.3)$$

LUMINOL REACTION

$$luminol + R \cdot OOH \xrightarrow[\substack{\text{peroxidase} \\ \text{metals, oxidants}}]{\text{haemin}} aminophtalate + N_2 + R \cdot OH + light \quad (Eq.4)$$

PYROGALLOL REACTION

$$pyrogallol + H_2O_2 \xrightarrow{\text{peroxidase}} various\ oxidation\ products + light \quad (Eq.5)$$

Recently, chemiluminescent reactions have been utilized in immunoanalytical work. The principle of these applications has been to label antigen or antibody with substances active in chemiluminescent reactions, using chemiluminescence as the final detection step. Most of these luminescence immunoassay (LIA) systems have been based on the commonly used solid phase, double-antibody precipitation or homogeneous techniques, originally developed for use with isotope or enzyme labels.

The luminescent labels have been various reactants from all the major chemiluminescent systems described above; for example luciferase enzymes, pyridine or adenine nucleotides, luminol, haemin, peroxidase.

In several instances analytical sensitivity equal to or better than that obtained in radioimmunoassay (RIA) or enzyme immunoassay (EIA) has been attained.

THE CHEMILUMINESCENCE ANALYTICAL TECHNIQUE

General considerations

Luminescent reactions can be measured in essentially any instrument sensitive to emission of visible light. The most commonly used instruments for chemiluminescence measurements are liquid scintillation counters, or more recently, the less expensive luminometers. Both instruments are based on photon detection by photomultipliers by which very low rates of photon emission can be detected. The measured light emission is related to concentration of reactant by referring to a sample with a known added level of the reactant.

Chemiluminescence measurements can usually be made in a few seconds since the light is often emitted as a short flash immediately following the mixing of reactants (Figure 9.1A). In some instances, however, the light can be

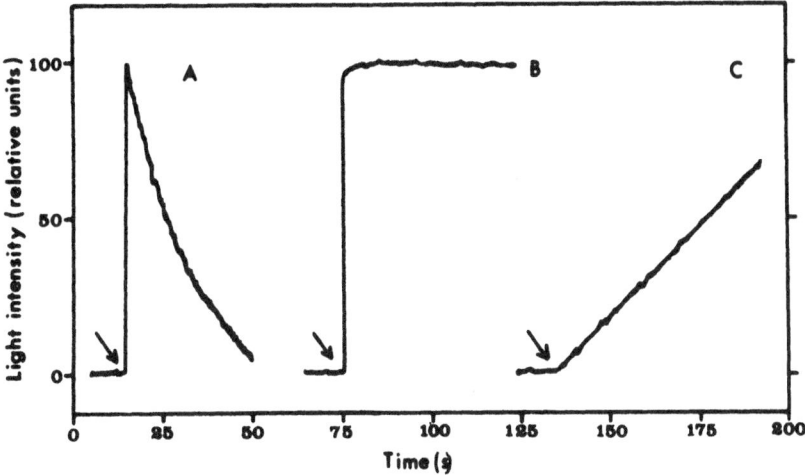

Figure 9.1 Time-courses of chemiluminescent reactions. The mixing of reactants initiating the chemiluminescent reactions takes place at the time indicated by arrows. (A) Time-course typical of for example the luminol reaction, reactions with crude firefly luciferase and other reactions with rapid depletion of one of the reactants. (B) Time-course obtainable with purified firefly luciferase of low activity with excess luciferin[5]. (C) Time-course obtainable, for example, with purified firefly luciferase reagent in the presence of an ATP-producing enzyme reaction, e.g. puruvate kinase or creatine kinase[4, 5]

made to appear as a prolonged emission of a more or less constant level of intensity. In principle this allows for higher sensitivity by accumulating for some time the number of impulses reaching the photomultiplier (Figure 9.1B).

When the chemiluminescent reaction is used to monitor an enzyme reaction producing, for example ATP, NADH or H_2O_2, the light emission is continually increased (Figure 9.1c) so that the sensitivity can be varied by choice of incubation time.

Practical aspects of chemiluminescence analysis

Although chemiluminescence analysis is normally a straightforward, simple procedure, some factors, concerning the physical and chemical requirements on the sample, should be noted.

The analysis

An analysis is usually performed by mixing the sample, containing the reactant to be analysed, with the chemiluminescent reagent, containing the remainder of the necessary reactants. If the reaction is fast (Figure 9.1A), the mixing has to be done with the sample in measuring position in order to be able to record the entire course of light emission.

Interference

Since measurements should be calibrated using the constant addition technique or, as for example in immunoanalytical work, suitable reference samples, interference with the measurement can usually be accounted for. Nevertheless it is obviously desirable to avoid strongly interfering conditions. Below is a summary of some commonly encountered conditions affecting chemiluminescence analyses.

Luminescence measurements are relatively insensitive to turbidity since most luminometers collect the total light emitted from the sample, regardless of scattering.

Strongly light-absorbing or fluorescent solutes in the sample may affect measurements, pH is usually an important variable since the colour of the emitted light, and thereby its effect on the photomultiplier, is often strongly dependent on pH. Chemiluminescent reactions are temperature-dependent with an optimum for luciferase reactions at 25–28 °C.

A potential source of interference in immunoanalytical work is components of serum such as adenine or pyridine nucleotides or enzyme reacting directly in the chemiluminescent reaction. This type of interference could be easily overcome, for example by washing in solid-phase immunoassays.

In luciferase reactions high concentrations of various salts and buffers are known to interfere by inhibiting the luciferase enzyme. This type of interference – as well as that observed with, for example, radical scavengers in the luminol system – should be minimized by, e.g., dilution and accounted for by constant addition calibration. For further general information concerning chemiluminescence analysis the reader is referred to one of several recent review articles[1-4].

APPLICATIONS OF CHEMILUMINESCENCE IN IMMUNOANALYSIS

The area is presently in a phase of rapid expansion and much work has been devoted to adaptation of chemiluminescence techniques to immunoassay. Many of the published studies concern model systems but several methods for analysis of clinically relevant substances have been published.

The general design of luminescence immunoassay systems is the same as used in other immunoassays. In most cases solid-phase or double-antibody precipitation techniques have been used. These systems require separation of bound and free label, for example by repeated washings. Some homogeneous systems have also been tested which do not require separation of labels. However, hitherto these assays are only suitable for low molecular weight antigens, e.g. steroids and drugs.

Below is a comprehensive survey of published applications, as well as some comments on problems associated with labelling, in particular the effects on chemiluminescence efficiency. It is beyond the scope of this paper to give details of coupling procedures; these problems have been discussed extensively in several recent reviews or bibliographies in connection with covalent coupling of enzymes or cofactors as used, for example, in enzyme immobilization or affinity chromatography[6-9].

Applications using luminescent reactions catalysed by firefly or bacterial luciferase

Reagents and chemiluminescent reactions

Firefly luciferase system[10, 11] – The reagents necessary for the firefly luciferase reaction are: firefly luciferase enzyme, firefly luciferin, and adenosine triphosphate (ATP). In principle any of these reagents can be used for labelling antigen or antibody. The chemiluminescent reaction is then initiated by addition of the other reagents. The resulting light emission is of high quantum yield (close to 90%) and has a maximum intensity at 562 nm. All reagents are commercially available in purified form from several biochemical firms.

For monitoring of ATP-producing (or ATP-consuming) enzyme reactions luciferase/luciferin analytical reagents are available in kit form.

Bacterial luciferase system[12, 13] – The reagents necessary for the bacterial luciferase reaction are: bacterial luciferase enzyme, flavin mononucleotide (FMN) and an aliphatic straight-chain aldehyde (usually decyl-, dodecyl- or tetradecyl-aldehyde). The chemiluminescent reaction is of relatively high quantum yield ($\sim 10\%$) and has a maximum intensity at about 490 nm.

The aldehydes and FMN are available as pure reagents from several biochemical and organic chemical firms. The luciferase is usually available as a crude mixture also containing NADH or NADPH/FMN oxidoreductase.

Such a preparation together with aldehyde and FMN has been used for sensitive monitoring of a commercially available glucose-6-phosphate dehydrogenase conjugate used in homogeneous immunoassay of phenytoin[14].

Conjugates and immunoassay

The luciferases, like other proteins, may in principle be covalently coupled to antigen or antibody, by activation of functional groups of their amino acids, e.g. lysine $(-NH_2)$ or cysteine $(-SH)$ (Figure 9.2) by bifunctional substances, e.g. glutaraldehyde. In practice loss of enzyme activity as a result of coupling has been the limiting factor for use of bacterial and firefly luciferase as IgG labels in solid-phase immunoassay[15, 16]. No conjugate suitable for practical work has yet been described. In principle, luciferin, ATP, NAD^+ or FMN may be covalently coupled by activation of $-NH_2$, $-COOH$ or $-OH$ groups (Figure 9.2) by bifunctional reagents, e.g. carbodi-imide.

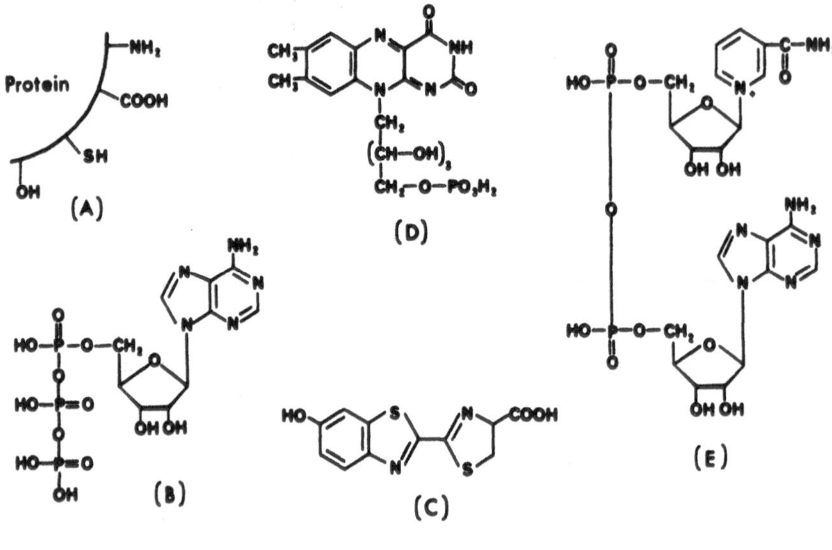

Figure 9.2 Chemical structure of reagents which may be used for labelling in immunoassays based on firefly or bacterial luciferase chemiluminescent reactions. Possible groups for attachment in coupling procedures are shown for luciferases (A). The cofactors in firefly luciferase reaction, ATP (B) and luciferin (C). Cofactors in bacterial luciferase reactions, FMN (D) and NAD^+ (E)

In practice, the choice of site of attachment will be limited, since luciferase specificity and activity, as well as colour of emitted light, are strongly dependent on the structure of the cofactor [17-19].

Derivatives of NAD^+ and ATP have been used as labels in two different homogeneous systems (Table 9.1). The NAD^+ derivative was active in the coupled oxidoreductase/bacterial luciferase reaction after enzymatic reduction[20]. The ATP derivative was active only after enzymatic liberation of ATP from the conjugate[21]. The enzyme(s) necessary for this liberation was present in the crude firefly luciferase reagent. In both cases very low levels of antigen could be detected in the chemiluminescence analysis[20,21].

Table 9.1 Immunoanalytical applications using conjugates active in firefly or bacterial luciferase chemiluminescent systems. The assays have been performed as homogeneous immunoassays

Quantitated substance	Sensitivity (g)	Conjugate/luminescent system	Ref.
Dinitrophenol-aminocaproate	1×10^{-8}	AENAD–Ag[a,b]/bacterial luciferase	20
Phenytoin	3×10^{-8}	G-6-PdH–Ag[b,c]/bacterial luciferase	14
Dinitrophenol-β-alanine	3×10^{-10}	ATP–Ag[b]/firefly luciferase	21

[a] AENAD, nicotinamide 6-(2-aminoethylamino) purine dinucleotide
[b] Ag, antigen
[c] G-6-PdH, glucose-6-phosphate dehydrogenase

An alternative approach to these direct applications of chemiluminescence has been published[14] (Table 9.1). It is based on one of the several commercial kits for homogeneous immunoassay using dehydrogenase enzyme as label and measuring formation of NADH spectrophotometrically. NADH may be monitored with increased sensitivity by the coupled oxidoreductase/bacterial luciferase reaction (equations 2–3). The increased sensitivity made it possible to perform the assay at less expense, using lower amounts of reagent.

Applications using luminescent reactions based on luminol or pyrogallol

Reagents and chemiluminescent reactions

Luminol system[22-24] – The luminol chemiluminescence results from the oxidation of luminol concomitant with catalytic decomposition of peroxide. The catalysts are any of several strong oxidants, metal complexes or enzymes containing haemin, such as peroxidase, microperoxidase, or their prosthetic group, i.e. protohaemin. The quantum yield is relatively low ($\leqslant 1\%$) and maximum light intensity is at about 425 nm.

The necessary reagents are: luminol, catalyst, e.g. haemin compounds, and peroxide, e.g. sodium perborate or hydrogen peroxide. All reactants are commercially available from several organic chemical and biochemical companies. It should be noted that one universally used immunoanalytical reagent, namely peroxidase–IgG conjugate, is in fact active in the luminol or pyrogallol chemiluminescent reactions, which may be used to quantitate the conjugate as an alternative to classical colorimetric tests for peroxidase activity[25-28].

Pyrogallol system[25, 26, 29] – The pyrogallol chemiluminescence results from the oxidation of pyrogallol catalysed by peroxidase. An intermediate product, purpurogallin, may be further oxidized in a similar chemiluminescent reaction[24, 29]. The total quantum yield is not defined, but that of purpurogallin is low $(10^{-5}-10^{-6}\%)$[24]. The maximum light intensity is at about 480 nm[26].

The necessary reagents are: pyrogallol, hydrogen peroxide and peroxidase and sometimes also purpurogallin or phenylenediamine[28, 29]. They may be obtained as pure reagents from several biochemical or organic chemical firms.

Conjugates and immunoassay

Luminol, pyrogallol or haematin may in principle be covalently coupled by activation of $-NH_2$, $-OH$ or $-COOH$ groups (Figure 9.3). In addition proteins containing haemin, e.g. peroxidase (cf. Figure 9.2), may be coupled by similar techniques as luciferases.

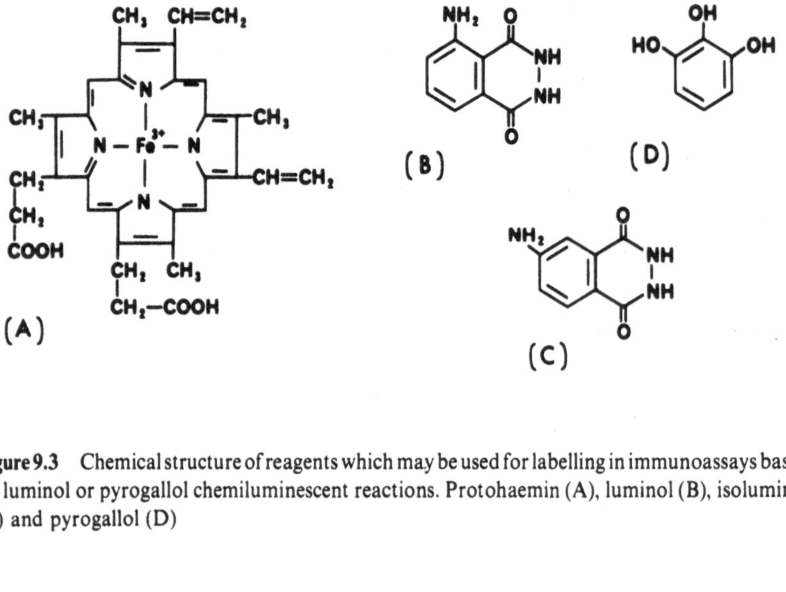

Figure 9.3 Chemical structure of reagents which may be used for labelling in immunoassays based on luminol or pyrogallol chemiluminescent reactions. Protohaemin (A), luminol (B), isoluminol (C) and pyrogallol (D)

In practice the $-NH_2$ group of luminol, or its derivative isoluminol, the $-COOH$ groups of haemin or suitable groups on proteins containing haemin, e.g. $-NH_2$ groups of peroxidase, have been used as attachment sites in coupling procedures[30]. Since peroxidase is a glycoprotein the sugar moiety may be activated by periodate and coupled to, e.g., $-NH_2$ groups of IgG[31]. The use of peroxidase in conjugates is well established, the enzyme activity being inhibited only to a minor extent by coupling. Commercial conjugates are prepared by glutaraldehyde or the sugar activation method, and the stability of the conjugates is very good.

Recently, in our own laboratory, conjugates with the prosthetic group of peroxidase, protohaemin (Figure 9.3), have been prepared[32]. Preliminary results indicate that these conjugates contain considerably higher specific luminescence than peroxidase conjugates, probably due to the increased labelling possible with the smaller haemin molecule.

Most applications using peroxidase conjugate have been performed under physiological conditions measuring the enzyme activity with luminol or pyrogallol and using solid-phase immunoassay systems (Table 9.2). Using alkaline pH, haemin could be solubilized from the protein moiety, catalysing the luminol reaction with increased efficiency, not limited by steric hindrance at the solid phase[27]. In all cases (Table 9.2) very low levels of antigen or antibody could be detected. Comparisons with RIA or EIA have demonstrated equal or better sensitivity[27, 28, 33, 35]. The luminol reaction catalysed by peroxidase has also been used to monitor H_2O_2, produced by a conjugate containing glucose oxidase[16].

Table 9.2 Immunoanalytical applications using conjugates catalysing the chemiluminescent luminol or pyrogallol reactions. The assays have been based on solid-phase or double-antibody precipitation techniques

Quantitated substance	Sensitivity (g)	Conjugate/luminescent system	Ref.
HSA[a]	5×10^{-9}	peroxidase–Ab[b]/luminol/perborate	27
Anti-HSA antibody	$\sim 10^{-9}$	peroxidase–Ab/luminol/perborate	27
Rabbit IgG	5×10^{-8}	protohaemin–Ab/luminol/perborate	32
Lymphocyte immunoglobulin	–[c]	peroxidase–Ab/luminol/H_2O_2	16
Cortisol	1×10^{-11}	peroxidase–Ag[d]/luminol/H_2O_2	33
Bacterial cell wall Ag	–[e]	peroxidase–Ab/pyrogallol/H_2O_2	34
Bacterial enterotoxin	$\sim 10^{-9}$	peroxidase–Ag/pyrogallol/H_2O_2	35
Viral particles	–[f]	peroxidase–Ab/pyrogallol/H_2O_2	28

[a] HSA, human serum albumin
[b] Ab, antibody
[c] About 10^5 lymphocytes
[d] Ag, antigen
[e] About 10^2 bacterial cells
[f] About 10^7 plaque-forming units

Labelling with luminol (Figure 9.3), the emitting species in the chemiluminescent reaction, presents special problems, since derivatization often partially or totally abolishes luminescent activity[36, 37]. Coupling to the $-NH_2$ group results in a relatively strong decrease of luminescent activity[37], possibly due to steric hindrance. However, such conjugates have been successfully used in immunoassays[38–41], since other factors have limited the assay, e.g. unspecific adsorption of conjugate.

The use of isoluminol (Figure 9.2), which by itself emits light considerably less efficient than luminol, may be an alternative. With isoluminol the conjugates may even have increased luminescent activity compared to that of free substance[37], possibly owing to the more favourable position of the $-NH_2$ group (cf. luminol).

Applications using luminol conjugates have been performed both with luminol and isoluminol derivatives (Table 9.3). Luminescent efficiencies of these conjugates have been 1–20% compared to that of free luminol. Conjugates have been prepared with more than 20 luminol molecules per IgG molecule[39]. Stability of the conjugates during storage has ranged from poor[38] to very good[39].

Table 9.3 Immunoanalytical applications using conjugates based on luminol derivatives active in chemiluminescent reactions. The assays have been based on solid-phase or double-antibody precipitation techniques if not otherwise indicated

Quantitated substance	Sensitivity (g)	Conjugate/luminescent system	Ref.
Testosterone	$\approx 10^{-9}$	luminol–Ag^a/Cu-acetate/H_2O_2	38
Rabbit IgG	5×10^{-9}	luminol–Ab^b/NaOCl/H_2O_2	39
Human IgG	5×10^{-6}	luminol–Ag/haemin/H_2O_2	40
Digoxin	8×10^{-11}	luminol–Ag/haemoglobin/$H_2O_2{}^c$	41
Insulin	2×10^{-9}	luminol–Ag/NAOCl/H_2O_2	41
Thyroxine	2×10^{-9}	isoluminol–Ag/haemin/$H_2O_2{}^d$	42
Thyroxine	4×10^{-9}	isoluminol–Ag/microperoxidase/$H_2O_2{}^d$	43
Progesterone	3×10^{-11}	isoluminol–Ag/microperoxidase/$H_2O_2{}^c$	44

^{a} Ag, antigen

^{b} Ab, antibody

^{c} Performed by homogeneous assay

^{d} Penetration of free label into gel beads followed by elution of bound label

Most applications have been performed with solid-phase or double-antibody systems. Homogeneous immunoassay of progesterone has also been performed using isoluminol conjugate and a proteolytic product of cytochrome c, microperoxidase, catalysing the luminescent reaction [44]. Catalytic activity is considerably increased, compared to peroxidase at the used pH, and the luminescent activity is comparable to that obtained under alkaline conditions with haemin[37]. However, interference caused by serum components is strong and solid-phase techniques may be preferable[43]. A point worthy of note is that in homogeneous assay, light intensity is enhanced when antibody binds to the conjugated label, probably due to establishment of a favourable hydrophobic environment for the emitting species, luminol[44, 45]. In all cases very low levels of antigen or antibody could be detected. Comparisons have been made with RIA or EIA demonstrating equal or better sensitivity[39, 43, 44].

In addition to the applications presented in Table 9.3 (and Table 9.2), it has been demonstrated that substances, i.e. biotin, could be quantitated using chemiluminescent labels in specific protein-binding reactions other than antibody–antigen interaction[20, 45].

CONCLUSIONS

The use of chemiluminescent reactions in immunoanalysis is currently being investigated in several laboratories. The present knowledge, although still limited, indicates that this new technique may have valuable properties compared to other immunoanalytical techniques. Some relevant properties of luminescence immunoassay (LIA) are listed in Table 9.4.

Table 9.4   Some properties of LIA, EIA and RIA

	LIA	EIA	RIA
Possibility of using low molecular labels	+	−	+
Possibility of employing catalysing labels for amplification	+	+	−
Possibility for homogeneous assay	+	+	−
No radioactivity hazards	+	+	−
Stable labels	(+)	(+)	−
Rapid detection procedure	(+)	−	+
Relatively cheap, compact instrumentation	+	(+)	−

Acknowledgments

This work was supported by the Swedish Board for Technical Development.

References

1. Whitehead, T. P., Kricka, L. J., Carter, T. J. N. and Thorpe, G. H. G. (1979). Analytical luminescence: its potential in the clinical laboratory. *Clin. Chem.*, **25**, 1531
2. Thore, A. (1979). Luminescence in clinical analysis. *Ann. Clin. Biochem.*, **16**, 359
3. Gorus, F. and Schram, E. (1979). Applications of bio- and chemiluminescence in the clinical laboratory. *Clin. Chem.*, **25**, 512
4. Thore, A. and Rawlings, T. (1980). *Chemiluminescent Analysis in the Life Sciences.* (SF-20101 Turku 10, Finland: Wallac OY)
5. Lundin, A., Rickardsson, A. and Thore, A. (1976). Continuous monitoring of ATP-converting reactions by purified firefly luciferase. *Anal. Biochem.*, **75**, 611
6. Wold, F. (1972). Bifunctional reagents. In Hirs, C. H. W. and Timasheff, S. N. (eds.) *Enzyme Structure (Part B), Methods in Enzymology*, Vol. 25, pp. 623–51. (New York: Academic Press)
7. Kennedy, J. H., Kricka, L. J. and Wilding, P. (1976). Protein–protein coupling reactions and the applications of protein conjugates. *Clin. Chim. Acta*, **70**, 1
8. Jacoby, W. B. and Wilcheck, M. (1974). *Affinity Techniques, Methods in Enzymology*, Vol. 34. (New York: Academic Press)
9. Mosbach, K. (1976). *Immobilized Enzymes, Methods of Enzymology*, Vol. 44. (New York: Academic Press)
10. DeLuca, M. (1976). Firefly luciferase. In Meister, A. (ed.) *Advances in Enzymology*, Vol. 44, pp. 37–68. (New York: John Wiley & Sons)

11. Thore, A. (1979). Technical aspects of the bioluminescent firefly luciferase assay of ATP. *Science Tools*, **26**, 30

12. Hastings, J. W. and Nealson, K. H. (1977). Bacterial bioluminescence. *Ann. Rev. Microbiol.*, **31**, 549

13. Stanley, P. E. (1978). Quantitation of picomole amounts of NADH, NADPH and FMN using bacterial luciferase. In DeLuca, M. (ed.). *Bioluminescence and Chemiluminescence, Methods in Enzymology*, Vol. 57, pp. 215–22. (New York: Academic Press)

14. Stanley, P. E. (1978). The application of analytical bioluminescence to the enzyme multiplied immunoassay technique for the assay of anticonvulsant drugs in plasma. In Crook, M. A. and Johnson, P. (eds.). *Liquid Scintillation Counting*, Vol. 5, pp. 79–84. (London: Heyden & Son)

15. Olsson, T., Thore, A., Carlsson, H. E., Brunius, G. and Eriksson, G. (1979). Quantitation of immunological reactions by luminescence. In Schram, E. and Stanley, P. E. (eds.). *International Symposium on Analytical Applications of Bioluminescence and Chemiluminescence, Proceedings 1978*, pp. 421–30. (Westlake Village, Cal. 91361: State Printing & Publishing Inc.)

16. Puget, K., Michelson, A. M. and Avrameas, S. (1977). Light emission techniques for the microestimation of femtogram levels of peroxidase. Application to peroxidase (and other enzymes)-coupled antibody–cell antigen interactions. *Anal. Biochem.*, **79**, 447

17. Lee, R. T., Denburg, J. L. and McElroy, W. D. (1970). Substrate binding properties of firefly luciferase II. ATP binding site. *Arch. Biochem. Biophys.*, **141**, 38

18. White, E. H., Rapaport, E., Hopkins, T. A. and Seeliger, H. H. (1969). Chemo- and bioluminescence of firefly luciferin. *J. Am. Chem. Soc.*, **91**, 2178

19. Mitchell, G. and Hastings, J. W. (1969). The effect of flavin isomers and analogues upon the color of bacterial bioluminescence. *J. Biol. Chem.*, **244**, 2572

20. Schroeder, H. R., Carrico, R. J., Boguslaski, R. C. and Christner, J. E. (1976). Specific binding reactions monitored with ligand–cofactor conjugates and bacterial luciferase. *Anal. Biochem.*, **72**, 283

21. Carrico, R. J., Yeung, K-K., Schroeder, H. R., Boguslaski, R. C., Buckler, R. T. and Christner, J. E. (1976). Specific protein-binding reactions monitored with ligand–ATP conjugates and firefly luciferase. *Anal. Biochem.*, **76**, 95

22. Roswell, D. F. and White, E. H. (1978). The chemiluminescence of luminol and related hydrazides. In DeLuca, M. (ed.) *Bioluminescence and Chemiluminescence, Methods in Enzymology*, Vol. 57, pp. 409–23. (New York: Academic Press)

23. Ewetz, L. and Thore, A. (1976). Factors affecting the specificity of the luminol reaction with hematin compounds. *Anal. Biochem.*, **71**, 564

24. Gundermann, K.-D. (1974). Recent advances in research on the chemiluminescence of organic compounds. *Top. Curr. Chem.*, **46**, 61

25. Ahnström, G., v. Ehrenstein, G. and Nilsson, R. (1961). The study of horseradish peroxidase catalyzed oxidations by means of chemiluminescence. *Acta Chem. Scand.*, **15**, 1417

26. Nilsson, R. (1964). On the mechanism of peroxidase catalyzed oxidations studied by means of chemiluminescence measurements. *Acta Chem. Scand.*, **18**, 389

27. Olsson, T., Brunius, G., Carlsson, H. E. and Thore, A. (1979). Luminescence immunoassay (LIA): a solid-phase immunoassay monitored by chemiluminescence. *J. Immunol. Methods*, **25**, 127

28. Velan, B., Schupper, H., Sery, T. and Halmann, M. (1979). Solid phase chemiluminescent immunoassay. In Schram, E. and Stanley, P. E. (eds.) *International Symposium on Analytical Applications of Bioluminescence and Chemiluminescence, Proceedings 1978*, pp. 431–7. (Westlake Village, Cal. 91361, USA: State Printing & Publishing Inc.)

29. Halmann, M., Velan, B., Sery, T. and Schupper, H. (1979). Peroxidase mediated chemiluminescence with phenol derivatives. Physicochemical parameters and uses in biological assays. *Photochem. Photobiol.*, **30**, 165

30. Avrameas, S. and Ternynck, T. (1971). Peroxidase labelled antibody and Fab conjugates with enhanced intracellular penetration. *Immunochemistry*, **8**, 1175

31. Nakane, P. K. and Kawaoi, A. (1974). Peroxidase-labeled antibody. A new method of conjugation. *J. Histochem. Cytochem.*, **22**, 1084

32. Olsson, T., Hallin, P. and Thore, A. (1980). Properties of a protohemin–antibody conjugate, prepared for luminescence immunoassay (LIA), monitored by luminol chemiluminescence. (In preparation)

33. Arakawa, H., Maeda, M. and Tsuji, A. (1979). Chemiluminescence enzyme immunoassay of cortisol using peroxidase as label. *Anal. Biochem.*, **97**, 248

34. Halmann, M., Velan, B. and Sery, T. (1977). Rapid identification and quantitation of small numbers of microorganisms by a chemiluminescent immunoreaction. *Appl. Environ. Microbiol.*, **34**, 473

35. Velan, B. and Halmann, M. (1978). Chemiluminescence immunoassay; a new sensitive method for determination of antigens. *Immunochemistry*, **15**, 331

36. White, E. H. (1961). The chemiluminescence of luminol. In McElroy, W. D. and Glass, B. (eds.) *A Symposium on Light and Life*, pp. 183–99. (Baltimore: Johns Hopkins Press)

37. Schroeder, H. R. and Yeager, F. M. (1978). Chemiluminescence yields and detection limits of some isoluminol derivatives in various oxidation systems. *Anal. Chem.*, **50**, 1114

38. Pratt, J. J., Woldring, M. G. and Villerius, L. (1978). Chemiluminescence-linked immunoassay. *J. Immunol. Methods*, **21**, 179

39. Simpson, J. S. A., Campbell, A. K., Ryall, M. E. T. and Woodhead, J. S. (1979). A stable chemiluminescent-labelled antibody for immunological assays. *Nature (London)*, **279**, 646

40. Hersh, L. S., Vann, W. P. and Wilhelm, S. A. (1979). A luminol-assisted, competitive-binding immunoassay of human immunoglobulin G. *Anal. Biochem.*, **93**, 267

41. Maier, C. L. (1978). Procedure for the assay of pharmacologically, immunologically and biochemically active compounds in biological fluids. (United States Patent 4,104,029)

42. Schroeder, H. R., Boguslaski, R. C., Carrico, R. J. and Buckler, R. T. (1978). Monitoring specific protein-binding reactions with chemiluminescence. In DeLuca, M. (ed.) *Bioluminescence and Chemiluminescence, Methods in Enzymology*, Vol. 57, pp. 424–45. (New York: Academic Press)

43. Schroeder, H. R., Yeager, F. M., Boguslaski, R. C. and Vogelhut, P. O. (1979). Immunoassay for serum thyroxine monitored by chemiluminescence. *J. Immunol. Methods*, **25**, 275

44. Kohen, F., Pazzagli, M., Kim, J. B., Lindner, H. R. and Boguslaski, R. C. (1979). An assay procedure for plasma progesterone based on antibody-enhanced chemiluminescence. *FEBS Lett.* **104**, 201

45. Schroeder, H. R., Vogelhut, P. O., Carrico, R. J., Boguslaski, R. C. and Buckler, R. T. (1976). Competitive protein binding assay for biotin monitored by chemiluminescence. *Anal. Chem.*, **48**, 1933

10
New Homogeneous Assay Methods for the Determination of Proteins

K. E. RUBENSTEIN

INTRODUCTION

This paper will describe three homogeneous immunoassay methods which are applicable to the determination of proteins in biological fluids. The term homogeneous, applied to immunoassays, indicates that no separation of bound from free label is required. One of these techniques utilizes an enzyme label, and the other two utilize fluorescent labels.

METHODS

The first technique is an adaptation of the EMIT® homogeneous enzyme immunoassay which until recently has been applied to the determination of small molecules. In the EMIT technique (Figure 10.1) a derivative of the analyte is linked covalently to an enzyme. When the resulting enzyme conjugate is complexed to an antibody, the enzyme is rendered inactive. Depending on the enzyme used, inhibition may result from steric exclusion of the enzyme substrate from the complex or from conformational changes in the enzyme. When a sample containing some analyte is present, a corresponding portion of the enzyme conjugate is freed from the complex and becomes active. Increasing analyte concentration leads therefore to increasing enzyme activity in the bulk assay mixture. Thus the separation of bound from free label, required in heterogeneous systems, becomes superfluous.

For larger analytes such as proteins, we might envisage complexes in which

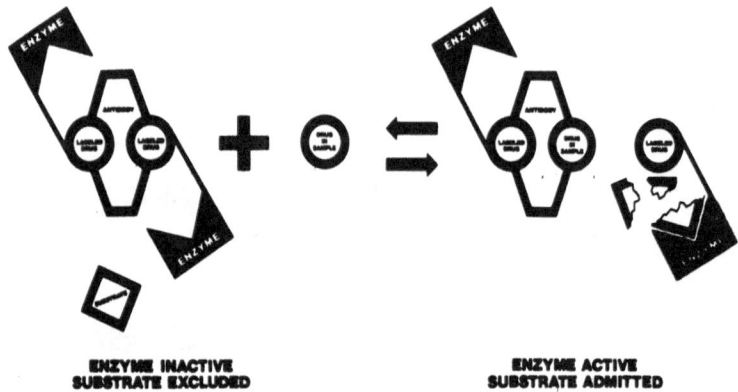

Figure 10.1 EMIT® homogeneous enzyme immunoassay

the antibodies are held too far away from the enzyme to have much of an effect on enzyme activity. In fact this is usually the case. We envisaged that an increase in the size of the enzyme substrate could improve this situation.

The development of an assay method utilizing such a macromolecular substrate is primarily the work of Gibbons et al.[1] and of Gushaw (unpublished). The enzyme chosen for this work is β-galactosidase from *Escherichia coli*. The enzyme has four active sites (Figure 10.2). Covalent

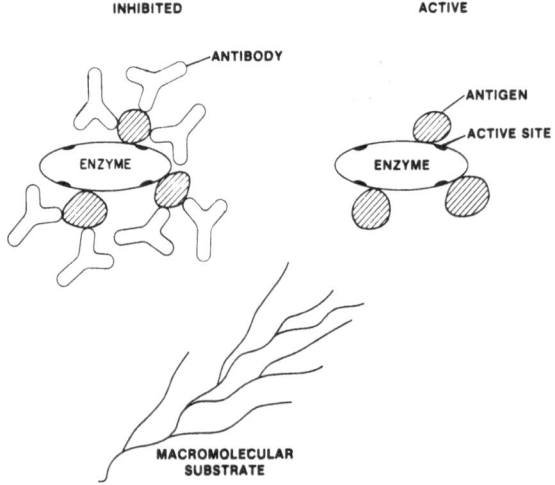

Figure 10.2 Inhibition of antigen-labelled enzyme by antibody binding

linkage of several antigen molecules to β-galactosidase results in the formation of enzyme conjugates possessing about one-half to one-third the specific enzyme activity of the native enzyme. In an antibody complex of such an enzyme conjugate, one might envisage that a small substrate could get to the active site while a macromolecular substrate would be sterically excluded.

The usual substrate for β-galactosidase assays is ortho-nitrophenyl-β-galactoside (ONPG) which is converted by the enzyme to a yellow nitro-phenolate ion with an absorption maximum at 420 nm. Gibbons et al.[2] synthesized a macromolecular substrate in which ONPG is attached to a polymeric dextran backbone via a hydrophilic spacer arm. About one ONPG has been incorporated for every five dextran monomer units.

β-galactosidase has been linked to antigens using a heterobifunctional coupling agent, meta-maleimidobenzoyl-N-hydroxysuccinimide ester. This agent permits the generation of relatively well-defined conjugates. The antigen may be linked first to the ester portion of the coupling agent followed by reaction of β-galactosidase, which couples to the maleimido portion via sulphhydryl groups. Thus conjugates containing up to seven molecules of antigen per molecule of enzyme were prepared and found to have essentially the same specific enzyme activity with ONPG as the unmodified enzyme. Addition of antibodies to the antigen results in no loss of activity with the small substrate, ONPG, whereas with ONPG-dextran enzyme activities are reduced by up to 90%. Thus with the macromolecular substrate, homogeneous enzyme immunoassays for several proteins have been demonstrated.

Preliminary data for a rapid IgG assay are presented. Operational parameters for this assay are shown in Table 10.1 in comparison to those for small molecule assays. Both procedures complete the measurement in less

Table 10.1   EMIT® assay parameters

	Small molecules	Proteins
Enzyme	lysozyme G-6PDH MDH	β-galactosidase
Temperature (°C)	37, 30	30
Wavelength (nm)	436, 340	410
Timing		
STAT	15 s delay 30 s read	15 s delay 30 s read
BATCH	up to 90 min	up to 2 h

than 1 min. The assay with macromolecular substrate is sensitive to about 5 μg IgG/ml. Comparative analysis data for the enzyme immunoassay for IgG versus radial immunodiffusion show a correlation coefficient of 0.98 and a slope of 1.01 for a small sampling ($n=21$).

This assay system has a broad range of applicability. Analytes for which assays have been demonstrated include large molecules such as IgM, negatively charged proteins such as albumin, basic proteins such as IgG, and small molecules such as theophylline.

The first of the two fluorescence techniques to be described is called fluorescence excitation transfer immunoassay and is based on the work of Ullman et al.[3] and Cobb (unpublished). The method is based on the increased efficiency of energy transfer from a fluorescer to a quencher when the two are brought into close proximity by virtue of an antigen–antibody reaction (Figure 10.3). The quencher, rhodamine, can accept energy from the excited fluorescer, fluorescein, with about 50% efficiency at a distance of 5 nm. The binding of fluorescein-labelled antigen to rhodamine-labelled antibody results in up to 90% quenching of fluorescence. Addition of analyte antigen results in displacement of tagged antigen which when free exhibits fluorescence emission. Therefore increased analyte in a sample results in increased fluorescence signal.

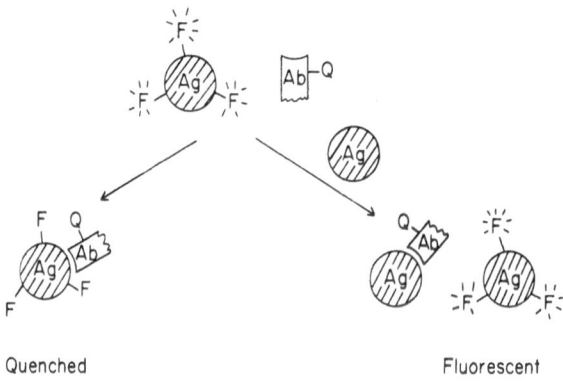

Figure 10.3   Fluorescence excitation transfer immunoassay

Both the antigen and the antibody are labelled with N-hydroxysuccinimide ester derivatives of the fluorescer and quencher. Typical degrees of labelling range from two to eight molecules of fluorescer or quencher per molecule of antigen or antibody.

The method is illustrated with preliminary information from an assay for IgM (Table 10.2). In addition to the fluorescein–rhodamine pair, synthetic dyes prepared in our laboratories have been used. A fluorescer called Khannacein$_{520}$ and a molecule called Quencher$_{539}$ have been employed. This pair operates at wavelengths about 30 nm greater than the fluorescein–rhodamine pair which helps to reduce matrix interferences. Measurements are rapid with total assay times of 30 s. Within-run precision studies involving 30 replicates typically resulted in coefficients of variation of 5–6%. Sensitivity to about 100 μg IgM/ml has been demonstrated.

Table 10.2 Fluorescent excitation transfer immunoassay (IgM assay operational parameters)

Fluorescer:	Fluorescein$_{490}$ (Khannacein$_{520}$)
Quencher:	Rhodamine$_{520}$ (Quencher$_{539}$)
Assay Time:	10 second delay, 20 second measurement
Assay Temperature:	30°C
Wavelength:	Excitation 490 (520) nm Emission 520 (539) nm
Sample Matrix:	Serum
Sample Volume:	35 μl of a 1 : 18 prediluted sample
Potential Sensitivity:	Approximately 100 μg/ml

Comparison has been made to a radial immunodiffusion method. A correlation coefficient of 0.98 was obtained. The slope of the regression line is 1.14 and the Y-intercept is $- 3.7$ mg/dl. Mean analytical concentrations were 167 mg/dl by the fluorescence method and 169 mg/dl for the immunodiffusion method.

The method is broadly applicable to proteins and small molecules. Proteins for immunization must be highly pure, but proteins for labelling need only be $> 50\%$ pure. Antibodies must be free from interfering cross-reactivities but need not in general be purified prior to labelling.

The final assay method to be discussed is the antigen-labelled fluorescence protection assay first described by Zuk et al.[4] This principle has been applied by Brinkley and co-workers[5] to the determination of reagin, the class of antibodies formed in response to syphilis infection which recognize the phospholipid, cardiolipin.

This technique utilizes a conjugate of fluorescein and cardiolipin. The conjugate is combined with cholesterol and lecithin in a 5/15/80 molar ratio, and the mixture is sonicated to produce liposomes with average diameters in the 200–250 Å range. These particles are small enough to act as a homogeneous solute and have been shown to bind strongly to serum reagin.

Addition of antifluorescein antibodies to a solution of vesicles results in rapid quenching of the fluorescence due to binding of the antibodies to exposed fluorescein groups (Figure 10.4). Preincubation of vesicles with reagin-positive serum results in inhibition of antifluorescein binding and quenching is inhibited.

The assay is performed by measuring the change of fluorescence over a defined interval of time. The quenching rate data are transformed by a least squares computation to a ΔF value. In the absence of reagin, there is little change in fluorescence during the measuring interval, since quenching is essentially complete when the measurement is initiated. Binding of reagin to the vesicles decreases the rate of change in the fluorescence signal so that a larger ΔF is seen during the measuring interval. Consequently increasing

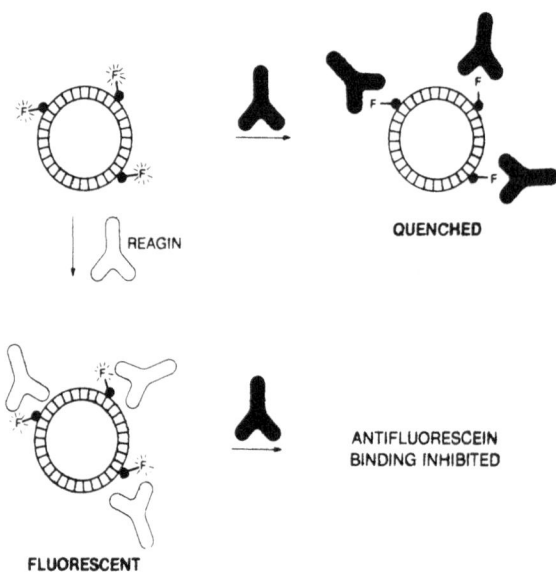

REAGIN

QUENCHED

ANTIFLUORESCEIN
BINDING INHIBITED

FLUORESCENT

Figure 10.4 Homogeneous fluorescence protection assay for syphilis

reagin concentration leads to an increased change in fluorescence, ΔF.

A preliminary assay has been developed and evaluated. The protocol is quite simple. Liposomes are incubated with serum for 15 min. Antifluorescein is then added, and the rate of decay of the fluorescent signal is immediately measured using a device which automatically controls the delay and measurement intervals. A serum blank must be determined for each sample.

A study involving 65 sera shows a reasonable correlation of 91% with the RPR card test. Five samples which assayed false-negative by the fluorescence protection method were only weakly positive by the RPR test. Further optimization of the procedure should eliminate these discrepancies. Relative to other available reagin tests, the present method has the advantage of giving an objective, quantitative result with only a single dilution of the sample.

References

1. Gibbons, I., Skold, C., Rowley, G. L. and Ullman, E. F. (1980). Homogeneous immunoassay for proteins employing β-galactosidase. *Anal. Biochem.*, **102**, 167
2. Gibbons, I., Skold, C., Rowley, G. L. and Ullman, E. F. (1979). Homogeneous enzyme immunoassay method for specific proteins. (Meeting abstract). *Clin. Chem.*, **25**, 1078
3. Ullman, E. F., Schwarzberg, M. and Rubenstein, K. E. (1976). Fluorescent excitation transfer immunoassay. *J. Biol. Chem.*, **251**, 4172
4. Zuk, R. F., Rowley, G. L. and Ullman, E. F. (1979). Fluorescence protection immunoassay: a new homogeneous assay technique. *Clin. Chem.*, **25**, 1554
5. Brinkley, J. M., Rowley, G. L., Singh, P. and Ullman, E. F. (1979). Homogeneous fluorescence protection assay for anti cardiolipin. (Meeting abstract). *Clin. Chem.*, **25**, 1077

11
Antisera in Immunoassays with special Reference to Monoclonal Antibodies to Human Immunoglobulins

D. CATTY, N. R. LING, J. A. LOWE AND C. RAYKUNDALIA

INTRODUCTION

When antisera are raised by the conventional means of injection of immunogen in adjuvant into animals, the antibodies are derived from many responding clones of cells and are consequently heterogeneous in structure, specificity, titre and binding properties to antigen. The performance characteristics of any single antiserum used in a particular immunoassay depend upon the balance of properties of the antibodies it contains, which may provide an overall 'good' or 'bad' rating. It is possible to define, partially at least in scientific terms, those properties of antisera that make them especially useful for a particular assay system. Thus the properties of antisera required for use in, for instance, gel precipitation assays, in nephelometry, in enzyme immunoassays and for radioimmunoassays can be described.

Experience in immunization methods reveals that there are certain 'ground rules' in the preparation of antisera for particular purposes; these come partially from an understanding of the nature of the immune response and partially from trial and error. Although there is no perfect recipe for antiserum production, following the 'rules' yields useful results in a large proportion of cases. In addition some final processing of antisera is usually essential before they can be adopted as specific reagents in sensitive assays.

Recently a novel method of producing antibodies has been developed[1, 2];

this entails the fusion *in vitro* of a single antibody-producing lymphocyte with a plasmacytoma cell to produce a dividing and potentially immortal, antibody-producing hybrid cell line (hybridoma) which secretes antibody homogeneous both in structure and in binding properties to antigen. As the specificity of these monoclonal antibodies is restricted to a single antigen determinant, these reagents are proving to be of enormous value and importance in the analysis of complex antigen systems that have not yielded easily to specific antiserum production by conventional means, for instance transplantation and other cell surface antigens[3-8]. However, in terms of routine immunoassays the possible advantages of homogeneous antibody reagents have not yet been properly explored.

A programme for the production of monoclonal antibodies to human immunoglobulins and immunoglobulin fragments is in operation in this Department. It is based on the Kohler and Milstein[1] technique for the production of antibody-secreting mouse hybridomas. After fusion of spleen and plasmacytoma cells the hybridomas are grown up in selective media and antibody produced is detected by examination of supernates of culture wells. It is essential that antibody is detected at an early stage of growth when comparatively few hybridoma cells are present, and hence it is important at the outset to have an assay system which is sensitive and reliable and, since very large numbers of tests must be made, it should also be simple and rapid.

In measuring antibody to a soluble antigen such as the one used here there are three main alternative techniques of adequate sensitivity; these are (a) passive haemagglutination using antigen-coated red cells; (b) ELISA; and (c) radioimmunoassay. We report here our findings on the performance of monoclonal antibodies to human immunoglobulin Fc (γ) chain and kappa and lambda light chains in relation to the above three tests.

PROPERTIES OF CONVENTIONAL ANTISERA

Antibody responses are normally heterogeneous at many levels; in the nature of classes and subclasses in which antibodies may be produced, in the specificity, titre and binding properties to antigen. In one antiserum there may be antibodies to a whole pattern of antigens (oligospecific) or to a single antigen ('monospecific') but in the latter case antibody is still not homogeneous as immunogens are multi-determinant structures which stimulate many clones of cells into response. The clonal products that finally appear in the serum differ greatly in specificity, titre, affinity and optimum conditions for binding to antigen. A single amino acid substitution difference between two molecules can give rise, in animals possessing the one form of molecule, and presented with the other as immunogen, to antibodies which exhibit extensive polyclonality. This is illustrated in Figure 11.1; on the left is shown the stained pattern of electrofocused immunoglobulins of a mouse immunized with an

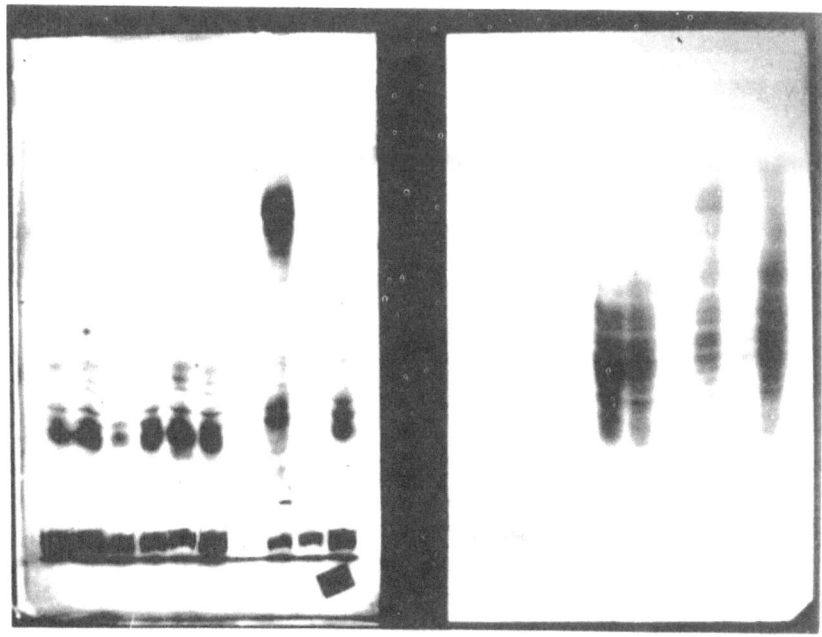

Figure 11.1 Isoelectric focusing with autoradiography of antiserum from a single Balb/c mouse (Ig-^{a}) immunized with the Ig-1^b heavy chain allotype of the C57BL/6 strain γ2a immunoglobulin molecule. The mouse antiserum samples have been focused on thin-layer polyacrylamide gel with an ampholite gradient of pH 5-9. The focused plate was incubated in radioiodinated immunoglobulin antigen and the autoradiograph of the focused antibody clones is seen on the right. The stained plate showing all the focused proteins is shown on the left

allotypically different Ig heavy chain, and on the right is the autoradiograph of the specific antibody clones as seen after incubation with iodinated antigen. There is clonal heterogeneity in this antibody system even though the number of antigen determinants on target molecules is insufficient to produce precipitation with antibody *in vitro*.

Complex antigens in concentrations down to about 5 mg/l can usually be measured by a range of precipitation assays in agar gel which includes radial immunodiffusion, 'rocket' and two-dimensional electrophoresis. Since precipitation depends upon efficient lattice formation between antibodies and several antigen determinants, both multiple specificity and a balance in the titre of the antibodies is important and probably of more relevance than affinity. For reasons of economy, and to give low backgrounds in stained plates, high-titre precipitating antisera that can be used in high dilution are always preferable. In 'rocket' and two-dimensional work it is essential to have antibodies in the agar of narrow isoelectric range for the broadest utilization of the techniques. Sheep IgG2 antibodies are especially useful in this respect and can be used to quantitate the widest range of human serum proteins.

Nephelometric assays are gaining in importance in the routine laboratories. They are useful for measuring the larger molecular weight antigens to concentrations of about 10 mg/l. As the system depends upon detection of rapidly formed multi-determinant immune complexes in fluid the antisera need to possess, in addition to multiple specificity, a combination of high average avidity and high average titre. The former seems essential to produce the appropriate size of immune complex to work well in the optical system; the latter is essential for allowing high working dilutions that give low background and sensitivity to the assay. It is our experience that only a small proportion of animals respond with the right balance of properties of antibodies for sensitive performance of nephelometric assays, so these reagents are very precious.

Antisera for enzyme immunoassays such as ELISA demand, in addition to certain intrinsic properties, further purification steps as a prelude to enzyme conjugation or use as 'coating' antibodies. ELISA is not normally applied in quantitative work but at its most sensitive it can detect antigen or antibody to about 5 μg/l. To achieve this, however, antiserum reagents need to be of the highest quality. Antiglobulin–enzyme conjugates give the least background activity if they are affinity-purified antibodies free of aggregates and soluble complexes and with avid binding properties. The conjugate should also be specific to the species (and to the class) of the intermediate (e.g. the patient's) antibody. Antibodies used as a 'coating' or 'sensitizing' layer on plastic should be affinity-purified where possible to reduce the non-specific binding of subsequent antibody layers; they should also ideally be of the same species as the enzyme-conjugated antiglobulin, but this often only works in practice when the antigen is large and multi-determinant.

The most important application of radioimmunoassays (RIAs) is that used to detect low molecular weight antigens present in low concentrations down to about 1 μg/l, such as the polypeptide hormones. The molecules, being small, have reduced numbers of antigen determinants, usually require coupling to larger protein carriers to make them immunogenic, and, as free haptens, they do not generate precipitates with antibody. It has been shown in many studies that antibodies to haptens, including hormones, display marked heterogeneity both in specificity and in affinity of binding[9]. In RIAs it is essential to select antisera that display high average affinity to obtain the sensitivity required for quantitative inhibition at low concentrations. However, many sera with high affinity characteristics contain antibodies that bind to chemically similar determinants (e.g. of related hormones) so there is always the risk of attaining maximal sensitivity at the expense of specificity. Thus very careful selection of antisera is needed to find those that achieve a suitable balance. A golden rule is always to immunize a panel of animals with each immunogen and test bleed each animal frequently, so that the best phase in the response, for balance of antibody properties, can be selected.

FACTORS INFLUENCING THE ANTIBODY RESPONSE

The immunogen

There is a great deal of basic information obtainable in textbooks of immunochemistry about the physicochemical properties of molecules that influence their immunogenicity; these can be only briefly mentioned here. In general molecules have to be bigger than about 5000 MW to be immunogenic without conjugation to a carrier. Large molecules with a high degree of conformation and structural rigidity tend to be strong immunogens with immunodominant regions and multiple antigenic determinants; there is, however, an overriding necessity for the molecule to be seen as foreign by the recipient animal. Mammalian serum proteins, although structurally complex in the main, are poor immunogens in closely related species, requiring the assistance of both adjuvants and T helper cells to stimulate antibody production. In relation to haptens, their size, charge and polar or non-polar properties are all important in inducing the antibody response. These properties can be influenced by the extent of uniformity and density of conjugation of hapten to carrier, and by the choice of carrier itself.

'Rules' about antibody responses

In considering antibody responses to proteins and haptens there are certain 'rules' that are followed by the responding animal which can be of considerable assistance in the preparation of antisera.

(1) Immunization with protein from a closely related species gives an antibody response that recognizes only the minor structural differences that exist between the same molecule in the two (and other) species.
(2) The broadest set of antibody specificities to a protein is produced in species that are phylogenetically distant to the immunogen source.
(3) Antibodies to native proteins are normally to surface determinants which can be sequential, conformational or haptenic sites.
(4) Antibodies to larger haptens each have specificity for only a portion of the total structure and this is predominantly away from the coupling site; the choice of coupling reaction, and to which group of the hapten, may then be critical for the final range of specificities achieved.
(5) Antibodies to smaller haptens may incorporate specificity to the link region and even into the carrier, so choice of carrier with small haptens may be critical.
(6) Antibodies to large hydrophobic haptens tend to have the highest average affinity.
(7) Antigen determinants and haptens vary in charge so antibodies have a range of pH optima for binding.

Preparation of immunogen

Animals can, and frequently do, respond by making disproportionate amounts of antibody to contaminants that have gone undetected in the antigen preparation; the removal of such antibodies represents often the major operation in the preparation of a specific antibody reagent. There is no doubt, then, that the preparation of an 'immunologically' pure immunogen solves one major problem in getting a satisfactory response. An approach which gives remarkable results in this respect exploits the existing antibody specificity of a serum to prepare immunogenic antigen-pure immune complexes that exist in the precipitation peaks developed by two-dimensional electrophoresis in agarose. Figure 11.2 shows the complex pattern of soluble

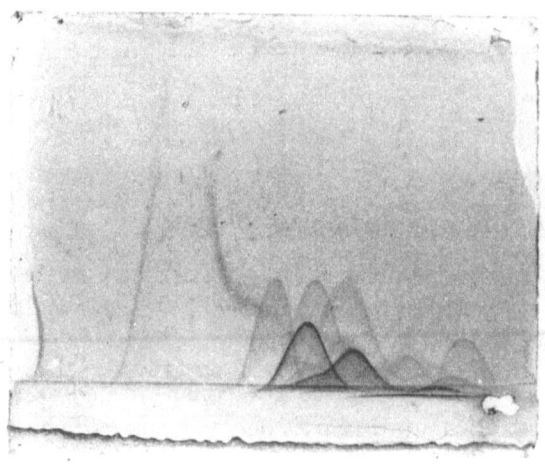

Surface memb./
homologous antiserum

Figure 11.2   Two-dimensional electrophoresis pattern of the soluble surface tegument antigens of *Schistosoma mansoni* developed with an oligospecific rabbit antiserum.

antigens released by the surface tegument of adult *Schistosoma mansoni*, to which an oligospecific rabbit antiserum has been raised and here used in the two-dimensional assay against the antigen mixture. Specific antibody to any one of these components of the tegument can, with care, be successfully prepared, without the need for physicochemical antigen separations. Figure 11.3 shows just such a monospecific antiserum to one antigen of the worm prepared by excision of the single precipitation peak and its use as an immunogen. This approach was first described by Bradwell *et al.*[10] for the production of specific antibodies to thyroxine-binding globulin.

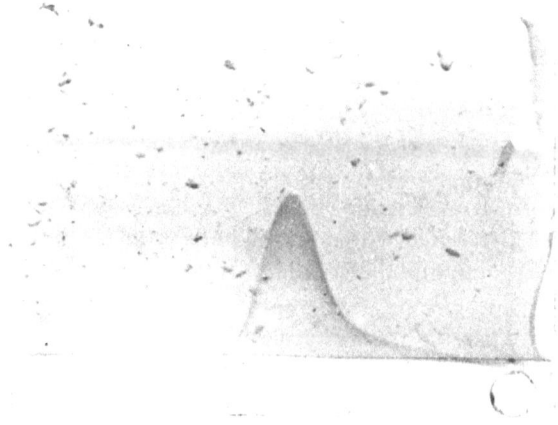

Monospecific antiserum
to an adult surface membrane
antigen

Figure 11.3 Two-dimensional electrophoresis of the same antigens as shown in Figure 10.2 but developed with an antiserum in the agarose obtained by injecting a rabbit with a single excised precipitation peak from plates run as in Figure 10.2. Antisera specific to single antigens of complex mixtures can be routinely raised under appropriate conditions (see text)

Immunization

High affinity antibodies of appropriate specificity can be produced in many animals although the rabbit, goat and sheep are favoured for the obvious reasons of economy, practicability and volumes generated. There are no methods of immunization that are guaranteed to provide the right result; molecules differ in immunogenicity and animals vary in the response they make to them, often by many orders of magnitude. Certain practices are known to influence the response in a universal manner, however. The application of Freund's complete adjuvant emulsified with immunogen serves to protect immunogen from rapid removal and breakdown in the body and attracts the right collection of host cells to the site to initiate and sustain a prolonged antibody response locally. Another influence is to reduce the optimum effective dose of immunogen to levels in which often nanogram quantities incorporated in immune complexes give vigorous responses of high affinity antibodies. This is particularly so if the emulsion is distributed subcutaneously in very small volume (0.1–1.0 ml) over many sites of the body. This immunization procedure frequently requires no boosting, but where further injections are needed they should be given after as long an interval as possible up to several months. Affinity of antibodies tends to increase with time and with greater intervals between boosts.

PROCESSING OF ANTISERA

Those engaged routinely with the preparation of antisera come to recognize
that the harvesting of sera from animals is only the start to obtaining a
working reagent. For most assays the only relevant fraction of the serum is the
immunoglobulin; the rest of the proteins can be conveniently removed. This
has the effect of increasing the ratio of antibody to total protein, reducing the
background staining of agar plates and increasing the sensitivity of most
assays. Ig separation is also the initial required step for fluorochrome and
enzyme labelling of antibodies, and is usual for affinity purification of
antibodies.

After the first tests on specificity it may be necessary to undertake an
absorption of antibodies as an alternative to affinity purification. Absorption
should, wherever possible, involve insolubilized antigen polymers as absorption in the fluid phase, with formation of soluble immune complexes in the
reagent, creates new problems of high backgrounds, etc. which are even
harder to solve. Apart from this consideration insoluble adsorbents offer the
advantages that they can be re-utilized, they do not dilute the antibody and
they add no passenger materials to the antibody under absorption. Once the
reagent is shown to be specific to the target antigen it should be calibrated
against working standards. These can be 'in-house' standards or commercial,
national or international standards as available. Often adjustments can then
be made to titre or affinity by prudent mixing of reagents, concentration etc.
Finally each reagent should be characterized for its performance and value
across a range of immunoassays to which it might be applied. As more
becomes known about the properties of antibodies in different immunoassays
so it becomes necessary to define antibodies beyond merely their specificity
and titre.

PREPARATION AND TESTING OF MONOCLONAL ANTIBODIES TO HUMAN IgG

Materials and methods

Hybridoma technique

This is based on the protocol of Galfré et al.[11]. Spleen cell suspensions are
prepared by injecting 20 ml of RPMI 1640 medium into the spleen. The
medium is injected through a fine-gauge needle inserted successively into
different parts of the body of the spleen so as to blow out the cells in that
region. The HAT-sensitive plasmacytoma line was the NS1 thioguanine-
resistant variant of the MOPC21 line which synthesizes (but does not secrete)
free light chains. It was a gift from Dr C. Milstein.

Immunization schedule

Balb/c mice were primed with antigen in complete Freund's adjuvant and boosted by i.p. and i.v. injections of soluble antigen until test bleeds showed an adequate response had been produced. A final i.v. plus i.p. injection was given 4 days before the fusion.

Collection of culture supernates

Cell suspensions from each spleen fusion were divided into 48 wells each of 2 ml volume in Linbro trays. A large part of the supernate of each well was removed at intervals over a 10-day period and replaced by a HAT-modifying RPMI 1640 medium containing 20% fetal calf serum. Subsequent supernates were collected for testing initially by direct passive haemagglutination.

Immunoassay procedures

Passive haemagglutination

Whole human IgG, the Fc fragment and free kappa and lambda chains were attached to sheep red cells by a modified chromic chloride technique[12]. The supernates are serially diluted in 0.05 ml volumes of Hepes-buffered RPMI medium containing 2% fetal calf serum and one drop of 0.5% antigen-coated red cells is added. The settled pattern end-point is read a few hours later. Maximal sensitivity with this technique is dependent upon achieving optimal coating with antigen and is of the order of nanograms per ml (micrograms per litre). If cells are coated under sterile conditions and stored at 4°C, the coated cells may be used for at least a month. Occasionally supernates were also tested by *indirect* passive haemagglutination as follows: three drops of culture supernate and one drop of 0.5% suspension of antigen-coated sheep red cells were added to one well of a U-shaped microtitre tray, duplicated wells being set up for each supernate. After 10 min the tray was centrifuged at low speed and the supernate discarded by sucking off at the pump with a very fine-tipped Pasteur pipette. The cells were washed by addition of three drops of medium (without resuspension of cells) and centrifuged. One drop of Hepes-buffered RPMI medium containing 2% fetal calf serum was added to each well, plus one drop of a 1:100 dilution of an anti-mouse IgG serum (preabsorbed with insoluble human IgG). After resuspension the cells were allowed to settle at room temperature and the settled end-point noted.

ELISA

The enzyme-linked immunosorbent assay was performed according to the description of Engvall and Perlmann[13]. Microtitre plates were sensitized with whole human IgG (purified from pooled human serum) or kappa or lambda free light chains (from single urinary Bence Jones proteins). This was achieved by overnight soaking at room temperature using 0.2 ml per well of solutions of 2 μg/ml of antigen in 0.05 mol carbonate/bicarbonate buffer pH 9.6 as described by Voller *et al.*[14]. Plates were washed the following morning in normal saline containing 0.05% Tween 20. Phosphate-buffered saline containing 0.05% Tween 20 was used to make serial dilutions of monoclonal antibodies in uncoated plates; 0.2 ml of each of these dilutions was then added to the washed, sensitized wells, with one or two rows of the plate per antibody. After 2 h the plates were again washed and 0.2 ml of a standard 1 : 100 dilution of alkaline phosphatase (Sigma)-conjugated IgG fraction of rabbit antiserum to mouse immunoglobulins was added to each well (including control wells that had contained normal mouse serum instead of monoclonal antibody). After a further 2 h the plates were again washed and *P*-nitrophenyl phosphate, dissolved in 0.1 mol diethanolamine buffer, pH 9.8; 0.2 ml, was added as the enzyme substrate. The colour reaction on substrate was stopped after 45 min by the addition of 3 mol NaOH. The end-point titres were determined by eye using the control wells for comparison.

Solid phase radioimmunoassay

In principle this assay is very similar to the ELISA (above), using the same antigens to sensitize microtitre plates and the same anti-mouse immunoglobulin antibody to quantitate bound monoclonal mouse antibody. In this assay, however, the IgG fraction of the rabbit antiserum was labelled, to high specific activity, with ^{125}I by the Chloramine-T technique of Greenwood *et al.*[15] and 0.05 ml of a 1 : 100 dilution was used to label the wells. These were then washed copiously, dried, cut into separate units and counted individually. Antigen-coating of the plates was performed with 0.05 ml of antigen at 5 μg/ml. In this assay three types of control well were used: those that were unsensitized, those without monoclonal antibody and those without either. As the first type of control well usually gave the highest background count this was the control used for deducting background binding for each sample tested.

Liquid phase radioimmunoassay

The microradioimmunoassay technique as described by Herzenberg and Herzenberg[16] for determination of mouse immunoglobulin allotypes utilizes the loss of counts in a standard small volume (0.05 ml) of supernatant that occurs when antigen is lost from solution and brought to the base of assay tubes by high-speed centrifugation of the immune complexes. The technique has since been modified by Catty and King[17] by the addition of polyethylene glycol (PEG, 6000 m.w.) which shortens the operation of the assay to a few hours and increases its sensitivity. As such, it is a form of radioassay that can be adapted for measurement of both antigen and antibody and is very useful for small samples and low antigen concentrations. Precipitation and inhibition curves achieved by diluting antibody or inhibitor give valuable information about antibody titre and affinity and about the identity and concentration of antigen inhibitors.

Assays are performed in 7×50 mm disposable polystyrene tubes. For precipitation analysis, as performed here, 0.05 ml of ^{125}I-labelled human IgG diluted 1 : 100 in a 3% bovine serum albumin (BSA) in 0.05 M Tris buffer, pH 7.5, is added by micropipette to 0.05 ml samples of serially diluted monoclonal mouse antibodies or polyclonal sheep antisera. To this is then added 0.05 ml of a 12% PEG solution in 0.9% NaCl (final PEG concentration 4%). The labelled antigen dilution is such as to provide 40 000–50 000 ct min^{-1} 0.05 ml^{-1} and contains 5–25 ng in this volume. The assays are incubated for up to 3 h at 37 °C and then brought to 4 °C and held there for another 2–3 h. The tubes are then centrifuged at 10 000 r/min (14 000 g) for 20 min and 0.05 ml of each supernatant is placed in 1 ml of saline and counted. Results are expressed as the percentage of total antigen counts precipitated against antibody dilution (see Figures 11.4–11.8). In one assay experiment reported here the effect of PEG concentration on antigen precipitation by monoclonal antibodies was investigated (see Figure 11.4 and Results).

Isoelectric focusing of antibodies

The technique of thin-layer polyacrylamide isoelectric focusing was first applied to immunoglobulins by Awdeh et al.[18]. Our investigation of mouse monoclonal antibodies (and the polyclonal anti-allotypic antibodies shown in Figure 11.1) used the LKB 2117 Multiphor Electrophoresis equipment and LKB Ampholine 1809 carrier ampholites incorporated in polyacrylamide gel over a pH gradient of 5–9. Samples of antibodies (4 μl) were applied to the anodic end of the gel and focused by application of a potential difference across the gel. During focusing the gel plate is cooled by the circulation of water at 4 °C through the supporting plate beneath. Autoradiographs of antibody clones are produced by incubation of focused plates in very dilute samples of ^{125}I-labelled antigen followed by extensive washing, and then leaving the dried plates in contact with photographic film. The plates can also be stained in 0.1% Coomassie Brilliant Blue to show the total pattern of focused proteins.

RESULTS AND DISCUSSION

Once the basic hybridoma technique has been established the major problem in the early stages of monoclonal antibody production is the development of an assay system for screening of culture supernates. The amount of antibody produced in the primary cultures of the hybridomas is very small so a sensitive technique is essential; it should also be simple and rapid to perform. The passive haemagglutination assay is the obvious first choice amongst the available systems for testing antibodies and was accordingly adopted for the initial screening of supernates. Once initial problems of the purity of the antigens used to coat the sheep red cells was overcome then the direct passive haemagglutination assay was found to be of adequate sensitivity to detect supernatant antibodies in very low concentrations (Table 11.1). As each monoclonal antibody exhibits specificity to a single antigen determinant that might be on any domain of the complex immunizing antigen, the matter of antigen purity for the demonstration of the specificity of the antibody to, for example, kappa or lambda light chain, as in Table 11.1, represents no small

Table 11.1 Direct and indirect haemagglutination assay of mono-clonal anti-light chain antibodies in primary culture supernates

Culture supernate	Kappa – SRBC		Lambda – SRBC	
	Direct	Indirect	Direct	Indirect
Anti-kappa	1 : 32	1 : 128	nil	nil
Anti-lambda	nil	nil	1 : 16	1 : 64

.SRBC = sheep red blood cells

problem in this and other binding assays. In practice much time and effort has to be expended to achieve sufficiently high degrees of antigen (or antigen subcomponent or fragment) purity to demonstrate the above specificities and those to the $Fc(\gamma)$ fragment (Table 11.2). Table 11.1 also compares the direct and indirect haemagglutination titres of anti-kappa and anti-lambda mono-clonal antibodies. The indirect assay, as also the ELISA and solid-phase radioimmunoassay, detects only antibodies of sufficiently high affinity to withstand the washing stages, whereas the direct haemagglutination test might be expected to detect antibodies, of any affinity, that are capable also of binding to a minimum of two of the same determinants coating the red cells. In practice the indirect test was always more sensitive, suggesting that all the monoclonal antibodies produced so far are of reasonably high affinity. For routine purposes, however, the direct test is much more convenient. As a sensitive one-stage screening procedure for the detection of antibody it offers the advantages of speed, simplicity and cheapness and is in addition capable of useful application for the determination of the specificity of the antibodies.

Once a hybridoma clone has grown up substantial quantities of monoclonal antibody can be harvested. At this stage it becomes useful to undertake a more detailed characterization of the product, not just in terms of specificity and titre, but also for other properties such as antigen binding capacity, precipitating capacity and affinity. In addition the monoclonality of the

Table 11.2 Characteristics of 25 monoclonal antibodies to human IgG Fc (γ)

Clone	Antigen-coated red cell agglutination titre (log₂)		Indirect ELISA titre (log₂)	Solid-phase RIA		Liquid-phase RIA (4% PEG)		
	IgG	Fc(γ)	IgG	Percentage binding IgG	Titre (10%:log₂) IgG	Percentage PPTN IgG	Titre (20%:log₂)	Slope
xlallP	4	34	19	100	>24	5	—	—
lal	30	29	10	73	21	—	—	—
G7cP	16	>24	17	66	16	35	6	10
x3a8P	17	22	17	86	22	43	12	8
8a4P	15	17	14	41	18	5	—	—
3e7P	13	10	13	ND	ND	ND	—	—
F10FP	12	>12	15	59	18	84	12	12
G1BP	8	>12	11	54	14	19	4	5
H1BP	7	12	10	36	14	—	—	—
E1gP	6	11	12	26	8	68	6	27
K1dP	2	8	9	41	20	51	6	10
F1d	4	6	9	14	5	—	—	—
9a6P	6	3	11	50	17	34	7	5
C4eP	4	2	7	11	5	—	—	—
7e9	2	2	8	13	7	—	—	—
x1e4	2	3	7	68	>24	—	—	—
A4cP	1	2	12	6	5	—	—	—
x6a7P	12	—	10	26	9	—	—	—
x1a2P	5	—	16	82	20	35	<7	16
E7d	4	—	7	21	9	—	—	—
AleP	1	—	8	16	6	17	—	—
J10dP	—	7	11	74	11	—	—	—
J3dP	—	3	9	55	10	—	—	—
H10eP	—	2	8	13	5	—	—	—
3a11P	—	—	ND	5	<4	—	—	—

ND = Not done   PPTN = precipitation

Footnote to Tables 11.2, 11.3 and 11.4

In the haemagglutination and ELISA assays in Tables 11.2–11.4, the log₂ titres define the last dilution that gives a positive reaction. In the solid-phase RIA the binding to antigen is expressed as a percentage of that obtained with the highest binding antibody (= 100%). The titre is the last dilution that gives above 10% binding, a point substantially above background. In the liquid-phase RIA the titre is the last dilution that gives above 20% precipitation of antigen. The slope is calculated from the linear part of the dilution curve and expresses the drop in percentage antigen precipitation that results from
one serial dilution of the antibody.

F

Table 11.3 Characteristics of six monoclonal antibodies to human Ig kappa light chain

| Clone | Antigen-coated red cell agglutination titre (log₂) | | Indirect ELISA titre (log₂) | Solid-phase RIA | | | | Liquid-phase RIA (4% PEG) | |
| | | | | Percentage binding | | Titre (10%:log₂) | | Percentage PPTN | Slope |
	IgG	Kappa	Kappa	IgG	Kappa	IgG	Kappa	IgG	
KA1	–	26	14	18	71	12	17	–	–
6e1	>24	>24	14	40	76	21	15	–	9
29/103P	<12	11	12	33	100	16	17	46	9
le9P	Pro	9	7	42	33	14	11	47	5
7a8P	Pro	8	7	32	43	14	7	45	5
2A5P	ND	ND	8	21	45	10	15	ND	ND

Explanation: see Table 11.2
Pro = prozone; titre not determined
ND = Not done

Table 11.4 Characteristics of two monoclonal antibodies to human Ig lambda light chains

| Clone | Antigen-coated red cell agglutination titre (log₂) | | Indirect ELISA titre (log₂) | Solid phase RIA | | | | Liquid-phase RIA (4% PEG) | |
| | | | | Percentage binding | | Titre (10%:log₂) | | Percentage PPTN | Slope |
	IgG	Lambda	Lambda	IgG	Lambda	IgG	Lambda	IgG	
C4	20	15	14	30	100	20	22	19	3
G4aP	9	13	13	20	76	17	19	9	3

Explanation: see Table 11.2

antibody needs to be confirmed and the class of immunoglobulin investigated. Suitable assays for these characterizations are ELISA, radioimmunoassays and isoelectric focusing. The results of the quantitative assays, including direct haemagglutination, for 25 monoclonal antibodies to human IgG, six to kappa and two to lambda light chains are summarized in Tables 11.2–11.4 and illustrated (radioimmunoassay results) in Figures 11.4–11.8.

In Table 11.2 the antibodies to IgG are placed in rank order of passive haemagglutination titre to Fc(γ)-coated cells. The titres do not correlate in all cases with IgG-coated cells, probably because some antibodies are directed to determinants only expressed on intact molecules (x6a7P) or exposed on the Fc fragment (xlallP). A second point to note is the more obvious lack of correlation, with many antibodies, between agglutination titres and the direct antigen-binding capacity in ELISA or solid-phase RIA. Thus, for instance, xle4 binds antigen to 68% of maximum in RIA but has a titre of only 3 in agglutination. One explanation for these inconsistencies might lie in steric considerations of poor availability of the antigen determinant for bivalent antibody seeking to bind by both combining sites and so to produce agglutination. Similar inconsistencies between binding assay titres can be observed in the anti-kappa and anti-lambda antibodies (Tables 11.3 and 11.4).

The performance of the monoclonal antibodies in a liquid-phase RIA gives an interesting insight into relationships between specificity and solubility of immune complexes. It became clear in preliminary assays that no precipitation could be achieved by any antibody in the PEG concentration of 2%, which is adequate to promote maximal precipitation with polyclonal sheep antisera to human IgG Fc. However, an increase to 4% optimized the precipitating capacities of the monoclonal antibodies which range from 5% to 84% of labelled IgG (Table 11.2). This is also illustrated in Figure 11.4. At PEG concentrations above 4% the background precipitation of antigen increases to unacceptable levels with both monoclonal and sheep antibodies. It should be noted that approximately one-half of the antibodies to IgG Fc and at least two out of six anti-kappa antibodies do not precipitate antigen specifically to any degree at all at any PEG concentration (Tables 11.2 and 11.3). In comparing precipitation of IgG by anti-kappa and anti-lambda samples it must be pointed out that the two forms of light chain are unequally represented on immunoglobulins in man. Thus the 19% precipitation of IgG produced by C4 anti-lambda represents 50–60% precipitation of the lambda-bearing IgG molecules and this coincides with the relatively high binding and agglutination titres of this antibody (Table 11.4).

The question of why some monoclonal antibodies precipitate and others do not cannot be entirely resolved without further study. It is clear, however, from the properties so far identified that precipitating capacity has no connection with absolute binding or agglutination titres of the antibodies (Table 11.2). The precipitation curves of all the positive anti-IgG Fc monoclonals are shown in Figure 11.5 and some selected ones compared with

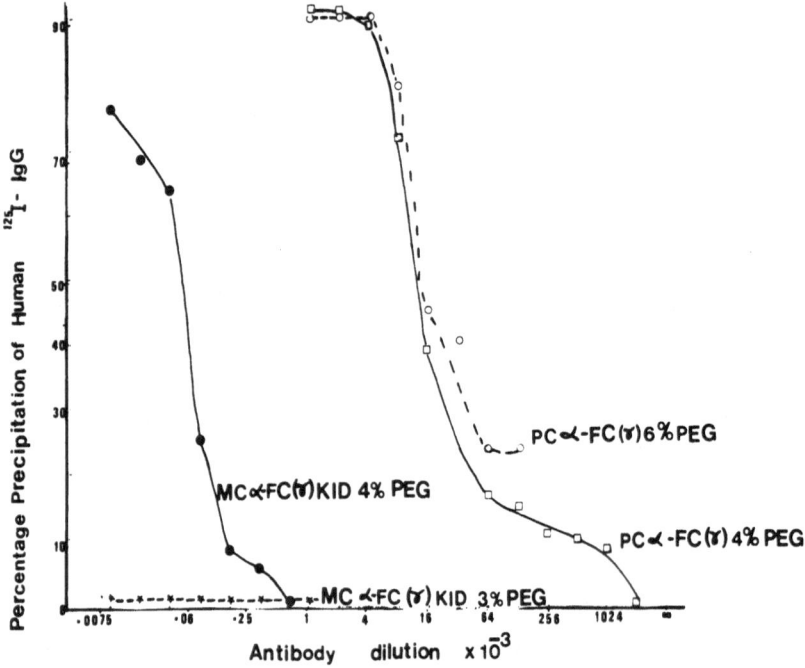

Figure 11.4   The effect of polyethylene glycol concentration on the precipitation of radiolabelled human IgG in liquid phase by monoclonal mouse antibodies and polyclonal sheep antiserum. RIA titrations of polyclonal (PC) sheep antiserum (ZDIIG) and monoclonal (MC) mouse antibody (KID) to Fc(γ) of human IgG at final concentrations of 6%, 4% and 3% PEG.

the polyclonal sheep antiserum in Figure 11.6. It is apparent that no monoclonal antibody has as adequate a precipitating capacity, nor as high a precipitating titre, as the sheep antiserum which works to advantage in this assay by virtue of multiple binding properties and high average affinity. It is notable, however, that the slope of the monoclonal antibody curve for EIgP (percentage loss in precipitation between two serial dilutions in the linear region) exceeds that for the polyclonal serum, and this is interpreted as indicating a greater affinity of this antibody than is average for the sheep antibodies. However there does not seem to be any obvious correlation between affinity and capacity to precipitate antigen as several monoclonal antibodies in this series demonstrate high affinity and poor precipitation. Precipitating activity is seen to be a very variable property in regard to the anti-kappa and anti-lambda light chain antibodies (Figures 11.7 and 11.8). There is also no obvious correlation between binding characteristics on solid-phase and precipitating properties. The dilution curves for the solid-phase RIA binding of all the IgG Fc-specific monoclonal antibodies is shown in

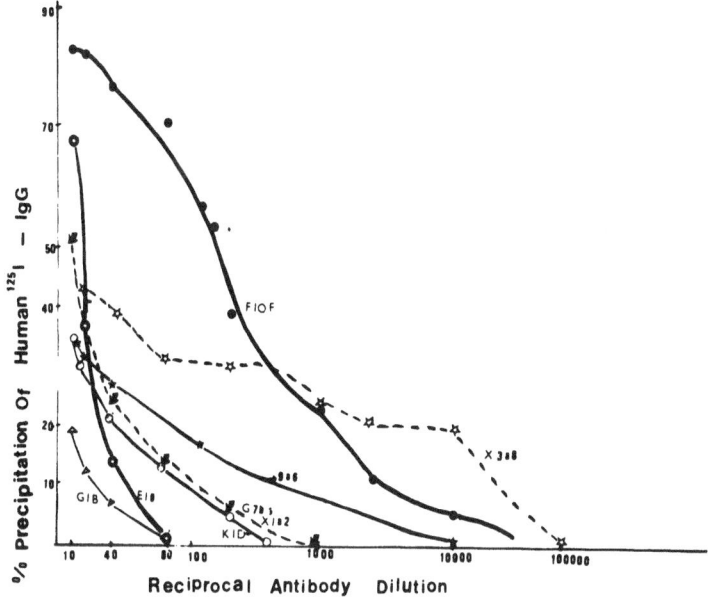

Figure 11.5 Liquid-phase radioimmunoassay dilution curves for precipitation of radiolabelled human IgG by monoclonal mouse antibodies. Note the very wide range of precipitating activities, affinities and titres of the samples

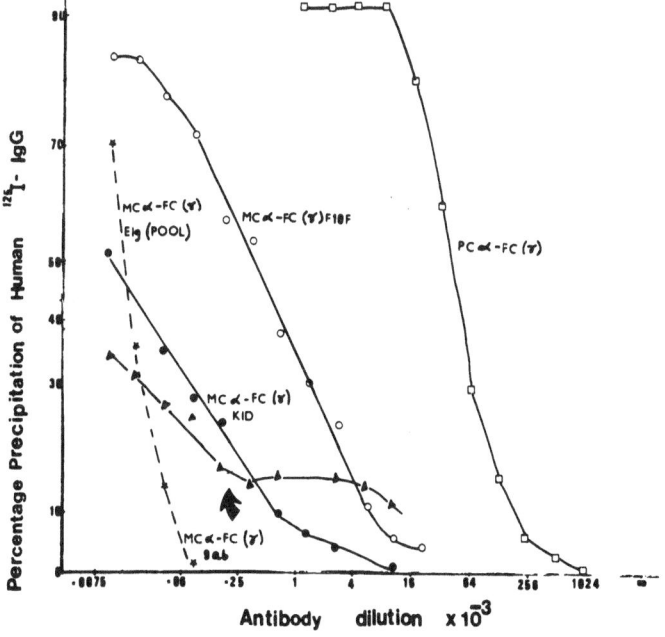

Figure 11.6 Liquid-phase radioimmunoassay dilution curves for precipitation of radiolabelled human IgG by a high titre, high average affinity, polyclonal sheep antiserum to human IgG Fc and by some selected monoclonal mouse antibodies with the highest precipitating activities so far produced. PC = polyclonal; MC = monoclonal

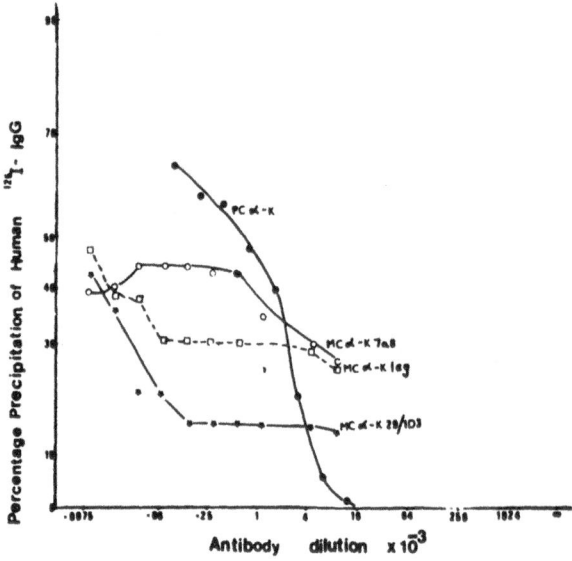

Figure 11.7 Liquid-phase radioimmunoassay dilution curves for precipitation of radiolabelled human IgG by a high average affinity polyclonal sheep antiserum to kappa light chain and by three precipitating monoclonal mouse antibodies with considerably lower affinity. Note that the sheep antibodies precipitate about 70% of the labelled antigen. This figure is close to the observed expression of kappa chain on human IgG. PC = polyclonal; MC = monoclonal

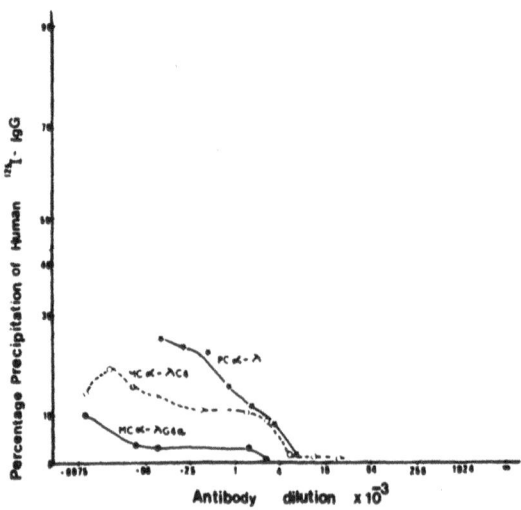

Figure 11.8 Liquid-phase radioimmunoassay dilution curves for precipitation of radiolabelled human IgG by a polyclonal sheep antiserum to lambda light chain and by two precipitating monoclonal mouse antibodies. Note that the sheep antibodies precipitate about 30% of the labelled antigen. This figure is close to the observed expression of lambda chain on human IgG. PC = polyclonal; MC = monoclonal

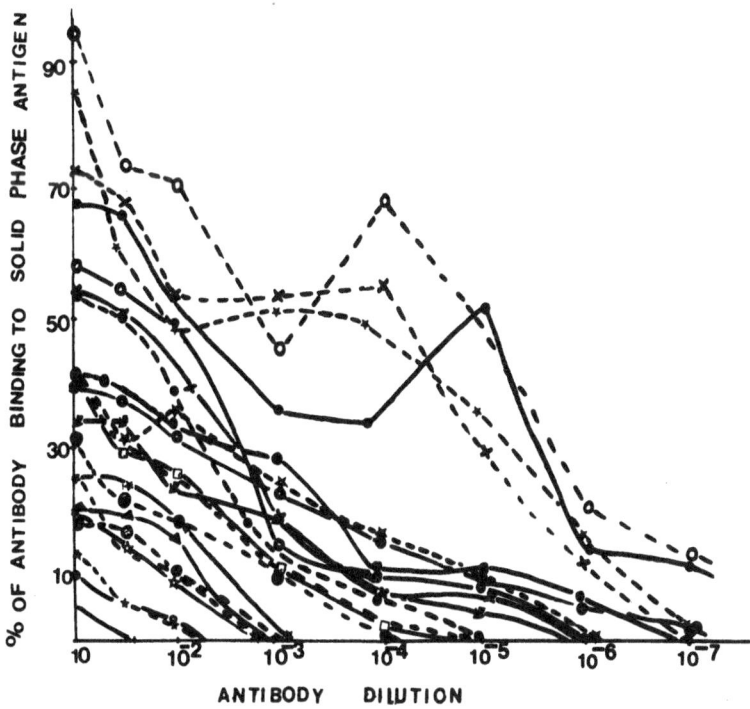

Figure 11.9   Solid-phase radioimmunoassay dilution curves for the binding of 25 monoclonal mouse antibodies to human IgG. Note the wide range of binding affinities and titres in this collection

Figure 11.9. The precipitating antibodies do not occupy a special high-binding, or high-affinity section of this profile and several non-precipitating antibodies have greater binding titres. The ability of a homogeneous antibody, specific to a single determinant of an antigen, to bring that antigen out of solution may depend more upon the availability of the antigen determinant than upon any intrinsic property of the antibody, other than a reasonable binding affinity – at least this would be the first and most obvious explanation to consider in future experiments.

For all the hybridoma-derived antibodies produced so far to human immunoglobulins we have confirmed the monoclonal nature of the cell products by isoelectric focusing and autoradiography. In Figure 11.10 the six anti-kappa and two anti-lambda antibodies, harvested in the ascitic fluids of mice growing the hybridomas as peritoneal tumours, have been focused and the plates then treated with radioiodinated human IgG. The autoradiograph (on the left) shows the antigen-binding single clone product (clonotype) of each sample that locates at an individual point (PI) on the ampholite pH gradient. On the right, for reference, is the same plate after protein-staining, which shows the complete pattern of focused proteins present in the ascitic

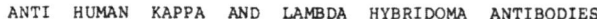

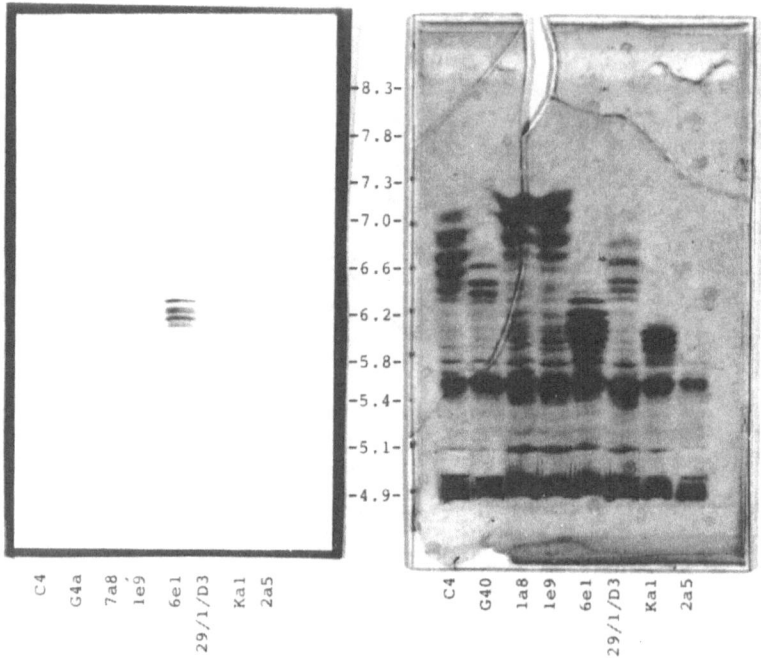

Figure 11.10 Isoelectric focusing with autoradiography of mouse monoclonal antibodies to human kappa and lambda light chains. The autoradiograph is shown on the left, the stained plate on the right. For conditions see text

fluid. It can be seen that each monoclonal antibody focuses into a cluster of bands which is assumed to represent minor charge differences that accumulate post-synthetically on the molecules. In view of the evenness of antigen binding across the bands of each clone it would seem unlikely that the banding could be due to charge differences caused by random linkage of NS1 light chain to the heavy chain carrying antibody specificity. This would give a range of labelling intensities across the bands as affinity would be variable within the molecules.

Acknowledgments

The work reported in this paper was supported by the Leukemia Research Fund and by United Africa Company International. We also thank Miss Debbie Hardie for expert technical assistance and Mrs F. O'Reilly for preparing the manuscript for publication.

References

1. Kohler, G. and Milstein, C. (1975). Continuous culture of fused cells secreting specific antibody. *Nature (London)*, **256**, 495

2. Kohler, G. and Milstein, C. (1976). Derivation of specific antibody-producing tissue culture and tumour lines by cell fusion. *Eur. J. Immunol.*, **6**, 511

3. Melchers, F., Potter, M. and Warner, N. L. (eds.). Lymphocyte hybridomas. *Current Topics in Microbiology and Immunology*, **81**, 1978

4. Truco, M. M., Stocker, J. W. and Ceppellini, R. (1978). Monoclonal antibodies against lymphocyte antigens. *Nature (London)*, **273**, 666

5. Goding, J.,W. Oi, V. T., Jones, P. P., Herzenberg, L. A.ıand Herzenberg, L. A.(1979). In Pernis, B. and Vogel, H. T. (eds.). *Cells of Immunoglobulin Synthesis*, pp. 309–334. (New York: Academic Press)

6. Gasse, D. L., Winters, B. A., Haas, J. B., McKearn, T. J. and Kennett, R. H. (1979). Monoclonal antibodies directed to a B cell antigen present in rats, mice and humans. *Proc. Natl. Acad. Sci.*, **76**, 4636

7. Kung, P. C., Goldstein, G., Reinherz, E. L. and Schlossman, S. F. (1979). Monoclonal antibodies defining distinctive human T cell surface antigens. *Science*, **206**, 347

8. Brodsky, F. M., Bodmer, W. F. and Parham, P. (1979). Characterisation of a monoclonal anti-β-2 microglobulin antibody and its use in the genetic and biochemical analysis of major histocompatibility antigens. *Eur. J. Immunol.*, **9**, 536

9. Parker, C. W. (1976). *Radioimmunoassay of Biologically Active Compounds*. Foundations in Immunology series. (New Jersey: Prentice Hall)

10. Bradwell, A. R., Burnett, D., Ramsden, D. B., Burr, W. A., Prince, H. P. and Hoffenberg, R. (1976). Preparation of a monospecific antiserum to thyroxine binding globulin for its quantitation by rocket immunoelectrophoresis. *Clin. Chim. Acta*, **71**, 501

11. Galfré, G., Howe, S. C., Milstein, C., Butcher, G. W. and Howard, J. C. (1977). Antibodies to major histicompatibility antigens produced by hybrid cell lines. *Nature (London)*, **206**, 550

12. Ling, N. R., Stephens, G., Bratt, P. and Dhaliwal, H. S. (1979). Attachment of antigens and antibodies to fixed red cells; their use in rosette and haemagglutination tests; a comparison with fresh red cells. *Molec. Immunol.*, **16**, 637

13. Engvall, E. and Perlmann, P. (1971). ELISA. Quantitative assay of immunoglobulin G. *Immunochemistry*, **8**, 871

14. Voller, A., Bidwell, D. E., Huldt, G. and Engvall, E. (1974). A microplate method of enzyme-linked immunosorbent assay and its application to malaria. *Bull. WHO*, **51**, 209

15. Greenwood, F. C., Hunter, W. M. and Glover, J. S. (1963). The preparation of ^{131}I-labelled human growth hormone. *Biochem. J.*, **89**, 114

16. Herzenberg, L. A. and Herzenberg, L. A. (1973). Mouse immunoglobulin allotypes: description and special methodology. In Weir, D. M. (ed.) *Handbook of Experimental Immunology*, Chap. 13. (Oxford: Blackwell Scientific Publications)

17. Catty, D. and King, T. D. (1974). The effect of polyethylene glycol (PEG) on precipitation of mouse and rabbit immunoglobulin allotypes in microradioimmunoassays. *Immunochemistry*, **11**, 615

18. Awdeh, Z. L., Williamson, A. R. and Askonas, B. A. (1968). Isoelectric focussing in polyacrylamide gel and its application to immunoglobulins. *Nature (London)*, **219**, 66

12
External Quality Assessment Schemes for Immunoassays

W. M. HUNTER, I. McKENZIE AND R. R. A. BACON

INTRODUCTION

Radioimmunoassays (RIAs) are complex and expensive procedures, yet when properly performed they yield information which has much greater clinical value than most of the simpler analyses in clinical chemistry. Thus, assays of T_3, T_4 and TSH together provide a very precise measure of the status of the pituitary–thyroid axis; in so doing, they replace much more expensive *in vivo* procedures. Serum growth hormone measurements are central in recognizing HGH-deficient dwarfism; they provide the best index of the severity of acromegaly, and their availability has permitted the introduction of medical treatment whose efficacy could not have been discovered (let alone monitored in individual patients) without the assay. In the management of patients with secondary amenorrhoea the FSH assay recognizes ovarian failure, e.g. due to early menopause. The second step is the recognition of hyperprolactinaemia for which specific treatment is available, and for the remaining patients basal LH and FSH values then help in the selection of the appropriate means of inducing ovulation.

This chapter describes schemes which are designed to assess the extent to which these new analyses are delivering the necessary information throughout the country. The schemes are also designed to seek remedial action by giving advice on assay design and management.

EXTERNAL QUALITY ASSESSMENT

International agreement on the term 'quality assessment' (EQAS) for what used to be called 'external quality control' is now likely. The new term brings out the distinction between their purpose and that of internal quality *control* which differs in (a) being used on every batch of analyses and (b) producing results which are immediately available to assist in deciding whether the individual batch of analyses is or is not acceptable. There is a further distinction which, as we shall see, has special importance for immunoassays and it is this: internal QC inevitably is designed to monitor the reproducibility of an assay system and it tends not to question the fundamental design of the assay. It is analogous to industrial QC in which the question being asked is 'do these replicates of our manufactured product meet the design specification?'. EQAS has an extra dimension: it can question the local assayist's specification against the broader consensus view of what should and can be specified.

This chapter will concentrate on the area of assay design assessment. In so doing it will reveal the one inadequacy of the term 'quality assessment' – at least as a description of our own activities; assessment sounds passive, whereas our schemes seek improvement in performance through an intensive dialogue with participants.

The evolution of our approach as applied to assays for growth hormone has been fully described[1, 2] and a generalized strategy based upon that experience has also been set out[3]. This chapter will touch upon three things:

(1) the evidence which suitable EQAS can produce on the adequacy of assay design;
(2) the precise nature of, and the mechanisms giving rise to, the technical deficiencies so revealed;
(3) some general technical directions which may be taken in seeking improvement.

The first two will be considered together and the deficiencies can be grouped by their symptoms.

BIAS: IMPORTANCE AND IDENTIFICATION

Perhaps the main formal demonstration which we owe to EQAS of RIAs is that, unlike the situation obtaining in mainstream clinical chemistry where imprecision is the principal problem[4], immunoassays frequently display unacceptable bias associated with acceptable precision. The mere use of the term 'bias' implies that there is a 'correct' value. For some substances these are provided by virtue of reference procedures for which the main current examples in RIA are the gas chromatography mass spectroscopy (GCMS) measurements used notably by the Tenovus group to provide target values for steroid assays[5-7] in their EQAS for oestradiol[8]. Hopefully such provision will spread throughout the range of hapten assays, but we shall have to remember that even well-defined physical methods may be prone to bias, and their precision too must be tested and displayed.

For 'biological' analytes, i.e. those whose structure is not fully defined – and notably for proteins – we cannot provide a 'correct' value. We can, however, provide a most useful 'target' value which may be either the overall mean value or the mean value from a reference group of laboratories (after suitable trimming – see, for example Healy[9] – in either case). We cannot demonstrate conclusively that such target values are unbiased. All we can do is to accumulate evidence for the absence of bias from each of several causes.

THE CAUSES OF BIAS

Problems related to standards

It is almost impossible to exaggerate the immense importance of suitable standards or the value of the activities of our colleagues in providing primary standards at National Institute for Biological Standards and Control (NIBSC). To quote but a single example, their prescience and professionalism have combined to ensure that human serum TSH measurements throughout the world have, almost from the outset, been expressed in terms of an agreed unitage based upon a common standard[10, 11].

EQAS have, thus far, revealed two kinds of problems relating to standards. First come the 'miscalibration' group, i.e. the incorrect dilution of the correct standard, the use of an incorrect activity for the correct standard, and the incorrect calibration of a secondary or in-house standard from the primary standard. These can be either 'coarse', e.g. one participant in the HGH scheme had miscalibrated by a factor of 2, or 'fine' – another required correction $\times$ 1.25[1]. The importance of encouraging kit manufacturers to calibrate in terms of the agreed International Standard or Reference Preparation requires emphasis. The manufacturer is better equipped to do this than is the kit user since he should know the appropriate diluent for cross-calibrating standards. Second are problems relating to the stability of stored solutions of standards. Our experience with HGH will illustrate this. An ampoule of the International Reference Preparation (IRP) contains sufficient material for some 10 000 assays, and our participants habitually distribute (some of) this material through stock and working dilutions, the former (at least) being stored, generally at $-20\,°C$, for many months. When they were asked to provide evidence for stability during such storage – not too difficult to do really, since native caution should surely have led some to assay stored solutions against standards from a fresh ampoule – very little was forthcoming. Not one participant provided confidence limits for such a comparison! We came to focus on this question following the discovery that the overall results on recovery pools made by adding the IRP to HGH-free material came out in the range 115–120%. [We had achieved good baseline performance by this time (see below) so bias was not due to lack of assay specificity.] Attempts to check local standards by distributing solutions of IRP in assay diluent came to grief because the latter lost activity during distribution. We therefore prepared some 2000 ampoules of freeze-dried 'working standards' from one ampoule of the IRP – but we distributed these unlabelled, merely asking participants to assay their contents. The mean value showed a bias of $+11\%$, which was close to that of recovery pools, suggesting strongly that the bias (in estimations on recovery pools) was due to losses in activity in locally stored standards. We recommended that all participants use the freeze-dried working standards, and Table 12.1 shows the success which followed. Our second UK working standard, again from a single ampoule of IRP, yielded 10 000 ampoules each containing 32 μU and suitable for a single assay. We have had to research the handling of this material – notably the carried used, but accelerated

Table 12.1 HGH external QAS: effect of provision of working standards on recovery

6 months ending	Pools	Distributions	Reference group	All laboratories
30 April 1977	1	3	126	132
25 July 1977	1	5	122	117
28 November 1977	2	3 and 4	121	118
June 1978 Working Standards distributed				
26 November 1978	1	1	97.3	110
30 June 1979	1	3	98.6	96.4
31 August 1979	2	3	99.8	100.0
20 November 1979	2	3	102.0	105.1

The pools consisted of HGH-free human serum to which HGH from a freshly opened ampoule of IRP (NIBSC preparation 66/217) was added.

degradation tests indicate that the stability of this second batch is good. It seems likely that the provision of working standards may improve the accuracy of other assays. The total expenditure of effort involved in such central provision is probably rather less than the sum of the local efforts otherwise required. However, a transfer of resources is implicit in central provision, and it will be necessary (a) to continue to provide evidence of improved accuracy, and (b) to convince the relevant authorities (the DHSS in the UK) of their importance. The National Institute for Biological Standards and Control would be the obvious institute to undertake this task for the UK or perhaps for the EEC. WHO should be encouraged to consider the logistics of providing working standards on an international basis – perhaps by defining and designating suitably sized regions.

Bias related to separation system

Differences between the protein content of standards and unknowns can give rise to systematic bias which may be either constant throughout the range, i.e. standards and unknowns are parallel; or may be range-related (standards not parallel to unknowns). The best example we have is an acutely embarrassing one since it occurred with a 'recommended procedure' which was designed by us. We chose the option of a double-antibody separation system which was intended to be indifferent to the variations in human serum content over the range 0–25%, standards and other reagents being made up in a diluent containing 2% horse serum. This worked well in our own laboratory, and in our hands was unbiased on recovery pools. Several participants using the procedure turned in results which revealed serious negative bias – but with good precision, i.e. the cumulative relationship to the reference group mean for 3 such laboratories was -25 ± 19 (SD)%, -19 ± 9 and -17 ± 9 based upon 25–30 determinations. Their bias for recovery and 'regular' pools at the same level of concentration was of similar magnitude[3]. At the present time the evidence suggests that the 2% horse serum which is present in the assay diluent must be just on the brink of a plateau for the precipitation of the double-antibody system. Its replacement by 5% bovine serum may bring the system into proper reproducibility, and this is being tested. Clearly we had not adequately checked our procedure for ruggedness.

Bias due to inappropriate 'scaling' and the assumption of over-wide working ranges

This is perhaps the most common cause of bias. It is most frequently encountered in assays which are operated down to their detection limits, i.e. assays for substances which (a) are secreted intermittently and for which many sera are analyte-free, or rather have analyte levels below an agreed threshold, e.g. HGH has such a threshold at 1 mIU/l, or (b) are readily measurable in certain patients, e.g. TSH in hypothyroids, FSH and LH in normal adults, but are below the detection limit of present assays in others, e.g. TSH in thyrotoxics, FSH and LH in some patients with secondary amenorrhoea and LH in prepubertal children. We have addressed this question of 'baseline performance' in the schemes run from Edinburgh for HGH, LH, FSH and prolactin and Figure 12.1 illustrates the problem encountered for these hormones as well as for TSH (by courtesy of Mr D. W. Schardt of the University Department of Medicine, Newcastle). In this figure the samples distributed had very low analyte concentrations which, on the basis of the evidence from assays with low detection limits, was somewhere within (or below) the shaded areas. Values above these were of two kinds:

(1) The participants reported < (say) 2 mIU/l (for HGH), < (say) 3.3 IU/l (for LH) or < (say) 2 mU/l (for TSH), in which cases he is correct and (on this

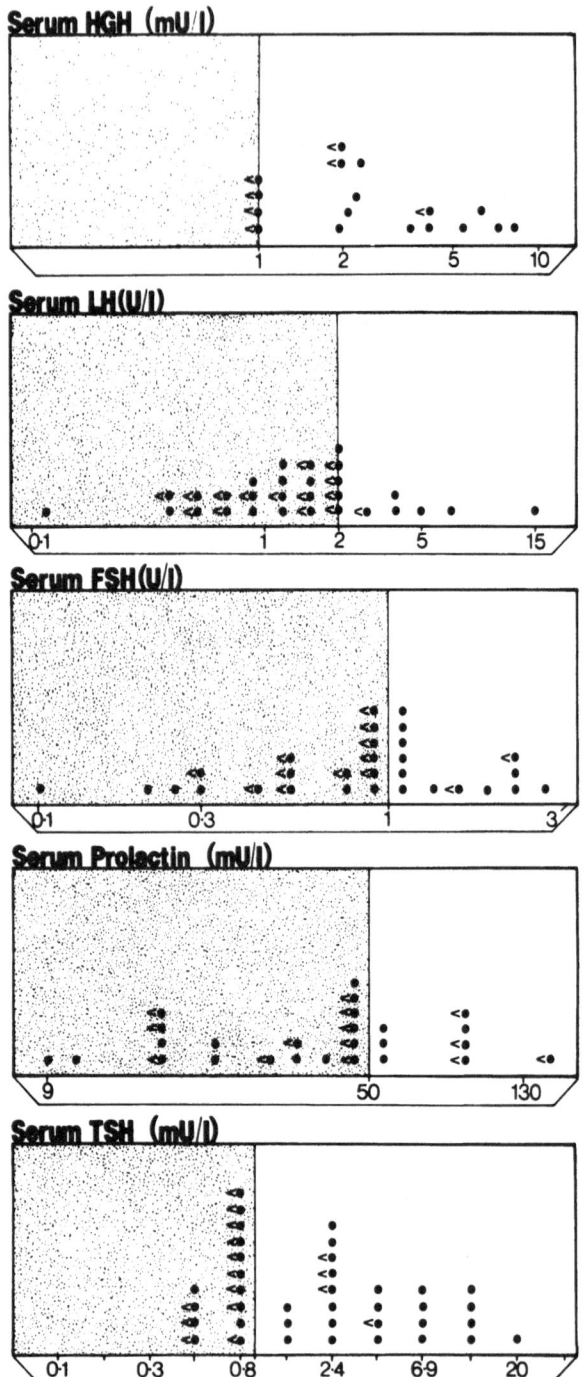

Figure 12.1　Hormone levels reported for samples which are analyte-free (or have very low concentrations of analyte). On the available evidence the correct values are within or below the shaded areas in each case

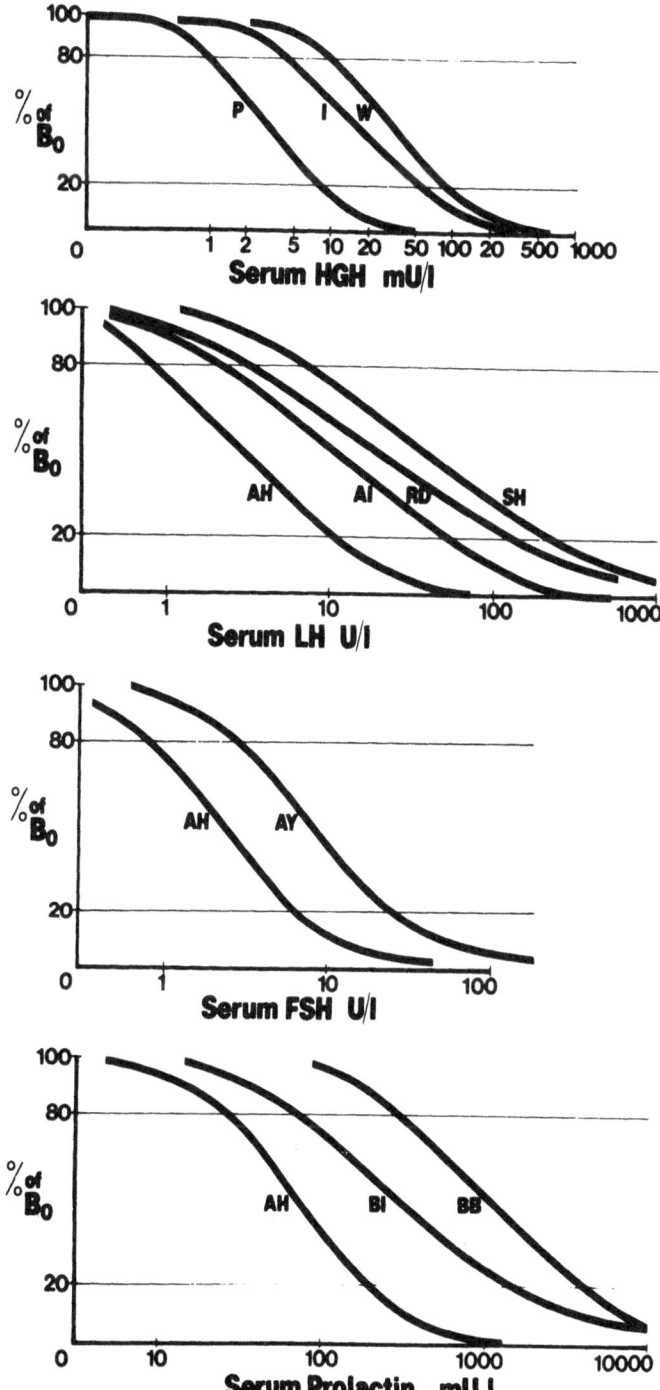

Figure 12.2 Variation in the 'scaling' of different participants' assays. The curves have been plotted from the returned method questionnaires which give the serum analyte concentrations required to give 20% and 80% inhibition of tracer binding. Serum is assumed to be present at the *lowest* dilution normally employed. The letters are participants' laboratory codes

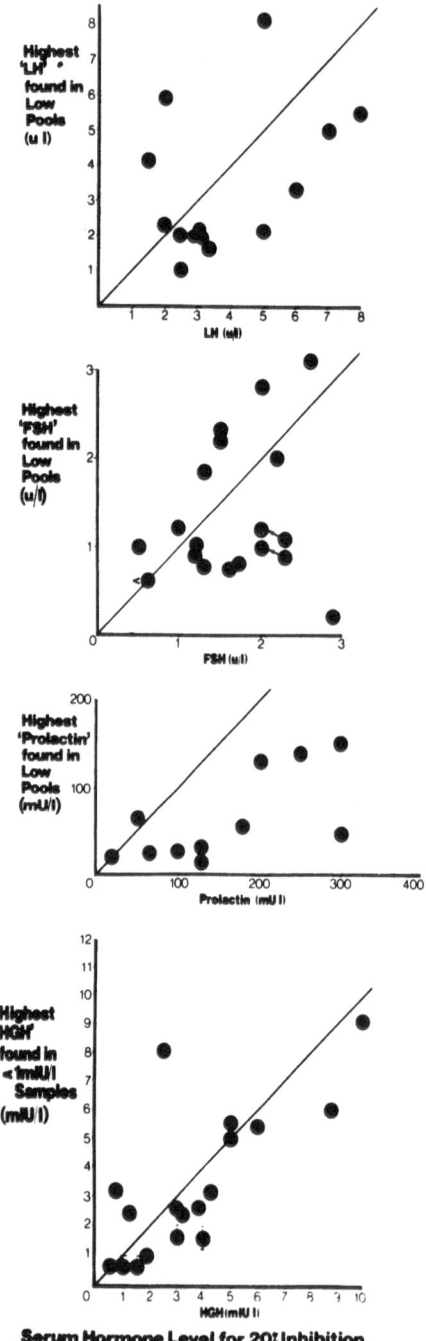

Figure 12.3   Relationship between 'false highs' in estimations carried out on analyte-free (or very low level) samples (Figure 12.1) and the 'scaling' of the assays (Figure 12.2)

evidence at least) he may have a realistic idea of his detection limit. One might suggest to him that a lower limit of detection might be desirable, but whether he accepts this will depend upon his aims and his capabilities.

(2) Other participants actually report *numerical values*, e.g. values in the region of 5–10 mIU/l for HGH where the correct value is < 1 mIU/l, up to 20 mIU/l for TSH where it should be < 1 mIU/l, up to 6 IU/l for LH and up to 2.5 IU/l for FSH where in reality the levels are < 2 and < 1 respectively.

This carries two implications: (a) there is very marked positive bias, and (b) since the participant has accepted and reported a value, he thinks his assay is operative on material for which in reality it is not. He therefore sees no reason for improving his sensitivity. For HGH we discovered (through the returns on detailed method questionnaires whose completion is a prerequisite for participation in our EQAS) that there was a marked difference in the 'scaling', i.e. in the target ranges over which different assays operated. Figure 12.2 shows this, and also that the same is true for the other hormones. For HGH we were able to demonstrate that the magnitude of false-positive determinations on analyte-free (or low-analyte) pools was correlated with the scaling of participants' standard curves, i.e. the further to the right the standard curve (Figure 12.2), the higher the false highs tended to be. This is illustrated in Figure 12.3.

The underlying mechanism is illustrated in Figure 12.4. The detection limit is determined on the basis of replicates in assay diluent. (There is a tendency to

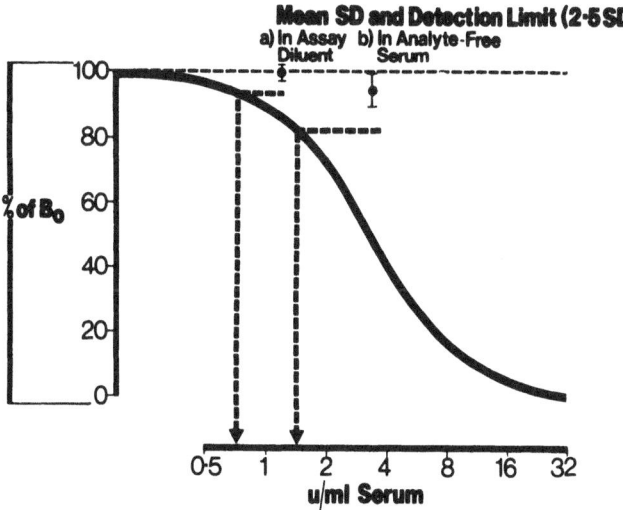

Figure 12.4 Difference in the detection limit of an assay when applied (a) to analyte in assay diluent when it is simply at (say) 2.5 SD, and (b) in serum when it becomes the mean displacement + 2.5 SD of the responses of (many) different analyte-free serum samples.

do this under optimum conditions – notably by putting the replicates close together rather than distributing them at random in large routine assays – but this is an aside!) However, if a collection of many different analyte-free samples is assayed the responses will generally display two extra effects: firstly the mean will generally not be the same as the diluent mean (typically it will have lower binding) and secondly the scatter of these replicates (in *different* analyte-free samples) will generally exceed the scatter of replicates in diluent. Clearly this has a major effect on our estimate of the lower limit of detection. Figure 12.4 provides an illustration which – on the basis both of our own experience as analysts, and strongly reinforced by our findings from EQAS – suggests that such differences between diluents and samples are frequently encountered. Nevertheless it may be possible to devise assays which do not so suffer – but the onus of proof rests on the analyst who should rigorously define the lower limit of his working range. For some substances the provision of even small (let alone substantial) numbers of analyte-free samples is difficult. In spite of this, however, our evidence argues strongly that more effort should be made in this direction. Sources of such material include:

(1) selection of subjects, e.g. prepubertal children for low LH, thyrotoxics for very low TSH;
(2) physiological manipulation, e.g. 2 h post-glucose (ideally in subjects tending to overweight for extra assurance) for very low HGH, T_3-suppression of normal TSH secretion for very low TSH, prolonged fasting (ideally of lean subjects) for low insulin;
(3) exploitation of species-specificity, e.g. non-primate growth hormones do not cross-react with HGH; and
(4) (less satisfactory) physical or chemical removal of analyte, e.g. by charcoal adsorption or immunosorption.

The second problem of range-related bias is the practice of accepting responses which are too near the lower asymptote (i.e at low percentage bound, high analyte levels). Figure 12.5 illustrates this: the Supraregional Assay Service (SAS) laboratories here show poor *between-laboratory* agreement on high level HGH pools. Yet when we examined *within-laboratory* reproducibility on these analyses they were no worse than at lower levels. Thus, bias rather than precision was the problem. Figure 12.6 illustrates one probable mechanism – it shows that in some assays (here LH) parallelism of unknowns with standards tends to break down as the lower asymptote is approached. Thus, bias, rather than precision may dictate our choice of a suitable upper cut-off.

RIAs have very limited working ranges, 10–30-fold being usual. Our evidence indicates that the assumption and use of unrealistically wide working ranges is common. Setting the requisite limits requires investigation of bias in addition to an assessment of precision. Many protein hormones have very wide pathophysiological ranges and these can be covered accurately only by operating the assay on several different dilutions of sample (see Figure 12.7).

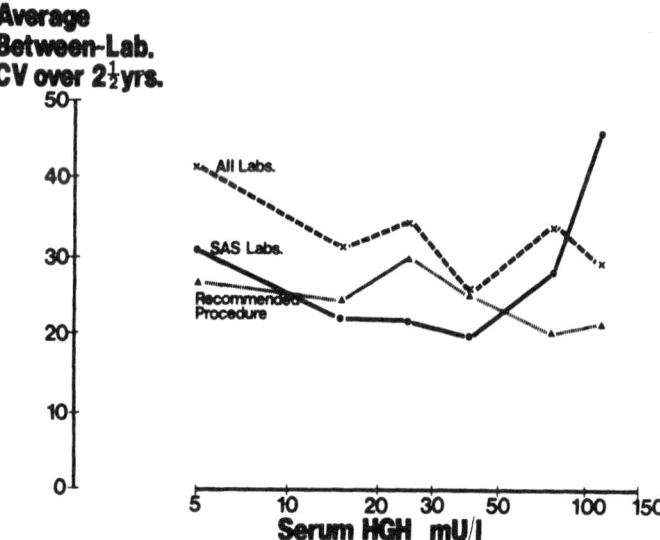

Figure 12.5 Variation in between-laboratory CV at different HGH concentrations. The results in the ranges 3–9.9, 10–19.9, 20–29.9, 30–49.9, 50–99.9 and > 100 mIU/l have been accumulated and their means plotted at the mid-points of their ranges.

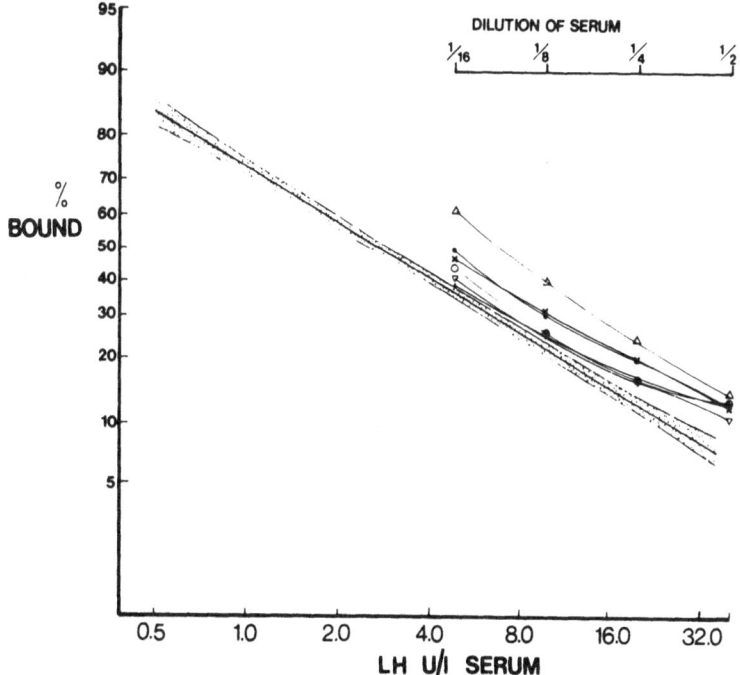

Figure 12.6 Deviation from parallelism in the response curves of serum from that of standards. The serum and standard curves are parallel in the middle of the response range but they deviate at high hormone (low binding) levels. If, as here, the deviations in different sera are reproducible and all in the same direction; the problem is one of *bias* and not *imprecision*. The effect here was due to higher and more variable NSB values in sera than in diluent. The stippled area represents the envelope encompassing ± 1 SD from the computed standard curve

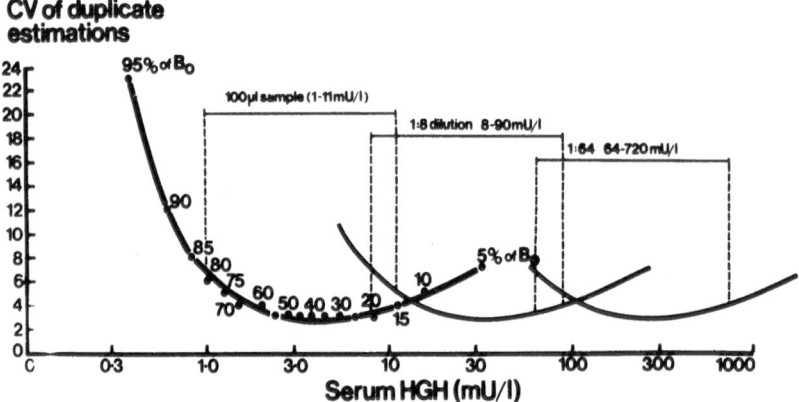

Figure 12.7 Precision profile and use of multiple dilutions which are necessary to cover the pathophysiological range of serum HGH concentrations. The figures alongside the left-hand curve (95% of B_0, 90, 80, ... 10, 5% of B_0) indicate percentage of tracer bound taking binding of tracer to antibody in the absence of added standard as 100%. Note that the CV at 80% of B_0 is twice that at 40% B, while at 90% it is four times the 40% B value. However, bias as well as precision must be considered in deciding the acceptability of estimations as the upper and lower asymptotes are approached

SUMMARY OF EQAS FINDINGS

We have described above some of the main imperfections in the use of RIAs. There are others which are peculiar to this specialty, e.g. problems of preparing and maintaining supplies of high-quality tracers and antisera, and distortions due to the use of oversimplified curve-fitting models for data processing. Still other problems are shared with other forms of analysis, e.g. the unrecognized occurrence of within-assay drift (which we suspect is not uncommon in RIA practice), and the perpetration of errors through switching samples and through clerical mistakes. Two points other than those detailed above deserve special mention.

(1) One of the main differences between the good and the bad radioim-munoassayist is that the former keeps his between-batch CV down to about 1.5 × within-batch CV, while the latter allows a 3–4-fold difference.
(2) Internal QC procedures must all too often either (a) be inadequate to assess performance or (b) yield the necessary evidence which is then ignored!

Before indulging in some well-informed speculation, we would like to suggest that the ability to deliver assays of adequate quality for widespread service be taken into account when choosing between different options. Thus follicular function, e.g. in secondary amenorrhoea, can be very accurately assessed if a good assay for serum oestradiol is available. However, these assays are difficult and on present evidence from the UK-EQAS an adequate nationwide service is not going to be available for some time unless new and more rugged methods are developed. Urinary oestrogen levels are no better. Indeed the DHSS Working Party set up to assess performance were so shocked that they very seriously considered recommending that these measurements be abandoned! Serum LH and FSH assays can yield some of the required information provided they are designed to measure levels *below*, as well as at and above, those found in normal adults. The assays used in the assessment of the pituitary – thyroid axis provide another example of the differences between the capabilities and the actual delivery of the assay service. The EQAS has revealed the sad truth that for TSH few of the widely used commercial kits and only about half of the SAS laboratories can actually provide the accuracy and precision which is required to cover the established clinical uses as set out in the SAS booklet.

TECHNICAL ADVANCES IN THE IMMEDIATE FUTURE

As a hedge against failure to obtain the necessary improvements in performance through gentle education and persuasion, we may expect the following technical advances to bring major advantages.

(1) With only three specialized reagents, viz. donkey antisera to each rabbit, sheep and guinea-pig IgG, which have been linked to Sepharose 4B, we can carry out the separation stage on any RIA using 30 min incubation and then a 'hands on' step which comfortably handles up to 1000 tubes per hour by means of the sucrose layering procedure[12]. This method has very high precision and is indifferent to variations in serum content over the range 2–50%. The equipment is very much less expensive than large refrigerated centrifuges. The magnetic particle separation system described by Professor Landon's group is a possible alternative.

(2) Computerized data processing is increasing, and although we may pass through a period in which the equipment is not powerful enough and/or the programs not sophisticated enough to handle the data without distortion, computers will rapidly get cheaper and will be able to handle more carefully designed programs such as that described by Raab and McKenzie[13]. This program is modular and it: (a) rejects results where replication is inadequate, (b) checks for drift, (c) examines the relationship between variance of the response metameter with dose, (d) offers alternative curve fitting models including asymmetric variants of the 4-parameter log. logistic and provides data on which model gives the best 'fit', (e) can fit standard curves for RIA and IRMA with or without inclusion of O standards and non-specific estimations, (f) sets out precision profiles from standards and from unknowns, (g) calculates detection limits at stated levels of confidence, (h) indicates the contribution made by counting error to the total error, (i) interpolates the

results for unknowns and includes checks for parallelism wherever more than one dilution is employed, and (j) produces summary statistics on precision and parallelism.

The program will shortly become widely available through the provision of a Department of Health and Social Security/Scottish Home and Health Department grant to further its implementation within the National Health Service.

(3) Finally, we have reason to believe that for proteins, immunoradiometric assays will steadily replace conventional RIA since they appear to offer lower detection limits for any given incubation time, much wider working ranges and they suffer relatively little from non-specific serum effects.

References

1. Hunter, W. M. and McKenzie, I. (1979). Quality control of radioimmunoassays for proteins: the first two and a half years of a national scheme for serum growth hormone measurements. *Ann. Clin. Biochem.*, **16**, 131

2. Hunter, W. M. and McKenzie, I. (1979). A national quality control scheme for serum HGH assays. In Bizollon, Ch. A. (ed.) *Radioimmunology 1979*, pp. 269–80. (Amsterdam: Elsevier/North Holland Biomedical Press)

3. Hunter, W. M., Bacon, R. R. A. and McKenzie, I. G. M. (1980). National quality control scheme for human growth hormone assays: a model for protein hormones. In Gaskell, S. J., Pike, A. W. and Finlay, E. M. H. (eds.) *Quality Control in Clinical Endocrinology*. VIII Tenovus Workshop. (Cardiff: Alpha Omega Publishing) (In press)

4. Whitehead, T. P. (1977). *Quality Control in Clinical Chemistry*, p. 115. (New York: Wiley)

5. Gaskell, S. J., Pike, A. W. and Finlay, E. M. H. (1980). New techniques in gas chromatography–mass spectrometry and their use in the validation of routine steroid assays. In Gaskell, S. J., Pike, A. W. and Finlay, E. M. H. (eds.) *Quality Control in Clinical Endocrinology*. VIII Tenovus Workshop. (Cardiff: Alpha Omega Publishing) (In press)

6. Riad-Fahmy, D., Read, G. F., Gaskell, S. J., Dyas, J. and Hindawi, R. (1980). A simple, direct radioimmunoassay for plasma cortisol featuring a ^{125}I-radioligand and a solid-phase separation technique. *Clin. Chem.*, **25**, 665

7. Hindawi, R. K., Gaskell, S. J., Read, G. F. and Riad-Fahmy, D. (1980). A simple, direct solid-phase enzyme-immunoassay for cortisol in plasma. *Ann. Clin. Biochem.* (In press)

8. Groom, G. V. (1980). A national quality control scheme for plasma, oestradiol-17β and progesterone in the United Kingdom. In Gaskell, S. J., Pike, A. W. and Finlay, E. M. H. (eds.) *Quality Control in Clinical Endocrinology*. VIII Tenovus Workshop. (Cardiff: Alpha Omega Publishing) (In press)

9. Healy, M. J. R. (1979). Outliers in clinical chemistry quality-control schemes. *Clin. Chem.*, **25**, 675

10. Bangham, D. R. and Cotes, P. M. (1971). Reference standards for radioimmunoassays. In Kirkham, K. E. and Hunter, W. M. (eds.) *Radioimmunoassay Methods*, p. 345. (Edinburgh and London: Churchill Livingstone)

11. World Health Organization (1975). Tech. Rep. Ser. No. 565, Geneva.

12. Hunter, W. M. (1978). A new automatable radioimmunoassay separation S stem. In Griffiths, K., Neville, A. M. and Pierrepoint, C. G. (eds.) *Tumour Markers: Determination and Clinical Role*. VI Tenovus Workshop, pp. 240–6. (Cardiff: Alpha Omega Publishing)

13. Raab, G. M. and McKenzie, I. G. M. (1980). A modular computer program for processing immunoassay data, or how to help a computer to handle assays intelligently. In Gaskell, S. J., Pike, A. W. and Finlay, E. M. H. (eds.) *Quality Control in Clinical Endocrinology*. VIII Tenovus Workshop. (Cardiff: Alpha Omega Publishing) (In press)

13
The Control of Performance in Immunoassays

J. S. WOODHEAD, HEATHER A. KEMP, A. B. J. NIX,
R. J. ROWLANDS, K. W. KEMP, D. W. WILSON AND
K. GRIFFITHS

INTRODUCTION

Immunological assays are inherently imprecise when compared with many of the chemical and physical techniques used in clinical biochemistry. Even when optimized, they are subject to errors arising from the instability of reagents and the involvement of complex manipulations as, for example, in assay separation. Nevertheless, the increasing involvement of immunoassays in the diagnosis of disease and the monitoring of patient treatment emphasizes the need for the adoption of control procedures, such that assay performance is maximized and then maintained within acceptable limits.

In order to assess performance of an assay it is, of course, necessary to understand the major sources of error in immunoassay systems. Errors may be random as in the case of pipetting errors. Alternatively they may be systematic. Within-batch drift can be produced by factors affecting the equilibrium of the reaction (e.g. temperature change) whereas between-batch variability may result from changes of methodology or reagents. Random errors result in poor precision while the systematic errors lead to the production of biased results. It is therefore necessary to monitor several aspects of assay performance if accurate results are to be produced consistently. During recent years a number of Department of Health and Social Security (DHSS) sponsored schemes have been developed to assess laboratory performance at a national level. The objectives of such schemes are not clearly defined. However, by distributing samples to laboratories for assay at regular intervals, the organizer seeks to gain information which will enable him to identify poor performance, and also monitor changes in performance with time. Such information should thus be of value to the laboratories concerned, as well as indicating where there exists a need for advice or further action from an objective assessor. In this chapter we draw attention to the relative insensitivity of schemes in operation at present and describe how simple procedures can be used within a laboratory to monitor several aspects of assay performance.

ASSESSMENT OF PERFORMANCE BY EXTERNAL MONITORING

A fundamental difficulty facing the organizer of an external monitoring scheme is that he is forced to base his assessment on extremely limited data. In practice, up to five samples of serum pools are distributed at monthly intervals in such a way that approximately six pools will be measured on average four times by each laboratory. Individual performance is assessed by obtaining a coefficient of variation (CV) for each pool (the standard deviation of the observations divided by the mean value). The limitation of this procedure is illustrated in Figure 13.1a, which plots the distribution of values for CV which would be obtained for a laboratory with a true CV of 10%, when that estimate is based on only four observations. Not only is the distribution wide, 95% of the estimates ranging from 2 to 18%, it is also skewed indicating a tendency to underestimate. As illustrated in the lower portion of Figure 13.1, the situation is noticeably improved by increasing the number of observations to 10. It is unfortunate, however, that for some assays CV is frequently greater than 10%. Figure 13.2a shows the distribution of CV estimates again based on four observations for a laboratory with a true CV of 15%. The distribution is wide, 95% of the observed values falling between 4 and 27%, and once again it is skewed. As before the situation is improved by increasing the number of observations to 10, though here the estimate still ranges from 8 to 22%.

The statistical confidence limits on a CV derived from 4 or 10 observations are illustrated in Figure 13.3. Based on only four observations, the 95% confidence limits on an estimated CV of 10% are 4–36%. Based on 10 observations these limits are 6–18%.

In an attempt to derive an index of overall performance of a laboratory, it has been common practice to combine the data obtained from all pools estimated during a 6-month period, thus yielding a 'running CV'. Since the pools assayed during that period cover a wide range of analyte concentrations, this approach is only valid if the error of the analyte estimation is proportional to the dose of analyte present. Calculation of precision profiles[1,2] indicates that this is not so, relative error being greater at the extremes of the dose range and in some cases constant only over a limited portion of the dose–response curve.

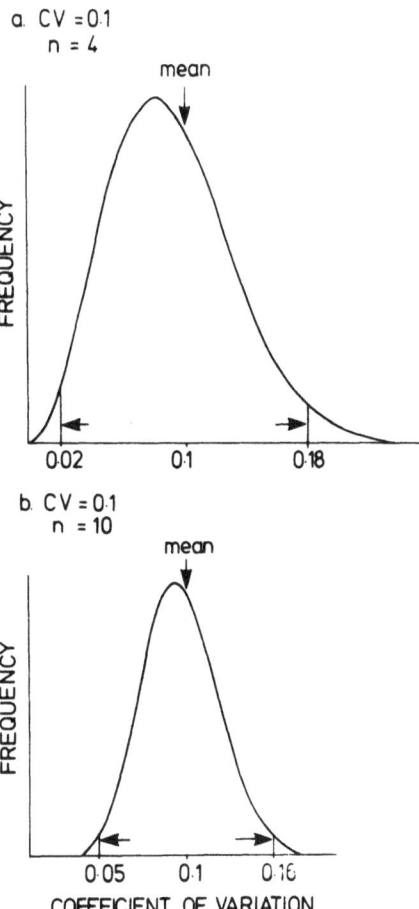

Figure 13.1 Sampling distribution of CV based on 4 or 10 observations for a laboratory with a true CV of 10%. Arrows indicate 2.5 and 97.5 percentiles

It is interesting to note that, in a situation where CV is dose-dependent, the distribution of the running CV based on a limited number of observations can be similar to that observed when the true CV is constant. Figure 13.4 shows the effect of combining data from three pools where the CV differs on the distribution of calculated CV.

An alternative approach to external assessment of certain steroid immunoassays has been the use of a variance index (VI), as developed by Whitehead[3] for application to monitoring in clinical chemistry laboratories. The principle of the method is to relate each observation to the method mean as given by the formula

$$\frac{x - \bar{x}_m}{\bar{x}_m} \times 100$$

where x is the observed value, and $\bar{x}_m$ the method mean.

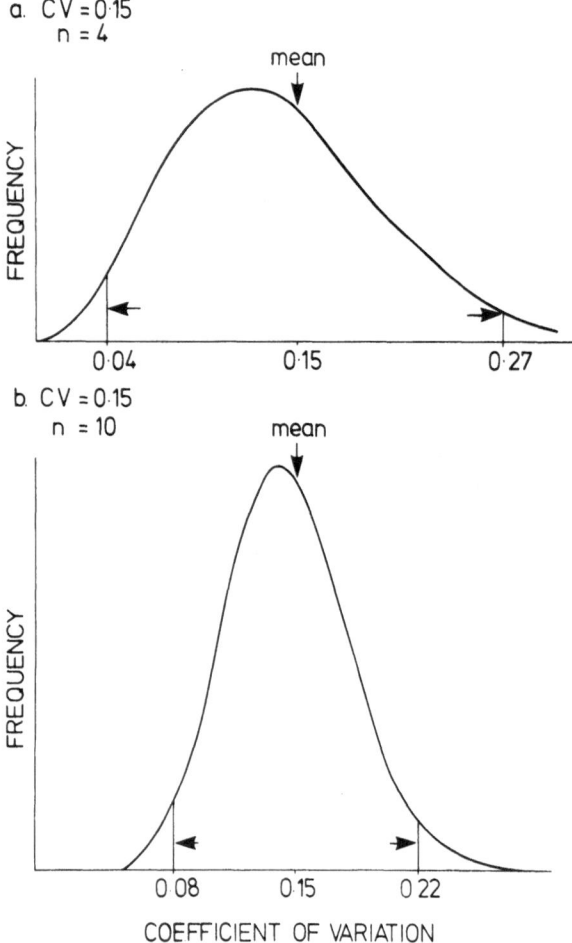

Figure 13.2   Sampling distribution of CV based on 4 or 10 observations for a laboratory with a true CV of 15%. Arrows indicate 2.5 and 97.5 percentiles

The VI is obtained by dividing this value by a chosen target coefficient of variation (CCV). Thus a high VI is taken as an indication of poor performance. In order to deal with the problems of wide fluctuations in VI based on individual observations, Whitehead introduced the principle of a running mean VI based on the most recent 40 observations. In this way long-term fluctuations could be distinguished from the background 'noise' level.

We have used computer-simulated data to study the performance of a relatively poor laboratory as assessed by calculation of VI. The data were simulated for a laboratory with a true CV of 23% when the CCV is 15%. Figure 13.5 shows a plot of 600 observations obtained for this laboratory using a running mean of 40. It is apparent that overall there is oscillation

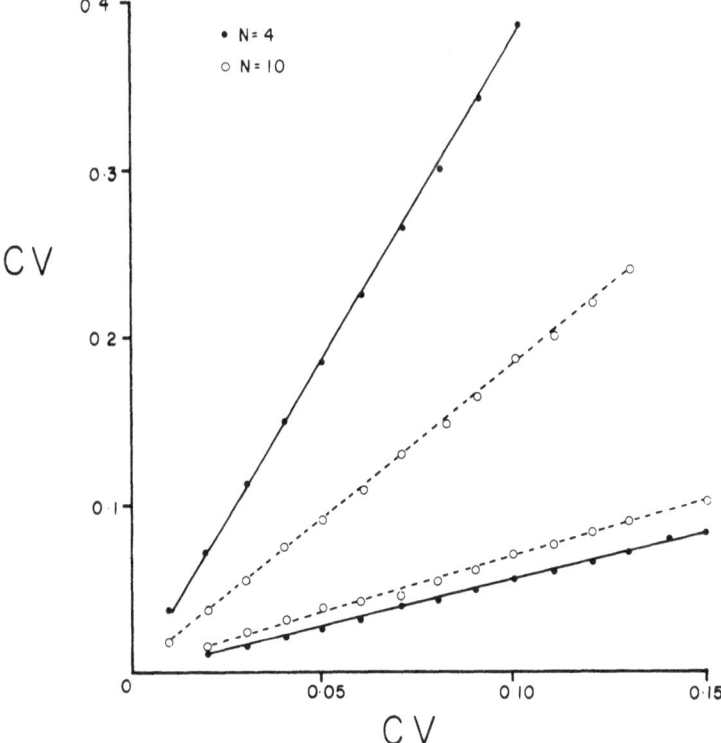

Figure 13.3   Confidence limits (95%) for a true CV (ordinate) given an observed CV (abscissa) derived from 4 or 10 observations

about the expected VI of 122. It is important to note, however, that these simulated data exhibit spurious trends. It would be tempting, for example, to interpret the early pattern (observations 40–70) as indicating an improvement in assay performance. Subsequently there appears to be a static period (observations 70–130) followed by an apparent deterioration in performance (observations 130–170). In fact there is no interpretation, since the true CV is constant at 23%.

However, the real danger in this system becomes apparent when, because of the limited observations available to organizers of external assessment schemes, a smaller running mean is used. Figure 13.6 shows the initial portion of the data from Figure 13.5 plotted using a running mean of 10. The marked downward trend in VI from 130 to 70 (observations 10–16) followed by a reversal (observations 17–26) implies dramatic improvement followed by equally dramatic deterioration when the system has in fact remained static. When the same data are plotted using a running mean of only four observations (Figure 13.7) these fluctuations assume ludicrous proportions. The ability to identify changes in laboratory performance against this background noise is clearly limited.

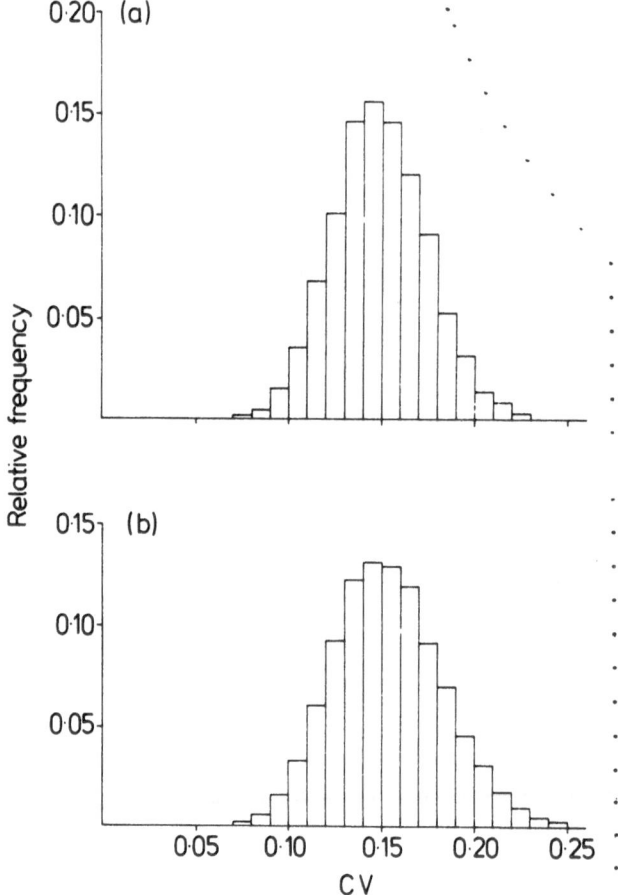

Figure 13.4 Simulated sampling distribution of running CV (four estimates on each of six pools) . for the situation where true CV is constant at 15% (a) or varied (b). In the latter case pools were assigned a CV as follows: 2 at 10%, 2 at 15% and 2 at 20%

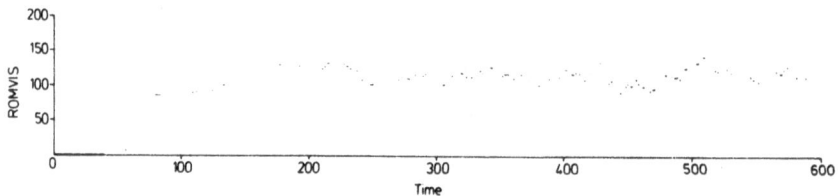

Figure 13.5 Simulated variance index for a laboratory with a true CV of 23% using a chosen CVV of 15%. The data plotted are derived using a running average of 40 observations (ROMVIS)

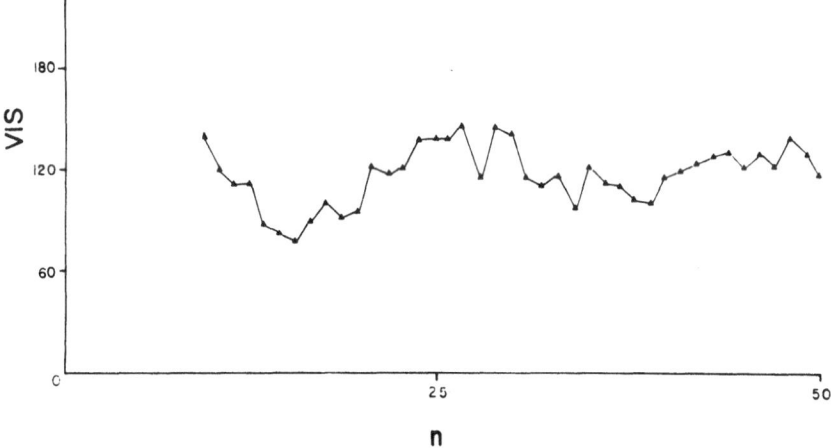

Figure 13.6   Simulated variance index for a laboratory with a true CV of 23% using a chosen CV of 15%. In this case the early part of the data used to construct Figure 13.5 have been plotted based on a running average of 10 observations

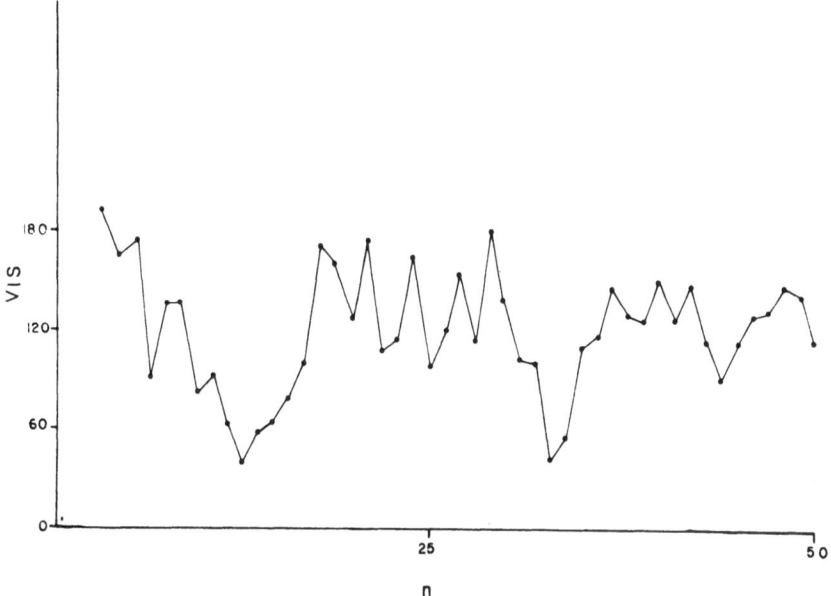

Figure 13.7   Simulated variance index for a laboratory with a true CV of 23% using a chosen CV of 15%. In this case the data used to construct Figure 13.5 have been plotted based on a running average of four observations

When assays are available at a limited number of centres, it is desirable that the results obtained in different centres agree as closely as possible. It is standard practice to use the relationship of observed values to the group mean

Table 13.1 Sample of values obtained for 22 laboratories for control pool of oestradiol-17β

Laboratory	Mean (pmol/l)	CV(%)
1	235	4
2	210	4
3	334	3
4	263	4
5	280	2
6	290	2
7	260	2
8	283	1
9	238	13
10	232	4
11	160	12
12	160	19
13	261	18
14	146	1
15	228	39
16	330	4
17	189	15
18	200	38
19	331	1
20	287	16
21	195	6
22	180	4

as an indication of the bias of a particular laboratory. In this situation, too, the limitations imposed by small samples are apparent. Table 13.1 lists data obtained for 22 laboratories on a pool used in the assessment of performance in the measurement of oestradiol-17β. We have used these data to study the effect on the performance of laboratory 1 of other laboratories. Relative to the group of the first eight laboratories (mean value 269), laboratory 1 shows a distinct negative bias. This bias disappears when the next seven laboratories are included since the group mean now becomes 238. The position remains similar when the final seven laboratories are included (mean 240). Because of the variation in estimates on the pool (CV = 4% for laboratory 1), the calculated bias will follow a distribution. Figure 13.8 illustrates the distribution of bias for laboratory 1 expressed as VI (CCV = 15%) when that laboratory is considered as part of a group of 8, 15 or 22 laboratories.

Assessment of bias by this procedure is thus limited by the problem of imprecision. When precision is low the calculated bias shows a wide distribution. This is illustrated in Figure 13.9, which plots the distribution of bias values calculated for laboratory 13 (CV = 18%) in relation to the overall group mean. Thus the effect of other laboratories in a group on individual performance, and the large error involved in calculating bias, emphasize the problems facing the organizer of a scheme which attempts to monitor changes in the performance of an individual laboratory.

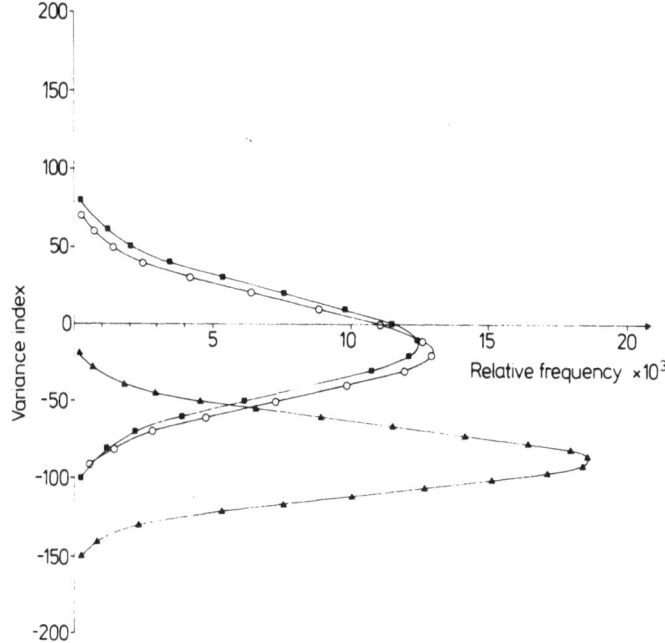

Figure 13.8   Relative frequency distributions of variance index for laboratory 1 as a function of group size. ($\triangle$——$\triangle$, Laboratories 1–8; $\square$——$\square$, Laboratories 1–15; $\bigcirc$——$\bigcirc$, Laboratories 1–22.) Note that the apparent mean bias and the distribution about that mean are both influenced by the performance of laboratories within the group

INTERNAL MONITORING OF ASSAY PERFORMANCE

It is universally accepted that if a laboratory wishes to maintain a satisfactory level of performance on a day-to-day basis, some form of internal monitoring system is essential. Ideally, it should be possible not only to recognize the out-of-control situation, but also to identify the nature of change which produced that situation and the point at which the change occurred. Such a procedure can be carried out by a system involving sequential monitoring based on established analyte pools. Suitable criteria for pool selection are:

(1) they should resemble as near as possible the type of sample used in the assay (e.g. patient serum);
(2) they should contain concentrations of analyte which correspond to patient values where critical interpretation is required; and
(3) they should be available in sufficiently large quantities for continuous monitoring over a reasonable period of time (i.e for several months).

G

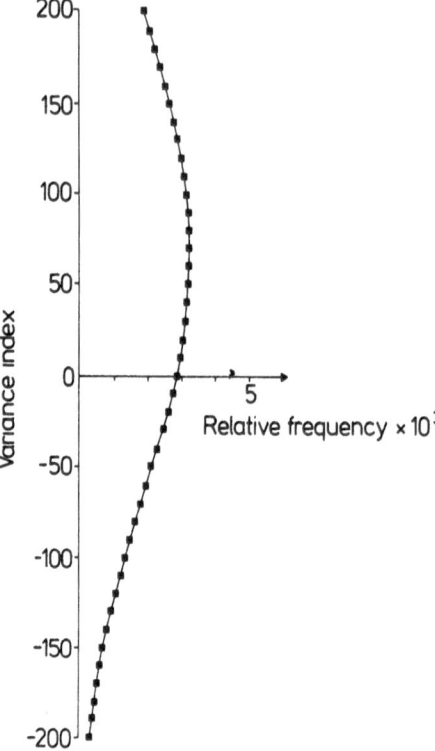

Figure 13.9   Relative frequency distribution of variance index for a laboratory (13) which has a true CV of 18% for a chosen CV of 15%

We have adopted the following scheme for monitoring the performance of an assay for human α-fetoprotein (AFP), used as a screening test on maternal blood for the antenatal diagnosis of neural tube defects. Three parameters were chosen for monitoring: (i) assay precision, (ii) batch variance (drift), and (iii) between-batch variation. Assessment was based on three sample pools prepared by adding purified AFP to 300 ml volumes of fresh sheep serum. Ideally of course analyte-free human serum should be used, so that care was taken to establish that the sheep serum produced no detectable interference in the assay. The procedure used was a radioimmunoassay which involved a 5 h reaction between rabbit antibody (Hoechst Pharmaceutical Company, Hounslow, Middlesex, UK), [^{125}I]AFP (supplied by Dr J. Young, Ninewells Hospital, Dundee, UK) and patient samples or standard (NIBSC, 72/227). Precipitation of the bound antigen was carried out overnight using sheep (anti-rabbit IgG) antibody. All assays were carried out using a computer-controlled, fully automated immunoassay system (Kemtek 3000, Kemble Instruments Limited, Burgess Hill, Sussex, UK). Sample pools were placed after the standard curve and then after each batch of 20 patient sera. All samples were assayed in duplicate.

Precision was monitored by calculating the error in each pair of observations at low, medium and high analyte concentrations. The batch variance was monitored by calculating the error between the mean concentration of each pool at the beginning and end of each assay. Drift was thus identified when the error exceeded that arising from random variation. Monitoring of between-assay variance was based on the mean value obtained for each pair of pool estimations. This type of analysis is considerably more sensitive to variation than that based on monitoring mean values for the complete assay. Sequential analysis of the data was provided by plotting each parameter in the form of a CUSUM. The application of this type of monitoring to internal control of immunoassay performance has been described previously[4, 5]. The formulae used to derive values for each of the parameters are listed in Appendix 1. Each pool was assayed ten times in duplicate in order to derive target values for precision and mean analyte concentrations. The V-masks used in monitoring were designed as described previously[4] with the objective of identifying a shift in excess of 1.5 times the standard deviation of the target values within an average of five estimations. Such a scheme would yield a false-positive rate of 1 in 200 observations.

The data derived from 17 sequential assays of α-fetoprotein can be used to illustrate the unique advantages of this type of monitoring system. Figure 13.10 shows a CUSUM plot of assay precision as indicated by the low pool (50 μg/l). The tendency for this sequential plot to rise indicates that the error obtained in repeated assays is marginally higher than the target value, though

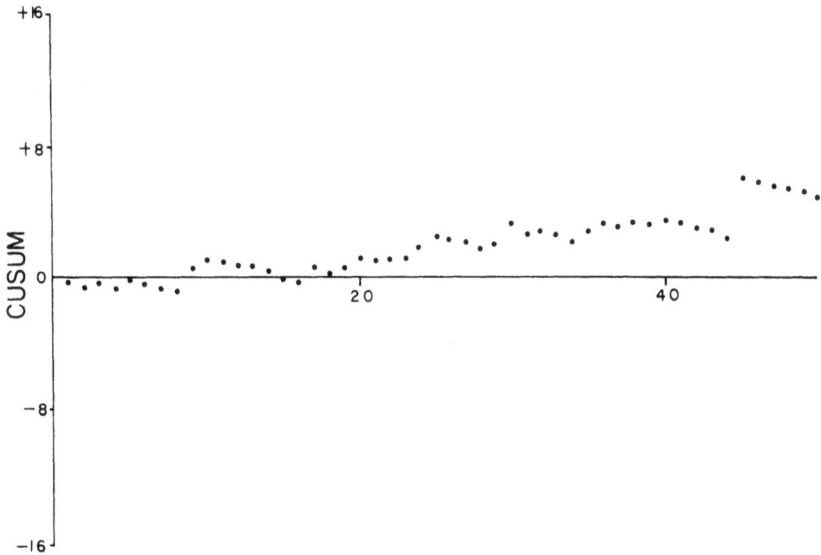

Figure 13.10 CUSUM plot for precision of serum AFP assays based on duplicate determinations of low pool

only once (observation 45) is an out-of-control situation identified. This situation was also identified by the medium pool, and it was noticeable that several samples in that region of the assay showed rather poor duplication. This problem, which occurred near the end of an assay, was traced to malfunction of a pump in the automated system.

Figure 13.11 shows a CUSUM plot for the batch variance based on data derived from the medium pool (79 μg/l). Each point is based on the difference between first and last estimates of that pool in each assay. No drift was detected up to assays 11 and 12 which were both flagged as out of control. There was no doubt that substantial drift had occurred in both these assays which were rejected on that basis. The problem appeared to be associated with overheating of equipment during assay separation. After correction of this problem no further drift occurred.

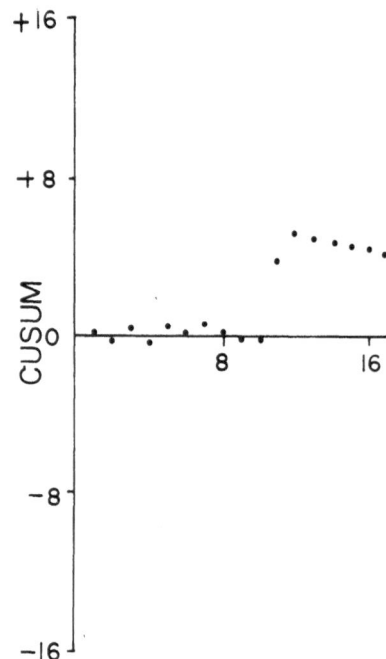

Figure 13.11 CUSUM plot for batch variance of serum AFP assays based on the difference between duplicate determinations of a medium pool placed at the beginning and end of each batch

A third type of out-of-control situation is illustrated in Figure 13.12 which shows a CUSUM plot based on mean values for the high pool (151 μg/l). Observations 36–40 show the appearance of a systematic error which produced high values for this pool within a single assay. The acute deviation of this CUSUM plot was flagged as out of control using the V-mask by the third

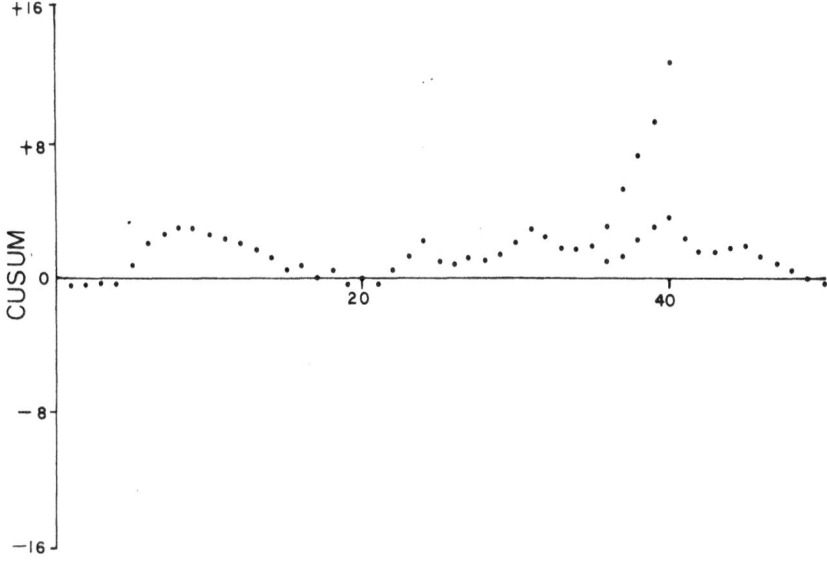

Figure 13.12   CUSUM plot of mean values of duplicate estimations obtained with a high pool in the serum AFP assay

observation within that assay. The error which produced this marked positive bias was traced to a batch of serum used as diluent for standards in this assay. The assay was repeated using a different batch of serum diluent and was subsequently in control. It is important to note that the situations illustrated in Figures 13.11 and 13.12 reflected systematic error, there being no loss of precision on either occasion.

DISCUSSION

These studies on control of α-fetoprotein assays serve to emphasize the fact that even with relatively straightforward immunoassay techniques there still exist many potential sources of error. By adopting a simple monitoring procedure, we have demonstrated how it is possible to identify some of these errors and treat them accordingly. Of particular value is the ability to distinguish the random errors caused by machine or operator failure from the more systematic errors introduced by methodological or reagent variability. Monitoring of precision, independent of other parameters, is of overwhelming importance[6] for if precision is poor it may be impossible to identify other sources of assay error.

A major drawback of external assessment schemes in operation at present is that they do not adequately assess assay precision. For example, as illustrated in Figure 13.9, there is little point in attempting to identify bias when the poor performance of a laboratory makes such identification impossible. Moreover, it is apparent that attempts to monitor the performance of a laboratory based on limited statistical data are only capable of identifying extreme situations, and are certainly not appropriate for assessing fluctuations in individual performance.

The computer simulation studies as shown in Figures 13.5–13.7 illustrate the problem that it is not possible to assume that a monitoring scheme, which has been applied successfully in certain areas of clinical biochemistry, is necessarily appropriate to the assessment of performance in immunoassay laboratories. In such cases the inherently high imprecision and infrequency of sampling combine to render VI monitoring virtually useless as a guide to assay performance.

If immunoassay performance in UK laboratories is to be improved, it can only be by attacking the sources of error directly. It is first necessary to understand the nature of the error in individual assay systems. Where these can be traced to reagent variability, a central supply of standardized reagents should be considered. Subsequent monitoring of the assay performance can be made only through effective internal control. We feel that the means for such control should be provided centrally in the form of advice, computer programs for data-handling and also serum pools for use in each assay. The data generated by such a scheme would enable an organizer to assess assay performance in a far more meaningful way than through existing schemes with their high inertia and low sensitivity. This direct approach to identification and elimination of error could only improve the quality of immunoassay techniques in this country.

Acknowledgments

We gratefully acknowledge generous financial support from Ciba-Geigy Ltd., The Welsh Office and the Tenovus Organization.

APPENDIX 1

Precision

Target standard deviation (σ_T) was calculated from 10 pairs of estimations on each pool using the formula:

$$\sigma_T = \sqrt{\frac{\Sigma (x_2 - x_1)^2}{2n}} \tag{1}$$

where x_2 = observation 2 } of each pair
      x_1 = observation 1
and n = number of pairs (10)

The value used for the CUSUM plot of precision was then calculated from the formula:

$$\frac{\left[\dfrac{Sp^2}{\sigma_T{}^2}-1\right]}{2\sqrt{2}} \tag{2}$$

where $Sp^2 = \dfrac{(x_2-x_1)^2}{2}$ \hfill (3)

Batch variance

Target standard deviation (σ_T) for each pool was calculated by the formula:

$$\sigma_T = \sqrt{\frac{\Sigma x^2 - n(\bar{x}^2)}{n-1}} \tag{4}$$

where $x =$ each single estimation
       $\bar{x} =$ mean of n estimations (target mean)
and $n =$ number of single estimations (20).

The value used for the CUSUM plot of batch variance was calculated from the formula:

$$\frac{\left[\dfrac{S_b{}^2}{\sigma_T{}^2}-1\right]}{2\sqrt{2}} \tag{5}$$

where $S_b{}^2 = (\bar{x}_e - \bar{x}_b)^2$ \hfill (6)
       $\bar{x}_e =$ mean of pair at the end of the batch
       $\bar{x}_b =$ mean of pair at the beginning of the batch.

MEAN

Target standard deviation (σ_T) for each pool was calculated from 10 pairs of observations from the formula:

$$\sigma_T = \sqrt{\frac{\Sigma x^2 - n(\bar{x}^2)}{n-1}} \tag{7}$$

where $x =$ individual estimation
       $\bar{x} =$ mean of n estimations (target mean)
and $n =$ number of single estimations (20).

The value of the CUSUM used for the mean of each pair of observations on each pool was calculated from the formula:

$$\frac{(\bar{x}_j - \bar{x})}{\sqrt{2\sigma_T}} \tag{8}$$

where $\bar{x}_j$ = mean of each pair of estimations
$\bar{x}$ = target mean

Note: these formulae were derived such that when the data are plotted one unit on the ordinate scale is one CUSUM unit, and an identical unit on the abscissa represents one observation of each parameter. The V masks used in each case were designed as described previously[4].

References

1. Wilson, D. W., Sarfaty, G., Clarris, B., Douglas, M. and Crawshaw, K. (1971). The prediction of standard curves and errors for the assays of estradiol by competitive protein binding. *Steroids*, **18**, 77
2. Rodbard, D. (1974). Statistical quality control and routine data processing for radioimmunoassays and immunoradiometric assays. *Clin. Chem.*, **20**, 1255
3. Whitehead, T. P. (1977). *Quality Control in Clinical Chemistry*. (New York: Wiley)
4. Kemp, K. W., Nix, A. B. J., Wilson, D. W. and Griffiths, K. (1978). Internal quality control of radioimmunoassay. *J. Endocrinol.*, **76**, 203
5. Wilson, D. W., Griffiths, K., Kemp, K. W., Nix, A. B. J. and Rowlands, R. J. (1979). Internal quality control of radioimmunoassays: monitoring of error, *J. Endocrinol.*, **80**, 365
6. Ekins, R. P. (1979). Assay design and quality control. In Bizollon, C. A. (ed.) *Radioimmunology 1979*, pp. 239–55. (Amsterdam: Elsevier/North Holland Biomedical Press)

14
Components in a Model for the Production of Reference Materials with special Reference to Immunoassays

M. HJELM

Reactions between antigens and antibodies are used for a wide variety of purposes in biology, e.g. to study:

(1) basic principles for the reaction between the two types of molecules;
(2) the structure and function of antigens and antibodies;
(3) the structure and function of cell membranes;
(4) the recognition of subclasses of cells.

The same type of reaction can be used for:

(1) the assay of the concentrations of antigens and antibodies in biological fluids;
(2) the assay of rates of synthesis and catabolism of the antigens of antibodies.

Numerous investigations of all the types mentioned above are already used routinely in the diagnosis and follow-up (of treatment) of an increasing number of disorders. This gives rise to a situation in clinical laboratory sciences, as in other areas of analytical chemistry, that enforces steps to be taken to ensure that results are comparable.

Comparability of results is essential in, e.g.:

(1) Epidemiological studies in the broader sense. Such studies could aim at establishing reference values for populations of healthy subjects or for

particular types of disorders or comparing subjects of different ethnic, geographic backgrounds, etc.

(2) Longitudinal studies of one or several individuals under physiological and pathophysiological conditions. Such studies could aim at establishing the intra-individual variation of a biomedical parameter during health and disease.

In both cases it is worthwhile to point out that small but significant systematic differences or trends might be of equal importance in indicating even a profound change of the homeostatic system, as large changes.

In general comparability of results can be achieved by introducing reference materials and well-defined methods, or both, in a particular measurement area.

Several attempts have been made to define a *reference material*, e.g. the recent provisional recommendations, by the International Organization for Standardization/Committee on Reference Materials[1] that:

reference materials are substances or materials one or more properties of which is sufficiently well established to be used for the calibration of an apparatus or for the verification of a measurement method.

It follows that properties of both analytes and reagents can be certified. The possibility of producing a reference material is dependent on the quality of the available methodology. The International Federation of Clinical Chemistry (IFCC) has recently suggested a system for the classification of methods[2], mainly used to assay the concentrations of a compound in biological fluids in clinical chemistry: definitive methods; reference methods; routine methods.

The definitions of the three types of methods are given in Table 14.1. There is, of course, no sharp distinction between definitive and reference methods or a reference method and a routine method. With the introduction of this classification system attention has, however, been drawn to the need for the development of definitive methods in the biomedical field.

With the recent introduction of quantitative mass spectrometry and use of stable labelled isotopes as internal standards, there is now the opportunity of

Table 14.1 IFCC classificatory system for analytical procedures in clinical chemistry

Term	Definition
Definitive method	a method which after exhaustive investigation is found to have no source of inaccuracy or ambiguity
Reference method	a method which after exhaustive investigation has been shown to have negligible inaccuracy in comparison with its precision
Routine methods	
of known bias	a method in which the direction and extent of bias has been established
of unknown bias	a method of unknown bias

developing definitive methods for the assay of low molecular mass compounds below, at present, about 1000 daltons.

Definitive methods can be used to produce biomedical matrix reference materials. Such a production has also been initiated by several international organizations including WHO, Geneva; The National Bureau of Standards (NBS), Washington and the Community Bureau of Reference (BCR), Brussels. As an example it can be mentioned that a reference material for cortisol and oestradiol-17β in human serum is soon to be expected from the BCR in Brussels. These two compounds are routinely assayed by many different types of immunoassays and are in need of standardization.

The development of definitive methods and the concomitant production of biomedical matrix reference materials for low molecular mass compounds will represent a considerable step forward in facilitating the improvement of the accuracy of measurements in clinical laboratory sciences. One fundamental quantity can be assayed, i.e. the number of molecules in a defined volume. Such a quantity is essential in calculating other quantities related to the function of the molecules such as activity coefficient, freely diffusible and bound fractions of the compound in matrix systems such as blood and tissues. Values of this type will, of course, be necessary to obtain in order to broaden our understanding of how homeostatic mechanisms work in health and disease.

The situation for high molecular mass compounds, e.g. proteins and antibodies, is far more complex and less developed as concerns the possibility to assay accurately the concentration of such compounds in biological fluid. It is also obvious that many different types of reference materials are needed, e.g. specificity seems to be the more important property to certify for an antibody preparation intended for the *classification* of cells. Accuracy in the sense that every antibody in the reference preparation reacted with membrane antigens would in this respect not be so important. If, however, such a preparation was used to assay the total number of binding sites, accuracy would become important again.

For all immunoassays used to determine the concentration of antigens and antibodies in biological fluids the same need for accuracy would principally apply as for any type of concentration measurement. This is easy to say but at present more than difficult to achieve even if it might not be impossible to develop appropriate methodology and reference materials based on technological and financial collaboration between interested countries.

The second best and at present more realistic alternative would be to go for *reference methods of proven transferability* for the certification of a matrix reference material and define specifications for the production and characterization of antigens, antibodies and reagents that will ensure *repeatability* of hopefully critical properties of successive batches of reference materials. This philosophy would also hopefully ensure that whatever bias exists between the immunological properties of the analyte in the reference materials and unknown specimens that bias remains constant. The same will be true for reference materials for antibodies.

There is a general model established for the production of reference materials for low molecular mass compounds in a biological matrix and the establishment of an acceptable analytical protocol for the method used to certify such materials[3, 4]. It should be possible to use the same approach for the production of reference materials for high molecular mass compounds in a biological matrix.

In the following, an attempt has been made to examine this general model (Table 14.2) for the production of a biomedical reference material with special

Table 14.2   The components in a general model for the production of certified biomedical matrix reference materials

The user's general specifications of the reference material related to its intended use

The pre-analytical handling of the matrix material and other materials

The analytical and statistical procedures

Storage and distribution

regard to the production of reference materials for antigens in biological fluids. Such reference materials would be used for the standardization of assays of high molecular mass compounds in biological fluids, e.g. the plasma proteins, the most frequently used application of the antigen–antibody reaction in clinical chemistry.

THE USER'S GENERAL SPECIFICATIONS FOR THE REFERENCE MATERIAL RELATED TO ITS INTENDED USE

The type of material

If the intended use of a matrix reference material is to detect and eliminate systematic errors in an analytical procedure due to matrix effects the reference material should be of the same type as the specimens to be assayed. This means that, e.g., human plasma might be preferred to animal materials.

It has in this respect often been argued that human material should not be used for this purpose. One argument in defence of human materials is, however, that in the end the patient will profit from the contribution made by the blood donor also in this case even to the extent that a transfusion of plasma proteins can be avoided.

The antibodies should also be well characterized. Specificity might not be the only important feature to the antibodies but also other parameters related to their general molecular properties, i.e. the primary, secondary and tertiary structure of the antibodies as macromolecules might be required in order to make comparisons between batches.

The allowable uncertainty of the certified value

Ideally objective clinical parameters should be used to define the allowable uncertainty of the certified value, e.g. the relationship between the magnitude of uncertainty and the frequency of erroneous decisions. In practice the allowable uncertainty will at present have to be based on some type of consensus value.

It should be remembered in this respect that the interlaboratory variation observed in a quality control scheme by using a certified reference material for standardization of an assay will not be better than the uncertainty of the certified value of the reference material.

The concentration of many plasma proteins shows a remarkable individual constancy over many years and even slight deviations from the individual level might be of clinical significance. The uncertainty of the certified value for such reference materials should most likely be much less than has previously been assumed and a coefficient of variation in the order of 1–2% might be desirable. This is an alternative approach towards defining uncertainty.

THE PRE-ANALYTICAL HANDLING OF THE MATRIX MATERIAL AND OTHER MATERIALS

In order to ensure transferability of properties, technical specifications for this component might include:

Conditions for specimen collection

These include the question of whether blood should be collected from fasting or non-fasting subjects, and at what time of the day? Such factors will, in the first instance, affect the composition and properties of the matrix. The properties of the antigen or antibody might also be affected due to reactions with ligands, the concentrations of which might vary over a 24 h period.

Conditions for the preparation of the reference material

These conditions cover the question whether the reference material should be available in liquid form (filtered or unfiltered) or after freeze-drying? Again, both the properties of the analyte and the matrix might differ from physiological conditions depending on preparatory procedure.

General characteristics used to ensure comparability of batches (certified compound and matrix)

Such characteristics might include physical measurements, e.g. patterns obtained by ultracentrifugation, chromatography, electrophoresis, equilibrium dialysis. Little experimental work has so far been done in this field but it might be rewarding to increase the efforts.

The handling of the reference material before certification

Improper handling of a matrix material before analysis might change the properties of both the analyte and the matrix, and introduce systematic deviations from the physiological state.

THE ANALYTICAL AND STATISTICAL PROCEDURE

A certified value for a reference material should preferably be based on assays carried out in several laboratories. It would be necessary for the participating laboratories to:

(1) establish detailed draft analytical protocols for the method(s) to be used – several methods are preferred to a single one;
(2) examine the protocol(s) for sources of systematic errors in collaboration with the other laboratories, usually at a series of meetings;
(3) test the transferability of the methods in a feasibility study;
(4) establish the final analytical protocol(s).

In this way, systematic errors related, for example, to pipetting, temperature, pH, mixing, and principles for the establishment of the calibration curve, can be identified and eliminated.

Based on the outcome of the feasibility study it will also be possible to make a choice of methods to be used for the certification of the reference material and the optimal statistical procedure to obtain a certified value within its predetermined acceptable uncertainty using a minimum of assays and participating laboratories. Improved statistical methods can also be achieved following this procedure for the control of stability of the reference material.

Few attempts to certify a high molecular mass compound based on immunoassays and following such a detailed procedure as the one described above have so far been carried out. It has, however, successfully been tried in another difficult area of clinical laboratory sciences in need of standardization – coagulation assays – in order to certify reference material for thromboplastins.

STORAGE AND DISTRIBUTION

It goes almost without saying that a tremendous amount of work to establish biological reference materials easily can be spoiled if storage and distribution conditions are not correct. However, accelerated degradation tests should give good guidance in this respect.

CONCLUSIONS

There will be an increasing need for standardization of quantitative immunoassays in the 1980s. This will involve the establishment of reference methodology and the production of reference materials.

References

1. Provisional definitions, ISO/REMCO, **34**, (1977)
2. Buttner, J., Borthe, R., Boutwell, J. H. and Broughton, P. M. G. (1975). Approval recommendation on quality control in clinical chemistry. Part 1: general principles and terminology. *Clin. Chim. Acta*, **63**, F25
3. Cali, J. P. (1976). Rationale for reference methods in clinical chemistry. *Pure Appl. Chem.*, **45**, 61
4. Hjelm, M. (1980). Components in a model for the production of certified biomedical reference materials. *Proc. Eighth Tenovus Workshop: Quality Control in Clinical Endocrinology*. (Cardiff): (In press)

15
Standardization of Immunological Reagents

I. BATTY

The International Union of Immunological Societies Standardization Committee and others have been working towards the standardization of immunological reagents. The primary aim of such standardization is to improve the quality of laboratory results and to provide a means to ensure uniformity in the designation of the concentration of clinically important substances in body fluids which cannot be adequately characterized by chemical and physical means.

Although immunology is a relatively young discipline the time has long since passed, at least in the major areas, when comparability and uniformity of results could be ensured by the interchange of materials between interested workers.

It might be thought that reagents which are used by scientists for tests in the laboratory, where expense, time and inclination are virtually the only factors which determine how well the performance of the test and the reagents are controlled, was the area least in need of standardization. This might be true if each test result could be regarded in isolation and there was no need to communicate results to others or to compare results obtained in different laboratories or even in one laboratory at different times.

It is fair to say that the basis for immunological standardization was laid down over 80 years ago by Ehrlich's classical work on the standardization of diphtheria toxin and Kraus' demonstration that when soluble antigen meets its homologous antiserum a visible precipitate often forms. So biological standardization has a long and honourable history.

The standardization of immunological reagents, however, only got under way some 15–20 years ago when immunological reagents and test systems became commercially available on a large scale and when immunological tests were being used in ever-increasing numbers and routinely performed by staff sometimes insufficiently aware of the basis of the tests, so that errors once introduced could go unchecked.

At this time, several groups of workers were becoming concerned at the quality of laboratory results as they found that there was no uniformity in the designation of the concentration of clinically important substances in body fluids. Two studies in particular highlighted these difficulties. Firstly, Bozoky's study[1] which found a 940-fold difference between the highest and the lowest concentrations of rheumatoid factor recorded by 19 expert laboratories using the Waaler Rose technique on the same sample, whilst a 310-fold difference (640–20 000) was found amongst those using the latex technique.

The second is illustrated in Figure 15.1; this uses information collected by Rowe and his colleagues in 1970[2] from a study on the measurement of human immunoglobulins by immunological methods. They found that the estimates of the immunoglobulin content of a single sample varied widely from laboratory to laboratory.

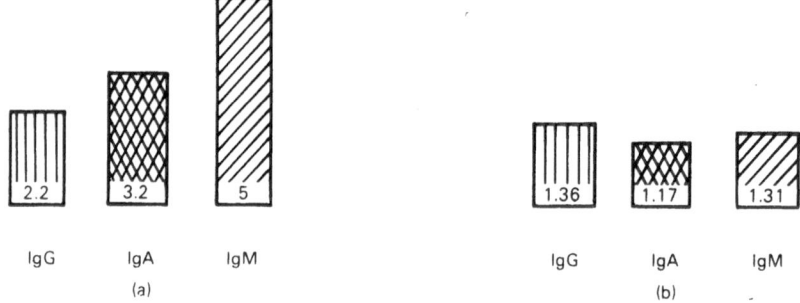

Figure 15.1 Ratio of the highest and lowest values obtained by expert laboratories measuring immunoglobulins in the same pathological serum: (a) using their own antisera and antigen standards; (b) using a common antigen standard of arbitrary unitage and different antisera

Results were recorded in mg/ml and the ratios between the highest and lowest results returned were 2.2-fold for IgG; 3.2-fold for IgA and 5-fold for IgM. The study was repeated but a common reference preparation with an arbitrary designated unitage was included in the test. All laboratories used different antisera but recorded their results in terms of the common reference antigen and the ratio of highest to lowest result was reduced to 1.36-fold for IgG, 1.18-fold for IgA and 1.31-fold for IgM. This study clearly demonstrated both the need for, and the value of, assessing the potency of complex substances in similarly complex matrices in terms of a common standard, particularly in situations where it is often difficult to reduce the number of variables in the test system at least to any significant degree, or to define the conditions sufficiently so that the test system has a high reproducibility (precision).

The primary concern has been with the activity rather than the purity of such a standard; although it is possible to produce many antigens in a highly purified form it is an unfortunate fact that highly purified such preparations are often lacking in stability and do not necessarily behave in the test system as do crude or native antigens, for example albumin. This may give rise to non-parallelism in the dose–response curves and thus invalid assays. Naturally, if it is possible to prepare a pure antigen in a stable form that behaves in exactly the same way in the test system as does the native antigen, then this is a situation eminently to be desired; though, this being said, one is immediately into a discussion as to the criterion of purity and some of the early confusion in the measurement of immunoglobulins and the more recent confusion in the measurement of α-fetoprotein stemmed from differences in purity of the so-called 'pure' antigen.

OPTIMAL TIME FOR THE INTRODUCTION OF STANDARDS

When is the optimal time for introducing an international standard? Imagine that you have discovered that an abnormal constituent or a change in level of a normal constituent of a body fluid or tissue can be used to diagnose or monitor a disease process, and you have devised a specific sensitive and reproducible test system to measure it. Before writing the paper that will help you towards your Nobel prize or at least a fellowship of some sort, you will have tested a number of samples from patients suffering from the condition and a similar or greater number of samples from subjects known by other criteria to be free from the disease. Being a careful worker you will have repeated your tests many times and you will have had the foresight to collect a reasonable volume of material from one or two patients whose samples gave the most clear-cut reproducible assay, or you will have made a pool of such samples to be used as your personal standard with which to compare subsequent samples and other batches of the necessary reagents. This is fine; you don't yet need a national or international standard. Your paper is published after what always seems an unconscionable period of time and you begin to receive letters from workers in the same field asking for further details; this is followed by requests for samples of your reagents and controls. There aren't too many of these so you send out small aliquots to your friends and other interested workers – there is still no need for a standard – if this small group gets variable or discrepant results you meet or you correspond – you exchange materials – you sort out the problems.

Then other papers appear confirming the usefulness of the test system, probably including some modification to make the test easier or quicker or using smaller samples. At this point, and rapidly if the papers or communications have reached a wide audience, more and more laboratories will try the test; some will devise different methods of test and eventually a manufacturer will begin to make the reagents and, if possible, put them together in kit form. Other manufacturers will follow; the test system will be promoted and if it has value, particularly for patient care, it will begin to be performed by laboratory workers who, although they may be technically better qualified, are not using the same reagents, and do not necessarily have an understanding of the basis of the test; neither do they have the time or interest to examine all components of the system critically. Then you begin to hear that laboratory X has abandoned the test because all samples appear to be in the abnormal range, or laboratory Y says the test doesn't work, whilst laboratory Z says the test system is OK but the original workers set the level of positivity at the wrong value. Ideally it is *now* that there should be an international standard available against which the various laboratories can check their results. A standard available at this time is particularly useful in setting up the normal range for the substance in the designated populations. Routine laboratories seldom have the time to set up their own normal or reference ranges but they have a very real need for them.

The impetus towards a standard for an immunological reagent, or test system, can come from many quarters; clinicians, individual research workers, scientific societies, national control or regulatory authorities or international or regional organizations. It usually happens when some group of workers become dissatisfied with variations in the results obtained by different laboratories on the same, or similar, populations or with the variability in performance of the reagents they use. The immunoglobulin standard is an example of the first, and the FITC conjugated anti-human Ig of the latter.

PRIORITIES

The number of immunological reagents and test systems is so large that each request for setting up a standard must be considered objectively and priorities decided on the basis of how much results would be improved by a standard; how important the results are to health care; what would be the cost of producing such a standard; and, not least important, is there the expertise available to write the specifications, produce and organize the collaborative assay of the standard?

CRITERIA FOR MATERIAL STANDARDS

A standard must ideally:

(1) have the same properties in the test system as the substance to be measured;
(2) be stable;
(3) be physically homogeneous;
(4) be free from bacterial contamination;
(5) be capable of accurate division into aliquots;
(6) be freeze-dried with minimal denaturation;

(7) have a uniform moisture content $< 1\%$;

(8) reconstitute completely to give a clear solution.

It is not always possible to fulfil all these requirements but every attempt should be made to do so.

PREPARATION OF STANDARDS

The most important stages in standard preparations are:

(1) *Determination of need.* The IUIS first circulated a questionnaire to some 150 clinical immunologists and laboratory-based immunologists in 30 countries to assess their priorities – on this basis and considering the state of the art, the availability of materials and expertise, determined the final priorities.

(2) *Writing of specifications.* This is best done by an international group of workers experienced in the test system and possibly better written by one or two experts and approved by such a group.

(3) *Procurement of material.* Source is not important if it fulfils specifications and detailed information on all aspects of its preparation is available. All the standards or reference preparations we are concerned with are freeze-dried according to the WHO specifications, partly for stability but mainly for ease of transportation internationally. Although these specifications were written some years ago they have not yet been superseded, but such methods should always be considered critically whenever a standard for a new antigen or antibody is being prepared, or when the preparation of a standard for an antigen or antibody for use in a different situation or test system is being undertaken. It is conceivable that changes take place during freeze-drying that, without necessarily affecting potency or stability, do affect the suitability of the material for a particular purpose. An instance of this is the present International Standard for immunoglobulins G, M and A which, though highly satisfactory for radial immunodiffusion, reconstitutes to give a slightly turbid solution unsatisfactory for nephelometric measurement by automated techniques, as it gives too high a blank reading. The WHO international reference preparation for six serum proteins, which was freon-treated before freeze-drying and reconstitutes to give a crystal-clear fluid has, therefore, been calibrated for immunoglobulins G, M and A in terms of first standard so that there is now a comparison material with values of G, M and A in international units which can be used in a nephelometric test.

(4) *Collection of stability data.* This starts as soon as the material is in its final form. A number of randomly selected ampoules proportional to the size of the batch are measured for dry weight and moisture content to ensure the accuracy of filling and the efficacy of the freeze-drying, and a further

number of samples undergo accelerated degradation tests usually at a range of temperatures from that of liquid nitrogen to 56 °C. It is important that a standard shall maintain its activity without detectable loss throughout its life; but the life which you believe is reasonable varies with the rate of change of the technologies involved. One should always be prepared to scrap a standard if a significantly better one can be provided; 'Biological' standards, e.g. tetanus antitoxin, are expected to last for 20 years. This being said, according to the Arrhenius plot on the serum protein standard, the complement component tested immunogically will retain its potency for 2000 years.

(5) *Collaborative assay.* The protocols for this are agreed if not actually written by experienced workers in the field with the advice of a statistician. Usually two or more candidate preparations (in the case of the serum protein standard it was five) are tested at the same time against several specimens using at least two methods – their own and a common recommended or defined method agreed as the best currently available for routine work (our Immune Complexes subcommittee spent its first 2 years on a field trial to determine this). Interestingly several studies have shown that there may be less variation in the results obtained with own method than with the defined method, largely because familiarity with a technique can compensate for its apparent deficiencies. When possible the protocols require the establishment of dose–response curves which should run parallel over the range of test with those of the preparations which are to be measured against it.

(6) *Statistical analysis of results.* This is really a part of the collaborative assay, and the aim is to establish linearity, parallelism and confirm the suitability of the material as a standard.

(7) *Acceptance as an international standard and allocation of unitage.*

A submission which gives all the information under headings (1)–(6) is made to The Chief, Biologicals WHO, who arranges its consideration by the expert panel on biological standardization. It is accepted or referred for further information or studies; it can be rejected on scientific grounds. If accepted then, with the agreement of the participants in the collaborative assay, a unitage is assigned.

Standards are very valuable assets resulting from a great deal of careful work, internationally and expertly validated, but before you can use them intelligently, it is important to be clear on the matter of units.

Units are defined in Table 15.1. It is important to appreciate that units as applied to biological materials are analogous to international physical units of length or mass which can be equally arbitrary (Table 15.1), where you see the unit of mass is simply the mass of an international prototype kilogram, although one would wish to move to definitions such as that of the metre as shown in the same table. However, for routine work the metre is still related to

Table 15.1 How to define units

(a) The international unit of biological material has by definition the specific biological activity contained in a defined weight of the current international standard

(b) The international unit of mass (kilogram) has by definition the mass of the international prototype of the kilogram

(c) The international unit of length (metre) has by definition the length equal to 1 650 763.73 wavelengths in a vacuum of the radiation corresponding to the transition between the levels $2p_{10}$ and $5d_5$ of the krypton-86 atom.

(d) The international unit of immunoglobulin G has by definition the same activity as 0.8147 mg of the dry powder present in an ampoule of the international research standard for human serum immunoglobulins

the distance between two points on a wall in Paris; that is to an international material standard just as is the international unit of human immunoglobulin G which has by definition the same activity as 0.8147 mg of the dry powder present in an ampoule of the international research standard for human serum immunoglobulins G, M and A. Of course, you would not try to weigh out this amount of hygroscopic powder, but reconstitute the total contents in a suitable volume of diluent in the knowledge that this volume now contains 100 units of IgG.

It must be remembered that there is no relationship between the unit of a specific antigen or antibody and the unit of a second antigen or antibody having a different specificity. The unit of IgE, for example, has the same activity as 0.006562 mg of the dry powder in the international reference preparation of IgE. A unit of IgG does not precipitate the same mass of specific antibody as does one unit of IgM or one unit of ANA.

CONTINUITY OF UNITS

Nevertheless, for any given substance the international unit is continuous and represents the same amount of activity in each succeeding standard – this is ensured by always comparing the new standard with the old in an international collaborative assay and assigning its unitage in terms of the old standard so the activity of one unit of material remains the same although the weight of dry material containing this activity is likely to be different.

USE

The prime function of an immunological standard is to enable the activity of a sample of unknown potency to be measured by immunoassay and expressed conveniently in international units to thus ensure the uniformity in measurement of normal or abnormal constituents of body fluids or tissue extracts in the hope that this will lead to a uniformity in the diagnosis of immune disorders. Its use should:

(1) enable a clear distinction to be made between healthy and diseased individuals and populations;
(2) provide a reliable basis for aetiological diagnosis and sound treatment;
(3) allow a meaningful intra- and inter-laboratory comparison of test results for medical follow-up, epidemiological investigations, health surveys and the better use of historical data;
(4) facilitate meaningful communications among laboratory staffs, clinicians and health administrators world-wide, rendered more necessary by the increasing mobility of populations.

A secondary function is to provide a benchmark against which users can assess the performance of reagents and test kits. But international standards are, as I have already said, expensive and difficult to produce so they should never be used as working reagents nor for general experimental purposes, but should be used for the calibration of secondary national or laboratory standards without which no laboratory can be assured of the quality of its performance. That being said, Table 15.2 lists the international immunological standards which are available to bonafide scientific workers from WHO free, on receipt of a letter from the scientist explaining his need.

Table 15.2 Standards available for immunological use (WHO)

Preparation	Quantity/ ampoule (IU)	Year of establishment	Weight containing one IU (mg)
Rheumatoid arthritis serum	100	1965	0.171
Antinuclear factor serum (homogeneous)	100	1970	0.186
Human serum immunoglobulins IgG, IgM and IgA	100	1970	0.8147
Human serum immunoglobulin IgD*	100	1971	
Human serum immunoglobulin IgE	11 500	1973	0.006562
α-fetoprotein, human	100 000	1975	0.0013991
Carcinoembryonic antigen (CEA) human	100	1975	0.0236
FITC conjugated sheep anti-human Ig	100	1976	0.0594
FITC conjugated sheep anti-human IgM (μ-chain)	100	1977	0.0447
Serum proteins (albumin, α-1-antitrypsin, α-2-macroglobulin, C3, ceruloplasmin and transferrin)	100	1977	1.1137
International reference preparation of human serum complement components C.1q, C4, C5 and Factor B	100	1980	–

* British Standard

On the way, but not yet through all the stages, are standards for enzyme-labelled human immunoglobulin, methods and candidate preparations selected, immune complexes and antibody to dsDNA are at a similar stage, various allergen extracts are now available for international collaborative assay and a standard for FITC conjugated human anti-LIgG (anti-γ-chain) are undergoing statistical analysis.

I have covered, in some cases very briefly, the history of standards, the studies demonstrating the value of standards, the optimal timing for introduction of standards, their importance in determining the normal or reference values of populations, the priorities for standards, the criteria for and the stages in their preparations, the nature and continuity of units, the function of standards, and listed those available or well on the way.

So far I have not mentioned methods because I believe that it is counter-productive to insist that a standard methodology be used in all immunology laboratories even if any regulatory authority was in a position to do this. What is required is a reference or recommended method which if followed closely should give the correct value within the agreed limits to the standard material and by inference to other like materials. Given this, the user can both control his own method and set up his own laboratory standard for day-to-day use. By this it is implied that the reference method if correctly applied will enable the user to obtain results which he/she can confidently state are inside or outside the agreed normal or reference ranges for the population under consideration.

It must be self-evident that quality control and quality assurance, most important tools in any clinical laboratory, are more meaningful if they include the use of laboratory standards calibrated in terms of the appropriate national or international standards. Indeed, the biggest abuse of standards is to leave them in store and not to use them whenever the immunological reagents that they are intended for are used. The other most common abuse arises from a failure to take account of the complex nature of the active material being studied. It is always important to ensure that you are comparing like with like.

References

1. Bozoky, S. (1963). The problem of standardization in rheumatoid arthritis serology. *Arthr. Rheum.*, **6**, 641
2. Rowe, D. S., Anderson, S. G. and Grab, B. (1970). The research standard for human serum immunoglobulins IgG, IgA and IgM. *Bull. WHO*, **42**, 535

Part II
Applications of
Immunoassays

16
Steroid Immunoassays in Endocrinology

D. RIAD-FAHMY, G. F. READ, B. G. JOYCE AND R. F. WALKER

INTRODUCTION

Biochemical assessment of endocrine function is critically dependent on the development of accurate analytical procedures having the sensitivity required for determining the picomolar concentrations of steroid hormones in peripheral plasma. High throughput in such assays is also vital if results are to be made available in time to influence clinical decisions. Since immunoassays provide a unique combination of sensitivity and specificity they are well suited to the determination of steroid hormone concentrations.

SPECIFICITY IN STEROID IMMUNOASSAYS

Specificity in immunoassays is largely, but not entirely, dependent on the quality of the antisera; fortunately it is currently possible to generate antisera having predictable, well-defined specificity. It is now well accepted that in assays for steroids, and other small molecules, if haptens are coupled to a carrier protein through their functional groups this will interfere with the expression of these groups as antigenic determinants; the specificity of the antisera will therefore be low. Thus if anti-progesterone sera are prepared using progesterone-20-OCMO conjugates they show marked cross-reactivity, not only to other C-21 steroids such as deoxycorticosterone, but also to C-19 steroids such as testosterone. If progesterone is coupled through the B or C rings (Figure 16.1) the antisera discriminate more efficiently between related steroids[1,2].

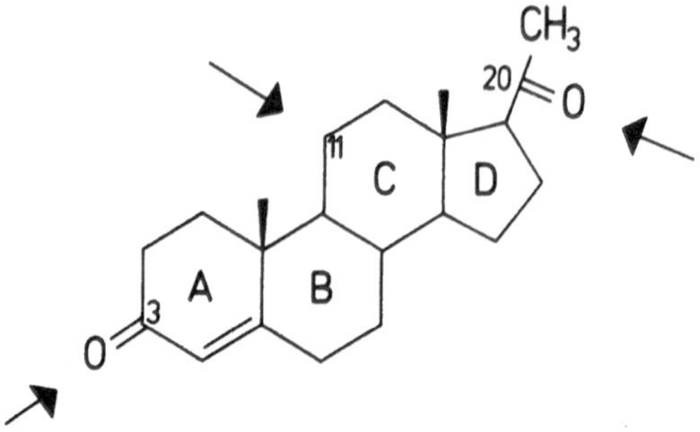

Steroid	Cross-reaction		
	P-20	P-3	P-11
Progesterone	100	100	100
Pregnenolone	1.1	13	0.5
17α-hydroxyprogesterone	98	4.6	1.2
Testosterone	95	0.05	0.04
11α-hydroxyprogesterone	7.1	13	34.5

Figure 16.1 Sites of conjugation of progesterone for generation of antisera, and specificity of antisera (data from ref. 8)

    While practically all possible sites for conjugation of steroids have been evaluated there is now a reasonable consensus on the optimum site to obtain specific antisera to the major steroid hormones. Thus most workers have successfully raised anti-progesterone sera using progesterone coupled through the 11α position, usually progesterone 11α-hemisuccinate. Specific antisera to oestradiol and oestriol have been conventionally obtained using 6-(O-carboxymethyl)-oxime derivatives[3] but equally specific sera may be obtained with the 3-(O-carboxymethyl) ether derivative[4] or with the 3-hemisuccinate providing the derivative is adequately purified[5].
    Antisera to cortisol have often been obtained using cortisol 21-hemisuccinate derivatives, but highly specific antisera are generated more reproducibly with cortisol 3-(O-carboxymethyl)-oxime conjugates[6, 7]. Specificity data are shown in Table 16.1. The immunoassay of testosterone raises interesting questions of specificity. Antisera are conventionally obtained using antisera to testosterone-3-(O-carboxymethyl)-oxime conjugates. Such antisera may cross-react with the major testosterone metabolite, 5α-dihydrotestosterone to an extent varying from 20 to 100%. This specificity is adequate to give accurate estimates of testosterone in male plasma but not in female plasma where the metabolite may be present in equimolar concentration[13]. Attempts to produce specific antisera reproducibly have utilized conjugation at 1, 6, 7, 15 and 18 but have not achieved outstanding success. Antisera with a cross-reaction of 10–30% with 5α-dihydrotestosterone may be generated repro-

Table 16.1 Relative specificities of various anti-cortisol sera

	Cross-reaction (%)				
	F-21-BSA[9]	F-21-BSA[10]	F-21-BSA[11]	F-21-BSA[12]	F-3-BSA[6]
Cortisol	100	100	100	100	100
11-Deoxycortisol (Reichstein's S)	–	9	10	100	7.1
Corticosterone	48	8	1.4	–	4
Cortisone	35	12	–	40	0.7
17-OH-Progesterone	–	2.5	–	56	<0.01
Progesterone	–	1.0	5.5	28	<0.01
Testosterone	7.5	0.3	–	13	<0.01

BSA: bovine serum albumin

ducibly to testosterone 11α-hemisuccinate conjugates. The major interference is then caused by 11β-hydroxy androgens, and these are readily removed by a simple, pre-assay, solvent partition stage[14].

An alternative approach is to use the available antisera but to separate the testosterone (T) and 5α-dihydrotestosterone (5αT). Obviously this may be achieved by chromatography but this is a slow, labour-intensive procedure. The Radiochemical Centre has pioneered an alternative approach in which the (T + 5αT) is estimated using a non-specific antiserum, then the testosterone is oxidized and the residual 5αT determined. The testosterone concentration may then be calculated. However the approach is theoretically unsound in that the cross-reaction of 5αT with a testosterone antiserum is not, and can not, be constant for all values of B/BO. It is theoretically more correct to construct a matrix using standards containing both T and 5αT[15] but the number of standards required makes the procedure impractical for routine use unless the assay is fully automated.

Another way of obtaining assay specificity is to incorporate a degree of sample purification prior to the immunoassay. In its simplest form this may be a solvent extraction which fulfils two functions: firstly it gives a uniform assay matrix free from serum-binding proteins, and secondly selection of a solvent of minimal polarity gives useful discrimination against more polar metabolites which may cross-react in the assay. The majority of anti-steroid sera require such a solvent extraction. Notable exceptions to this general rule are assays for cortisol. The specificity achieved in these direct assays is due partly to the specificity of the antiserum but mainly to the fact that circulating cortisol concentrations are high, and cross-reacting steroids are present in only low concentrations. In the absence of solvent extraction steroid-binding proteins are deactivated by low pH[16, 17] heat treatment[18, 19], enzyme digestion[20] or addition of ANS, that is 8-anilino-1-naphthalenesulphonic acid[21].

Choice of a suitable solvent is particularly critical in the assay of progesterone, where the use of petroleum ether from a different supplier may give significantly greater values, and the use of a polar solvent such as ethanol may give results up to three times higher. However it has been possible to develop a direct, non-extraction assay for 'progestins'. 'Progesterone' concentrations determined by the direct assay, at pH 4, and by an assay incorporating extraction with petroleum ether provided the data presented in Figure 16.2. While the direct assay gave results which were significantly higher than those obtained in the specific assay the same pattern of results was obtained.

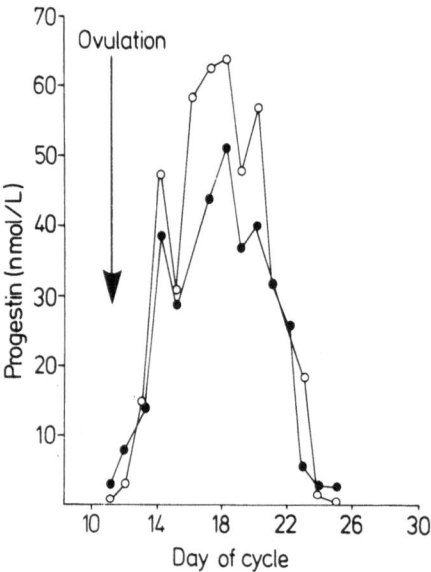

Figure 16.2 Progesterone levels throughout the menstrual cycle as determined by a routine solid-phase EIA (●) and the total 'progestin' EIA (○)

It is possible to use this simple, direct, readily automated EIA to determine 'total progestin' concentration in plasma samples obtained from women attending infertility clinics[22]. It may be argued that total progestin values, from samples taken every other day, will give a more useful indication of ovarian function than two accurate progesterone determinations, at approximately the same cost. The difference between the direct and extraction assays for progesterone is not totally explicable in terms of the known metabolites and their cross-reactions, although pregnenolone conjugates have been implicated[23]. The sacrifice of specificity to achieve high sample throughput will undoubtedly remain a serious drawback to the acceptance of fully automated procedures for most steroid hormones. It may be that exceptionally specific antisera, obtained by cloning of selected lymphocytes[24], may resolve this problem.

The use of chromatography for pre-assay purification will usually give accurate results, even with non-specific sera. Such techniques, whether column chromatography, thin-layer chromatography, or the more modern HPLC, are too time-consuming for routine clinical use. However the combination of a single chromatography step with determination of several related steroids has been advocated as an effective way of determining a steroid profile[25].

SEPARATION PROCEDURES IN STEROID IMMUNOASSAYS

The majority of assays in routine use continue to use dextran-coated charcoal for the separation of antibody-bound and free steroid in spite of the well-documented disadvantages of this technique. These include the restriction to small batch sizes inherent to this time-dependent procedure and the difficulties occasioned by batch-to-batch variation in commercially supplied charcoal. Also popular are second-antibody procedures, using sera raised in a second species to immunoglobulins taken from the species used to raise the primary serum. The possible presence of non-specific binding proteins in the second antibody, used at comparatively high concentration, and in the normal serum added to bulk up the precipitate, may be disadvantageous. The importance of ensuring that the second antibody has an affinity for the complete spectrum of immunoglobulins present in the first antibody has usually been neglected[26]. Less widely used techniques are precipitation of the bound fraction with polyethylene glycol and ammonium sulphate[27] and extraction of the free fraction with scintillant. The latter is obviously only applicable in a RIA and since the free and bound are not physically separated the procedure is again time-dependent.

LABELS USED IN STEROID IMMUNOASSAYS

Data provided by Supraregional Assay Centres and other laboratories in the United Kingdom indicate that most routine, clinical chemistry laboratories use RIAs featuring liquid-phase antisera and tritiated radioligands for determining steroid hormone concentrations. Few laboratories use ^{125}I-labelled steroids, and in only one centre is an EIA in routine use (Table 16.2). The RIAs using liquid-phase antisera and [^3H]-radioligands have the general format illustrated in Figure 16.3 and are the least cost-effective assay procedures. The steadily rising demands made on service laboratories indicate a pressing need for the introduction of more cost-effective procedures that do not require expensive new equipment.

The major disadvantages of radioimmunoassays featuring ^3H-labelled steroids include the high and ever-increasing cost of scintillant, the difficulties in automating such procedures, and the fact that β-scintillation counters are

H

Table 16.2   Steroid immunoassays in the United Kingdom: a 1980 overview

	Assay			
	T	*Prog.*	*E₂*	*17α-OH-Prog.*
Number of laboratories	35	44	35	9
Number using:				
RIA				
³H	30	40	35	9
¹²⁵I	5	3	0	0
EIA	0	1	0	0

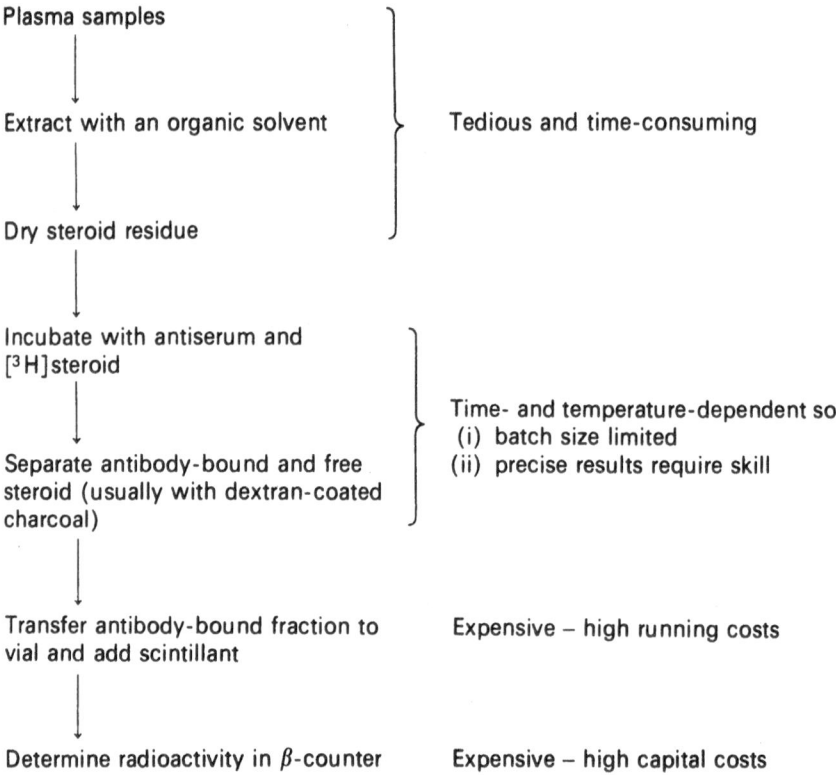

Figure 16.3   General format of conventional steroid RIAs and their disadvantages

single-channel instruments, and comparatively expensive. The latter restricts
the number of counts which may be economically accumulated, and makes
this the most time-consuming area of the assay procedure. The introduction of
relatively cheap, multi-channel γ-scintillation counters has effectively minimized the counter problem when using [¹²⁵I]-radioligands.

[125I]-RADIOLIGANDS

The introduction of reliable techniques for the preparation of [125I]-iodohistamine radioligands[28,29] has substantially reduced the cost of certain steroid assays including cortisol[17,30] and testosterone[31]. The high affinity of many anti-steroid sera for these radioligands[32] restricts their current usefulness, since it prevents development of sensitive equilibrium assays. This limitation may well be only temporary for the development of fully automated procedures with accurate time control may facilitate development of disequilibrium assays in which the high avidity of these labels may confer a considerable advantage. In certain instances a sensitive assay may be achieved by reducing the affinity of the antiserum for the radioligand by introducing a limited degree of heterology. Thus if antisera are generated using a progesterone-11α-chloroformate conjugate and a radioligand synthesized from progesterone-11α-hemisuccinate a sensitive assay can be developed[33].

In steroids lacking the angular methyl group at C-10 such as oestrone and oestradiol, the C-11 position is less sterically hindered, facilitating the synthesis of 11β-substituted derivatives. Thus an antiserum may be raised to a 11β-hemisuccinate derivative of oestradiol and [125I]iodinated oestradiol 11α-hemisuccinate tyrosine methyl ether used as label. The assay incorporating this 11α/11β heterology has adequate sensitivity (3.25 pg) for routine determinations of circulating levels of oestradiol in women[34]. The 11α-hydroxy derivatives of oestradiol are not available commercially, which has perhaps prevented the wider adoption of this procedure. It is, perhaps, surprising that these authors were able to iodinate the preformed conjugate since this will normally lead to iodination in the A-ring of the oestrogen with consequent loss of immunoreactivity[35,36].

In most laboratories limited counting facilities restrict the useful shelf-life of [125I]radioligands to about 60 days. This disadvantage, coupled with the health hazard in preparing the label and the general problems associated with disposing of radioactive waste, make alternative non-isotopic labels particularly attractive.

NON-ISOTOPIC STEROID IMMUNOASSAYS (NIIA)

An important advantage of NIIAs is that the end-point detection time may be extremely short, and that such assays may not require separation of antibody-bound and free antigen. These assays, not requiring a separation step, are known as *homogeneous* assays[37]; conversely assays requiring such a separation are known as *heterogeneous*.

Homogeneous assays have generally lacked adequate sensitivity to estimate circulating steroid levels, and their practical use has been restricted to the assay of drugs. An early homogeneous technique was that of Leute *et al.*[38] for morphine, based on the broadening of lines in the electron spin resonance spectrum when a morphine nitroxide label was bound to antiserum, so that the maximum peak height dropped significantly and only the free drug was detected. The most widespread homogeneous assays are undoubtedly the EIAs developed by the Syva corporation, termed EMIT. As yet the technique has not shown the sensitivity required for most steroid assays but it would appear to have the potential to determine circulating levels of cortisol and DHA sulphate, and oestriol in the pregnant female.

FLUORESCENT LABELS

Other homogeneous assays are based on the enhancement or quenching of fluorescence. Polarization fluorescence immunoassay has been applied to the estimation of oestradiol[39]. If a small, fluorescent molecule is irradiated by polarized light it will rotate freely during the lifetime of the excited state, and the polarization of the emitted light will be low. If the molecule is bound to a large antibody molecule, free rotation will be reduced, and the signal correspondingly enhanced. Dandliker and his co-workers synthesized a fluorescent oestradiol derivative, tentatively characterized as N-(oestradiol-6-imino-oxyacetyl)-fluorescein amine, and presented data (Figure 16.4) indicating binding of this label to an anti-oestradiol serum, this binding being

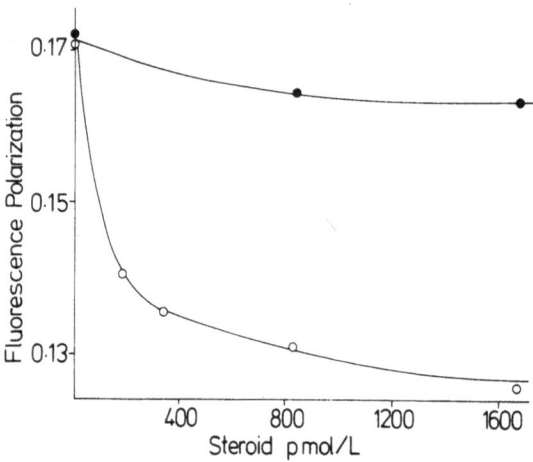

Figure 16.4   Fluorescent polarization inhibition curves of oestradiol (○) and progesterone (●) with an oestradiol/fluorescein conjugate. Taken from Dandliker et al.[39]

reduced by oestradiol and stilboestrol, but not by progesterone. The sensitivity of the procedure featuring fluorescence polarization may approximate to that achieved in RIAs but, as yet, practical assays have only been

reported for the determination of serum levels of gentamicin[40] and phenytoin[41]. Polarization FIA has a major disadvantage in that there is, at present,
no commercially available, relatively inexpensive instrument suitable for the
technique.

Heterogeneous FIA are essentially similar in format to RIA, and if solid-
phase antisera are used, have the advantage that non-specific fluorescent
compounds in the plasma can be removed by washing. Fluoroimmunoassays
for 5α-dihydrotestosterone and oestradiol have been reported with sensitivities comparable to those of the corresponding RIAs[42, 43]. Sensitivity in
these assays was achieved by the high molar incorporation (25 : 1) of the
fluorophore (4-methylumbelliferone-3-acetic acid) into the polylysine residue
of the steroid conjugates used as labels. These labels have long shelf lives and
are not associated with the 'quenching effect' observed in labels having a high
molar incorporation of fluorescein[44]. Difficulties involved in the tedious and
time-consuming preparation of these labels may restrict the use of these
otherwise excellent assays.

CHEMILUMINESCENT LABELS

Chemiluminescent molecules, like fluorescent molecules and enzymes, have
the advantage of prolonged shelf life and rapid end-point determination with
no radiation hazard. Luminol (5-amino-2,3-dihydrophthalazin-1,4-dione) is
a widely used chemiluminescent label and on oxidation in alkaline conditions
may be detected[45] at a sensitivity of 10^{-18} mol/l. This sensitivity of end-point
detection has not been reflected in the sensitivity of well-validated assays for
small molecules. One major difficulty has been that diazotization of the 5-
amino group leads to a reduction in the quantum yield. It is possible that
development of a second-generation luminescent label with greater tolerance
to substitution will overcome this problem. A more severe limitation is the
nature of the reagent blank effect. Simpson et al.[45] have stated: 'chemiluminescence offers a major advantage, particularly with respect to sensitivity, . . . in that detection is made against a background which is theoretically zero'. While the instrument background may be made insignificant, the
assay blank is several orders of magnitude higher. This is inevitable since the
luminol system contains alkaline hydrogen peroxide and this will react with
the amino groups of the antibody, and, more importantly, of the carrier
protein invariably required in dilute antisera solutions. Thus an extremely
sensitive chemiluminescent assay for a hapten would appear to require
development of a new class of chemiluminescent label or a modified assay
system.

The immunometric, or labelled-antibody assay using luminol appears to be
practical for proteins such as IgG[45], but the difficulties in applying the
radioimmunometric assay to steroids[46] make this approach unpromising.

Pratt *et al.*[47] have coupled a luminol derivative – provisionally 8-(4'-carboxymethylphenyl) - azo - 5 - amino - 1, 2, 3, 4 - tetrahydrophthalazine - 1, 4 - dione – and the hapten, testosterone 7α-carboxymethyl thioether, to ovalbumin. This complex then competes with testosterone for antibody, and following a second antibody separation chemiluminescence in the pellet is determined by addition of H_2O_2. The assay appears to lack adequate sensitivity but this would undoubtedly be improved by better instrumentation.

ENZYME LABELS

Enzyme labels are undoubtedly the most widely used of all non-isotopic tracers, and there are several recent reviews[48-52] and an international symposium[52] devoted to this topic. As noted by Schuurs and van Weemen[50], no single enzyme is ideal for use in all immunoassays but it was recently suggested (*Enzyme-Linked Immunospecific Assay for Infectious Agents*, National Institutes of Health, Bethesda, MD, USA, September 1979) that horseradish peroxidase is the most suitable enzyme currently available. The factors governing the choice of enzyme are listed in Table 16.3 and the enzymes most commonly used to prepare steroid conjugates are listed in Table 16.4.

In the pioneering studies of the group at Organon[53] horseradish peroxidase/steroid conjugates were used as enzyme labels, *o*-phenylenediamine/H_2O_2 being the substrate for colour development. This novel technique met with only limited success[54], for oestrone, oestradiol and oestriol EIAs lacked the sensitivity required for determining low steroid concentrations. Introduction of varying degrees of bridge site heterology into these assay systems improved sensitivity in some instances but only at the cost of decreased specificity. Although heterologous EIAs may allow better cross-matching of the affinity constants of the enzyme labels and the antigenic

Table 16.3 Criteria for choice of an enzyme label

---

(1) Availability of pure, low-cost, homogeneous enzyme preparations

(2) High specific activity

(3) Presence of residues through which the enzyme can be cross-linked to other molecules with minimal loss of both enzyme and antigen activity

(4) Stable enzyme conjugates

(5) Enzyme absent from biological fluids

(6) Assay method that is simple, cheap, sensitive, precise, and not affected by factors present in biological fluids

(7) Enzyme, substrate, cofactors, etc. should not pose a potential health hazard

---

Data from ref. 51

Table 16.4   Enzymes used as labels in EIA

Enzyme	Reference
Acetyl cholinesterase	59
Alkaline phosphatase	60
Carbonic anhydrase	Exley and Abuknesha (unpublished).
β-D-Galactosidase	61
Glucoamylase	62
Glucose oxidase	63
Glucose-6-phosphate dehydrogenase	64
Horseradish peroxidase (HRP)	54, 65
Lysozyme	37
Malate dehydrogenase	66

steroid[55] recent studies at the Tenovus Institute indicate it is possible to develop homologous EIAs having sensitivities equal to or better than the corresponding RIAs for both naturally occurring and synthetic steroids.

Early work at 'Tenovus' was very largely concerned with the factors influencing sensitivity in EIAs. These investigations featured a progesterone-11α-hemisuccinate/HRP conjugate as the enzyme label and a Sepharose-coupled antiserum raised in rabbits against a progesterone-11α-hemisuccinyl/BSA conjugate[56]. The lower limit of sensitivity[57] achieved in this system (200 pg/assay tube) was poor compared with the corresponding RIA using a tritiated radioligand. Decreasing the molar incorporation of the steroid into the enzyme label caused a marked improvement in sensitivity[26] (see Table 16.5). Other workers[58] have also noted that enzyme labels having

Table 16.5   Comparison of sensitivity data for RIA and EIA

Steroid		RIA (DCC)	EIA (Sepharose)	
E$_2$	MIR	–	11.0	2.2
	Sensitivity (pg)	2	62	17
P	MIR	–	7.0	37
	Sensitivity (pg)	1.9	200	105

MIR = molar incorporation ratio
DCC = dextron-coated charcoal

low molar incorporation ratios are required for the development of sensitive EIAs. It is therefore surprising that Comoglio and Celada[61] were only able to develop an EIA for cortisol using an enzyme conjugate having a high molar incorporation ratio (10:1).

Reports in the literature suggested that introduction of a liquid-phase separation procedure might well facilitate the development of sensitive assays[67, 68]. A liquid-phase sheep anti-rabbit second-antibody precipitation procedure was therefore used in the EIA for progesterone. This alternative separation procedure provided an assay having a sensitivity equal to that of the corresponding RIA[69] (see Table 16.6). Although suitable for determining

Table 16.6 A comparison of sensitivity data from RIA and various EIA procedures

	Separation procedure			
Steroid	RIA (DCC)	EIA		Cellulose
		Sepharose	Ab$_2$	
Oestradiol (pg)	0.7	17	2.0	–
Progesterone (pg)	1.9	105	1.8	4.0

DCC = dextran-coated charcoal; Ab$_2$ = second antibody.

progesterone concentrations in small plasma aliquots ($30\,\mu l$) this EIA required prolonged centrifugation times and this limited throughput. Later studies indicated that microcrystalline cellulose was a more suitable solid-phase support than Sepharose[22]. A system incorporating a cellulose-coupled anti-progesterone serum allowed development of a high-throughput EIA having a sensitivity comparable with that of the RIA (Table 16.6). A further advantage of assays featuring cellulose-coupled antisera is that magnetic particles can be incorporated into the solid-phase support and this facilitates mixing and obviates the need for centrifugation[70]. Theoretically a good separation procedure should not disturb the equilibrium between antibody-bound and free steroid; therefore all well-optimized systems should be equivalent. It is therefore difficult to reconcile the influence of the separation procedure on assay sensitivity, but this discrepancy has been noted by other workers[58,61]. A possible hypothesis would be that different solid-phase matrices alter the reaction rate, insensitive assays being caused by antibody and antigen reactions failing to approach equilibrium in a reasonable time unless high concentrations of reactants are used.

The solid-phase, homologous EIA for progesterone, using the cellulose matrix, provided results in good agreement with those of the RIA (Figure 16.5) and internal and external quality control data (Figures 16.6 and 16.7) suggest that the performance of this EIA is adequate for routine clinical use. External quality control questionnaires indicate that this is the only NIIA in current use in the UK for the routine determination of plasma steroid concentrations (Table 16.2). An alternative EIA for progesterone has been reported[71], but this procedure is difficult to evaluate and has not, to our knowledge, been used in clinical studies.

The development of an 'in-house' EIA for plasma oestradiol[72] followed very similar lines to those which had proved to be successful for progesterone

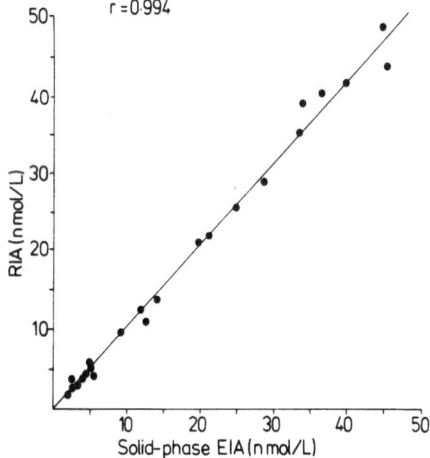

Figure 16.5 Comparison of results obtained by the solid-phase EIA and a RIA in routine use (n = 22)

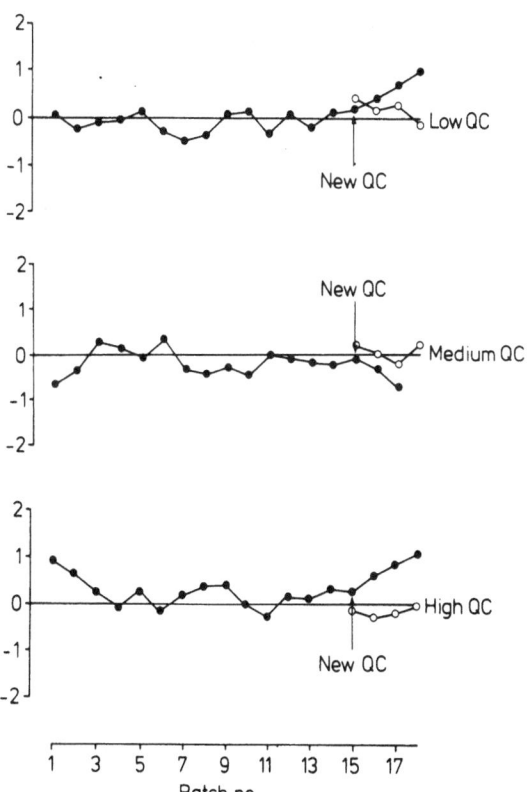

Figure 16.6 Internal quality control of the progesterone EIA

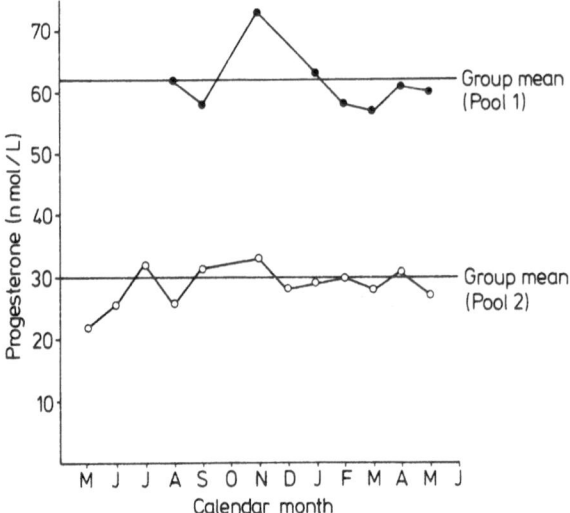

Figure 16.7 External quality control of the progesterone EIA

(Tables 16.5 and 16.6). In these studies an oestradiol-6-OCMO/horseradish peroxidase conjugate was used as the label and the immunogen used for raising the antiserum was oestradiol-6-OCMO/bovine serum albumin conjugate. This antiserum was coupled to cellulose and shown to be specific (Table 16.7). Use of this solid-phase antiserum and an enzyme label having a low

Table 16.7 Cross-reaction of structurally related steroids as determined by EIA and RIA

Steroid	Cross-reactions (%)	
	RIA	EIA
Oestradiol	100	100
6-Oxo-oestradiol	200	200
Oestrone	4.2	5.1
Oestriol	0.05	0.02
Dehydroepiandrosterone		
Testosterone	< 0.01	< 0.01
Progesterone		
Cortisol		

molar incorporation ratio allowed development of a standard curve covering the range (0–200 pg/assay tube) and precision was good. When this assay was used to determine concentrations of oestradiol in plasma samples having target values determined by GC-MS or by RIA the results obtained by the EIA were from two to five times greater than the target values. This discrepancy was not caused by lack of specificity of the antiserum but is believed to be due to the horseradish peroxidase of the label acting as a binding protein for oestradiol. It has proved possible to develop a dose–response curve for oestradiol using horseradish peroxidase as the binding agent since oestradiol and sodium azide compete for binding on horseradish peroxidase and when sodium azide is bound enzyme activity is very much reduced (Figure 16.8). This binding may only be significant in the development of sensitive assay systems because assays using horseradish peroxidase labels have been reported for total oestrogens[53] and oestradiol[73] in pregnancy plasma. In this context the studies of Exley and his co-workers are particularly relevant because they have focused attention on an alternative label, prepared using *E. coli* β-galactosidase, in immunoassays for oestradiol[74]. The oestradiol-6-OCMO/β-galactosidase conjugate was purified by affinity chromatography prior to use (Figure 16.9). Although this purification removed non-conjugated enzyme these workers noted that non-enzymatic protein conjugates would remain as contaminants in the label and these could have an adverse effect on sensitivity. The influence of heterology in this system was also investigated using anti-oestradiol sera raised against the homologous oestradiol-6-OCMO/BSA and heterologous oestradiol-3-glucuronide/BSA and oestradiol-3-hemisuccinyl/BSA conjugates. It was noted[55, 74] that sensitivity and specificity varied according to the antiserum used (E_2-3HS/BSA > E_2-3g/BSA > E_2-6-CMO/BSA). The heterologous combination

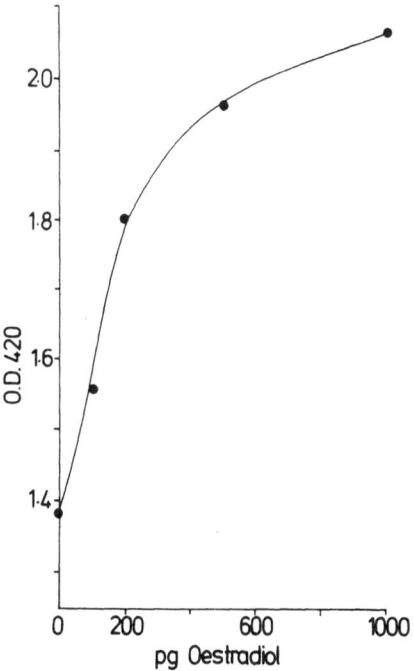

Figure 16.8 The effect of oestradiol on the activity of horseradish peroxidase in the presence of sodium azide (HRP-25 ng/tube; NaN_3-150 μmol/tube)

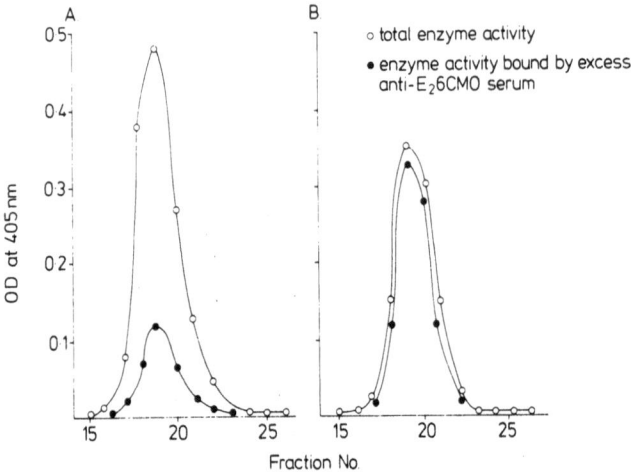

Figure 16.9 Sephadex G-25 column chromatograms before (A) and after (B) affinity chromatography of the *E. coli* β-galactosidase-$E_2$6–CMO conjugate[75]

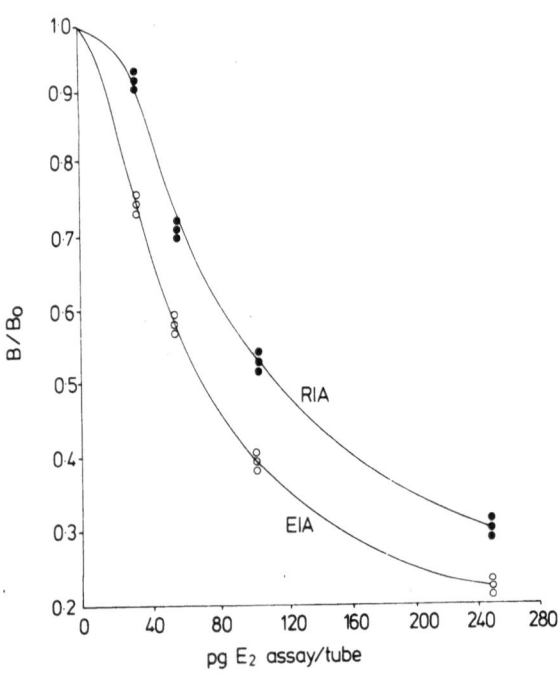

Figure 16.10 EIA and RIA standard curves for E_2

of anti-oestradiol-3-hemisuccinate serum and oestradiol-6–CMO enzyme label provided sensitivity and also retained specificity probably because the bridge/site difference occurred at a position not 'recognized' by the antiserum[5]. It will be interesting to see whether this sensitive system which features a dose–response curve covering the range 0–280 pg (Figure 16.10) when used for assay of plasma samples will provide results in agreement with target values determined by reference techniques. Arakawa et al.[58] in an extensive study of sensitivity vs. homology and heterology in EIAs for cortisol have also noted that bridge/site heterology at C-3 and C-6 provides a system having optimal sensitivity. The slight change in configuration in the system featuring cortisol-6β hemisuccinate/horseradish peroxidase and an antiserum raised against cortisol-6α hemisuccinate/BSA was found to be less sensitive than that using C-3/C-6 heterology.

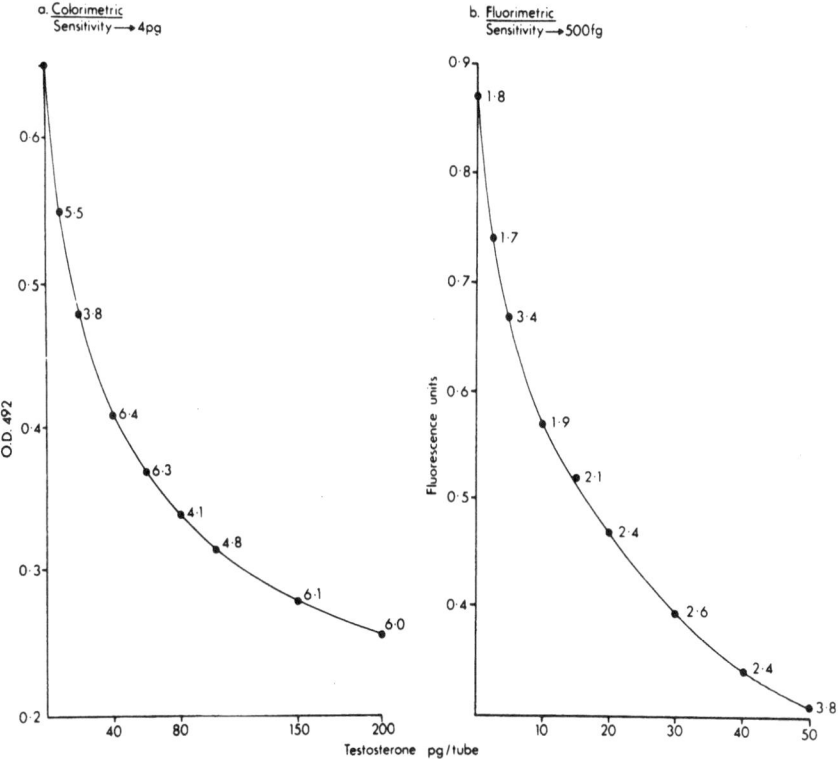

Figure 16.11 Composite standard curves for the EIA of testosterone by procedures incorporating colorimetric and fluorimetric end-points

Recent studies by the group at Organon[76, 77] suggest that the balance between sensitivity and specificity is best achieved in EIAs for testosterone using a heterologous system featuring an antiserum raised against an 11α-hydroxy-testosterone-11-succinyl/BSA conjugate and a testosterone-3CMO/horseradish peroxidase conjugate as label. This is in marked contrast to our findings and those of other workers[78, 79] which indicate that homologous EIAs have the sensitivity and specificity required for accurate determination of plasma testosterone concentrations. In the homologous EIA developed at Tenovus the cellulose-coupled antiserum was raised against a testosterone-11-hemisuccinate/BSA conjugate, and testosterone-11-hemi-succinate/horseradish peroxidase was used as label[80]. The dose–response curve in this procedure covered the range 0–200 pg and had a lower limit of sensitivity of 4 pg/assay tube (Figure 16.11) which compared favourably with other published procedures (Table 16.8). EIA of plasma samples provided results in good agreement not only with the RIA in routine use but also with a GLC-MS technique (Figure 16.12).

Table 16.8   EIA procedures for testosterone

Reference	Label	Volume of plasma (μl)	Range of standard curve	Sensitivity (pg)
81	T-3-Glucoamylase	500 ♂	0–10 ng	250
82	T-3-HRP	1000 ♂	0–2 ng	?
76	T-3-HRP	1000 ♂	0–2 ng	?
78	T-3-Penicilinase	100–500 ♂	0–800 pg	10–15
79	T-3-HRP	200 ♂, 500 ♀	0–300 pg	12
80*	T-11-HRP	20 ♂	0–200 pg	4
83*	T-11-HRP	100 ♀	0–50 pg	0.5

T-3: testosterone-3-O-carboxymethyl-oxime
T-11: testosterone-11α-hemisuccinate
HRP: horseradish peroxidase
  *: currently used at the Tenovus Institute

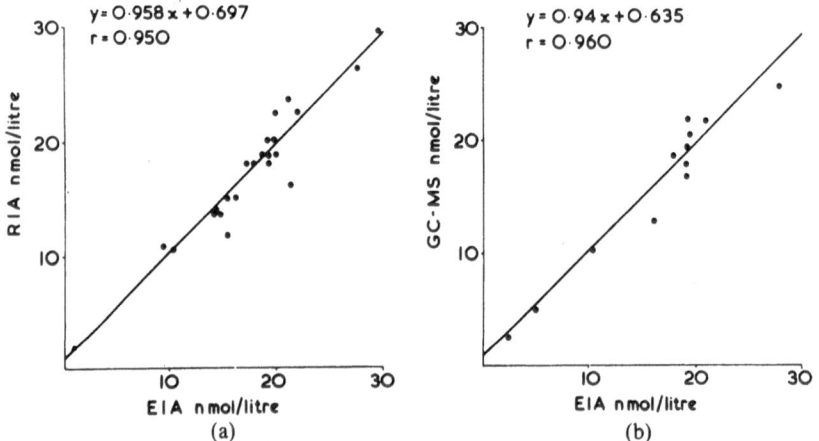

Figure 16.12 Correlation between results obtained in assays for plasma testosterone by (a) EIA and RIA; (b) EIA and GC-MS techniques ·

The sensitivity of the 'in-house' EIA for testosterone was improved by using a fluorimetric rather than a colorimetric end-point determination. In developing the fluorescence end-point three possible substrates were considered; tyramine hydrochloride, p-hydroxyphenlyacetic acid and homovanillic acid. The fluorescence produced by equivalent concentrations of tyramine hydrochloride and p-hydroxyphenylacetic acid were investigated: since the latter substrate gave greater fluorescence it was used in these studies. Homovanillic acid, reported to have approximately the same relative fluorescence as p-hydroxyphenylacetic acid[84], proved too costly for routine use. In this fluorimetric EIA (FEIA) the dose–response curve covered the range 0–50 pg, had good precision and a lower limit of sensitivity of 0.5 pg/assay tube (Figure 16.11). Testosterone concentrations in plasma and saliva samples collected by healthy women were determined by the FEIA[83] and a well-validated RIA[14]. The results obtained had the excellent correlation shown in Figure 16.13.

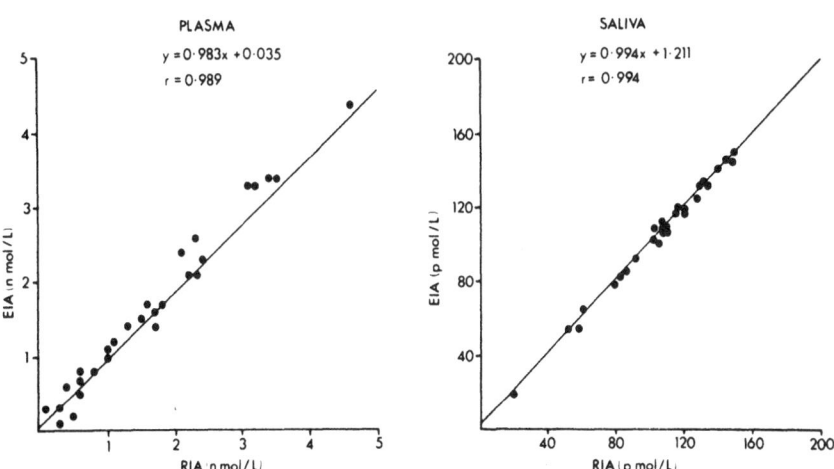

Figure 16.13 Correlation between results obtained by a RIA and EIA for plasma and salivary testosterone concentrations

The possibility of increasing the sensitivity of EIAs by using alternative end-point determinations is certainly attractive. In the study of Arakawa et al.[58], cortisol concentrations were determined by RIA and by EIAs having spectrophotometric, fluorophotometric and chemiluminescent end-points. The spectrophotometric EIA was found to have a sensitivity comparable with that of the RIA but EIAs having fluorimetric and chemiluminescent end-points had considerably better sensitivity (Table 16.9). In these EIAs the ligand used was a cortisol/horseradish peroxidase conjugate; the substrates for development of fluorescence and chemiluminescence being tyramine and luminol/H_2O_2 respectively. Other EIAs featuring alternative enzyme labels have been reported (Table 16.10). The homologous EIA for cortisol developed

Table 16.9 Sensitivity in cortisol EIAs[58]

End-point determination	Sensitivity (pg)
Spectrophotometric	100
Fluorophotometric	25
Chemiluminescence	5

Table 16.10 EIA procedures for cortisol

Reference	Label	Volume of plasma (µl)	Range of curve (ng)	Sensitivity (pg)
61	β-D-galactosidase	100	0–20	100/150
60	alkaline phosphatase	10	0–8	100
88	alkaline phosphatase	10	0–8	?
58	HRP	10	–	100
89	β-D-galactosidase	20	0–10	200
85	HRP	100	0–20	120

at Tenovus used a cellulose-coupled antiserum raised against a cortisol-21 hemisuccinate/ovalbumin conjugate and a cortisol-21 hemisuccinate/HRP conjugate as enzyme label[85]. It provided results, on assay of pathological samples, which were in excellent agreement with those of a reference GLC-MS procedure[17].

Consideration has recently been given to the nomenclature of NIIAs[86,87]. The EIA described above using luminol/H_2O_2 as substrate for the end-point determination would, using the Whitehead scheme, be known as LEIA. The signal derived from the luminol/H_2O_2 is weak, so alternative procedures featuring enzyme-linked luminescent systems (LEMIT) are attractive, as are those discussed earlier which involve labelling of steroid with suitable luminol derivatives (LIA). Development of these luminescent assays will not be hampered by lack of suitable equipment because a wide range of instruments is currently available[90].

EIAs, whatever their end-point, could well reduce running costs and increase throughput in routine clinical chemistry laboratories. 'In-house' immunoassays at Tenovus using [^{3}H]radioligands and liquid-phase antisera allow processing of only 30 samples/day and cost 30p/sample. Solid-phase EIAs, on the other hand, have twice this throughput and cost/sample is considerably reduced to only 10p. Sensitive specific EIAs for nearly all naturally occurring steroids of clinical value in assessing endocrine function have now been developed. Their more widespread use in routine practice will undoubtedly help to make results available in time to influence patient treatment.

The success achieved by EIA of naturally occurring steroids has encouraged the development of similar procedures for synthetic steroids. Such high-

Table 16.11 Antisera and labels used in EIAs for synthetic steroids

	Norethisterone (NE)	*Ethynyloestradiol* (EE$_2$)
Immunogen	NE-11α-hemisuccinyl/BSA	EE$_2$-6-(*O*-carboxymethyl)-oxime/BSA
Label	NE-11α-hemisuccinyl/HRP	EE$_2$-3-(*O*-carboxymethyl)-ether/HRP

BSA: bovine serum albumin; HRP: horseradish peroxidase.

throughput assays are required for processing the large sample numbers generated by fertility-control programmes and pharmacokinetic studies of synthetic steroids. EIAs for norethisterone and ethynyl oestradiol have been established at Tenovus since these synthetic steroids are widely used in contraceptive formulations. Details of the antisera and enzyme labels used in these EIAs are given in Table 16.11.

The data derived from cross-reactivity studies indicated that the norethisterone antiserum was specific, but that of ethynyl oestradiol showed unacceptably high cross-reactivity with the synthetic gestagens lynestrenol, *d*-norgestrel and norethisterone which could well be co-administered with ethynyl oestradiol (Tables 16.12 and 16.13). The conventional procedures for developing specific assays using non-specific antisera usually involve chromatographic purification. This time-consuming procedure, which precludes high throughput, was avoided in the assay for ethynyl oestradiol by using a solid-phase immunoadsorbent 'extraction' procedure[91]. A non-specific oestradiol antiserum having high cross-reactivity with ethynyl oestradiol but not with interfering gestagens was coupled to cellulose. Excess solid-phase antiserum was then used to 'extract' ethynyl oestradiol from plasma samples at pH 4. Following centrifugation the bound ethynyl oestradiol was removed from the antiserum with ethanol and assayed. This extraction procedure not only eliminated interference from cross-reacting steroids but also avoided the

Table 16.12 Cross-reactions of various steroids with anti-11α-hydroxynorethisterone-11-hemisuccinyl-BSA serum

Steroid	*Percentage cross-reaction*
Norethisterone	100.0
Norethisterone oenanthate	0.15
Norethisterone acetate	2.25
3α, 5α-Tetrahydronorethisterone	0.61
3α, 5β-Tetrahydronorethisterone	0.2
3β, 5α-Tetrahydronorethisterone	3.0
3β, 5β-Tetrahydronorethisterone	1.8
5α-Dihydronorethisterone	24.0
5β-Dihydronorethisterone	1.76
Oestradiol	<0.001
Testosterone	<0.1

'high blank' problems commonly associated with assays for synthetic steroids[83]. The specificity finally achieved in the EIA for plasma ethynyl oestradiol is indicated in Table 16.13.

Table 16.13 Specificity of the EIA for EE_2 with (+) and without (−) pre-assay solid-phase immunoadsorbent purification

Steroid	Percentage cross-reaction	
	−	+
Ethynyl oestradiol	100	100
Lynoestrenol	8.45	0.012
Norethisterone	8.45	0.015
Norgestrel	1.17	0.019
Mestranol	3.57	0.138
Oestradiol	0.059	0.007

− Cross-reactions determined by criteria of Abraham[92]
+ Cross-reactions following solid-phase immunoadsorbent purification

Table 16.14 Immunoassay procedures for norethisterone and ethynyl oestradiol

Reference	Label	Volume of plasma (μl)	Range of standard curve (pg)	Sensitivity
Norethisterone				
93	[^{125}I]NET	100	0–200	3 pg/tube
94	[^{125}I]NET	100	0–500	5 pg/tube
95	[^{3}H]NET	100	0–800	12.5 pg/tube
96	[^{125}I]NET	20–500	0–500	50 pg/ml
121	HRP-NET	10	0–150	3 pg/tube
Ethynyloestradiol				
97	[^{3}H]EE$_2$	?	0–2000	25 pg/tube
98	[^{3}H]EE$_2$	1000	0–500	25 pg/ml
91	HRP-EE$_2$	300	0–100	2 pg/tube

NET: norethisterone
EE_2: ethynyloestradiol
HRP: horseradish peroxidase

The dose–response curves used in the EIA for norethisterone and ethynyl oestradiol (Figures 16.14 and 16.15) had good precision, and lower limits of sensitivity were 3 and 2 pg/assay tube respectively. These sensitive EIAs for synthetic steroids provide results in agreement with well-validated 'in-house' RIA procedures (Figures 16.16 and 16.17). They also compare favourably with other recently published procedures using tritiated and iodinated radioligands (Table 16.14).

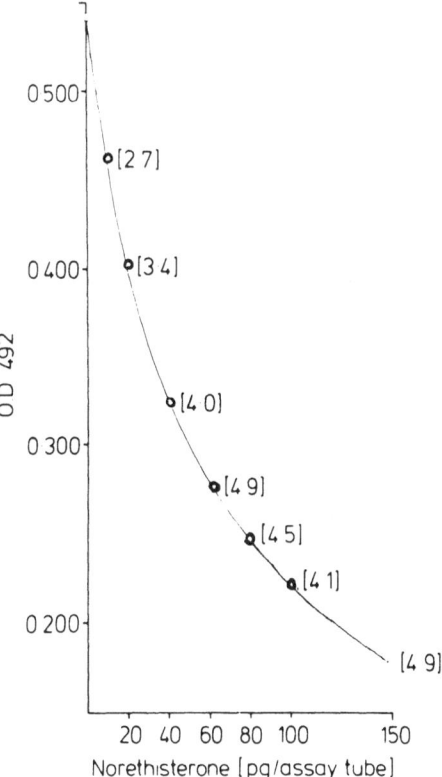

Figure 16.14 Composite standard curves for the EIA norethisterone

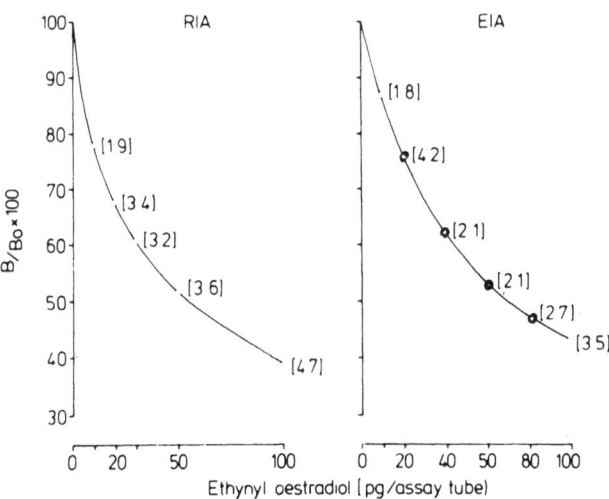

Figure 16.15 Replicate standard curves ($n = 12$) for ethynyl oestradiol used in the RIA and EIA

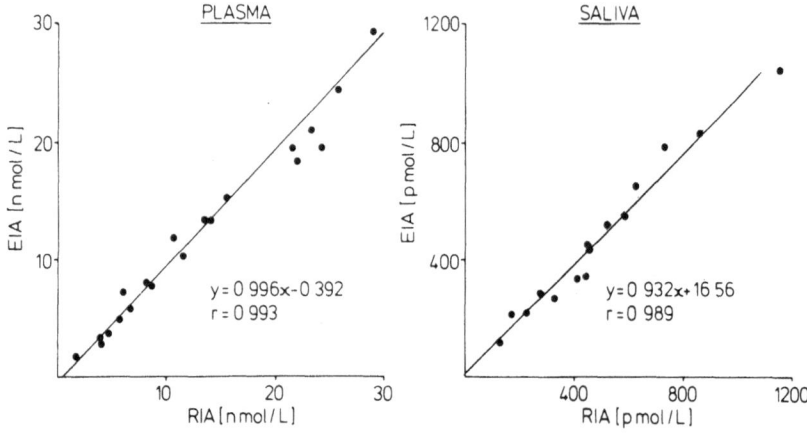

Figure 16.16   Norethisterone EIA: correlation between EIA and RIA for plasma and saliva

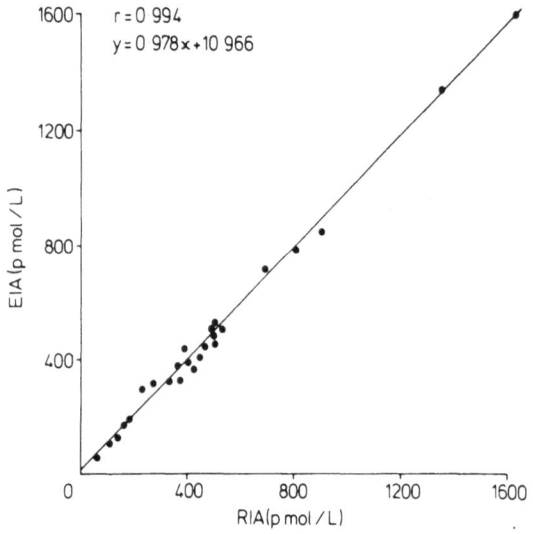

Figure 16.17   Correlation of ethynyl oestradiol concentrations in plasma determined by RIA and EIA

   In developing countries in which family planning is accepted as an essential factor in primary health care there is the need to establish simple assay procedures for synthetic steroids. Immunoassays featuring [³H] or [¹²⁵I]radioligands which have comparatively short working lives are not applicable since delays in long supply lines may well make such labels unusable on receipt. The stability of enzyme labels – coupled with the need for simple equipment, easily serviced and maintained by local technicians – make EIA the method of choice in such situations. A further problem in developing countries is the reluctance of subjects to agree to plasma sampling regimens. Assay of naturally occurring and synthetic steroids in saliva rather than plasma is therefore an attractive alternative.

SALIVARY STEROIDS FOR ASSESSING ENDOCRINE FUNCTION

The functional integrity of endocrine systems is currently assessed by collecting plasma samples before, during and after a variety of stimulation and suppression tests. Since plasma steroid concentrations fluctuate widely, multiple sampling regimens are required for accurate determination of 'basal' endocrine function. These sampling procedures are time-consuming for clinicians and may be disturbing for patients. Assay of steroids in saliva therefore has many advantages, in particular saliva samples can be easily collected at frequent intervals by patients themselves, and they find no difficulty in salivating directly into small glass tubes providing volumes of 3 ml in about 10 min. Salivary sampling regimens would also appear to be cost-effective since by saving clinician time and the cost of a syringe and needle the overall cost/sample ratio is considerably reduced.

Steroid concentrations in saliva appear to be independent of flow rate since the results obtained on assay of samples collected at normal and maximal flow rates were in excellent agreement (Figures 16.18 and 16.19). In these studies

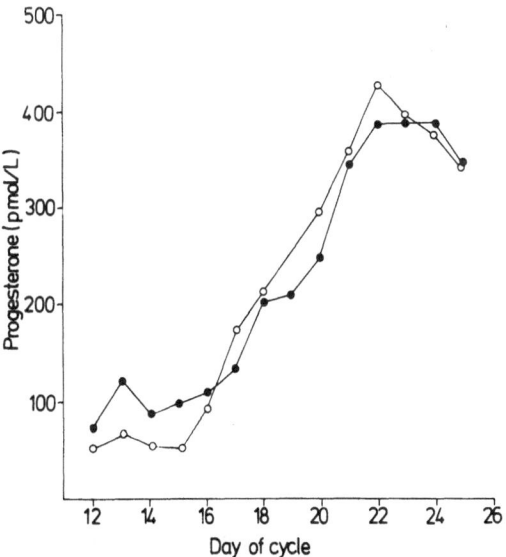

Figure 16.18 Progesterone concentrations in matched samples of parotid fluid (O——O) collected under citric acid stimulation, and of mixed whole saliva (●——●) collected with no stimulation, from a normal woman

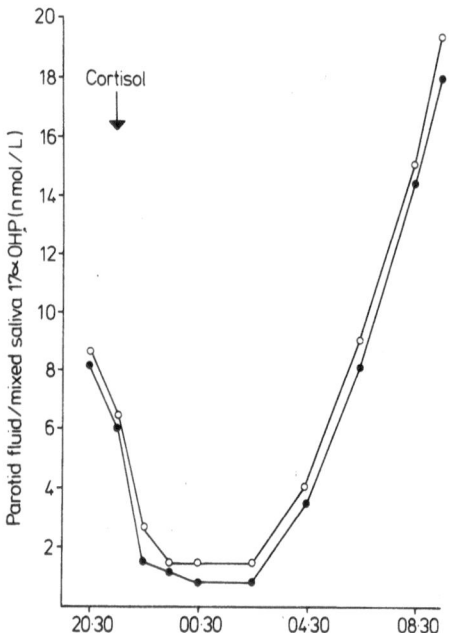

Figure 16.19 Concentrations of 17α-hydroxyprogesterone in matched samples of parotid fluid (●———●), collected under citric acid stimulation, and of mixed saliva (○———○) collected with no stimulation, from a CAH patient

maximally stimulated salivary flow rates were achieved by dropwise addition of a citric acid syrup to the tongue, problems of contamination being avoided by collecting parotid fluid using a modified Carlsen–Crittenden device[99]. This device, manufactured from moulded plastic, consists of an inner and outer well (Figure 16.20). Fine-bore metal tubes connect these wells to lengths of

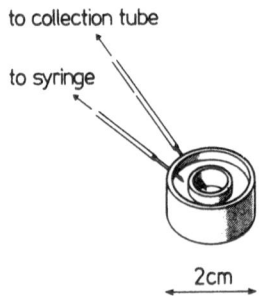

Figure 16.20 Modified Carlson–Crittenden device

lightweight plastic tubing. The tubing connected to the outer well is attached to a syringe (10 ml). The inner well is placed over the duct of the parotid gland and the device is held in place by applying slight negative pressure to the outer well by means of the syringe. The opening of the duct is easily located, appearing as a small white spot on the inner surface of the cheek near the upper second molar. Following dropwise addition of the citric acid to the tongue the parotid fluid drains from the central well through the plastic tube and is collected in a small glass tube.

Recent studies by New and her co-workers[100] on the determination of aldosterone concentrations in saliva indicate that salivary concentrations of this steroid are independent of flow rate provided that the volume of saliva collected is less than 4 ml. Other workers have also called attention to the need for small salivary sample volumes so that equilibrium between plasma and salivary steroid concentrations is maintained[101].

Steroid concentrations in matched samples of plasma and saliva show good correlation (Figures 16.21 and 16.22) and suggest that salivary steroids may

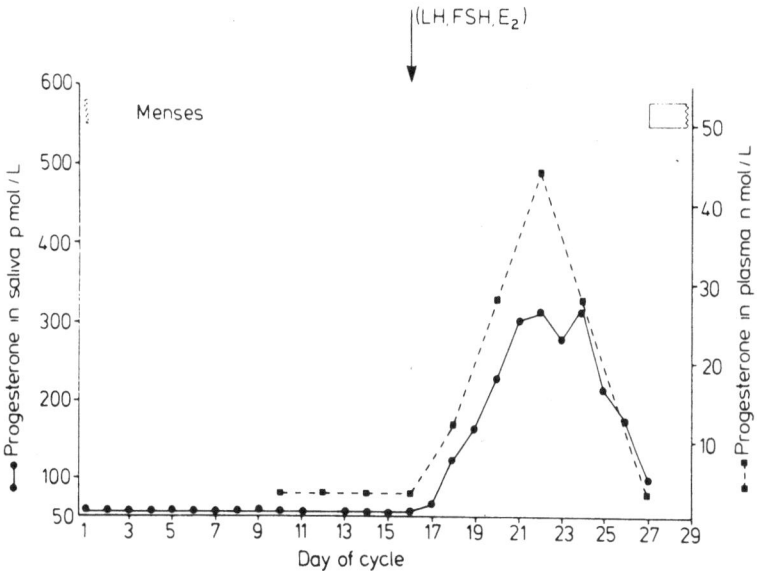

Figure 16.21 Progesterone concentrations in matched samples of plasma and saliva collected from a normal woman throughout the menstrual cycle

have a role to play in assessing endocrine function. Steroid concentrations in saliva are low, being only 2–10% of plasma values. Immunoassays suitable for determining the low concentrations of naturally occurring and synthetic steroids in small aliquots of saliva (10–500 μl) have now been established (Table 16.15). The clinical usefulness of salivary progesterone and testosterone concentrations for assessing gonadal function[91, 102, 103] and of salivary cortisol and 17αOH-progesterone in studies of hypo-thalamo–pituitary–adrenal defects has recently been determined[104, 105] Since this interesting new approach is proving to be of value a brief overview is presented in the following sections. In this context it is noteworthy that steroid

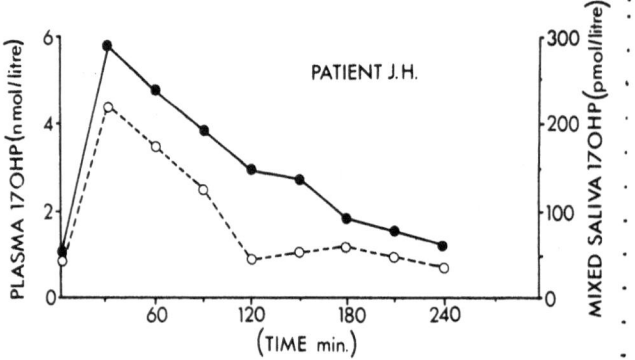

Figure 16.22 Concentrations of 17α-hydroxyprogesterone in matched samples of plasma (●—
—●) and saliva (○----○) collected from a CAH patient during the course of stimulation with
Synacthen (250 μg; i.m.)

Table 16.15 Immunoassays for salivary steroids

Steroid	Saliva volume (μl)	Sensitivity (pg/tube)	Current procedure
Cortisol	10	4	RIA
17α-OH progesterone	200	4	RIA
Progesterone	400	7	RIA
Testosterone	200	0.5	EIA
Norethisterone	100	3	EIA
d-Norgestrel	500	1	RIA

concentrations in saliva samples have shown no significant change when
stored at $-20\,°C$ for periods of at least 6 months.

Salivary progesterone

The routine biochemical investigation of women attending infertility clinics is
generally restricted to the determination of steroid concentrations in plasma
samples collected at fortnightly intervals; and these results, together with basal
body temperature (BBT) charts, are usually the only parameters available to
clinicians[106, 107]. It is now generally accepted that BBT charts are not a
particularly reliable guide to ovulation. The data presented in Figure 16.23
support this observation since in a healthy volunteer the BBT chart showed no
evidence for ovulation, but a normal preovulatory surge in plasma LH/FSH
was noted and progesterone concentrations in matched samples of plasma
and saliva were within the normal range in the luteal phase of the cycle.

The normal range for salivary progesterone concentrations (Figure 16.24)
was established by assaying the daily saliva samples collected by a group
($n=15$) of healthy women. These women, aged 18–34, also provided matched
plasma samples so dating of the cycle by the conventional method of

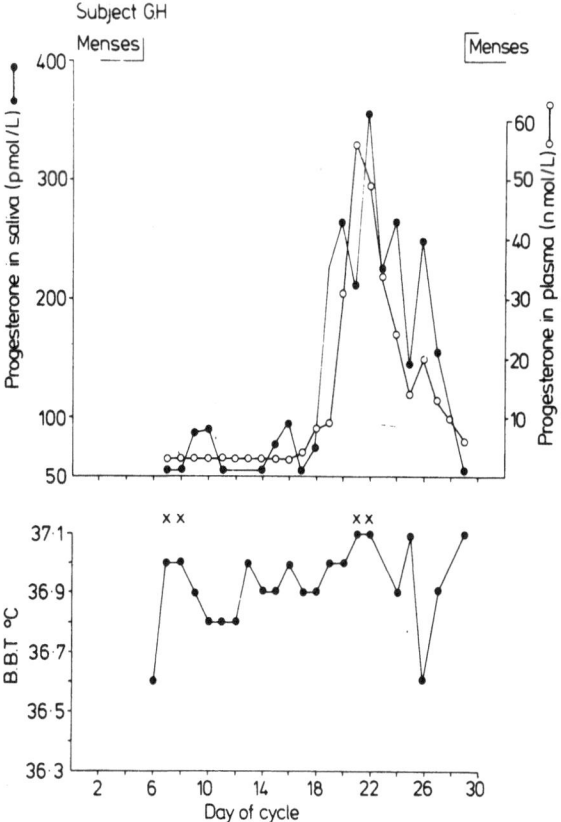

Figure 16.23 Plasma and salivary progesterone concentrations throughout the menstrual cycle of a normal female, and the corresponding basal body temperatures (BBT)

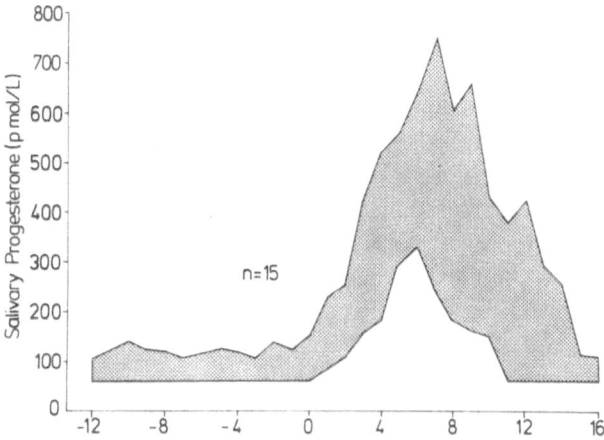

Figure 16.24 Salivary progesterone concentrations throughout the menstrual cycle in a group of normal women ($n = 15$). Day 0 represents the maximum LH/FSH level determined in corresponding plasma samples

determining polypeptide (LH/FSH) and steroid (oestradiol/progesterone) concentrations was possible. In the follicular phase of the cycle, salivary progesterone levels rarely exceeded 100 pmol/l, but in the early luteal phase salivary progesterone concentrations increased and peak values ranging from 300 to 800 pmol/1 were observed in the mid-luteal phase of the cycle. Progesterone levels declined just prior to menstruation[102] and at menses were usually less than 150 pmol/l. Another group of women ($n = 10$) aged 21–41 who were menstruating normally agreed to collect daily saliva samples but refused venepuncture. Progesterone concentrations in these saliva samples were within the normal range (Figure 16.25).

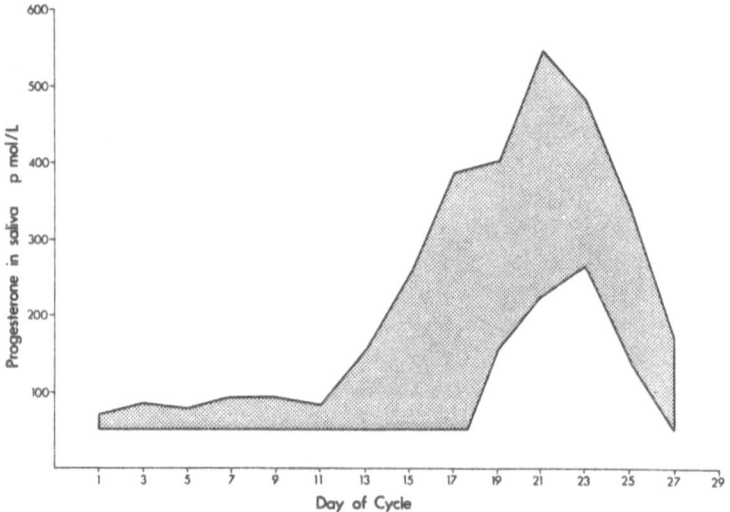

Figure 16.25 Salivary progesterone concentrations throughout the menstrual cycle determined in ten normal women

Assay of daily saliva samples collected for not less than 30 days by patients attending an infertility clinic provided interesting data (Figure 16.26). Consistently low levels were observed in a patient (P.D.) with primary amenorrhoea. In another patient (L.D.) with the suspected luteal phase syndrome salivary progesterone levels were consistent with this diagnosis, being well below the normal range in the latter part of the cycle. A third patient (I.C.) had a bizarre pattern, progesterone levels being high at the beginning and end of her so-called cycle. This odd pattern was only revealed by serial sampling: it would most probably have remained undetected by the standard procedure of collecting one or at most two plasma samples per month.

Salivary progesterone concentrations may be used to monitor treatment of infertile women with bromergocryptine and clomiphene (Clomid; Merrell); representative data from such patients being presented in Figures 16.27–16.29.

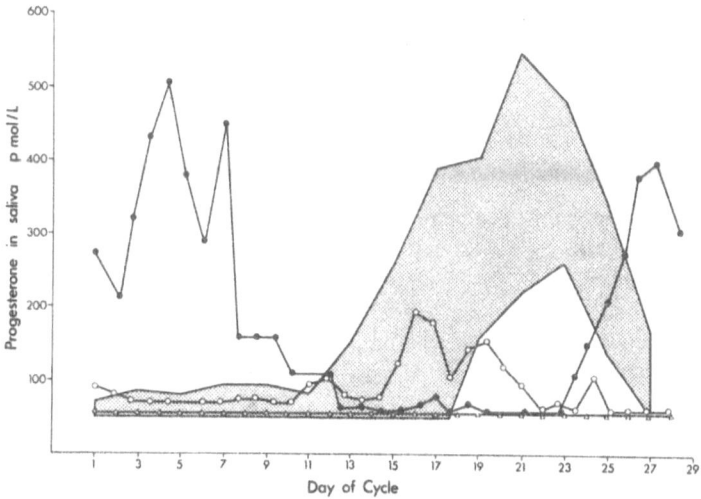

Figure 16.26 Salivary progesterone concentrations determined throughout the menstrual cycle in women attending an infertility clinic: the dotted area shows the normal range; Δ——Δ, subject P.D.; ○——○, subject L.D.; ●——●, subject I.C.

In one hyperprolactinaemic patient circulating prolactin concentrations were 183 mIU/ml: it was therefore not surprising to find that the woman was amenorrhoeic and had consistently low salivary progesterone concentrations prior to treatment (Figure 16.27).

Following treatment with gradually increasing doses of bromergocryptine (Parlodel; Sandoz), prolactin concentrations fell to about 35 mIU/ml; the rising salivary progesterone concentrations associated with normal prolactin levels indicated the improved ovarian function in this patient. In the luteal phase of the cycle which followed a short interval of bleeding, salivary progesterone concentrations rose steadily and were within the normal range. Subsequent routine investigations revealed that this patient conceived during this cycle.

In another infertile patient (Figure 16.28) salivary progesterone levels were below the normal range during the luteal phase of the pretreatment cycle, suggesting that this patient had the luteal phase deficiency syndrome. Following menstruation, clomiphene (50 mg) was administered for five consecutive days and in the luteal phase of this cycle salivary progesterone concentrations were within the normal range. It is interesting to note that in other infertile patients administration of an increased dose of clomiphene (100 mg) may well cause excessive stimulation since luteal phase salivary progesterone concentrations were considerably greater than those observed in normal women, values (Figure 16.29) ranging from 1200 to 2000 pmol/1 in the mid-luteal phase. Elevated plasma progesterone concentrations have also been reported in patients given high doses of clomiphene[108].

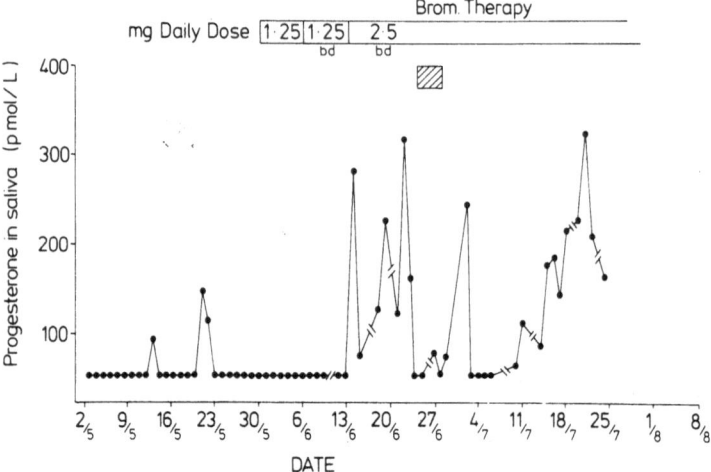

Figure 16.27 Salivary progesterone concentrations in a hyperprolactinaemic woman before and during treatment with bromergocryptine

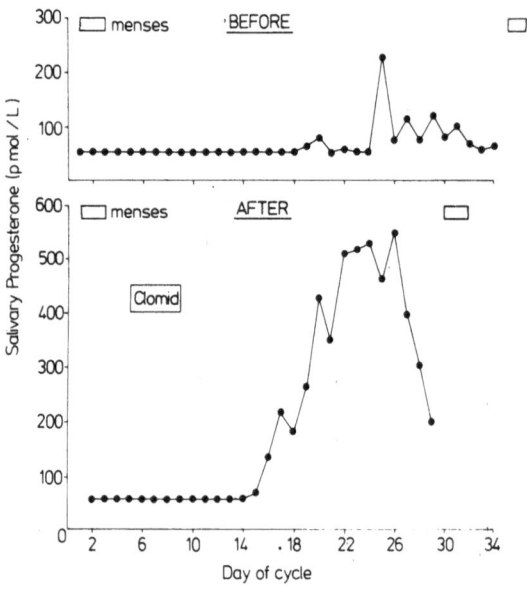

Figure 16.28 Daily salivary progesterone concentrations in a female subject before and after clomiphene treatment (50 mg/day)

In this context an assay for salivary oestradiol would obviously be of value but problems of sensitivity are restricting development of this assay. Present evidence would suggest that an assay having a lower limit of sensitivity of 50 fg/assay tube would be required to determine E_2 concentrations in small

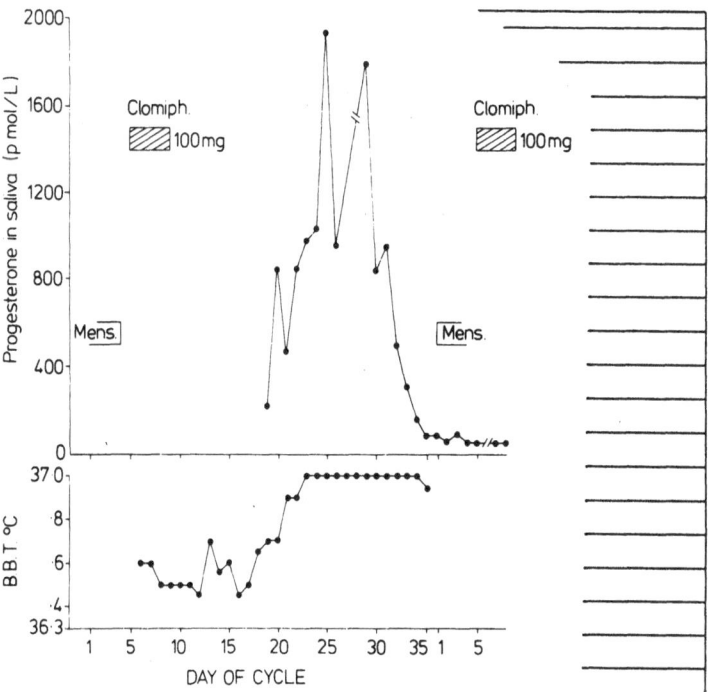

Figure 16.29 Characteristic salivary progesterone concentrations in an infertile patient during treatment with clomiphene (100 mg/day)

volumes (1 ml) of saliva; since the relatively low levels of E_2 circulating in plasma are largely bound by plasma proteins[109] and little free steroid is available for uptake by the salivary gland.

Salivary testosterone

Reports in the literature suggest that plasma 'free' testosterone[110, 111] may provide information of greater diagnostic significance than that of 'total' hormone concentrations in infertile hirsute women. Since the determination of plasma 'free' steroid concentrations is technically difficult such assays are not suitable for routine service needs. Testosterone concentrations in saliva which could well reflect the free fraction in plasma may therefore be particularly useful in these patients[83].

The normal range for salivary testosterone concentrations throughout the menstrual cycle was established by assaying the daily samples provided by a group ($n = 10$) of healthy women aged 21–34 who were known to be menstruating regularly (Figure 16.30). Since matched plasma samples were also available it was possible to date the cycles by conventional procedures. In the follicular phase of the cycle salivary testosterone concentrations were about 120 pmol/l. Just prior to ovulation levels increased and at ovulation

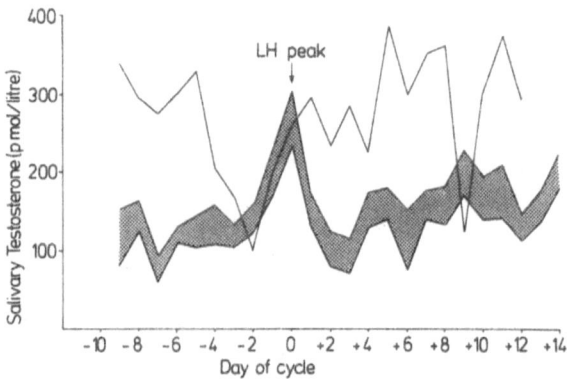

Figure 16.30 Salivary testosterone concentrations (mean + SEM) in a group of normal females (*n* = 10). Comparative data from an infertile hirsute patient (H.D.) are also shown

reached maximum values ranging from 220 to 300 pmol/1. Levels declined after ovulation, and in the luteal phase of the cycle were approximately 150 pmol/1. These results are in keeping with those of Abraham[112] who also noted a marked rise in plasma testosterone concentrations just prior to ovulation (Figure 16.31).

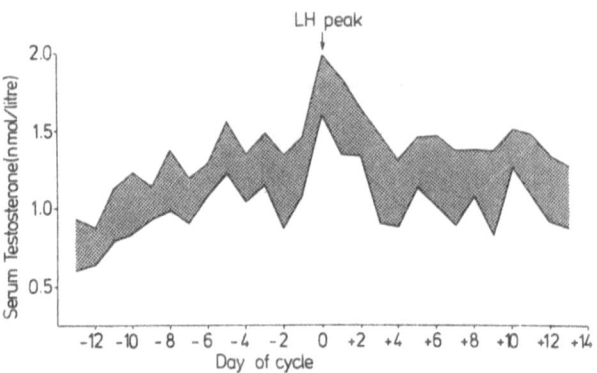

Figure 16.31 Serum testosterone concentrations (mean + SEM) during two consecutive cycles in normal females (*n* = 6). Redrawn from data of Abraham[112]

In four infertile hirsute patients plasma testosterone concentrations were within the normal range (0.3–2.5 nmol/l). In only one of these four patients were salivary testosterone levels above the normal range (patient H.D.; Figure 16.30). This woman was amenorrhoeic so it was not surprising to find that the rhythmic changes in testosterone levels which characterize normal cycles were lacking. Since salivary steroid concentrations reflect the 'free' fraction in plasma this patient may well have elevated plasma 'free' testosterone concentrations due to reduced binding by sex hormone binding globulin[113]

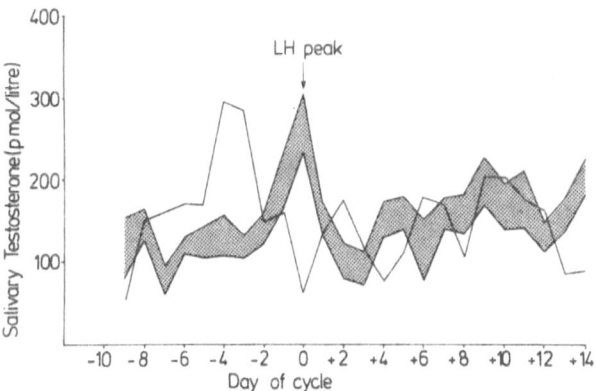

Figure 16.32   Salivary testosterone concentrations (mean + SEM) in normal females ($n = 10$) and an infertile, hirsute patient (S.B.)

Data derived on assay of samples provided by patient S.B. (Figure 16.32) are representative of 3 patients having normal plasma and salivary testosterone concentrations. In this patient, who collected saliva samples daily for 27 consecutive days following an interval of bleeding, the mean testosterone concentration was 150 pmol/l. These three patients all had oligomenorrhoea so the rhythmic pattern in salivary testosterone concentrations was absent. Hirsutism in these women may well be caused by increased activity of the 5α-reductase enzyme system or of receptor proteins in target tissues[13]. In this context it is interesting to note that Smith *et al.*[101], have reported the value of determining the 'androgenic status' of hirsute women based on salivary sampling regimens. These workers have noted that the ratio of 5α-dihydrotestosterone/testosterone has greater clinical significance in these patients than testosterone alone.

The determination of salivary testosterone levels may also be useful in studies of male infertility since in a group of normal men undergoing a typical 3-day stimulation test with human chorionic gonadotrophin (HCG) (5000 IU/day) the rising levels of testosterone in plasma were accurately reflected in saliva (Figure 16.33). The true value of this assay in investigations of male infertility remains to be assessed. In this context it is interesting to note that testosterone assays most probably have only a minor role to play in such investigations. The close juxtaposition of the testosterone-producing (Leydig) cells and the target (Sertoli) cells occurring in testicular tissue is unique. Circulating testosterone concentrations need not of necessity reflect those in the environment of the Sertoli cells[114]; assays for plasma and salivary testosterone may therefore be of little diagnostic significance in male infertility studies.

The assay for salivary testosterone has proved to be of value in demonstrating a well-defined circadian rhythm in testosterone secretion in normal

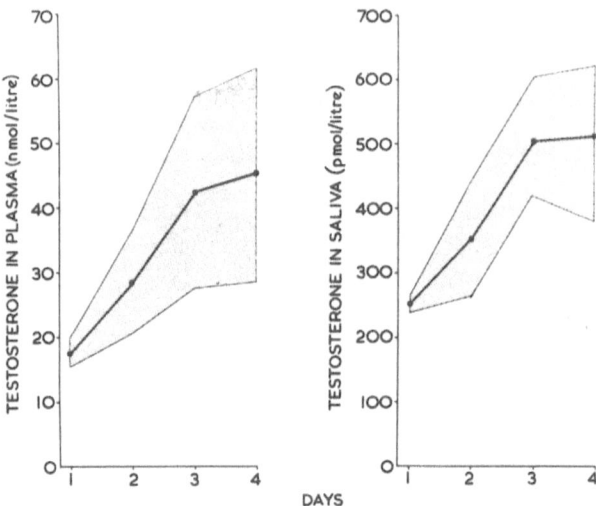

Figure 16.33 Response of testosterone in plasma and saliva to stimulation with HCG (5000 IU/day) for 3 days in a group of normal males

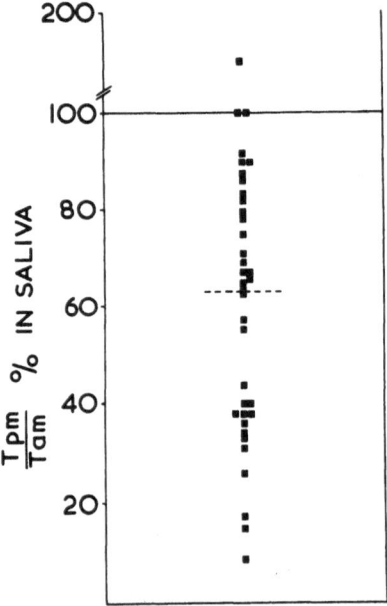

Figure 16.34 Changes in testosterone concentrations in saliva from 36 normal males – levels of testosterone in evening samples (Tpm) are expressed as a percentage of the matched morning samples (Tam)

men[103]. A group of 36 healthy men collected saliva samples on waking and just prior to sleeping. Salivary testosterone levels showed a well-defined circadian rhythm in all but three cases; the mean testosterone concentration in evening samples being about 60% of that observed in early morning samples (Figure 16.34). In a more detailed study a group ($n=9$) of healthy men collected saliva samples at 2 h intervals during waking hours. The mean testosterone concentration in early morning samples was approximately 300 pmol/l, levels declined during the day and in late evening samples were around 150 pmol/l (Figure 16.35).

The influences of a change in activity patterns on the rhythm of testosterone secretion has recently been investigated. Four men who were on a normal day/night schedule collected saliva samples at 2 h intervals during waking hours. They then changed their schedule and for 4 days they got up at

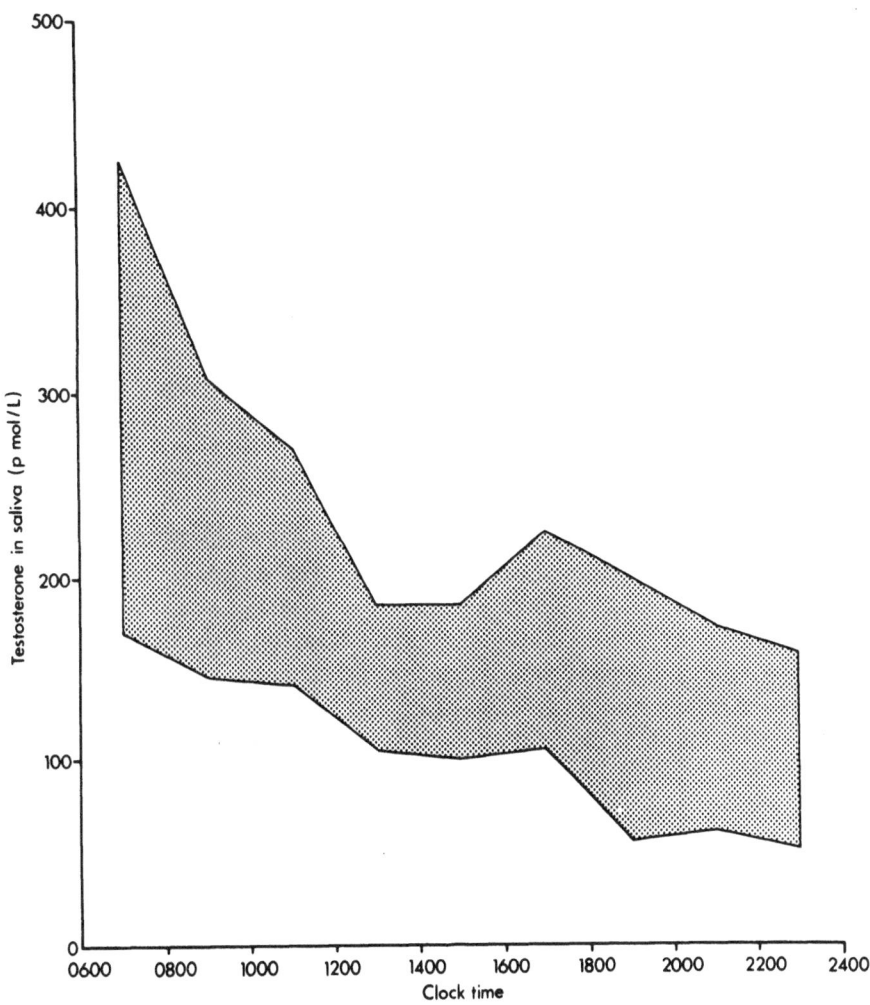

Figure 16.35 Concentrations of testosterone in saliva collected from six normal males at 2 h intervals: shaded area represents mean + SD

I

midnight and went to bed at 4 p.m. Representative data from one of these men (Figure 16.36) indicate that on the normal day/night schedules testosterone

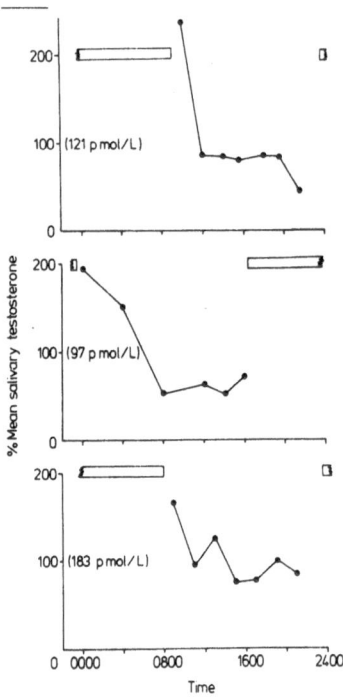

Figure 16.36 Circadian variation in salivary testosterone concentrations in a normal male, illustrating the effect of an altered activity cycle. Horizontal column indicates sleep period

levels were high at 9 a.m. When the schedules were altered testosterone levels at this time were low. This phase shift in testosterone secretion occurred on all 4 days of the altered schedule in all four participants. It was interesting to find that the circadian rhythm in salivary F shows little if any phase shift during this 4-day altered schedule. The men participating in this study were members of an expedition to Spitzbergen and while on this trip they were exposed to continuous daylight and ambient temperatures of 5–10 °C. The samples they collected together with QC samples taken from the UK were stored in ice-cold streams until their return to base camp[115]. It is possible that this assay, which can detect clear-cut changes in the rhythm of testosterone secretion, may also prove useful in research programmes designed to detect any subtle differences in secretion rates in normal men and prostatic cancer patients[103].

Salivary cortisol

It is interesting to note that the radioimmunoassay used for determining salivary cortisol concentrations differs from other salivary steroid assays in that the additional specificity conferred by solvent extraction is not required. It has proved possible to develop a direct assay for cortisol in saliva and since cortisol-binding proteins in saliva are lacking this direct assay can be performed at pH 7.4[116]. The direct assay for salivary cortisol was shown to be specific since samples assayed by this procedure and by a reference GC-MS technique provided results which were in excellent agreement.

In a group of healthy volunteers ($n = 10$) salivary cortisol concentrations showed a well-marked circadian rhythm (Figure 16.37); maximum levels of

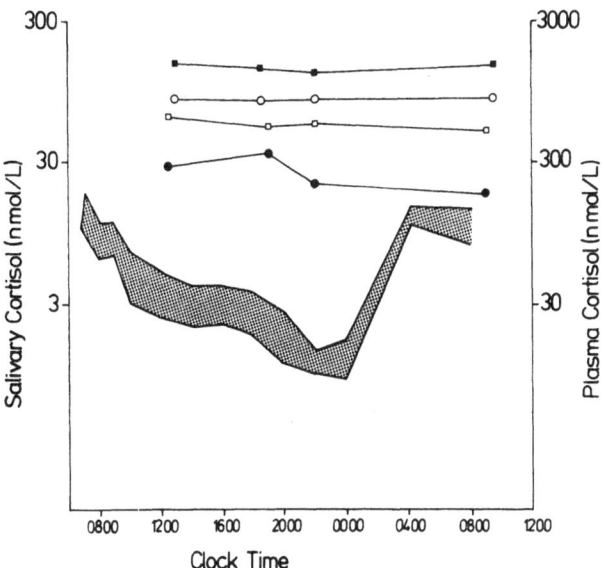

Figure 16.37 Diurnal variates in salivary cortisol concentrations in a group of normal subjects ($n = 10$). Also shown are plasma and salivary cortisol concentrations in two Cushingoid subjects. Patient A □ = saliva, ■ = plasma; Patient B ● = saliva, ○ = plasma

around 15 nmol/l being observed in early morning samples. These levels fell during the day and in the late evening were only 1 nmol/l. In two Cushingoid patients this rhythm was absent and levels of cortisol were high in both plasma and saliva. Patient A had an ectopic ACTH-producing tumour so it is not surprising to find high cortisol concentrations in plasma (1500 nmol/l) and saliva (80 nmol/l). Another devoted volunteer provided matched samples of plasma and saliva at 15 min intervals from 8 a.m. to 8 p.m. The falling cortisol concentrations in plasma were accurately reflected in saliva. The bursts of adrenal secretory activity causing lower amplitude fluctuations are seen equally well in saliva as plasma (Figure 16.38).

Normal volunteers who gave informed consent for a typical Synacthen stimulation test (Figure 16.39) had baseline cortisol concentrations in plasma

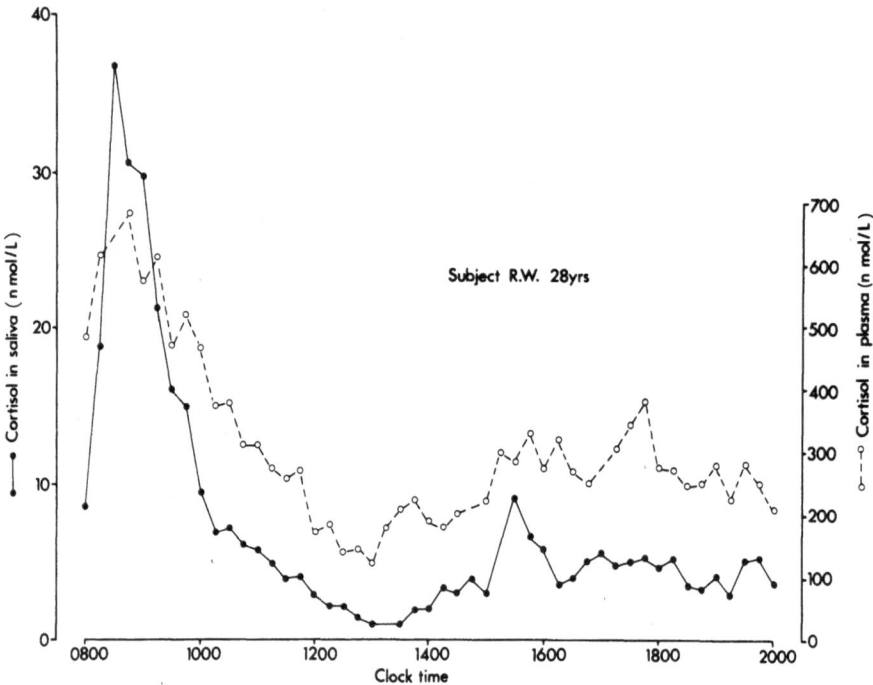

Figure 16.38 Cortisol concentrations in matched plasma and saliva samples collected from a normal male at 15 min intervals throughout a 12 h period

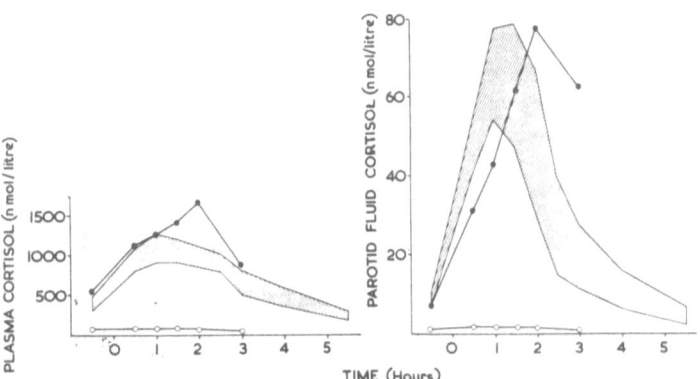

Figure 16.39 Response of plasma and salivary cortisol concentrations in a group of normal volunteers ($n = 7$) to adrenal stimulation with Synacthen (250 μg; i.m.). Also shown are the response of a patient with adrenal atrophy and a subject taking an oestrogen-containing contraceptive preparation. ○ Subject with adrenal atrophy, ● subject taking oestrogen contraceptive preparation, ▨ normal plasma cortisol response mean $\pm$ SD $n = 7$ ▨ normal parotid fluid cortisol response mean $\pm$ SD; $n = 7$

of 450 nmol/l; those in saliva were much lower, being only 10 nmol/l. Following Synacthen stimulation cortisol concentrations rose, reaching peak values in both plasma and saliva after 1 h. Plasma cortisol concentrations rose 3-fold but those in saliva showed an 8-fold rise. This difference probably occurred because the high circulating cortisol levels saturate available binding sites on transcortin. A disproportionate rise in the 'free' steroid fraction therefore occurs in plasma, which is reflected in the saliva concentration.

Oestrogens, both naturally occurring and synthetic, are known to increase circulating transcortin concentrations[117]. It is therefore not surprising to find that, in women taking an oestrogen-containing contraceptive preparation, baseline plasma cortisol levels are slightly elevated and a greater than normal response is observed on Synacthen stimulation. In marked contrast matched samples of saliva had baseline cortisol concentrations within the normal range and following Synacthen stimulation a normal, but slightly delayed, response occurred. A patient with secondary adrenal atrophy showed no response to Synacthen stimulation since plasma and salivary cortisol levels remained consistently low.

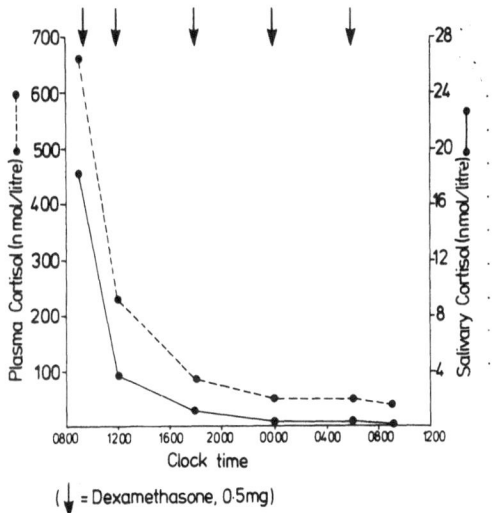

Figure 16.40 Cortisol concentrations in plasma and saliva samples collected from a normal volunteer following adrenal suppression with dexamethasone

The data presented in Figure 16.40 were obtained on assay of matched samples of plasma and saliva before and after administering a standard dose of dexamethasone to a healthy volunteer. Cortisol concentrations in saliva reflected those in plasma, suggesting that decreased adrenal function following dexamethasone treatment could be monitored equally as well in saliva as plasma.

A Cushingoid patient known to have an adrenal tumour provided matched plasma and saliva samples before and after administering metyrapone. This compound, by inhibiting the 11β-hydroxylase enzyme system, causes a marked reduction in the biosynthesis of cortisol by adrenal tissue. The decreased adrenal secretion of cortisol in this patient was indicated by the falling concentrations in both plasma and saliva (Figure 16.41). Cortisol levels

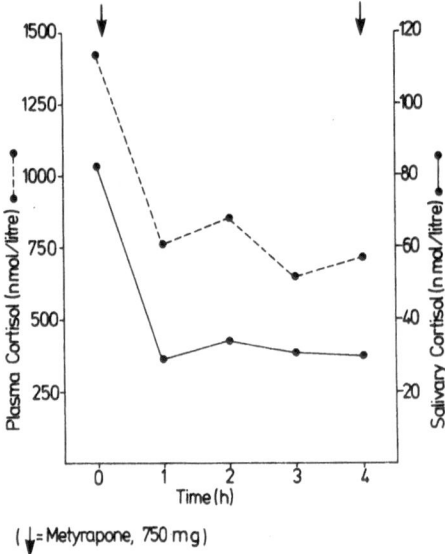

(↓ = Metyrapone, 750 mg)

Figure 16.41   Cortisol concentrations in plasma and saliva samples collected from a patient with Cushing's syndrome following administration of metyrapone

in plasma and saliva show excellent correlation, suggesting that the response to metyrapone could be monitored by salivary sampling regimens. It is noteworthy that this patient collapsed after 4 h and the full dose of metyrapone could not be administered. These results would suggest that salivary cortisol concentrations not only reflect basal adrenal function but also the change in adrenal secretory activity following a variety of stimulation and suppression tests.

Salivary 17α-hydroxyprogesterone

In patients having congenital adrenal hyperplasia (CAH) adrenal function is usually defective due to a C-21 hydroxylase enzyme deficiency (Figure 16.42).

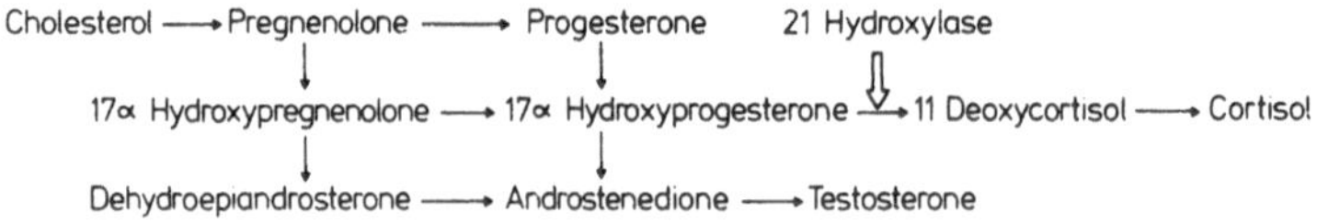

Cholesterol ⟶ Pregnenolone ⟶ Progesterone   21 Hydroxylase

17α Hydroxypregnenolone ⟶ 17α Hydroxyprogesterone ⤵ 11 Deoxycortisol ⟶ Cortisol

Dehydroepiandrosterone ⟶ Androstenedione ⟶ Testosterone

Figure 16.42   Adrenal steroid biosynthesis

The adrenal gland in these patients secretes little cortisol but secretion of cortisol precursors including 17α-hydroxyprogesterone is high. Such patients are usually treated with orally active glucocorticoids; these compounds feed back at the hypothalamo–pituitary level and inhibit the secretion of ACTH. Adrenal activity is thereby reduced and 17α-hydroxyprogesterone levels fall[118]. It is, however, noteworthy that normal 17α-hydroxyprogesterone concentrations may only be achieved after at least 1 week of treatment[119]. It is possible to utilize the determination of 17α-hydroxyprogesterone concentrations to monitor the efficacy of glucocorticosteroid replacement therapy in CAH patients. Data derived on assay of matched samples of plasma and saliva provided by a CAH patient are presented in Figure 16.43. This 12-

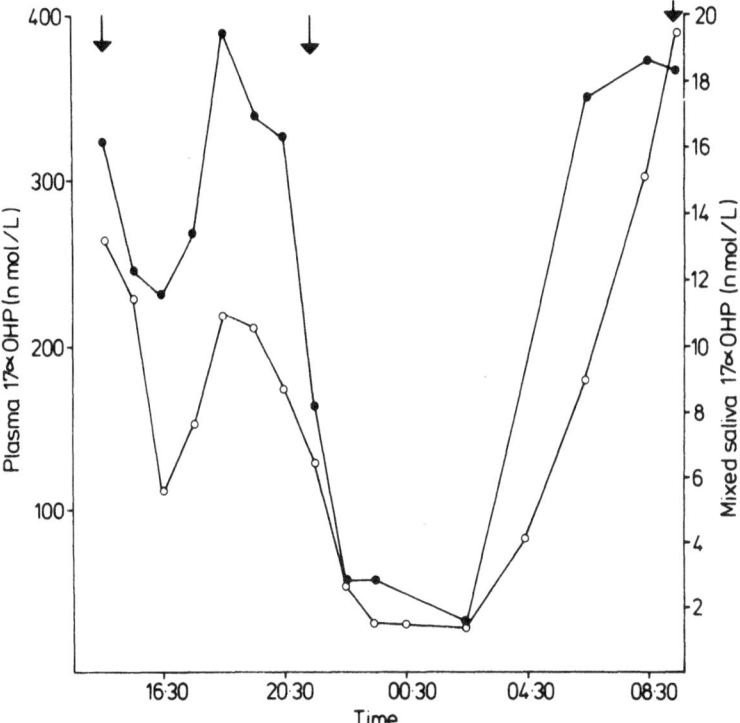

Figure 16.43 Concentrations of 17α-hydroxyprogesterone in matched plasma and mixed saliva samples collected from a CAH patient over a 24 h period; the arrows indicate the times of cortisol administration

year-old-girl was receiving daily doses of glucocorticosteroids at the times indicated. The concentrations of 17α-hydroxyprogesterone in plasma were accurately reflected in saliva, suggesting that salivary sampling regimens could well be used for monitoring treatment in these patients[105, 120]. The ease and frequency of saliva collections is particularly attractive in the long-term management of these patients. Paediatricians have experienced no difficulty in collecting saliva samples from children over 4 years of age. In babies and infants, however, saliva is sucked from the floor of the mouth using a wide-bore plastic tube attached to a syringe.

The normal range for salivary 17α-hydroxyprogesterone concentrations was established by assaying samples provided by a group ($n = 32$) of children age-matched with the CAH patients. In these normal children aged 9 months to 17 years the mean salivary 17α-hydroxyprogesterone was 500 pmol/l, ranging from 100 to 1500 pmol/l (Figure 16.44). In saliva samples from a

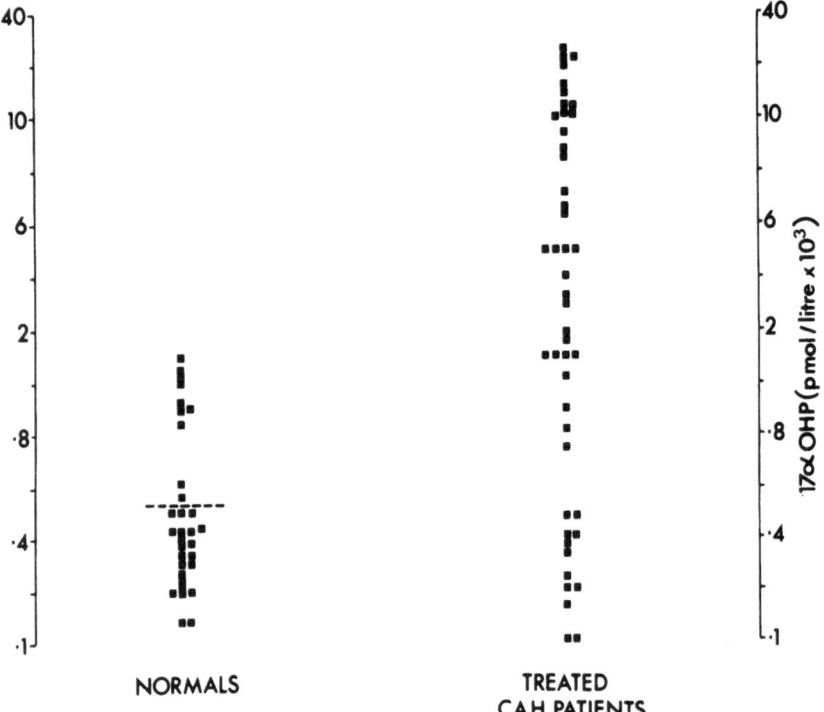

NORMALS   TREATED
                           CAH PATIENTS

Figure 16.44 Concentrations of 17α-hydroxyprogesterone in mixed saliva collected from normal subjects ($n = 32$) and patients with congenital adrenal hyperplasia

group of 16 treated CAH patients 17α-hydroxyprogesterone levels showed considerably greater variation. The values observed ranged from 70 to 26 000 pmol/l; high levels were invariably associated with inadequate treatment.

Synacthen stimulation tests are sometimes used in studies of CAH, particularly when there is some doubt about the diagnosis. It was therefore interesting to find (Figure 16.45) that the increased 17α-hydroxyprogesterone concentrations occurring in response to Synacthen (250 μg, i.m.) in two well-controlled CAH patients (J.H. and C.B.) were similar to those observed in healthy volunteers. In patient J.H., who was a 10-year-old boy, baseline

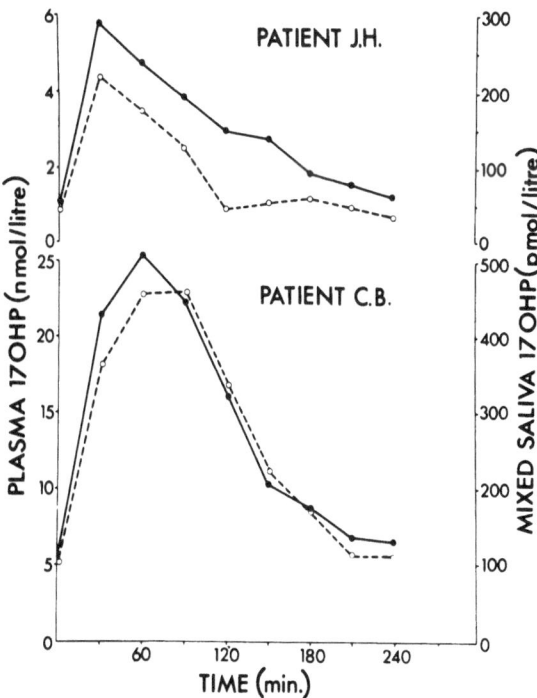

Figure 16.45 Response of 17α-hydroxyprogesterone to Synacthen stimulation (250 μg; i.m.) in matched plasma (●——●) and saliva (○----○) samples collected from CAH patients

salivary 17α-hydroxyprogesterone concentrations were only 50 pmol/l, but in patient C.B. baseline levels were higher (100 pmol/l), possibly because this 14-year-old girl provided samples during the luteal phase of the menstrual cycle and at this time 17α-hydroxyprogesterone concentrations are known to be increased.

Several of the older girls in the group attending an outpatient CAH clinic at the University Hospital of Wales at Cardiff have started to menstruate, and it is interesting to compare the steroid profiles through the cycle in these girls with those of normal women. The rhythmic changes in salivary progesterone concentrations which characterize the normal menstrual cycle have been described earlier; but, as the data presented in Figure 16.46 show, salivary 17α-hydroxyprogesterone concentrations also vary through the normal cycle. In the follicular phase levels are low but following ovulation concentrations of salivary 17α-hydroxyprogesterone, like those of progesterone, increase, reaching maximum values in the mid-luteal phase. In a well-controlled 14-year-old CAH patient (C.B.) who was having regular intervals of bleeding, the pattern of salivary 17α-hydroxyprogesterone concentrations closely approximated to that of normal women (Figure 16.47). In marked contrast salivary progesterone concentrations, although higher in the luteal phase than in the follicular phase of the cycle, were nearly all below the

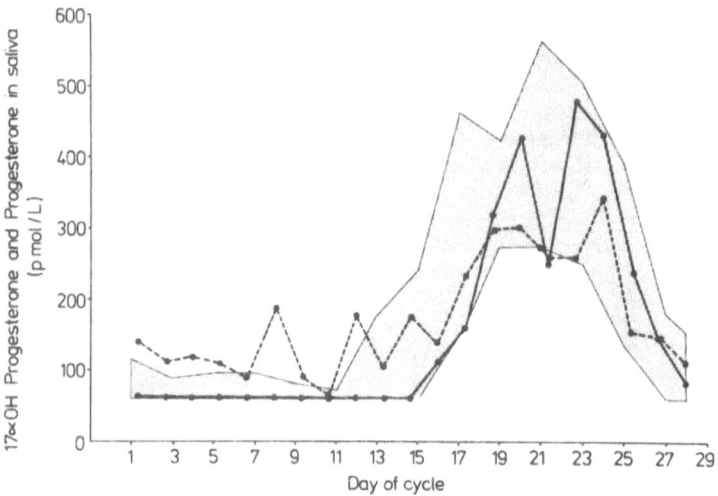

Figure 16.46 Variations throughout the menstrual cycle of salivary progesterone in a group of normal volunteers (dotted area); and of progesterone (●——●) and 17α-hydroxyprogesterone (●----●) in saliva samples in a normal female

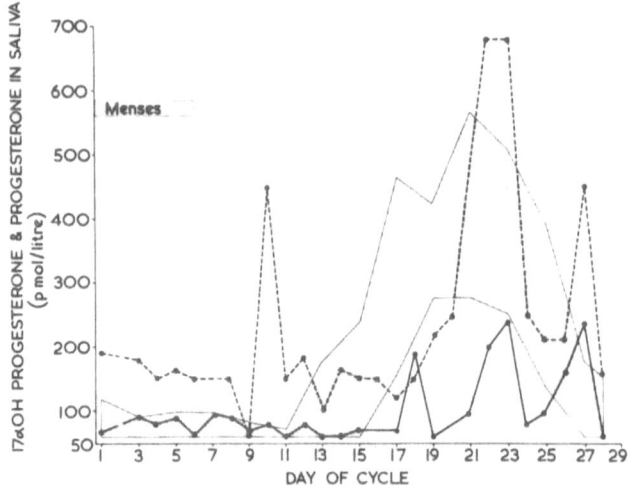

Figure 16.47 Variation throughout a 30-day study between menses of salivary progesterone (●——●) and 17α-hydroxyprogesterone (●----●) in a well-controlled patient (C.B.) with CAH. Also shown is the normal range throughout a menstrual cycle of salivary progesterone concentrations

normal range. The pattern of salivary progesterone concentrations in this patient was very similar to that observed in infertile women having the luteal phase deficiency syndrome. In a poorly controlled CAH patient (C.H.) aged 14, bleeding occurred at irregular intervals. It was therefore not surprising to find (Figure 16.48) that in this patient the normal pattern in salivary progesterone and 17α-hydroxyprogesterone was absent. Levels of 17α-hydroxyprogesterone were consistently high and progesterone concentrations fluctuated widely. It is very likely that in this patient these steroids are largely adrenal in origin, whereas in normal women these steroids originate very largely in ovarian tissue.

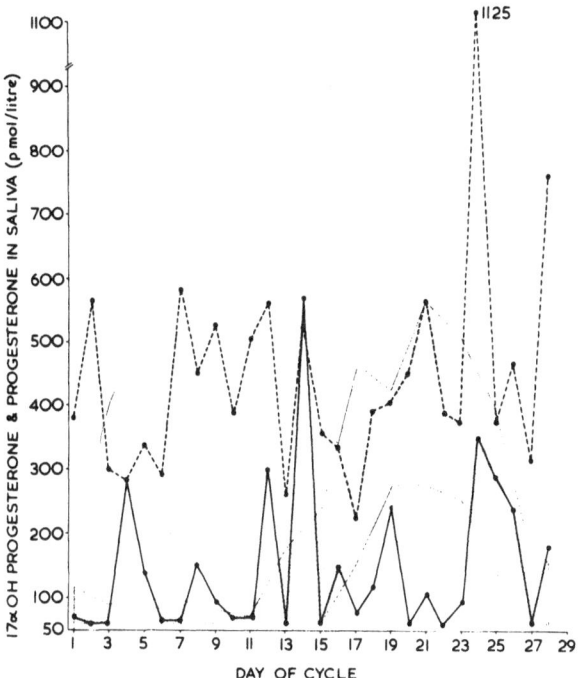

Figure 16.48 Variation throughout a 30-day study of salivary progesterone (●——●) and 17α-hydroxyprogesterone (●- - - -●) in a poorly controlled subject (C.H.) with CAH. The dotted area corresponds to normal range of salivary progesterone concentrations

The studies reported here would suggest that the determination of steroid concentrations in saliva could well replace those in plasma. Salivary assays may therefore have an important role to play not only in assessing gonadal and adrenal function but also for monitoring treatment in patients having endocrine dysfunction. An interesting new development widely applicable in fertility control studies is the assay of synthetic steroids in saliva. Salivary sampling regimens are particularly attractive in these studies since they avoid ethical or religious taboos associated with the collection of plasma samples.

Salivary norethisterone (NET) concentration

Fertility control programmes are frequently undertaken in developing countries and, because in these countries trained laboratory staff and/or equipment may be lacking, the assay developed was simple, featuring a solid-phase antiserum and an enzyme label[121]. The colorimetric end-point could therefore be determined using a simple spectrophotometer. This enzyme immunoassay had a lower limit of 3 pg/assay tube and the dose–response curve covered the range 0–150 pg (Figure 16.14). NET concentrations in plasma and saliva samples determined by a reference radioimmunoassay and by this enzyme immunoassay showed excellent correlation (Figure 16.16).

In matched samples of plasma and saliva provided by three healthy women NET levels increased rapidly following oral administration of a capsule containing 500 μg NET and 35 μg ethynyloestradiol (EE). Peak values were observed 30–90 min after taking the capsule, levels falling precipitously thereafter (Figure 16.49). The maximum concentrations of NET achieved in

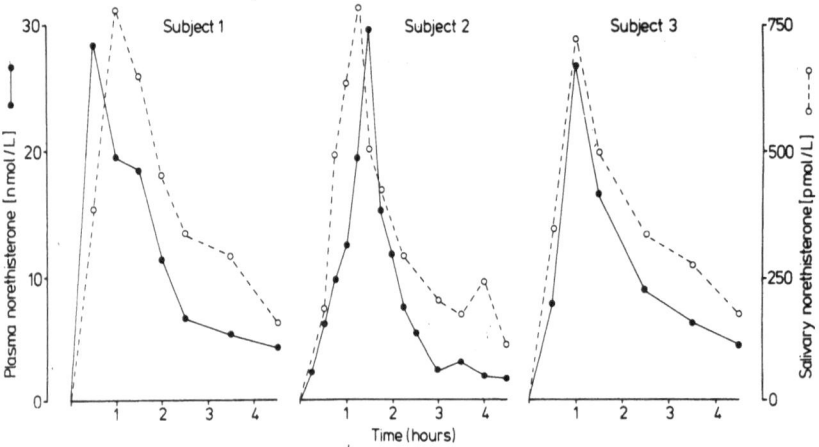

Figure 16.49   Norethisterone EIA pharmacokinetics following an oral NET capsule (NE 500 μg; EE$_2$ 35 μg)

plasma and saliva varied from one subject to another; the mean peak value observed in plasma was 28 nmol/l, whereas that in saliva was 720 pmol/l.

The data presented in Figure 16.50 illustrate a particular difficulty common to all salivary studies. A healthy woman took a NET-containing tablet which was crushed before swallowing. Despite rigorous brushing of the teeth and rinsing of the mouth before collecting saliva, the NET concentrations in early samples were markedly elevated, suggesting gross oral contamination. This difficulty was overcome by administering a non-crushable capsule to the same volunteer. This problem of contamination of saliva samples is not restricted to studies of NET but is common to all studies using salivary sampling regimens for determining concentrations of orally administered compounds.

The ease and frequency with which saliva samples can be collected make salivary sampling regimens ideal for subject compliance and pharmacokinetic studies. The data presented in Figure 16.51, obtained on assay of saliva samples provided by healthy women after a NET-containing capsule (500 μg

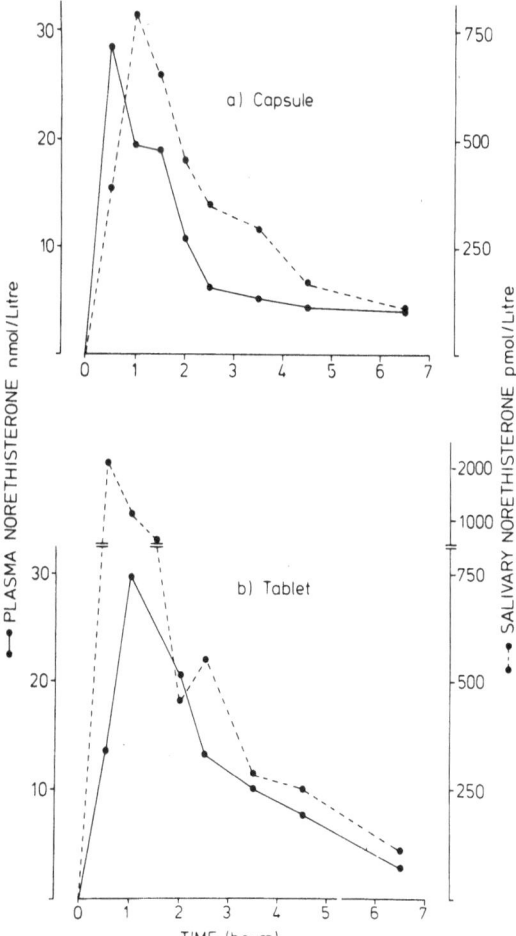

Figure 16.50 Plasma and salivary NET concentrations achieved after swallowing a NET-containing capsule and chewing a tablet

NET), indicate that peak values were achieved within 90 min and that NET is detectable for at least 6 h.

Salivary studies which allow frequent, easy, pain-free sample collection are therefore attractive not only in the routine investigation of hormonal abnormalities[122] but also in pharmacokinetic studies and fertility control programmes. Patients and volunteers participating in these studies have found collection of saliva samples preferable to venepuncture. This cost-effective procedure may therefore come into use. However, since studies involving salivary sampling regimens generate large numbers of samples, an essential prerequisite is the development of cheap, sensitive, specific, high-throughput procedures.

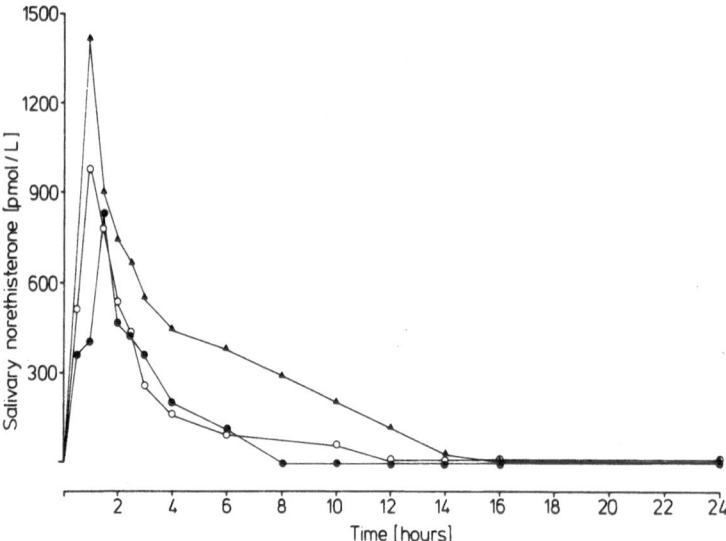

Figure 16.51   Norethisterone EIA: pharmacokinetics following an oral NET capsule (NET 500 μg: EE$_2$ 35 μg). ●——● = Patient R.B.; ▲——▲ = I.R.; ○——○ = D.R.

HIGH-THROUGHPUT ASSAYS

Many congruent factors have led to the current upsurge of interest in developing high-throughput steroid immunoassays, the most important being the ever-increasing number of samples submitted. The determination of steroid hormones in saliva rather than plasma has accentuated this problem. Further factors include the desire to devolve assays to peripheral laboratories or to less experienced staff, and attempts to improve intra-assay, inter-assay and inter-laboratory precision. A serious difficulty in automating any immunoassay is the need for separating free and bound antigen. Most major systems have abolished centrifugation although the Centria System (Union Carbide) is built around a centrifuge and uses centripetal force for reagent transfer and mixing. Other systems have used either filtration or some form of column. The latter may add markedly to the unit cost of an assay if commercial pre-packed columns are used. In Britain, at least, the high initial and running costs of commercially available automated equipment, combined with the relative inflexibility of these systems, has led to development of various in-house systems. These are usually based on continuous-flow techniques, using commercially available peristaltic pumps and dilution/sampling modules[123]. Such systems are comparatively cheap to acquire, particularly as the installation of large, fully automated clinical chemistry modules such as the SMA-12 (Technicon) has made modular continuous flow apparatus surplus to current requirements in many laboratories. These modular systems offer great flexibility and the possibility of using in-house antisera and radioligands, with corresponding cost reduction.

An alternative approach is to establish a simple, robust assay procedure in a central laboratory and then supply the necessary reagents, including solid-phase antisera and labelled steroids, which require fairly sophisticated preparative techniques, to other smaller centres. Thus a group of laboratories can use identical reagents and methodology and thereby reduce inter-laboratory variance. This approach has been followed at Tenovus and has led to the development of a reagent pack for determining plasma cortisol concentrations which, when used in other laboratories, provides results having inter-laboratory coefficients of variation not exceeding 15%[17].

In our opinion the next decade is likely to see immunoassays featuring tritiated radioligands increasingly replaced by those using non-isotopic labels. Low instrumentation costs are likely to make EIAs the predominant NIIA during this period. Finally the determination of salivary steroids, although still confined to relatively few centres, is likely to become increasingly popular.

References

1. Lindner, H. R., Perel, E. and Friedlander, A. (1970). In Finkelstein, M., Conti, C., Klopper, A. and Cassano, C. (eds.) *Research on Steroids*, Vol. IV, p. 197. (Oxford: Pergamon Press)
2. Niswender, G. D. and Midgely, A. R. (1970). Hapten-radioimmunoassay for steroid hormones. In Peron, F. and Caldwell, B. V. (eds.) *Immunologic Methods in Hormone Determination*, pp. 149–173. (New York: Appleton-Century-Crofts)
3. Dean, P. D. G., Exley, D. and Johnson, M. W. (1971). Formation of 17β-oestradiol-6-(O-carboxymethyl) oxime–bovine serum albumin conjugate. *Steroids*, **18**, 593
4. Rao, P. N. and Moore, P. H. (1977). Synthesis of new steroid haptens for radioimmunoassay. IV. 3-(O-carboxymethyl) ether derivatives of estrogens. Specific antisera for the assay of estrone, estradiol-17β and estriol. *Steroids*, **29**, 461
5. Exley, D. and Woodhams, B. (1976). The specificity of antisera raised by oestradiol-17β 3-hemisuccinyl bovine serum albumin. *Steroids*, **27**, 813
6. Fahmy, D. R., Read, G. F. and Hillier, S. G. (1975). Some observations on the determination of cortisol in human plasma by radioimmunoassay using antisera against cortisol-3-BSA. *Steroids*, **26**, 267
7. Dash, R. J., England, B. G., Midgely, A. R. and Niswender, G. D. (1975). A specific, non-chromatographic radioimmunoassay for human plasma cortisol. *Steroids*, **26**, 647
8. Niswender, G. D. (1973). Influence of the site of conjugation on the specificity of antibodies to progesterone. *Steroids*, **22**, 413
9. Nieschlag, E., Usadel, K.-H., Kley, H.K., Schwedes, U., Schöffling, K. and Kruskemper, H. L. (1974). A new approach for investigating hypothalamic-pituitary, gonadal and adrenal feedback control mechanisms: active immunisation with steroids. *Acta Endocrinol. (Kbh)*, **76**, 556
10. Abraham, G. E., Buster, J. E. and Teller, R. C. (1972). Radioimmunoassay of plasma cortisol. *Analyt. Letters*, **5**, 757
11. Vecsei, P., Penke, B., Katzy, R. and Baek, L. (1972). Radioimmunological determination of plasma cortisol. *Experientia*, **8**, 1104
12. Ruder, H. J., Guy, R. L. and Lipsett, M. B. (1972). A radioimmunoassay for cortisol in plasma and urine. *J. Clin. Endocrinol. Metab.*, **35**, 219
13. Vermeulen, A. (1979). The androgens. In Gray, C. H. and James, V. H. T. (eds.) *Hormones in Blood*, pp. 355–416. (London: Academic Press)

14. Joyce, B. G., Fahmy, D. and Hillier, S. G. (1975). Specific determination of testosterone in female plasma by radioimmunoassay: a rapid and reliable procedure for the routine clinical laboratory. *Clin. Chim. Acta*, **62**, 231

15. Llewellyn, D. E. H., Hillier, S. G. and Read, G. F. (1976). The use of multivariable standard curves in the radioimmunoassay of testosterone and 5α-dihydrotestosterone. *Steroids*, **28**, 339

16. Rolleri, E., Zannino, M., Orlandini, S. and Malvano, A. (1976). Direct radioimmunoassay for plasma cortisol. *Clin. Chim. Acta*, **66**, 319

17. Riad-Fahmy, D., Read, G. F., Gaskell, S. J., Dyas, J. and Hindawi, R. (1979). A simple, direct radioimmunoassay for plasma cortisol, featuring a ^{125}I radioligand and a solid-phase separation technique. *Clin. Chem.*, **25**, 665

18. Foster, L. B. and Dunn, R. T. (1974). Single antibody technique for radioimmunoassay of cortisol in unextracted serum or plasma. *Clin. Chem.*, **20**, 363

19. Donohue, J. and Sgoutas, D. (1975). Improved radioimmunoassay of plasma cortisol. *Clin. Chem.*, **21**, 770

20. Hasler, M. J., Painter, K. and Niswender, G. D. (1975). An ^{125}I-labelled cortisol radioimmunoassay in which serum binding proteins are enzymatically denatured. *Clin. Chem.*, **22**, 1850

21. Wong, P. Y., Mee, A. V. and Ho, F. F. K. (1979). A direct radioimmunoassay of serum cortisol with in-house ^{125}I-tracer and pre-conjugated double antibody. *Clin. Chem.*, **25**, 914

22. Joyce, B. G., Othick, A., Read, G. F. and Riad-Fahmy, D. (1980). A sensitive, specific, solid-phase enzyme immunoassay for plasma progesterone. (In preparation)

23. Allen, R. M. and Redshaw, M. R. (1978). The use of homologous and heterologous ^{125}I radioligands in the radioimmunoassay of progesterone. *Steroids*, **32**, 467

24. Kohler, G. and Milstein, C. (1975). Continuous culture of fused cells secreting antibody of pre-defined specificity. *Nature (London)*, **256**, 495

25. Abraham, G. E., Odell, W. D., Swerdloff, R. S. and Hopper, K. (1972). Simultaneous radioimmunoassays of plasma FSH, LH, progesterone, 17α-hydroxyprogesterone and estradiol-17β during the menstrual cycle. *J. Clin. Endocrinol. Metab.*, **34**, 312

26. Joyce, B. G., Read, G. F. and Riad-Fahmy, D. (1978). Enzymeimmunoassay for progesterone and oestradiol: a study of factors influencing sensitivity. In *Radioimmunoassay and Related Procedures in Medicine*, pp. 289–95. (Vienna: IAEA)

27. Edwards, C. R. W., Taylor, A. A., Baum, C. K. and Kurtz, A. B. (1975). Evaluation of two new techniques for steroid radioimmunoassays. In Cameron, E. H. D., Hillier, S. G. and Griffiths, K. (eds.) *Steroidimmunoassay*, pp. 229–34. (Cardiff: Alpha Omega)

28. Hunter, W. M., Nars, P. W. and Rutherford, F. J. (1975). Preparation and behaviour of ^{125}I-labelled radioligands for phenolic and neutral steroids. In Cameron, E. H. D., Hillier, S. G. and Griffiths, K. (eds.) *Steroidimmunoassay*, pp. 141–52. (Cardiff: Alpha Omega)

29. Hillier, S. G. and Read, G. F. (1975). Radioimmunoassay for plasma norethisterone and testosterone using antisera raised against C-11 conjugated haptens and radio-iodinated ligand. *J. Endocrinol.*, **67**, 5P

30. Seth, J. and Brown, L. M. (1978). A simple radioimmunoassay for plasma cortisol. *Clin. Chim. Acta*, **86**, 109

31. Dyas, J., Read, G. F. and Riad-Fahmy, D. (1979). A simple, robust assay for testosterone in male plasma using an ^{125}I-radioligand and a solid-phase separation technique. *Ann. Clin. Biochem.*, **16**, 325

32. Ekins, R. P. (1975). Discussion. In Cameron, E. H. D., Hillier, S. G. and Griffiths, K. (eds.) *Steroidimmunoassay*, pp. 172–4. (Cardiff: Alpha Omega)

33. Niswender, G. D. (1975). Discussion. In Cameron, E. H. D., Hillier, S. G. and Griffiths, K. (eds.) *Steroidimmunoassay*, pp. 47–8. (Cardiff: Alpha Omega)

34. England, B. G., Niswender, G. D. and Midgely, A. R. (1974). Radioimmunoassay of estradiol-17β without chromatography. *J. Clin. Endocrinol. Metab.*, **38**, 42

35. Abraham, G. E. and Odell, W. D. (1970). Solid-phase radioimmunoassay of serum estradiol-17β: a semi-automated approach. In Peron, F. and Caldwell, B. V. (eds.) *Immunologic Methods in Steroid Determination*, pp. 87–112. (New York: Appleton-Century-Crofts)

36. Jeffcoate, S. L., Gilby, E. D. and Edwards, R. (1973). Preparation and use of ^{125}I-steroid albumin conjugates as tracers in steroid radioimmunoassay. *Clin. Chim. Acta*, **43**, 343

37. Rubenstein, K. E., Schneider, R. S. and Ullman, E. F. (1972). 'Homogenous' enzyme immunoassay. A new immunochemical technique. *Biochem. Biophys. Res. Commun.*, **47**, 846

38. Leute, R. K., Ullman, E. F., Goldstein, A. and Herzen, L. A. (1972). Spin immunoassay technique for determination of morphine. *Nature (New Biol.)*, **236**, 93

39. Dandliker, W. B., Hicks, A. N., Levison, S. A. and Brown, R. J. (1977). Fluorescein-labelled estradiol: a probe for anti-estradiol antibody. *Res. Commun. Chem. Path. Pharmacol.*, **18**, 147

40. Watson, R. A. A., Landon, J., Shaw, E. J. and Smith, D. S. (1976). Polarisation fluoroimmunoassay of gentamicin. *Clin. Chim. Acta*, **73**, 51

41. McGregor, A. A., Crookall-Greening, J. O., Landon, J. and Smith, D. S. (1978). Polarisation fluoroimmunoassay of phenytoin. *Clin. Chim. Acta*, **83**, 161

42. Ekeke, G. I. and Exley, D. (1978). The assay of steroids by fluoroimmunoassay. In Pal, S. B. (ed.) *Enzyme Labelled Immunoassay of Hormones and Drugs*, pp. 195–205. (Berlin: Walter de Gruyter)

43. Ekeke, G. I., Exley, D. and Abuknesha, R. (1979). Immunofluorimetric assay of oestradiol-17β. *J. Steroid Biochem.*, **11**, 1597

44. Hassan, M., Landon, J. and Smith, D. S. (1979). Multi-fluorescein-substituted polymers as potential labels in fluoroimmunoassay: a system for improved detection sensitivity. *FEBS Letters*, **103**, 339

45. Simpson, J. S. A., Campbell, A. K., Ryall, M. E. T. and Woodhead, J. S. (1979). A stable chemiluminescent-labelled antibody for immunological assays. *Nature (London)*, **279**, 646

46. Woodhead, J. S., Evans, J., Scarisbrick, J. J., Read, G. F., Hillier, S. G. and Cameron, E. H. D. (1975). Discussion. In Cameron, E. H. D., Hillier, S. G. and Griffiths, K. (eds.) *Steroidimmunoassay*, pp. 269–71. (Cardiff: Alpha Omega)

47. Pratt, J. J., Woldring, M. G. and Villerius, L. (1978). Chemiluminescence-linked immunoassay. *J. Immunol. Methods*, **21**, 179

48. Wisdom, G. B. (1976). Enzyme-immunoassay. *Clin. Chem.*, **22**, 1243

49. Scharpe, S. L., Cooreman, W. M., Blomme, W. J. and Laekeman, G. M. (1976). Quantitative enzyme immunoassay: current status. *Clin. Chem.*, **22**, 733

50 Schuurs, A. H. W. M. and van Weemen, B. K. (1977). Enzyme-immunoassay. *Clin. Chim. Acta*, **81**, 1

51. O'Sullivan, M. J., Bridges, J. W. and Marks, V. (1979). Enzyme immunoassay: a review. *Ann. Clin. Biochem.*, **16**, 221

52. Pal, S. B. (1978). *Enzyme Labelled Immunoassay of Hormones and Drugs*. (Berlin: Walter de Gruyter)

53. Bosch, A. M. G., van Hell, H., Brands, J. A. M., van Weemen, B. K. and Schuurs, A. H. W. M. (1975). Methods for the determination of total estrogens (TE) and human placental lactogen (HPL) in plasma of pregnant women by enzyme-immunoassay (EIA). *Clin. Chem.*, **21**, 1009

54. van Weemen, B. K. and Schuurs, A. H. W. M. (1974). Immunoassay using antibody-enzyme conjugates. *FEBS Letters*, **43**, 215

55. Exley, D. (1978). The influence of heterology and homology on enzyme immunoassay. In Pal, S. B. (ed.) *Enzyme Labelled Immunoassay of Hormones and Drugs*, pp. 207–19. (Berlin: Walter de Gruyter)

56. Joyce, B. G., Read, G. F. and Fahmy, D. R. (1977). A specific enzyme immunoassay for

progesterone in human plasma. *Steroids*, **29**, 761

57. Kaiser, H. and Specker, H. (1956). Bewertung und Vergleich von Analysenverfahren. *Z. Anal. Chem.*, **149**, 46

58. Arakawa, H., Maeda, M. and Tsuji, A. (1979). Chemiluminescence enzyme immunoassay of cortisol using peroxidase as label. *Analyt. Biochem.*, **97**, 248

59. van der Waart, M., and Schuurs, A. H. W. M. (1976). Towards the development of radioenzyme-immunoassay. *Z. Analyt. Chem.*, **279**, 142

60. Ogihara, T., Miyai, K., Mishi, K., Ishibashi, K. and Kunahara, Y. (1977). Enzyme-labelled immunoassay for plasma cortisol. *J. Clin. Endocrinol. Metab.*, **44**, 91

61. Comoglio, S. and Celada, F. (1976). An immuno-enzymatic assay of cortisol using *E.coli* β-galactosidase as label. *J. Immunol. Methods*, **10**, 161

62. Ishikawa, E., (1973). Enzyme immunoassay of insulin by fluorimetry of the insulin-glucoamylase complex. *J. Biochem. (Tokyo)*, **73**, 1319

63. Holder, G. (1978). The estimation of serum cortisol by enzyme immunoassay. In Pal, S. B. (ed.). *Enzyme Labelled Immunoassay of Hormones and Drugs*. pp. 221–32. (Berlin: Walter de Gruyter)

64. Chang, J. J., Crowl, C. P. and Schneider, R. S. (1975). Homogeneous enzyme immunoassay for digoxin. *Clin. Chem.*, **21**, 967

65. van Weemen, B. K. and Schuurs, A. H. W. M. (1971). Immunoassay using antigen–enzyme conjugates. *FEBS Letters*, **15**, 232

66. Ullman, E. F., Blakemore, J., Leute, R. K., Eimstad, W. and Jaklitsch, A. (1973). Homogeneous enzyme immunoassay for thyrozine. *Clin. Chem.*, **21**, 1011

67. Kitagawa, T. and Aikawa, T. (1976). Enzyme coupled immunoassay of insulin using a novel coupling agent. *J. Biochem. (Tokyo)*, **79**, 233

68. Kato, K., Hamaguchi, Y., Fukui, H. and Ishikawa, E. (1973). Enzyme-linked immunoassay. 1. Novel method for synthesis of the insulin β-galactosidase conjugate and its applicability for insulin assay. *J. Biochem. (Tokyo)*, **78**, 235

69. Joyce, B. G., Wilson, D. W., Read, G. F. and Riad-Fahmy, D. (1978). An improved enzyme-immunoassay for progesterone in human plasma. *Clin. Chem.*, **24**, 2099

70. Nye, L., Forrest, G. C., Greenwood, H., Gardner, J. S., Jay, R., Roberts, J. R. and Landon, J. (1976). Solid-phase magnetic particle radioimmunoassay. *Clin. Chim. Acta*, **69**, 387

71. Dray, F., Andrieu, J.-M. and Renaud, F. (1975). Enzyme immunoassay of progesterone at the picogram level using beta-galactosidase as label. *Biochem. Biophys. Acta*, **403**, 131

72. Joyce, B. G. (1979). Enzyme immunoassay for steroid hormone analysis. *Ph.D. thesis*, University of Wales

73. Numazawa, M., Haryu, A., Kurosasa, K. and Nambara, T. (1977). Picogram order enzyme immunoassay of oestradiol. *FEBS Letters*, **79**, 396

74. Exley, D. and Abuknesha, R. (1978). A highly sensitive and specific enzymeimmunoassay method for oestradiol-17β. *FEBS Letters*, **91**, 162

75. Abuknesha, R. and Exley, D. (1978). Design and development of oestradiol-17β enzyme-immunoassay. In Pal, S. B. (ed.) *Enzyme Labelled Immunoassay of Hormones and Drugs*, pp. 139–52. (Berlin: Walter de Gruyter)

76. Bosch, A. M. G., van Hell, H., Brandts, J. and Schuurs, A. H. W. M. (1978). Specificity, sensitivity and reproducibility of enzyme-immunoassays. In Pal, S. B. (ed.). *Enzyme Labelled Immunosssay of Hormones and Drugs*, pp. 175–87. (Berlin: Walter de Gruyter)

77. Bosch, A. M. G., Stevens, W. H. J. M., van Wijngarden, C. J. and Schuurs, A. H. W. M. (1978). Solid-phase enzyme-immunoassay (EIA) of testosterone. *Z. Anal. Chem.*, **290**, 98

78. Joshi, U. M., Shah, H. P. and Sudhama, S. P. (1979). A sensitive and specific enzymeimmunoassay for serum testosterone. *Steroids*, **34**, 35

79. Osterman, T. M., Juntunen, K. O. and Gothoni, G. D. (1979). Enzymeimmunoassay of testosterone in plasma, with use of polyethylene glycol to separate antibody-bound and free hormone. *Steroids*, 34, 575

80. Turkes, A., Turkes, A. O., Joyce, B. G., Read, G. F. and Riad-Fahmy, D. (1979). A sensitive, solid-phase enzymeimmunoassay for testosterone in plasma and saliva. *Steroids*, **33**, 347

81. Tateishi, K., Yamamoto, H., Ogihara, T. and Hayashi, C. (1977). Enzyme immunoassay of serum testosterone. *Steroids*, **30**, 25

82. Rajkowski, K. M., Cittanova, N., Desfosses, B. and Jayle, M. F. (1979). The conjugation of testosterone with horseradish peroxidase and a sensitive enzyme assay for the conjugate. *Steroids*, **29**, 701

83. Turkes, A. O., Turkes, A., Joyce, B. G. and Riad-Fahmy, D. (1980). A sensitive enzymeimmunoassay with a fluorimetric end-point for the determination of testosterone in female plasma and saliva. *Steroids*, **35**, 89

84. Guilbault, G. C., Brignac, P. J. and Juneau, M. (1968). New substrates for the fluorimetric determination of oxidative enzymes. *Anal. Chem.*, **40**, 1256

85. Hindawi, R. K., Gaskell, S. J., Read, G. F. and Riad-Fahmy, D. (1980). A simple, direct, solid-phase enzymeimmunoassay for cortisol in plasma. *Ann. Clin. Biochem.*, **17**, 53

86. Landon, J., Hassan, M., Pourfarzaneh, M. and Smith, D. S. (1979). Non-isotopic immunoassay of hormones in blood. In Gray, C. H. and James, V. H. T. (eds.) *Hormones in Blood*, 3rd edn, Vol. III, pp. 1–40. (London: Academic Press)

87. Whitehead, T. P., Kricka, L. J., Carter, T. J. N. and Thorpe, G. H. G. (1979). Analytical luminescence: its potential in the clinical laboratory. *Clin. Chem.*, **25**, 1531

88. Kobayashi, Y., Ogihara, T., Nishitani, Y., Watanabe, F. and Kumahara, Y. (1979). Enzyme immunoassay of corticosterone. *J. Steroid Biochem.*, **11**, 1223

89. Monji, N., Gomez, N. O., Kawashima, H., Ali, H. and Castro, A. (1980). Practical enzymeimmunoassay for plasma cortisol using β-galactosidase as enzyme label. *J. Clin. Endocrinol. Metab.*, **50**, 355

90. Gorus, F. and Schram, E. (1979). Applications of bio- and chemiluminescence in the clinical laboratory. *Clin. Chem.*, **25**, 312

91. Turkes, A., Dyas, J., Read, G. F. and Riad-Fahmy, D. (1980). A sensitive enzyme-immunoassay for ethynyl oestradiol in plasma. *J. Endocrinol.* (In press)

92. Abraham, G. E. (1969). Solid phase radioimmunoassay of oestradiol-17β. *J. Clin. Endocrinol. Metab.*, **29**, 866

93. Warren, R. J. and Fotherby, K. (1974). Radioimmunoassay of synthetic progestogens: norethisterone and norgestrel. *J. Endocrinol.*, **62**, 605

94. Hillier, S. G., Jha, P., Griffiths, K. and Laumas, K. R. (1977). Long term contraception by steroid-releasing implants. VI. Serum concentrations of norethindrone in women bearing a single silastic implant releasing norethindrone acetate. *Contraception*, **15**, 473

95. Laumas, V., Malik, B. K., Jamal, K., Seth, U., Agarwal, N., Hingorani, V. and Laumas, K. R. (1978). Radioimmunoassay of norethindrone: serum levels of norethindrone in lactating women after insertion of a silastic implant releasing norethindrone acetate. *Contraception*, **18**, 595

96. Stanczyk, F. Z., Brenner, P. F., Mishell, D. R., Ortiz, A., Gentzschein, E. K. E. and Geobelsman, U. (1978). A radioimmunoassay for norethindrone (NET): measurement of serum NET concentrations following ingestion of NET-containing oral contraceptive steroids. *Contraception*, **18**, 615

97. Rao, P. N., de la Pena, A. and Goldzieher, J. W. (1974). Antisera for radioimmunoassay of 17-alpha-ethynylestradiol and Mestranol. *Steroids*, **24**, 803

98. Nilsson, S. and Nygren, K. G. (1978). Ethynyl estradiol in peripheral plasma after oral administration of 30 micrograms and 50 micrograms to women. *Contraception*, **18**, 469

99. Shannon, I. L., Prigmore, J. R. and Chauncey, H. H. (1962). Modified Carlson–Crittenden device for the collection of parotid fluid. *J. Dent. Res.*, **41**, 778

100. McVie, R., Levine, L. S. and New, M. I. (1979). The biologic significance of the aldosterone concentration in saliva. *Pediatr. Res.*, **13**, 755

101. Smith, R. G., Besch, P. K., Dill, B. and Buttram, V. C. (1979). Saliva as a matrix for measuring free androgens: comparison with serum androgens in polycystic ovarian disease. *Fertil. Steril.*, **31**, 513

102. Walker, R. F., Read, G. F. and Riad-Fahmy, D. (1979). Radioimmunoassay of progesterone in saliva: application to the assessment of ovarian function. *Clin. Chem.*, **25**, 2030

103. Walker, R. F., Wilson, D. W., Read, G. F. and Riad-Fahmy, D. (1980). Assessment of testicular function by the radioimmunoassay of testosterone in saliva. *Int. J. Andrology*, **3**, 105

104. Walker, R. F., Riad-Fahmy, D. and Read, G. F. (1978). Adrenal status assessed by direct radioimmunoassay of cortisol in whole saliva or parotid saliva. *Clin. Chem.*, **24**, 1460

105. Walker, R. F., Read, G. F., Hughes, I. A. and Riad-Fahmy, D. (1979). Radioimmunoassay of 17α-hydroxyprogesterone in saliva, parotid fluid and plasma of congenital adrenal hyperplasia patients. *Clin. Chem.*, **25**, 542

106. Fotherby, K. (1979). Progesterone: clinical aspects. In Gray, C. H. and James, V. H. T. (eds.) *Hormones in Blood*, 3rd edn, Vol. III, pp. 439–91. (London: Academic press)

107. Doring, G. R. (1973). Detection of ovulation by the basal body temperature method. In *Conference on Human Family Planning*, pp. 171–89. (Washington: Human Life Foundation)

108. Ross, G. T., Cargille, C. M., Lipsett, M. B., Rayford, P. L., Marshall, J. R., Strott, C. A. and Rodbard, D. (1970). Pituitary and gonadal hormones in women during spontaneous and induced ovulatory cycles. *Recent Prog. Horm. Res.*, **26**, 1

109. Speight, A., Hancock, K. W. and Oakey, R. E. (1979). Non-protein-bound oestrogens in plasma and urinary excretion of unconjugated oestrogens in non-pregnant women. *J. Endocrinol.*, **83**, 385

110. Rosenfield, R. L. (1971). Plasma testosterone binding globulin and indexes of the concentration of unbound plasma androgens in normal and hirsute subjects. *J. Clin. Endocrinol. Metab.*, **32**, 717

111. Vermeulen, A., Stoica, T. and Verdonck, L. (1971). The apparent free testosterone concentration, an index of androgenicity. *J. Clin. Endocrinol. Metab.*, **33**, 759

112. Abraham, G. E. (1974). Ovarian and adrenal contribution to peripheral androgens during the menstrual cycle. *J. Clin. Endocrinol. Metab.*, **39**, 340

113. Wieland, R. G., Zorn, E. M., Hallberg, M. C. and Furst, B. (1974). Testosterone and metabolites in women using radioimmunoassay techniques. In Curry, A. S. and Hewitt, J. V. (eds.) *Biochemistry of Women: Methods for Clinical Investigation*, pp. 181–9. (Cleveland: CRC Press)

114. Steinberger, E. (1979). Management of male reproductive dysfunction. *Clin. Obstet. Gynecol.*, **22**, 187

115. Campbell, I. T., Walker, R. F., Fahmy, D. R., Wilson, D. W. and Griffiths, K. (1980). Effects of continuous daylight on circadian rhythms of testosterone and cortisol in saliva. (In preparation)

116. Walker, R. F., Hughes, I. A., Riad-Fahmy, D. and Read, G. F. (1978). Assessment of ovarian function by salivary progesterone. *Lancet*, **2**, 585

117. Mills, I. H., Schedl, H. P., Chen, P. S. and Bartter, F. C. (1960). The effect of estrogen administration on the metabolism and protein binding of hydrocortisone. *J. Clin. Endocrinol. Metab.*, **20**, 515

118. Riad-Fahmy, D., Read, G. and Hughes, I. A. (1979). Corticosteroids. In Gray, C. H. and James, V. H. T. (eds.) *Hormones in Blood*, 3rd edn, Vol. III, pp. 179–262. (London: Academic Press)

119. Hughes, I. A. and Winter, J. S. D. (1976). The application of a serum 17-OH-progesterone radioimmunoassay to the diagnosis and management of congenital adrenal hyperplasia. *J. Pediatr.*, **88**, 766

120. Price, D. A., Astin, M. P., Chard, C. R. and Addison, G. M. (1979). Assay of

hydroxyprogesterone in saliva. *Lancet*, **2**, 368

121. Turkes, A., Dyas, J., Read, G. F. and Riad-Fahmy, D. (1980). A sensitive, solid-phase enzymeimmunoassay for norethisterone (norethindrone) in saliva and plasma. *Steroids*, **35**, 445

122. Seaton, B. and Riad-Fahmy, D. (1980). The use of salivary progesterone assays to monitor menstrual cycles in Bangladeshi women. *J. Endocrinol.* (In press)

123. Ismail, A. A., West, P. M. and Goldie, D. J. (1978). The 'Southmead System', a simple, fully-automated, continuous-flow system for immunoassays (appendix: application to serum thyroxine radioimmunoassays). *Clin. Chem.*, **24**, 571

17
Immunoassays in Pharmacology and Toxicology

V. MARKS

INTRODUCTION

Pharmacology is one of the oldest of the medical sciences. For much of its history, however, pharmacology was concerned almost exclusively with pharmacodynamics, i.e. what drugs do to the body – rather than with pharmacokinetics, i.e. what the body does to drugs. This aspect of pharmacology can, to a large extent, be said to date from the studies by Williams on drug metabolism and the appearance of his classic monograph on detoxication mechanisms. Studies on pharmacokinetics were hindered, even in those rare instances in which they might have been considered necessary, by the lack of suitable methods for measuring drugs in biological fluids and for following their metabolism and secretion.

In the wake of the thalidomide disaster, the whole subject of pharmacokinetics, drug safety and metabolism sprang into prominence. With it came an interest in measuring the concentration of drugs in blood and other body fluids – not only in experimental animals, as a means of increasing fundamental knowledge, but also as an aid to the more effective use of drugs in treatment[1]. These two important applications of drug measurements have much in common, but also many differences. Techniques that are suitable for one may be unsuitable for the other because of their potential danger, time requirement or, simply, feasibility.

Immunoassay was first used to measure drugs in blood and other biological fluids in 1968. It was, however, not until 1974 or thereabouts that its full potential for pharmacology was realized[2]. Since that time its growth has been truly phenomenal, and still far from complete[3-7].

DRUG IMMUNOASSAY

There are for drugs, as with all other immunoassays, four essential ingredients:

(1) a high-avidity, highly specific antibody;
(2) a high-specific activity label;
(3) a pure standard;
(4) appropriate instrumentation.

Each will be considered in turn.

The antibody

Most drugs have a molecular weight of less than 500 daltons and consequently are not naturally immunogenic. They can, however, generally be rendered so by linking them covalently to a protein, preferably one foreign to the species in which it is intended to raise the antibody[2]. A great number of proteins have been employed as the carrier – probably the commonest being bovine serum albumin (BSA). Latterly, however, we have tended to favour the use of chicken γ-globulin as there is some evidence that conjugates made with it are more immunogenic in rabbits and sheep than conjugates made with BSA. Some drugs contain functional groups which enable them to be joined to the carrier protein by direct conjugation; others require initial derivatization.

Various chemical reactions have been used to effect the conjugation of the hapten to protein, the most suitable depending upon the nature of the reactive group through which the linkage is to be made and its ability to enter into chemical reactions. Several reviews of the most commonly employed techniques are available[2,8,9]. Sometimes it may be necessary to use a closely related derivative of the drug, rather than the drug itself, as the starting material for making a conjugate in order to achieve the requisite specificity[10]. Only very rarely should a natural metabolite of the parent drug be used, however – despite its apparent attractions – since the antibody raised in response to it may favour the metabolite rather than the parent drug whose concentration it is intended to measure when both occur together in solution.

Our experience[11], and that of many other investigators, is that even where direct coupling is possible, immunogenicity with respect to the hapten (i.e. drug) can generally be increased by interposing a 'spacer-group' between it and the protein. The optimum spacer-group is four carbon atoms long. In many cases it can conveniently be provided by using a hemisuccinate derivative of the drug to make the conjugate.

Relative concentrations of hapten and carrier must be controlled in order to prevent over- or under-substitution, since either can diminish the immuno-genicity of the resultant conjugate. The optimum number of haptenic sub-stituents, using BSA as carrier, appears to be between 20 and 40, though antibodies have been raised successfully against immunogens containing as few as one or two haptens per carrier molecule[12, 13]. For proteins larger than BSA, a greater number of haptenic substituents per molecule might be expected to produce optimum immunogenic conjugates, but little factual information is currently available.

The immunogenic conjugate, however prepared, must be purified before it is injected into the animal. Purification can be achieved either by extensive dialysis or by gel filtration, and serves to rid the conjugate of unattached hapten or hapten that is only absorbed, rather than bound, to the protein and which may interfere with antibody production.

In order to evoke a good immune response the aqueous solution of the immunogenic conjugate must be dispersed in an oil containing adjuvant to form a stable emulsion. Whilst most investigators have used commercially available Freund's adjuvant for this purpose, we have for the past 6 years used a non-ulcerogenic adjuvant*. This is equally, if not more, effective in evoking an immunogenic response and is infinitely more humane. Its use has permitted us to use the highly effective multiple intradermal site technique[14] without causing pain or distress to the animal and, consequently, ensures its prolonged survival.

Even using the best conjugates and immunological techniques it is unusual, in our experience with drugs, to get as high titre antisera as are commonly obtained with proteins and steroids. Consequently we have tended to use sheep and other large animals for raising antisera for use in drug immunoassays. This ensures a uniformity of supply which could not otherwise be achieved, since it is our experience that antisera raised in different animals against the same conjugate, and even in the same animal from time to time, can vary quite markedly in their specificity and other binding characteristics.

The label

Contrary to our expectations when we entered the field of drug immunoassay, it has generally proved more difficult in practice to obtain the high specific activity labels necessary in order to achieve maximum sensitivity than to produce suitable antibodies.

During the course of developing a new drug, most manufacturers make a small amount of ^{14}C-labelled material to enable them, amongst other things, to trace its metabolism in experimental animals. Such material can be used – indeed it is ideal – for demonstrating the presence of specific antibodies to the drug in an antiserum but it rarely, if ever, has a sufficiently high specific activity to enable it to be used as the label in a quantitative radioimmunoassay (RIA). Tritiated derivatives of a sufficiently high specific activity to be used in

---

* Obtainable from Guildhay Antisera: Department of Biochemistry, University of Surrey, Guildford, Surrey, UK.

RIA can generally be prepared but usually only at great expense which can usually only be justified when a need for it has already been established. Like those made from ^{14}C, tritium labels have the advantage of an almost identical immunoreactivity with the antiserum as the native drug. They do, however, necessitate the use of scintillation counters and, contrary to expectation, have a limited shelf life, seeming often to undergo a rapid and catastrophic breakdown into non-immunoreactive components within a year or less of their manufacture.

Some of the ways adopted to try and overcome these difficulties have included the production of [125]I- or ^{75}Se-labelled derivatives; either by direct introduction of the label into the drug molecule itself[15] or, more commonly, by conjugating the drug to a compound such as tyrosine, tyramine, histidine or histamine which can itself be iodinated[16]. Enzyme[17] and fluorescent[18] labelled drugs have been used in immunoassays, these non-isotopic techniques have already established themselves as the labels of choice[19] for 'routine' clinical work. Usually, however, they represent an even greater investment in development costs than isotopic labels. This makes them less suitable for use in assays used exclusively for research into the pharmacokinetics of drugs which are no longer covered by patents, or for compounds, the clinical value of whose measurement has not yet been established.

Standards

The necessity of using standards identical to the substance to be measured is no less for drug than for other immunoassays. Generally this provides no special problems, but may do under certain circumstances such as when the pure drug is very unstable in dilute solution, for example, adriamycin; or when the native drug is a mixture of closely related compounds, all with slightly differing immunological and biological properties, and whose proportions are not necessarily constant from batch to batch, as in the case of bleomycin. Another problem of standardization which, though not unique to drugs, is highlighted by them, is the interference by metabolites. These are always present to a greater or lesser extent in biological fluids obtained from subjects treated with a drug, and they always react to some extent with the antiserum. The amount of distortion produced may be so small as to have no serious effect upon the validity of the result obtained. It may, on the other hand, completely invalidate it unless steps are taken to eliminate the interference by introducing a preliminary preparative step which may be as simple as differential extraction of the drug into a solvent or as complicated, and absolute[20,21], as its separation by high-performance liquid chromatography (HPLC).

Instrumentation

Instrumentation used for drug immunoassay is no different from that used for other types of immunoassay and must be appropriate. For RIA this means using either a scintillation or gamma counter according to the nature of the label; for assays using an enzyme label a highly sensitive and thermostatically controlled spectrophotometer is required, whilst those which use fluorescent labels depend upon the availability of a stable and sensitive fluorimeter. All of these pieces of equipment are available in a well-furnished clinical or research laboratory and therefore do not usually impose any restriction on the use of drug immunoassays once they have been developed.

ADVANTAGES AND DISADVANTAGES OF IMMUNOASSAY

Immunoassays have several advantages over the more conventional methods for measuring drugs in blood and other biological fluids[22,23], but also some minor disadvantages. Undoubtedly, the greatest single advantage of immunoassay techniques is their sensitivity. This is unrivalled by any other readily available analytical technique and can generally be achieved without prior extraction and concentration. Because of this it is often possible to carry out an immunoassay on as little as 10 μl of plasma – or less – making it ideal for work on small laboratory animals or clinically, for children in whom only capillary blood is available. Immunoassays can be applied almost universally to any substance with a molecular weight of more than 150 daltons. Class specificity is relatively easy to achieve, whilst specificity for the native drug itself can often be obtained by careful attention to the chemical methods used to prepare the immunogen used for making the antibody. By manipulating the conditions, e.g. pH, ionic strength of buffer and timing of reactions, under which an assay is performed, the 'specificity' of an antiserum can often be radically altered, thereby throwing considerable doubt upon the value of so-called 'cross-reactivity data' for antisera which are published without reference to the conditions under which they are actually used.

The combination of TLC or HPLC – as a preparative separation stage – with immunoassay detection and quantitation, provides a technique for measuring drugs in biological fluids with a specificity and sensitivity unsurpassed by any other. It is only equalled by the combined use of GLC and mass spectrometry; but is generally much easier to perform.

The HPLC-immunoassay combination has the added advantage that it permits quantitation not only of the native drug, but also of its immunoreactive metabolites[20,21] provided that suitable standards are available.

Conditions under which immunoassays are performed are generally mild, seldom requiring separation of the analyte from protein and other potential interfering substances present in the sample. Consequently, they can usually be carried out with the minimum of sample preparation, thus adding speed to its many other advantages. Most immunoassays are amenable to full, or at least partial, automation, making it possible for one person to perform large numbers of repetitive assays in a relatively short time. Such requirements generally exist during therapeutic drug trials, pharmacokinetic studies, screening patients for drug abuse and sometimes even in busy clinical units performing therapeutic drug monitoring.

The main disadvantages of immunoassay are the high initial costs of producing the reagents – which are necessarily unique for each drug; the possibility of interference by known, or even more important, by unknown or rarely formed metabolites of the parent drug and, in some cases, the technical complexity of the assay itself.

TYPES OF IMMUNOASSAY

Most immunoassays for drugs have used a radiolabelled hapten as the tracer. These are generally more useful for research and development than for clinical use where simplicity of performance and speed are at a premium. Nevertheless, RIA is still the most popular method for measuring cardiac glycosides, e.g. digoxin, digitoxin, in blood – mainly because of its sensitivity, precision and accuracy at the low levels normally encountered clinically. RIAs suffer from the overwhelming disadvantage that they necessarily incorporate a phase-separation stage. This not only introduces an important source of error, but also causes delays. Whilst these difficulties can largely be overcome by the use of automatic equipment, such as the Union Carbide Centria, with which it is possible to measure methotrexate by RIA at a rate of 30 samples in 30 min using a ^{125}I label, their existence has encouraged the search for more convenient techniques which can be used in the clinic or even at the bedside. Some are already on the market and their commercial availability is, in no small measure, responsible for the enormous upsurge of interest in therapeutic drug monitoring, currently the most active growth area in clinical laboratory medicine. Therapeutic drug monitoring has recently been the subject of extensive review[24, 25].

The first homogeneous immunoassay to be applied to the detection and measurement of drugs in a biological fluid was the FRAT[R] system introduced by the Syva Corporation[26]. Brilliant in concept, the technique was only sufficiently sensitive to permit detection and semiquantitation rather than the accurate measurement required for most clinical pharmacological studies. The next homogeneous immunoassay technique introduced by the same company, and sold as EMIT[R], overcame many of these difficulties. Other homogeneous immunoassay techniques for measuring drugs in blood plasma are now available, based on a variety of detection systems, e.g. fluorescence[18] and steric hindrance[27], but like the EMIT[R] system they are, generally, insufficiently sensitive to measure drugs used in very low doses and which therefore produce really low plasma concentrations, i.e. the low nmol/l range. This has not yet proved to be a serious disadvantage in therapeutic drug monitoring since, apart from digoxin, none of the drugs for which plasma measurements are indicated are used in such small doses.

USES OF DRUG IMMUNOASSAYS IN PHARMACOLOGY AND TOXICOLOGY

The applications of immunoassay in pharmacology can, broadly speaking, be considered under three heads:

(1) experimental pharmacokinetics and clinical pharmacology;
(2) therapeutic drug monitoring;
(3) epidemiology, forensic and toxicological medicine.

Experimental pharmacokinetics and pharmacology

During the development stages of a new drug it is generally possible to carry out preliminary pharmacokinetic and metabolism studies in experimental animals by conventional techniques. These including the use of ^{14}C or ^{3}H radiolabelled drugs. This latter approach is, however, seldom applicable even to human volunteer studies, let alone large-scale clinical trials. Other analytical techniques must therefore be used. Those most commonly employed are spectrophotometry and fluorimetry, gas-liquid chromatography (GLC), high-performance thin-layer chromatography (HPTLC) and high-performance liquid chromatography (HPLC) respectively. Bioassays are still extensively used for measuring antibiotics and antineoplastic agents. In cases where the concentration of the drug to be measured is very low, or where the utmost specificity is required, it may be necessary to resort to GC–MS or mass fragmentography. The tremendous advantage offered by RIA, and other types of immunoassay for measuring drugs during pharmacokinetic and pharmacodynamic studies has only been recognized comparatively recently and is still far from fully exploited.

RIAs have been used, to great advantage, to study the pharmacokinetic correlates of such old and well-used drugs as morphine[28] and digoxin[29] which could not reliably be measured in blood before the introduction of immunoassay. Because of its extreme sensitivity it is possible with RIA to trace both the appearance in the blood of a drug following ingestion of smaller doses than was hitherto possible[13], and to follow its disappearance. In this way new light may be thrown on the pharmacokinetics of a drug, thereby disturbing firmly entrenched theories which were based upon inadequate and imprecise data obtained by the use of insensitive analytical techniques.

In comparison with the GC–MS, its only serious rival for analytical sensitivity and specificity, RIA, is easier to perform, once the reagents have been prepared, and can be carried out on much smaller samples. Generally only a few microlitres or less of blood are required, making it especially useful for measuring drugs during serial studies on small laboratory animals.

By employing a 'group-specific' antiserum as detector and HPTLC or HPLC as the separator, immunoassay can be used to reveal the presence of previously unsuspected metabolites, provided that they retain at least some of the physical and immunological properties of the parent drug[20,21]. The chemical nature of the metabolites can subsequently be determined by conventional techniques should this be considered necessary.

Table 17.1 Steps in the developing and setting up of a drug immunoassay

(A) Consideration of the indications for developing and/or using an immunoassay

(B) Production of key reagents:
  (1) production of various immunogens
  (2) selection of species and number of animals to be used for antibody production, and decision on immunization schedule
  (3) nature, source and purity of label
  (4) choice of phase separation (if any)

(C) Technical validation of the immunoassay:
  (1) investigation of the dynamics of the antibody–antigen reaction and optimization of the assay
  (2) characterization of the specificity and sensitivity of the final assay
  (3) reproducibility and quality control

(D) Application of the immunoassay:
  (1) study of the absorption, pharmacokinetics and metabolism of the drug in volunteers and patients
  (2) investigation of clinical and toxicological problems
  (3) establishment of optimum therapeutic range in subjects receiving the drug therapeutically
  (4) recognition of the limitations of the assay

Table 17.2 Antisera prepared and used in drug immunoassays at the University of Surrey, 1973/79

Adriamycin	Methotrexate
Amitriptyline	Methyl prednisolone
Bleomycin	Morphine
Bromocriptine	Nortriptyline
Cannabis	
Codeine	Pepleomycin
	Pethidine
Cytosine arabinoside	Pethidine
Dexamethasone	Phenytoin
Diazepam	Prednisolone
Digoxin	Propranolol
Digitoxin	
Etorphine	Vinblastine
5-Fluoruracil	Vincristine
Gentamicin	VP16
Glibenclamide	
Imipramine	

Until now, immunoassays for some 200 drugs have been developed. For most of them, publication has been limited to a description of the technique, its sensitivity, specificity and applicability and the results of one or two pharmacokinetic experiments, usually in animals. The full impact on experimental pharmacology of immunoassay has, therefore, still to be felt. The procedure adopted at Surrey for developing a drug assay is outlined in Table 17.1 and described in greater detail elsewhere[2,8]. Antisera to drugs prepared using this procedure are shown in Table 17.2.

Therapeutic drug monitoring

It is undoubtedly in the field of therapeutic drug monitoring – itself probably the most rapidly growing branch of laboratory medicine – that drug immunoassays have had their greatest impact. This is due mainly to the introduction by the Syva Corporation of the EMIT® range of homogeneous drug immunoassays but other manufacturers, both of heterogeneous and homogeneous immunoassays, as well as a few hospital and university departments active in this field, have undoubtedly contributed to it. Compared with other methods of drug measurement homogeneous immunoassay techniques are generally simpler and quicker, and at least as accurate and precise[30,31]. Moreover, because they often do not require any equipment more complicated than a dilutor, temperature-controlled spectrophotometer or fluorimeter, they can be performed in the clinic or at the patient's bedside. This may be lifesaving when a decision on whether to give a further dose of a drug, such as digoxin, methotrexate, gentamicin or lignocaine – whose toxic effects cannot easily be predicted by any other methods -- is wholly dependent upon the result of the assay and must be made quickly.

Immunoassays, apart from those utilizing homogeneous assay principles, also have a place in therapeutic monitoring – especially during the 'work-up' stages in which investigations are undertaken to determine whether drug measurements improve therapeutic results[24]. RIAs and substitutional type enzyme immunoassays[17,32,33], because they are easier and cheaper to develop in the first place, generally become available for clinical use before market forces make it economical to develop a homogeneous assay. This may not always be the case, however, as new homogeneous immunoassay technologies make their appearance. Indications and reasons for developing and introducing an immunoassay for use in therapeutic drug monitoring have recently been discussed in detail[24,25] and will not be further considered here.

Epidemiological, forensic and toxicological uses

Semiquantitative immunoassays have, because of their sensitivity, 'group specificity' and ease of performance, found widespread application in detecting drug use and abuse in populations at large[34] as well as in those especially at risk[35]. Urine is the body fluid most favoured for such purposes but others, such as blood and saliva, may also be used, especially in sporting events involving the use of animals – particularly horses – when the question of doping arises.

Immunoassays intended for detecting drug use and abuse in urine must be capable of detecting most, if not all, of the metabolites of the drug suspected of being used, as well as with the parent compound. In the case of cannabis, for example, the 'native' drug, tetrahydrocannabinol (THC) is not actually excreted into the urine. Immunoassay that was 'specific' for THC would fail to detect even the recent use, let alone its use some time before. Such an 'assay' would be of limited clinical or toxicological value but would be extremely useful for studying THC pharmacokinetics. A diazepam antiserum raised in our laboratory is an example of one which does not cross-react to any significant extent with any of the diazepam metabolites or analogues. Whilst this makes it very useful for bioavailability studies and therapeutic drug monitoring in patients who are known to be taking diazepam (in whom interference by metabolites might constitute a major disadvantage), it makes it virtually worthless for screening for diazepine use and abuse, which is the major clinical indication for diazepine detection and measurement at the present time.

It can confidently be expected that by applying immunoassay techniques to the investigation of selected, or even of unselected, populations it will be possible to accumulate 'hard data' about the prevalence of drug use in that community. This should put paid to much of the idle speculation abounding in the scientific and lay literature which is, at best, based upon information obtained by verbal questionnaires and drug seizures. We have in our own laboratory recently embarked upon a project to try and determine, using immunoassay, the true incidence of caffeine toxicity in the community which has almost certainly been set too high.

It has been said, or at least implied, that immunoassays do not have the requisite specificity to make them suitable for forensic use, except as screening procedures. This view is based more upon false assumptions about the specificity of alternative methods of analysis – which are seldom as selective as their advocates suggest – than upon the non-specificity of immunoassay. As already mentioned, the combination of HPLC and immunoassay provides an analytical system with a sensitivity and specificity[20,21] unrivalled by any except GC–MS and compared with which it is both cheaper and simpler to use.

Interpretation of urine analysis by immunoassay is complicated by the fact that, because of its sensitivity, it is often possible to detect the presence of drug metabolites days, or even weeks, after the last occasion on which the drug was used and long after its pharmacological effects had worn off.

OUTLOOK FOR THE FUTURE

Despite what has already been achieved, the application of immunoassays to pharmacology and toxicology is just beginning. Assays have been developed for only a tiny fraction of the drugs currently employed and few of them are in a form suitable for clinical use. Homogeneous immunoassays as simple, or simpler than those already available, but more sensitive[36], will undoubtedly become available with the development of better enzyme, fluorescent, bio- and chemiluminescent[37] labels. Much work remains to be done to determine which drugs are worth monitoring in order to prove their clinical efficacy[24]. Effort put in now into the measurement of antineoplastic drugs in blood, and correlating the results with clinical improvement and the appearance of toxic side-effects, will pay handsome dividends. Other classes of drugs that lend themselves to monitoring include those that are used mainly for prevention of disease or for prophylaxis, e.g. the antimigraine, antidepressant and anti-schizophrenic drugs as well as lifesaving drugs such as antibiotics and antiarrhythmic agents with a narrow therapeutic index.

The impact of immunoassay upon toxicology has barely been felt. Its extension into the detection and measurement of toxic substances in food, the environment and even medicines and surgical appliances, can confidently be expected[38]. The use – especially – of the FAb fractions of antibodies raised against drugs and other toxic materials for which there are no known antidotes at present, may offer hope for patients who might otherwise die from their accidental or deliberate ingestion. Preliminary work with digoxin has already proved this feasible. It is only a matter of time before the principle is applied to other substances such as nortriptyline, dextropropoxyphine and paraquat, which are currently responsible for many potentially avoidable deaths.

In emergent nations where laboratory facilities are limited a start has already been made on the use of semiquantitative visually readable enzyme-linked immunosorbent (ELISA) techniques, employing disposable plastic microtitre plates, for determining compliance amongst patients prescribed drugs, such as dapsone, prophylactically or therapeutically. The extension of this principle into other areas such as the screening of milk for contamination by antibiotics can easily be foreseen.

References

1. Marks, V., Lindup, W. E. and Baylis, E. M. (1973). Measurement of therapeutic agents in blood. *Adv. Clin. Chem.*, **16**, 47
2. Marks, V., Morris, B. A. and Teale, J. D. (1974). Pharmacology. *Br. Med. Bull.*, **30**, 80
3. Landon, J. and Moffat, A. C. (1976). The radioimmunoassay of drugs: a review. *Analyst*, **101**, 225

K

4. Butler, V. P. (1975). Drug immunoassays. *J. Immunol. Methods*, **7**, 1

5. Mould, G. P., Aherne, G. W., Morris, B. A., Teale, J. D. and Marks, V. (1977). Radioimmunoassay of drugs and its clinical application. *Eur. J. Drug Metab. Pharmacol.*, **4**, 171

6. Marks, V. (1979). New developments in immunoassays for therapeutic drug monitoring. In Schonfield, H., Brockman, R. W. and Hahn, F. E. (eds.) *Antibiotics and Chemotherapy*, pp. 16–26. (Basel: Karger)

7. Marks, V., Mould, G. P., O'Sullivan, M. J. and Teale, J. D. (1980). Monitoring of drug disposition by immunoassay. In Bridges, J. W. and Chasseaud, L. F. (eds.) *Progress in Drug Metabolism*, Vol. 4, (Chichester: Wiley)

8. Erlanger, B. F. (1973). Principles and methods for the preparation of drug protein conjugates for immunological studies. *Pharmacol. Rev.*, **25**, 271

9. Aherne, G. W. and Marks, V. (1979). Radioimmunoassay techniques. In *Techniques in Metabolic Research*, pp. B215, 1–19. (Amsterdam: Elsevier)

10. Morris, B. A., Robinson, J. D., Piall, E., Aherne, G. W. and Marks, V. (1974). Development of a radioimmunoassay for morphine having minimal cross-reactivity with codeine. *J. Endocrinol.*, **64**, 6P

11. Robinson, J. D., Morris, B. A., Piall, E. M., Aherne, G. W. and Marks, V. (1975). The use of rats in screening of drug protein conjugates for immunoreactivity. In Pasternak, G. A. (ed.) *Radioimmunoassay in Clinical Biochemistry*, pp. 101–11. (London: Heyden)

12. Mould, G. P., Stout, G., Aherne, G. W. and Marks, V. (1978). Radioimmunoassay of amitriptyline and nortriptyline in body fluids. *Ann. Clin. Biochem.*, **15**, 221

13. Mould, G. P., Clough, J., Morris, B. A., Stout, G. and Marks, V. (1980). Radioimmunoassay of propranolol in plasma. *Biopharmaceutics and Drug Disposition*. (In press)

14. Vaitukaitis, J., Robbins, J. B., Nieschlag, E. and Ross, G. T. (1971). A method for producing specific antisera with small doses of immunogen. *J. Clin. Endocrinol. Metab.*, **33**, 988

15. Teale, J. D., Clough, J. M. and Marks, V. (1977). Radioimmunoassay of bleomycin in plasma and urine. *Br. J. Cancer*, **35**, 822

16. Kamel, R. S., Landon, J. and Smith, D. S. (1979). Novel ^{125}I-labelled nortriptyline derivatives and their use in liquid phase or magnetizable solid-phase second-antibody radioimmunoassays. *Clin. Chem.*, **25**, 1997

17. Al-Bassam, M. N., O'Sullivan, M. J., Gnemmi, E., Bridges, J. W. and Marks, V. (1978). Double-antibody enzyme-immunoassay for nortriptyline. *Clin. Chem.*, **24**, 1590

18. Miller, J. N., Lim, C. S. and Bridges, J. W. (1980). Fluorescamine and fluorescein as labels in energy-transfer immunoassay. *Analyst*, **105**, 91

19. Bastiani, R. J. (1979). The EMIT® system: a commercially successful innovation. In Schonfeld, H., Brockman, R. W. and Hahn, F. E. (eds.) *Antibiotics and Chemotherapy*, pp. 89–97. (Basel: Karger)

20. Marks, V. and Teale, J. D. (1979). The radioimmunoassay of cannabinoids: its clinical, pharmacological and forensic applications. In Nahas, G. G. and Paton, W. D. M. (eds.) *Marihuana: Biological Effects. Analysis, Metabolism, Cellular Responses, Reproduction and Brain*, pp. 81–88. (Oxford and New York: Pergamon Press)

21. Williams, P. L., Moffat, A. C. and King, L. J. (1978). Combined high-pressure liquid chromatography and radioimmunoassay method for the quantitation of delta-9-tetra-hydrocannabinol and some of its metabolites in human plasma. *J. Chromatogr.*, **155**, 273

22. De Graeve, J. (1980). Some considerations regarding drug determinations in biological fluids with physico-chemical methods. In Siest, G. and Young, D. S. (eds.) *Drug Measurement and Drug Effects in Laboratory Health Science*, pp. 2–19. (Basel: Karger)

23. Reiss, W., Brechbuhler, S. and Dubois, J. P. (1979). Rational analysis of drugs in biological fluids with particular reference to the tricyclic antidepressants. In Bridges, J. W. and Chasseaud, L. F. (eds.) *Progress in Drug Metabolism*, Vol. 3, pp. 115–49. (Chichester: Wiley)

24. Marks, V. (1979). Clinical monitoring of therapeutic drugs. *Ann. Clin, Biochem.*, **16**, 370

25. Richens, A. and Marks, V. (1981). *Therapeutic Drug Monitoring* (Edinburgh: Churchill Livingstone)

26. Schneider, R. S., Bastiani, R. J., Leute, R. K., Rubenstein, K. E. and Ullman, E. F. (1974). Use of enzyme and spin-labelling in homogeneous immunochemical detection method. In Mule, S. J., Sunshine, I., Braude, M. and Willette, R. E. (eds.) *Immunoassays for Drugs Subject to Abuse*, pp. 45–74. (Cleveland: CRC Press)

27. Wong, R. C., Burd, J. F., Carrico, R. J., Buckler, R. T., Thoma, J. and Boguslaski, R. C. (1979). Substrate-labelled fluorescent immunoassay for phenytoin in human serum. *Clin. Chem.*, **25**, 686

28. Aherne, G. W., Marks, V., Morris, B. A., Piall, E. M., Robinson, J. D. and Twycross, R. G. (1975). The measurement of serum morphine levels by radioimmunoassay following oral administration of diamorphine or morphine. *Br. J. Pharmacol.*, **54**, 228P

29. Baylis, E. M., Hall, M. S., Lewis, G. and Marks, V. (1972). Effects of renal function on plasma digoxin levels in elderly ambulant patients in domiciliary practice. *Br. Med. J.*, **1**, 338

30. Juel, R. (1979). The 1978 College of American Pathologists Therapeutic Drug Monitoring Interlaboratory Survey Program. *Am. J. Clin. Pathol.*, **72**, 306

31. American Association for Clinical Chemistry (1980). *Therapeutic Drug Monitoring: Continuing Education and Quality Control Program.* (Washington: AACC)

32. Marks, V., O'Sullivan, M. J., Al-Bassam, M. N. and Bridges, J. W. (1978). A double antibody enzyme-immunoassay for methotrexate. In Pal, S. B. (ed.) *Enzyme Labelled Immunoassay of Hormones and Drugs*, pp. 419–28. (Berlin: De Gruyter)

33. Ngowi, F. (1979). Development of an enzyme immunoassay for measuring 6-alpha-methylprednisolone in biological fluids. *MSc Thesis*, University of Surrey

34. Teale, J. D., Clough, J. M., King, L. J., Marks, V., Williams, P. L. and Moffat, A. C. (1977). The incidence of cannabinoids in fatally injured drivers: an investigation by radioimmunoassay and high pressure liquid chromatography. *J. Forens. Sci. Soc.*, **17**, 177

35. Marks, V. and Fry, D. E. (1977). Detection and measurement of drugs in biological fluids: their relevance to the problem of drug abuse. In Glatt, M. M. (ed.) *Drug Dependence: Current Problems and Issues*, pp. 295–327 (Lancaster: MTP Press)

36. Morris, D. L., Rawson, D., Ellis, P. B., Hornby, W. E., Schroeder, H. R., Boguslaski, R. C. and Carrico, R. J. (1979). Specific binding assays with a prosthetic group as label. *Ann. Clin. Biochem.*, Suppl. 1, 25

37. Schroeder, H. R., Vogelhut, P. O., Carrico, R. J., Boguslaski, R. C. and Buckler, R. T. (1976). Competitive protein binding assay for biotin monitored by chemiluminescence. *Anal. Chem.*, **48**, 1933

38. Luster, M. I., Albro, P. W., Chase, K., Clark, G. and McKinney, J. D. (1978). Radioimmunoassay for mono-(2-ethylhexyl) phthalate in unextracted plasma. *Clin. Chem.*, **24**, 429

18
Immunoassays in Autoimmune Disease

E. J. HOLBOROW, G. D. JOHNSON, R. MARCH and
J. REEBACK

In the diagnosis and management of autoimmune diseases, a major role for the clinical immunology laboratory is to identify and, where possible, measure the levels of circulating autoantibodies.

Autoantibodies occurring in disease fall under two headings. The first includes antibodies that are known to be involved in producing lesions by one or other of the humoral mechanisms of immune tissue damage. Well known examples of this class are the anti-red cell and platelet antibodies of autoimmune blood disease, the anti-DNA antibodies of systemic lupus erythematosus, the rheumatoid factors of rheumatoid arthritis and its variants, and the antibodies to nicotinic acetylcholine receptors which seem to produce the post-synaptic muscle membrane changes of myasthenia gravis. The second class of autoantibodies (smooth muscle antibodies and several other antibodies against intracellular antigens are examples) are those which seem to play no part in immunopathology, evidently owing their appearance to the workings of often obscure aetiological factors, but having diagnostic relevance to a greater or lesser degree. It may be noted that, with better understanding of the nature of the various diseases in question, antibodies in the second group have not infrequently found themselves reclassified as belonging to the first.

Developments in the methodology of measurement of autoantibodies have to a considerable extent been influenced by the historical fact that much autoantibody serology has been based upon indirect immunofluorescence. With this technique cryostat sections of normal tissues, or sometimes monolayers of tissue culture cells, are reacted on slides with the patients' serum, and the binding of any antibody present is revealed on fluorescence microscopy after a second treatment with fluorochrome-conjugated anti-globulin antibody. The specificity of autoantibodies detected in this way is inferred from recognition of the characteristic patterns of fluorescent staining seen under the microscope. It is the considerable diagnostic significance for a range of diseases of various distinguishable patterns of cell or tissue staining that has established indirect IF as an indispensable screening test for autoantibodies, with the added advantage that the complement-fixing properties of antibodies detected are readily determined by including fresh guinea-pig or human serum in the test and using anti-complement conjugate as the detector reagent.

Sera may, of course, be titrated by indirect IF, and this is widely done to obtain a measure of their autoantibody content, which may be of considerable clinical import. There are several factors which influence titration of antibodies by immunofluorescence, however. Among these are the presence of low avidity antibodies which may cause false negatives due to prozones[1], or give lower titres than the same weight of high-avidity antibodies; and washing out of particularly soluble antigens (e.g. some extractable nuclear antigens) from tissue sections during processing.

THE LIMITATIONS OF IMMUNOFLUORESCENCE

The essentially screening role of immunofluorescent tests for autoantibodies, however, needs to be emphasized. Indirect IF suffers from the limitation that it can indicate only the topography, i.e. the localization in tissues or cells, of the reaction of a given patient's serum with a tissue antigen, and does not necessarily distinguish between different antigens in the same location, nor tell us anything of the nature or specific determinants of the antigen in question.

The sensitivity and reproducibility of immunofluorescence techniques is variable, especially between laboratories, and the availability of reference sera containing defined Ig classes and levels of common human autoantibodies would do much to validate immunofluorescent immunoassay by titre, a very necessary requirement. At present, only a WHO 'homogeneous antinuclear factor' reference preparation (66/233) is available for such quality control, and others are needed.

Quality control is also of paramount importance in establishing the satisfactory performance of fluorescent anti-Ig conjugates. WHO issues a fluorescein conjugated sheep anti-human immunoglobulin international standard (48 00 10) and an anti-IgM international standard conjugate (M18L), and an anti-IgG international standard conjugate is in preparation. These conjugate quality control reagents find their most useful place as manufacturers' yardsticks[2] and as checks on the class specificity and performance of commercial conjugates, and are especially useful when unexpected results encountered in routine tests require validation.

ANTIGEN-SPECIFIC ASSAYS

Much painstaking effort has been and is being devoted to identifying more precisely the sub-cellular organelles, membrane components and extracellular structures which carry antigenic determinants reactive with organ-specific or non-organ-specific autoantibodies routinely screened for by immunofluorescence. These, it goes without saying, are extremely heterogeneous in nature, ranging from mitochondria, microsomes, ribosomes, nuclear antigens and cell membrane antigens and receptors on the one hand, to collagen and reticulin fibrils and intercellular cement substance extracellularly, and cytoskeletal filaments and tubules intracellularly, on the other. The 1980s may expect to see a considerable extension of assay procedures for autoantibodies based on reactions with purified antigenic components derived from these various materials. So far, however, attempts to use autoantigenic moieties to develop immunoassay procedures practicable for the clinical immunologist have in only relatively few instances succeeded in supplanting immunofluorescence as the pathologist's method of choice. One which has is the passive haemagglutination test for autoantibodies against thyroid microsomal antigen, which were initially distinguished from anti-thyroglobulin autoantibodies by immunofluorescence[3] and until recently were usually looked for by this technique. The practical reason for this change is that the immunofluorescent test for anti-microsomal antibody requires for its best performance cryostat sections of fresh thyroid tissue obtained surgically from patients with Graves' disease, in which microsomal antigen is prominent in the hypertrophic epithelium. The restricted availability of such surgical material has favoured the development of a simple alternative passive haemagglutination test adaptable to commercial supply (the Fujizoki test) so that now both commonly looked-for thyroid autoantibodies, anti-microsomal and anti-thryoglobin, can be assayed without immunofluorescence[4].

ASSAYS FOR ANTIBODIES TO NUCLEAR ANTIGENS

Interest in antinuclear antibodies, initially sparked off by the discovery of the LE cell phenomenon, led investigators to use many different methods for their detection, some of them indicated in Table 18.1. Of the different anti-DNA specificities encountered in human sera, so called anti-double-stranded (ds) antibodies commonly recognize sites on the phosphate deoxyribose chain shared by both ds and single-stranded (ss) DNA; much rarer are antibodies reactive only with ds-DNA. Anti-ds-DNA antibodies of both sorts have been repeatedly shown to be, with a few exceptions, restricted to patients with SLE, and immunoassays to measure primary binding of these antibodies to radio-labelled ds-DNA as antigen consequently now play an important part in the diagnosis and management of these patients. The validity of results of such assays depends upon the use of ds-DNA without single stranded regions as

Table 18.1 Assay methods for antinuclear antibodies

Antibody specificity	Occurrence in disease	Antigen specificity	Assay methods
Anti-deoxyribonucleoprotein (DNP)	SLE Drug induced LE	DNA-histone combination	RIA, ID, Latex, HA bentonite, LE cell
Anti-ds-DNA	SLE (rarely)	ds-DNA only	RIA, ID, CIE, HA, CF, *Crithidia* IF
Anti-ds ss-DNA	SLE (diagnostic) occ. RA and other CI diseases CAH	Ribophosphate backbone determinants and others common to ds and ss-DNA	RIA, ID, CIE, HA, CF
Anti-ss-DNA	Rheumatic and some other diseases	Nucleic acid bases and nucleotides	RIA, ID, CIE, HA, CF
Histone	Rheumatoid arthritis ? Other diseases	? Multiple	CF, special IF
Sm	30% SLE	Glycoproteins	ID, CIE, HA, CF (thymus extract contains Ag)
RNP	MCTD high titres Lower titres ± in other rheumatic diseases	RNA protein	ID, CIE, HA, CRF (thymus extract)
SS-A	Sjögren's disease and sicca syndromes ± in other rheumatic diseases	Unknown	ID, CIE (lymphoblastoid cell line extract)
SS-B	Sjögren's disease and sicca syndromes ± in other rheumatic diseases	Extractable, chemistry unknown	ID, CIE (thymus extract, lymphoblastoid cell lines)
Sel-1	Scleroderma	Extractable, chemistry unknown	ID (thymus extract)
RAP	Rheumatoid arthritis Sjögren's with RA	Chemistry unknown	ID (lymphoblastoid extract)
RANA	Rheumatoid arthritis Sjögren's with RA	Chemistry unknown	IF (lymphoblastoid cell lines)
Nucleolar	Scleroderma Sjögren's syndrome	4–6s RNA	IF

CF = Complement fixation
CIE = Counter immunoelectrophoresis
ID = Double immunodiffusion in gel
IF = Immunofluorescence
HA = Passive haemagglutination
RIA = Radioimmunoassay

Modified from Nakamura and Tan[5]

antigen since sera from diseases other than SLE may contain antibodies reacting with nucleic acid bases and nucleotide sequences accessible only in single-stranded DNA (anti-ss-DNA antibodies). This requirement demands rigorous tests of the antigen to establish lack of binding with anti-ss-DNA. Aarden et al.[6] have successfully used circular DNA from bacteriophage PM_2 to ensure unimpaired double-strandedness. Such a restriction, however, means that radio-immunoassays for anti-ds DNA antibodies are difficult to arrange and expensive to perform.

Another completely different method for anti-ds DNA devised by Aarden et al.[7] is an immunofluorescent test with the haemoflagellate Crithidia luciliae as substrate. This organism contains a giant mitochondrion in which ds-DNA is concentrated in a single large network, the kinetoplast. A correlation was found in SLE sera between ability to stain crithidial kinetoplasts in indirect immunofluorescence and to bind PM_2 circular DNA in the Farr immunoassay[6].

We have been interested in the suggestion of Barnett[8] that since most SLE sera containing anti-ds-DNA antibodies also contain as much or more antibody with specificity for ss-DNA only, measurement of the latter might give useful information both for diagnosis and management of SLE and perhaps also other rheumatic diseases in which antinuclear antibodies occur. We have carried out a preliminary study on the sera of patients for whom anti-DNA antibody tests were requested by the clinician in charge.

The object was to compare titres by immunofluorescent ANA, Crithidia luciliae, by anti-ds-DNA as measured by a Farr radioimmunoassay kit (Radiochemical Centre, Amersham) and checked against a reference standard serum, and by an anti-ss-DNA ELISA assay in microtitre trays coated with freshly boiled and cooled (ss) DNA. The ELISA test was standardized against a reference serum included with each assay. The results of this study, which will be reported in detail elsewhere, have confirmed that the majority of SLE sera have significantly raised levels of anti-ss as well as anti-ds-DNA antibodies (Figure 18.1), although the levels of the two types of antibody show little correlation (Figure 18.2). We also find that sera with immunofluorescent ANA levels of less than 25 IU/ml (in our hands 25 IU is equivalent to a titre of 1/40) seldom show significantly increased levels of antibody to ds-DNA (Figure 18.3). We conclude that only sera containing 25 IU of ANA or more qualify for further testing for specific anti-DNA antibodies. This is a useful guide for the clinical immunology laboratory screening sera diagnostically for anti-ds-DNA. Our findings also indicate, however, that the four tests – IF ANA, anti-ds-DNA, anti-ss-DNA and Crithidia – measure different properties of sera, and none of them can be substituted for any of the others.

The extent to which anti-DNA antibody reflects disease activity, or changes in level reflect changes in activity, is still controversial. Swaak et al.[9] have pointed out that although high levels of anti-ds-DNA antibody are a good diagnostic indicator of SLE, it is often a sudden fall in antibody levels rather

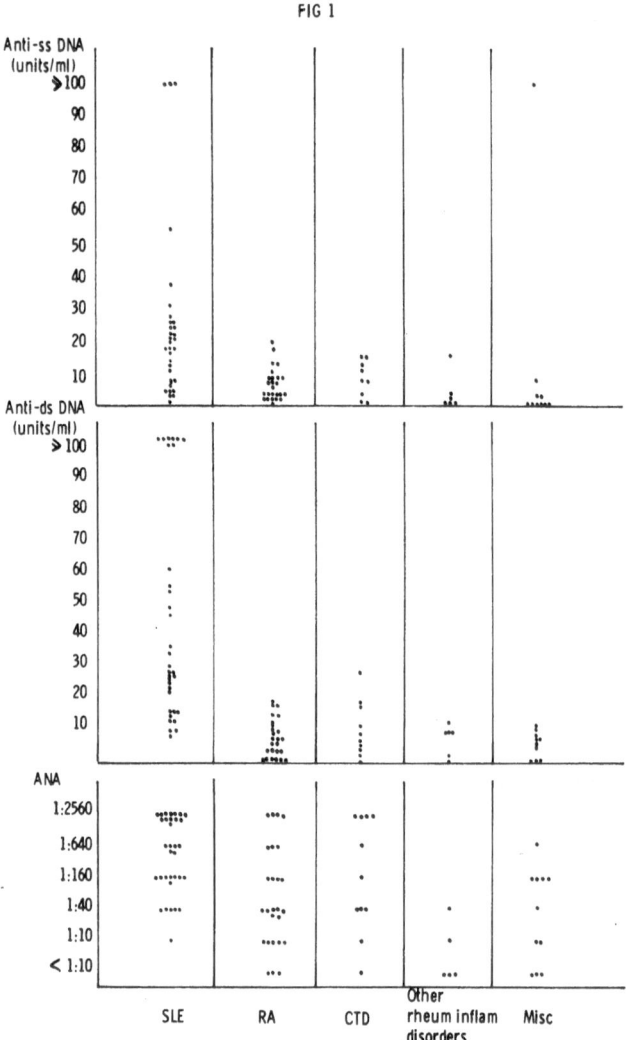

Figure 18.1   Immunofluorescent ANA levels with ss-DNA and ds-DNA binding levels in sera from patients for whom a DNA binding test was requested. Each point is one patient's serum. The final diagnoses are shown on the horizontal axis

than a rise that heralds a recrudescence of renal disease activity, and the role of immune complex deposits in promoting the latter no doubt explains this. Most rheumatologists, moreover, recognize that high DNA antibody levels do not necessarily indicate clinically active disease[10]. The Farr test, which uses a high salt concentration to precipitate DNA-bound antibody, selects in this way for antibody of higher affinity, and it may well be argued that assays for lower affinity antibody ought to give results relating more closely to activity[11, 12]. It must also be remembered, however, that experiments with

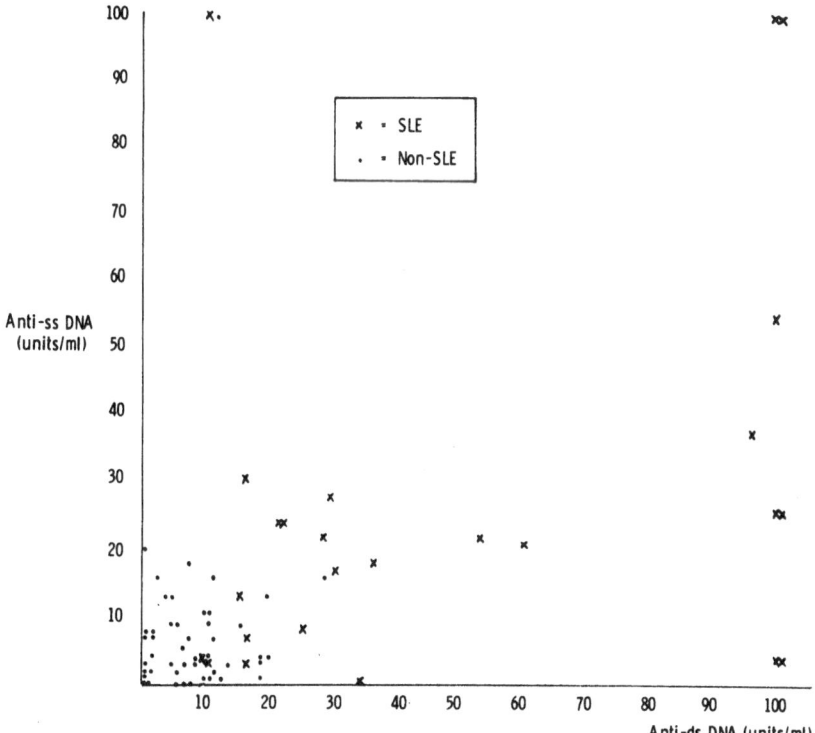

Figure 18.2 The anti-ds-DNA and anti-ss-DNA binding levels of the sera in Figure 18.1 compared

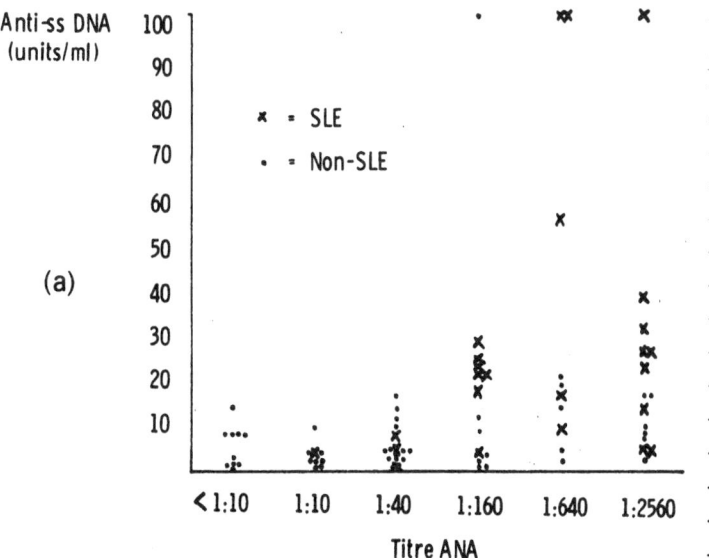

Figure 18.3 ANA titres of the sera in Figure 18.1 compared with (a) anti-ss-DNA and (b) anti-ds-DNA binding levels

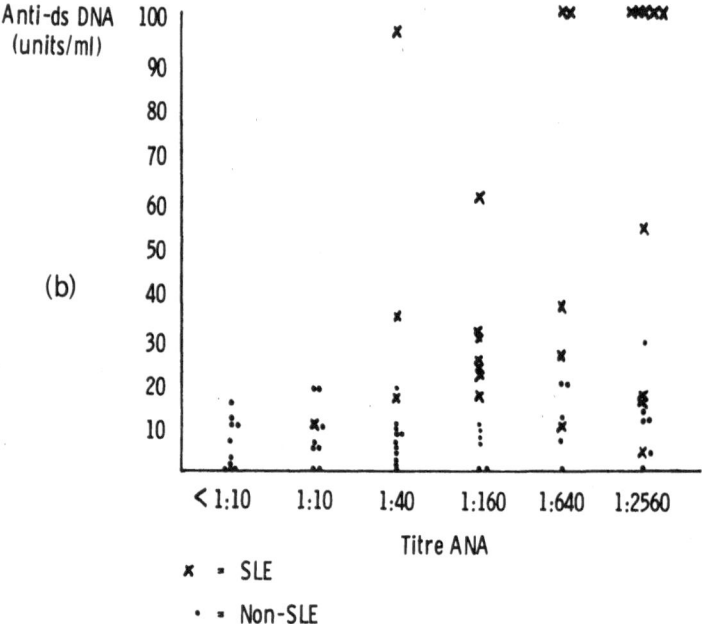

renal biopsy material from lupus kidneys have demonstrated only ss-DNA as the antigen component of the immune complex deposits[13]. There seems reason therefore to investigate separately the relationship of anti-ss-DNA antibody levels to disease activity in SLE, especially as a simple and reproducible ELISA test is available for this purpose.

Assays for antibodies against nuclear antigens other than DNA are hampered by lack of definition of the antigens concerned. An exception is the RNP antigen against which patients with mixed connective tissue disease are reported to have consistently very high titre antibodies[5], whose specificity is confirmed by the effects of RNase on the reactivity of the antigen. The recent demonstration of anti-RANA antibody[14] and anti-histone antibody[15] in rheumatoid arthritis sera is a stimulus to characterize both antigens more precisely.

ASSAYS FOR RHEUMATOID FACTORS

The concept of rheumatoid factors (RFs) as anti-immunoglobulin antibodies directed at human IgG as antigen occupies a central position in hypotheses of the autoimmune basis of rheumatoid arthritis. Tests which detect serum rheumatoid factors through their agglutination or flocculating action on coated erythrocytes or particles are selective for RFs of the multivalent IgM antibody class, and in this way identify patients with 'seropositive' rheumatoid disease.

There is much evidence to support interpretation of rheumatoid synovitis as a form of localized extravascular immune complex disease[16] in which a significant contribution to the inflammation-inducing immune complexes in question is made by IgG rheumatoid factor with its self-associating property[17]. In 'seropositive' patients, IgM rheumatoid factor, which likewise can undergo a complement fixing interaction with IgG, is clearly also involved in inducing and maintaining the chronic synovitis. The fact that extra-articular complications, due also, it is thought, to immune-complex-mediated vasculitis, are more likely in seropositive patients underlines the role of IgM RF.

What is less clear, however, is the significance of circulating IgG RF, which is reported to be present in the sera of most patients with rheumatoid arthritis, whether seropositive or seronegative for IgM RF[18, 19]. IgG RF in both serum and synovial fluid has been assayed by a number of different methods (reviewed by Pope and McDuffy[20]), which have been criticized as either laborious or insensitive or non-specific. There is still a lack of agreement whether, or to what extent, IgG RF levels are raised in seronegative rheumatoid arthritis, whether in either seropositive or seronegative patients IgG RF levels have any diagnostic significance, or whether changes in IgG RF serum levels reflect disease activity or drug action any better than changes in IgM RF.

One possibility for future investigation of the role of serum RFs of different classes is to use a red cell marker system of the sort described by Professor Coombs (this volume), and we are investigating this possibility jointly with him. The principle of the test is shown in Figure 18.4. The antigen – in

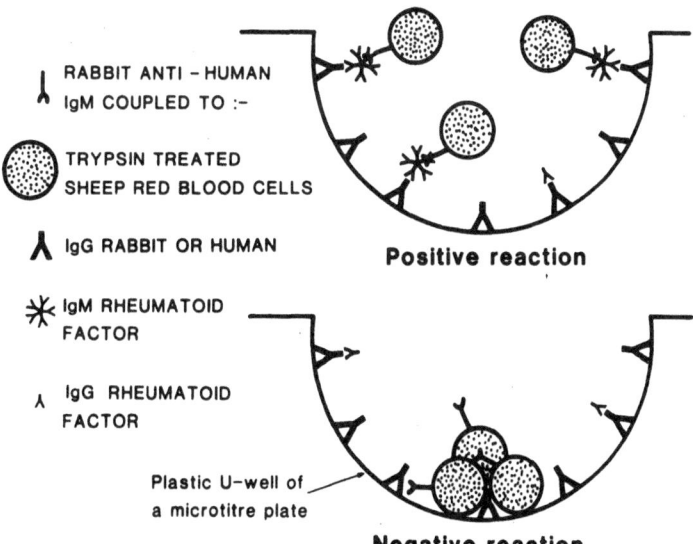

Figure 18.4 Diagram of MRSPAH test for rheumatoid factors of different classes

preliminary tests, rabbit IgG – is allowed to bind, in solution, to the plastic wells in a microtitre plate. The coated wells next receive the sera under test for rheumatoid factor, and are then washed. The indicator system is sheep red cells, trypsinized and then coupled with rabbit anti-Ig of defined specificity for human IgG, IgA or IgM. The antiglobulin used is adjusted so that although the cells are fully coated, when added to wells without human serum, they settle on standing to form a compact button. If rheumatoid factor of IgM class, for example, has bound to the rabbit IgG coating the well, sheep cells coated with anti-IgM antibody adhere to the plastic well surface and form a visible carpet. The test is therefore a mixed reverse solid-phase passive antiglobulin haemadherence (MRsPAH). For measurement of IgG RF, it is necessary first to inactivate accompanying IgM RF by mercaptoethanol or dithiothreitol treatment of the serum. This obviates the possibility of false ascertainment of IgG RF due to IgM RF binding to the coated well and at the same time binding non-RF IgG from the serum with its free valencies.

Preliminary studies with the MRsPAH system show that it may be used to detect IgM IgA and IgG RF separately, and to measure them by titration.

The MRsPAH reaction is simpler than other methods used for measuring RFs of different classes such as ELISA and radioimmunoassay, and does not

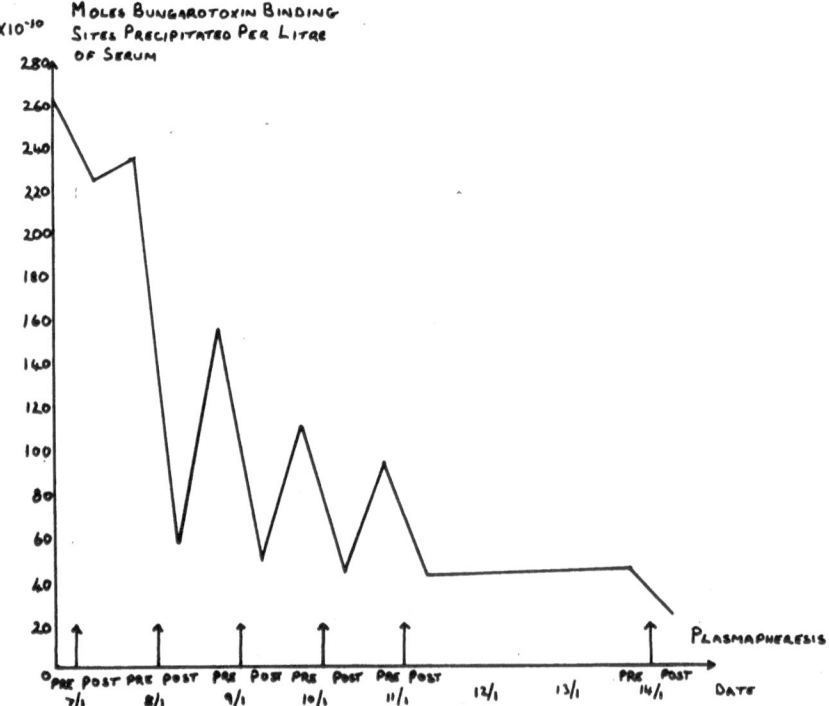

Figure 18.5   Effect of repeated plasma exchanges on the level of anti-acetylcholine receptor antibody in a patient with myasthenia gravis'

require expensive counting or measuring apparatus, the results being read visually. As with other methods, the antiglobulin reagents have to be carefully standardized and coupled. The sensitivity appears to be higher than that seen with the Rose–Waaler or latex methods.

The MRsPAH reaction may also prove suitable for study of other autoantibodies, at least in cases where the tissue antigens concerned are known and can be prepared in purified or enriched form. Another promising candidate might be the tissue specific antibodies in myasthenia gravis which are directed at antigenic sites on nicotinic acetylcholine receptors (AChR) of the post-synaptic membrane of muscle. At present, such antibodies are detected by a method which makes use of the fact that α-bungarotoxin, a snake venom polypeptide, binds specifically to AChRs. In a crude muscle membrane extract, radiolabelled α-bungarotoxin will thus act as a marker of AChRs, so that when serum containing anti-AChR antibody is added, and then, in turn, specific anti-human IgG antibody, the radioactivity in the specific precipitate will be a measure of the anti-AChR antibody present[21]. This is a laborious and complicated assay procedure. AChR autoantibodies appear to be specific for myasthenia gravis, and their removal by plasma exchange (Figure 18.5) produces a clinical remission[22]. A simpler assay method is needed for monitoring long-term as well as short-term changes in antibody levels, and we are investigating the practicability of a MRsPAH technique.

SUMMARY

Most advances relating autoantibodies more precisely to the diagnosis and management of the diseases in which they occur have followed more precise identification of the antigens concerned, improvement of methods for their isolation, and the development of standard simple immunoassay procedures. Autoantibody determinations are among the most frequently requested investigations performed by clinical immunology laboratories. The development of simple solid phase assays, avoiding difficulties arising from antigen solubility and requirements for radioisotopes, may be expected to enhance the clinical usefulness of such tests.

References

1. Linder, E. and Miettinen, A. (1976). Prozone effects in indirect immunofluorescence. *Scand. J. Immunol.*, **5**, 513
2. Johnson, G. D., Chantler, S., Batty, I. and Holborow, E. J. (1978). Use and abuse of international reference preparations in immunofluorescence. Ch. 11. In Dumonde, D. C. and Steward, M. W. (eds.) *Laboratory Tests in Rheumatic Diseases* (Lancaster: MTP Press)
3. Holborow, E. J., Brown, P. C., Doniach, D. and Roitt, I. M. (1959). Cytoplasmic localisation of 'complement-fixing' auto-antigen in human thyroid epithelium. *Br. J. Exp. Pathol.*, **40**, 583

4. Perrin, J. and Bubell, M. A. (1974). Assessment of a haemagglutinating test for thyroid microsomal antibody. *Med. Lab. Tech.*, **31**, 205

5. Nakamura, R. M. and Tan, E. M. (1978). Recent progress in the study of autoantibodies to nuclear antigens. *Hum. Pathol.*, **9**, 85

6. Aarden, L. A., Lakmaker, F. and Feltkamp, T. E. W. (1976). Immunology of DNA II: The effect of size and structure of the antigen on the Farr assay. *J. Immunol. Methods*, **10**, 39

7. Aarden, L. A., de Groot, E. R. and Feltkamp, T. E. W. (1975). Immunology of DNA III: *Crithidia luciliae*, a simple substrate for the determination of anti-ds DNA with the immunofluorescence technique. *Ann. NY Acad. Sci.*, **254**, 505

8. Barnett, E. V. (1970). Anti-DNA antibodies: Perspectives and perplexities. *J. Immunol. Methods*, **27**, 1

9. Swaak, A. J. G., Aarden, L. A., van Eps, S. and Feltkamp, T. E. W. (1979). Anti-ds DNA and complement profiles as prognostic guides in systemic lupus erythematosus. *Arthritis Rheum.*, **22**, 226

10. Hughes, G. R. V. (1979). The treatment of SLE: The case for conservative management. In Huskisson, E. C. (ed.) *Clinics in Rheumatic Diseases*, Ch. 15, Vol. 5, No. 2. (London: W. B. Saunders)

11. Steward, M. W., Glass, D. N., Maini, R. N. and Scott, J. T. (1974). Role of low avidity antibody to native DNA in human and murine lupus syndromes. *J. Rheumatol.*, Suppl. 1, **1**, Abstract No. 75

12. Smeenk, R. and Aarden, L. (1980). The use of PEG precipitation to detect low avidity anti-DNA antibodies in SLE. *J. Immunol. Methods* (In press)

13. Andres, G. A., Accini, L., Beiser, S. M., Christian, C. L., Cinotti, G. A., Erlanger, E. G., Hsu, K. C. and Seegal, B. C. (1971). Localisation of fluorescein-labelled antinucleoside antibodies in glomeruli of patients with active systemic lupus erythematosus nephritis. *J. Clin. Invest.*, **49**, 2106

14. Alspaugh, M., Jensen, F., Rabin, H. and Tan, E. M. (1978). Lymphocytes transformed by Epstein-Barr virus. Induction of nuclear antigen reactive with antibody in rheumatoid arthritis. *J. Exp. Med.*, **147**, 1018

15. Aitcheson, C. T., Peebles, C., Joslin, F. and Tan, E. M. (1980). Characteristics of antinuclear antibodies in rheumatoid arthritis: Reactivity of rheumatoid factor with a histone-dependent nuclear antigen. *Arthritis Rheum.*, **23**, 528

16. Zvaifler, N. J. (1974). Rheumatoid synovitis. An extravascular immune complex disease. *Arthritis Rheum.*, **17**, 297

17. Pope, R. M., Teller, D. C. and Mannik, M. (1974). The molecular basis of self association of antibodies to IgG (rheumatoid factors) in rheumatoid arthritis. *Proc. Natl. Acad. Sci.*, **71**, 517

18. Hay, F. C., Nineham, L. J. and Roitt, I. M. (1975). Routine assay for detection of IgG and IgM antiglobulins in seronegative and seropositive rheumatoid arthritis. *Br. Med. J.*, **3**, 203

19. Carson, D. A., Lawrence, S., Catalamo, M. A., Vaughan, J. H. and Abraham, G. (1977). Radioimmunoassay of IgG and IgM rheumatoid factors reacting with human IgG. *J. Immunol.*, **119**, 295

20. Pope, R. M. and McDuffy, S. J. (1979). IgG rheumatoid factor. Relationship to seropositive rheumatoid arthritis and absence in seronegative disorders. *Arthritis Rheum.*, **22**, 295

21. Vincent, A. (1979). Tissue specific antibodies in myasthenia gravis. *J. Clin. Pathol.*, **32**, Suppl. R. Coll. Pathol., **13**, 97

22. Pinching, A. J., Peters, D. K. and Newsom-Davies, J. (1976). Plasma exchange in myasthenia gravis. *Lancet*, **2**, 1373

19
Radioimmunoassays in Allergy

T. A. E. PLATTS-MILLS, M. D. CHAPMAN and E. TOVEY

INTRODUCTION

In 1873 Charles Blackley published his proof that pollen grains cause hay fever. He also developed techniques for counting pollen grains in the air and made the earliest estimates of the quantity of pollen necessary to cause symptoms. The quantities were so low (0.032 μg pollen/h) that Blackley became President of the British Homeopathic Society[1]. It was well known that allergic patients would give immediate skin reactions to allergen extracts. In 1921 Prausnitz and Küstner demonstrated that serum from an allergic person could passively sensitize the skin of a non-allergic person[2]. Using this P–K test it was possible to show that the active principle or reagin was antigen-specific, but the quantities of reagin were very low and they could not be detected by any other technique. Finally in 1967 Ishizaka and his colleagues demonstrated that the substance responsible for P–K activity belonged to a separate class of immunoglobulin – IgE[3]. This discovery led to detailed studies on the biology and structure of IgE and to the development of techniques for measuring total IgE and IgE antibodies[4, 5]. These techniques established that the quantity of IgE in serum is normally less than 1 μg/ml, while the quantity of IgE antibody to an individual allergen is generally less than 0.1 μg/ml. Thus all the important aspects of immediate hyper-sensitivity, i.e. allergens, IgE and specific antibodies, are normally found in such small quantities that they can only be detected or measured by bioassays or immunoassays. Many different immunoassays have been used in allergy but at present the most widely used assays depend on radiolabelled proteins. Both human and animal immunoglobulins label very well and so do most purified allergens using the modified Chloramine T technique[6]. Total serum IgE and some allergens can be measured using a classical double-antibody inhibition radioimmunoassay

(RIA). Many of the other assays used in allergy take unusual forms which have not been adopted in other branches of medicine. The reasons why these unusual assays work appear to reflect some of the important biological features of immediate hypersensitivity. Some of these assays use reagents which are very poorly defined and which cannot at present be standardized. Curiously, although assays used in allergy need to be very sensitive, great accuracy is often not required. This is because the range of results found is very wide, e.g. total serum IgE levels range from < 0.2 IU/ml to > 10 000IU/ml.

MEASUREMENTS OF IgE ANTIBODIES

The radioallergosorbent technique – RAST

The original studies on IgE demonstrated by radioimmunoelectrophoresis that IgE antibodies could bind radiolabelled allergens *in vitro*. However this technique is slow and only semi-quantitative. When the first IgE myeloma (ND) was discovered it became possible to prepare rabbit anti-IgE and also to specifically purify anti-IgE. Using radiolabelled anti-IgE, Wide *et al.* developed the radioallergosorbent technique (RAST)[7]. This technique has been of great importance in the diagnosis and study of allergy, but has no real parallel outside allergy. RAST is usually carried out using crude allergen extract linked by the cyanogen bromide technique to a solid-phase particle, either Sepharose beads, microfine cellulose beads or cellulose discs[8]. The particles are incubated with serum overnight and washed before adding radiolabelled anti-IgE (Figure 19.1). It may seem very surprising that crude allergen extracts, e.g. aqueous extract of pollen, house dust or dust mite culture can be used for the RAST. It might be maintained that because the particle has a range of proteins on it there is no indication from the result as to which protein is acting as the allergen. Despite this RAST can give very useful results, and correlates well with other *in vivo* and *in vitro* methods for diagnosing immediate hypersensitivity[9-11].

The quantity of allergen molecules available for binding IgE antibodies depends on:

(1) how much allergen is added to the activated particles;
(2) the capacity of the particle to bind proteins;
(3) the proportion of the protein in the extract which is allergen (Figure 19.2).

If the quantity of allergen on a particle is low because of any or several of these factors then the IgE antibody in a serum may not be fully bound. If a serum contains high levels of IgE antibody this problem may arise in sera from untreated patients. The problem is more likely to occur after desensitization treatment when there is a selective rise in IgG antibody (see Figure 19.2). The next problem with RAST is that the background binding of radiolabelled anti-IgE is primarily dependent on the non-specific binding of IgE. This non-

(a) Serum + antigen on bead   (b) Add radiolabelled Anti-IgE   (c) Wash particles

Count radioactivity
on beads

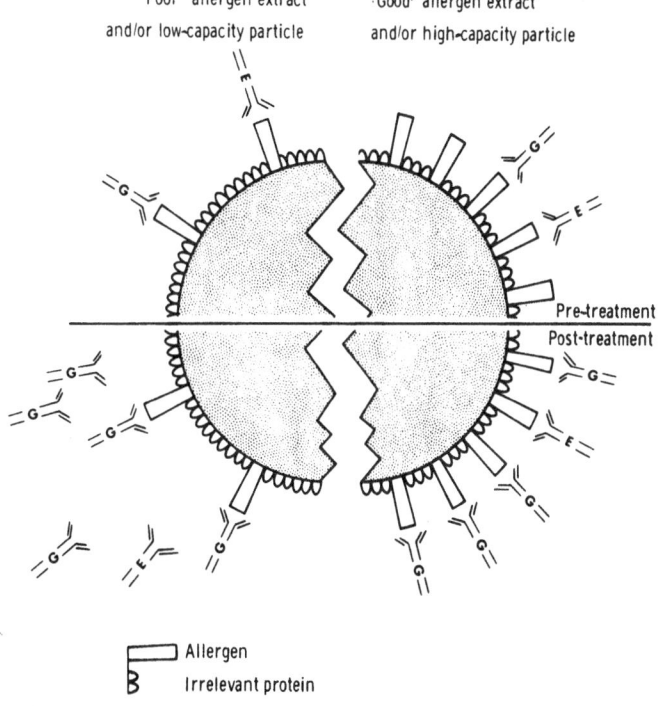

Figure 19.1 Radioallergosorbent technique (RAST). Allergens (Ag) are linked to a disc or Sepharose particle using the cyanogen bromide technique. The serum added includes specific IgE (= E ⪡) and non-specific IgE (= E ⪡) as well as specific (⪡) and non-specific (⪡) antibodies of other classes. Radiolabelled goat anti-IgE (*Anti-IgE ⪡) will detect specific IgE antibodies bound to allergen, but will also detect any other IgE that is bound non-specifically to the particle (not shown in figure)

'Poor' allergen extract
and/or low-capacity particle

'Good' allergen extract
and/or high-capacity particle

Pre-treatment
Post-treatment

☐ Allergen
β Irrelevant protein

Figure 19.2 With a 'poor' allergen extract or a low capacity particle (e.g. cellulose discs), the quantity of specific allergen molecules (☐) may be limiting. Accurate RAST results may be obtained with sera from patients who have not received desensitizing injections and who have modest levels of IgE antibodies (⟩ E=). Desensitizing injections (and some allergens) may give rise to high levels of IgG antibody (⟩ G=), i.e. 50 times more than the IgE antibody, and consequently binding of IgE antibodies may be reduced. This problem is unlikely to arise with high-capacity particles (e.g. Sepharose) or with 'good' extracts in which a high proportion of the protein is allergen

specific binding represents approximately 0.1–0.5% of the IgE present in a serum and can be demonstrated using IgE myeloma proteins which have no known antibody activity. This background increases as total IgE increases and may become a problem with sera containing over 1000 IU IgE/ml. The nature of the binding is not clear; however, it is known to vary from one particle to another and may also vary with different allergens on the same type of particle[12]. All classes of human immunoglobulin show similar non-specific binding (i.e. $\sim 0.2\%$) to solid-phase particles. The quantity of IgE in most sera is $< 1 \mu g/ml$ so that non-specific binding represents ~ 1 ng and it should be possible to measure levels of IgE antibody > 1 ng/ml. By contrast, normal serum contains 10 mg of IgG so that background binding might well be equivalent to 1 $\mu g/ml$ and levels of IgG antibody much less than this would be difficult to detect by RAST. The binding results observed with a series of sera from dust mite allergic patients are shown in Figure 19.3, using RAST discs linked to extract of *D. pteronyssinus* culture. It is clear that only for IgE are

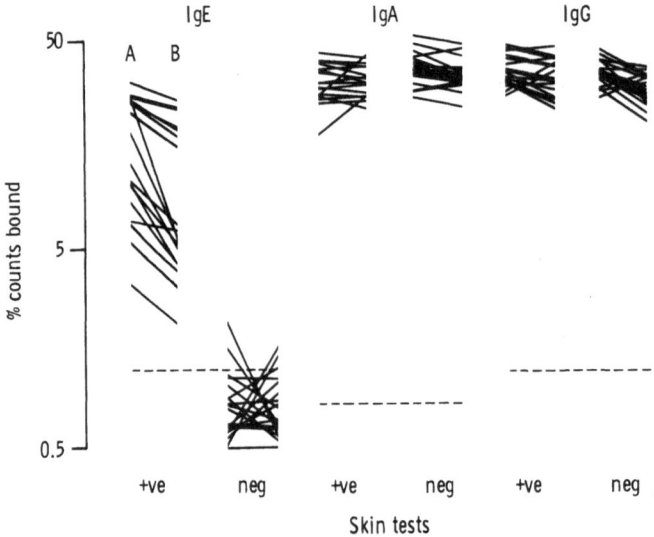

Figure 19.3 Attempts to modify RAST for IgA and IgG antibodies to *Dermatophagoides pteronyssinus*. Sera from 17 skin-test-positive and 17 skin-test-negative individuals were assayed at two dilutions 1/6 (A) and 1/12 (B). *D. pteronyssinus* extract was linked to cyanogen bromide-activated cellulose discs; after incubation with serum the discs were washed extensively and were incubated with ^{125}I-labelled anti-IgE, anti-IgA or anti-IgG. For IgE there was a consistent relationship between the two dilutions of allergic sera and the negative serum background was low enough for the assay to be useful. For the other classes the background binding was so high that no useful information could be obtained. The background binding using bovine serum albumin instead of human serum is also shown (----)

meaningful results obtained; the IgG and IgA binding values are very similar to results obtained with equivalent levels of IgG of IgA myeloma proteins. It is possible to reduce background binding by adding a large excess of protein and it is also possible to detect bound IgG by using radiolabelled staphylococcal protein A[13]. Despite many modifications solid-phase assays for classes of antibody other than IgE have generally proved unsatisfactory.

The success of RAST for IgE antibodies suggests that

(1) crude allergen extracts contain a reasonable proportion of allergen;
(2) the quantity of IgG antibody against allergens in sera from 'untreated' patients must be similar to the quantity of IgE antibody against allergens; and
(3) that IgE antibody responses must in most cases represent more than 1% of the total serum IgE.

The last point has now been established clearly by absorption experiments and other techniques[14-16]. Those studies showed that IgE antibodies to a single major allergen often represent as much as 30% of the total IgE and may average between 5 and 10%[17]. Before leaving RAST assays it is worth commenting on the methods of quantitation used. A standard serum can be chosen (which has high levels of IgE antibody to the relevant allergen) and serial two-fold dilutions of this serum can be assayed to produce a control curve. By referring results from at least two dilutions of serum to the standard curve, accurate results ($\pm 11\%$) can be obtained which correlate well with results of P–K testing or other assays[18-20]. Although accurate results can be obtained, RAST is often carried out using a single positive reference serum, and results are given as a percentage of this value or on a 0; +; + +; to + + + basis. Worse still, results for many different allergens are referred to the same positive reference. Assaying sera where total IgE levels are not known, 'one plus' RAST values may not be significant while + + and + + + values cannot be distinguished because different immunosorbents have different maximum binding values. Thus RAST can easily be reduced to a non-quantitative technique which is less reliable than skin testing.

Antigen-binding assays for IgG, IgA and IgE antibodies

The first attempts to use fluid-phase antigen-binding assays to measure antibodies to allergens were made using ammonium sulphate to precipitate immunoglobulins[21]. At this time radiolabelling of allergens was poor, the background on the assay was very high (20% of the radioactivity was precipitated non-specifically), and it was not clear which classes of immunoglobulin were precipitated. Subsequently Osler et al.[22] and Newcomb et al.[23] showed that individual classes of immunoglobulin could be precipitated by using specific antisera against IgG, IgM or IgA. Class-specific assays have been applied successfully to measuring IgG antibodies to allergens in sera from patients with ragweed hay fever[24,25]. Similar assays were used to measure IgG and IgA antibodies to ragweed antigen-E in nasal secretions[26] (Figure 19.4). To carry out class-specific assays it is essential that

Antigen Binding Radioimmunoassay

Serum sample
+
Allergen * (Radiolabelled with ^{125} Iodine)
+
Carrier Protein if necessary (e. g. IgE myeloma serum)

~ 4 hours ~

Goat anti-IgG (or anti-IgA or anti-IgE)

~ Overnight to precipitate ~

Wash, precipitate and count Radioactivity

Counts directly related to the quantity of specific IgG
(or IgA or IgE) antibody in the serum.

Figure 19.4   Protocols for allergen-binding assay

the antigen should be in excess, so that no cross-linking occurs between different classes. Antibodies which bind antigens in excess do not precipitate with another class. However, if there is a shortage of free antigen, mixed complexes could form which might 'coprecipitate' with a precipitate of another class (Figure 19.5). In order to ensure antigen excess at least 80% of the added radioactivity must not be bound by any class of antibody. The quantities of radiolabelled allergens used in these assays have varied from 100 μg albumin[22] to 1 μg antigen E[24] to ~ 10 ng antigen E[26]. Osler *et al.*[22] found that full saturation of all the antibodies in a hyperimmune rabbit serum required very high levels of antigen. Using very small quantities of allergens, saturation of all antibodies is probably not achieved but antigen excess can be[16,27]. The reason for this discrepancy between saturation and antigen excess is that many antibodies of low affinity will not bind antigens which are only present at concentrations of a few ng/ml. The reason for using low concentrations of allergens is that the background on these assays is directly related to the quantity of allergen added (Figure 19.6). Consequently the sensitivity of the assay increases with lower concentrations of allergen. Antibodies in nasal secretions or in sera from patients who have not received desensitizing injections can only be detected using low concentrations of allergen[26,28]. Thus all antigen-binding assays represent a compromise between complete saturation of the antibodies present and sensitivity.

In order to precipitate a class of immunoglobulin there must be sufficient protein to create a precipitate which can be washed (i.e. ~ 5–20 μg). Normal human serum contains ~ 10 mg IgG/ml (so that 0.1 ml of a 1/50 dilution of serum contains ~ 20 μg IgG protein). By contrast very few sera contain sufficient IgE to create a precipitate even if they are used undiluted. Despite the low levels of total IgE, the results of RAST absorption experiments suggested that allergic sera often contained levels of IgE antibody that should

Class-specific precipitates using Anti-IgE to precipitate

(i) Antigen excess - all antibodies of high enough affinity are in the state Ab(Ag)₂

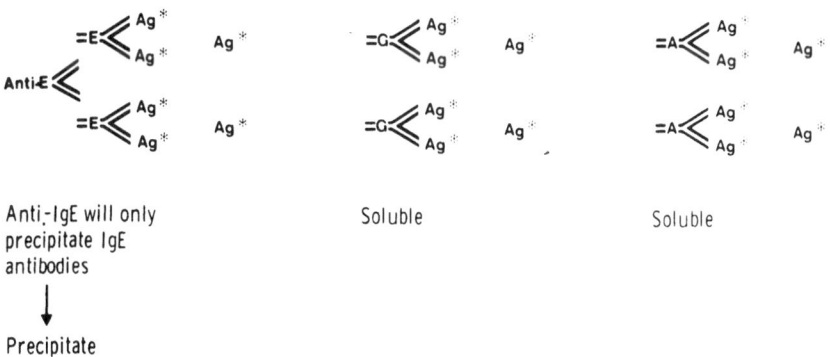

Anti-IgE will only   Soluble   Soluble
precipitate IgE
antibodies

↓

Precipitate

Counts in the precipitate accurately reflect the quantity of specific antibody of the class precipitated

(ii) Without antigen excess:

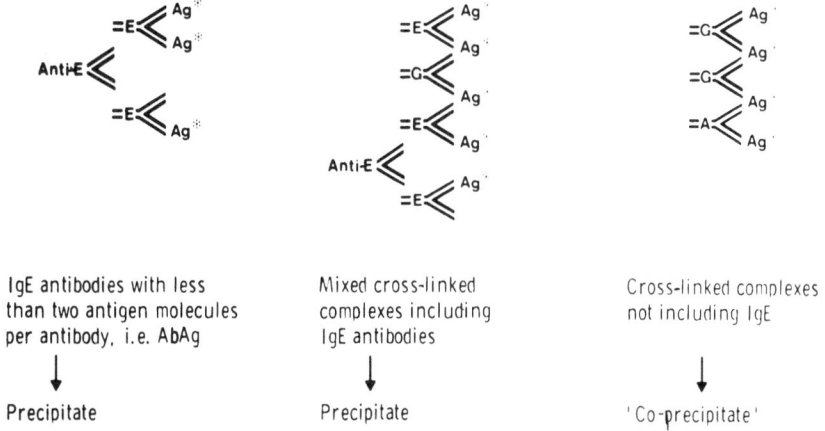

IgE antibodies with less   Mixed cross-linked   Cross-linked complexes
than two antigen molecules   complexes including   not including IgE
per antibody, i.e. AbAg   IgE antibodies

↓   ↓   ↓

Precipitate   Precipitate   'Co-precipitate'

Counts in the precipitate may underestimate or overestimate the quantity of specific antibody of
each class

Figure 19.5 Ideally all the allergen-specific antibodies will bind two separate radiolabelled allergen molecules (Ag*), i.e. they will be in the state Ab(Ag)₂. If there is a shortage of allergen two opposite effects can occur; (i) some of the antibody will be in the form AbAg*, or Ab, and the counts bound will be reduced, or (ii) some of the complexes will become cross-linked, in this case Ag* bound by specific antibodies of other classes may precipitate with IgE and so increase the counts bound

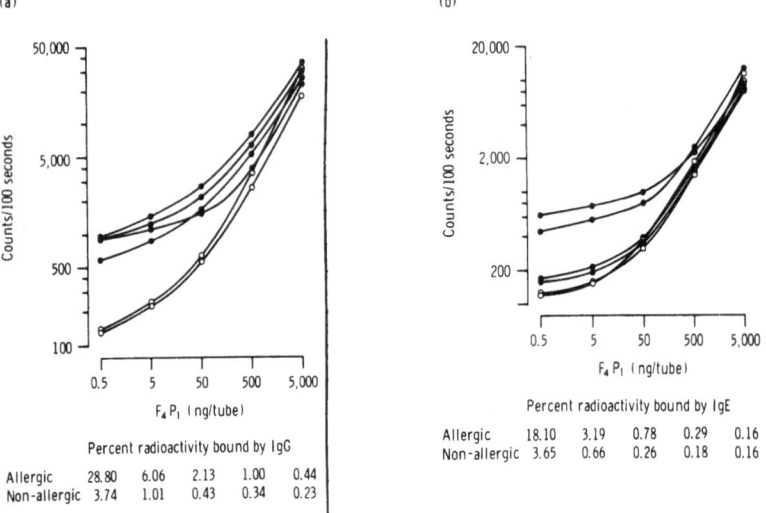

Figure 19.6 Antigen binding by IgG (a) and IgE (b) antibodies in allergic sera, in the presence of increasing concentrations of a radiolabelled mite allergen (F_4P_1). With low concentrations of allergen (< 20 ng) the binding by allergic sera (●——●) is much higher than that by non-allergic sera (○——○). As the concentration of allergen added increases the background rises, so that there is no significant difference between allergic and non-allergic (from ref. 27 by permission of *Clin. Exp. Immunol.*)

be easily measurable by antigen-binding techniques[14]. Several indirect approaches have been used to stabilize precipitates containing IgE, including agarose[3], anti-IgE on a solid phase[29], or the addition of a third antibody, i.e. rabbit anti-IgE followed by goat anti-rabbit IgG[30]. A more direct and simpler approach is to add IgE myeloma protein to provide sufficient irrelevant IgE to create a precipitate[16]. Clearly this technique is unlikely to be used for routine diagnostic purposes; however, 1 ml of myeloma serum will provide sufficient IgE for 1000 assays. The quantities of specific IgE antibodies are often high relative to total serum IgE, but are nonetheless low, i.e. < 0.1 μg IgE Ab/ml. It is not surprising that antigen-binding assays for IgE antibodies can only be carried out using low quantities of radiolabelled allergen[16,31,32]. In several situations antigen-binding assays for IgE antibodies have great advantages over RAST:

(1) Antibodies of IgG, IgA and IgE classes can be assayed in parallel using directly comparable units and single control curve. This is of special advantage in studying antibodies in nasal secretions and also for studying the relationship between IgG and IgE antibodies during desensitization treatment[33,34] (Figure 19.7).

(2) The assays require very little radiolabelled allergen and may be the only technique for measuring antibodies to highly purified allergens which are only available in small quantities.

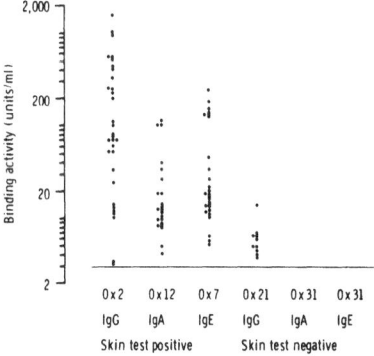

Figure 19.7 IgG, IgA and IgE binding activity for the mite allergen (F_4P_1) in sera from patients with positive or negative skin tests to *D. pteronyssinus* extract. The sera are directly comparable with those used in Figure 19.3 (from ref. 27 by permission of *Clin. Exp. Immunol.*)

(3) Because the background of the assays is unaffected by the total quantity of IgE in a serum, these assays are particularly suitable for measuring IgE antibodies in sera with high total IgE. This has already proved to be a great advantage in assaying sera from patients with atopic eczema.

The results of these assays have led to several conclusions[35] about the nature of the antibody response to inhalant allergens:

(1) That IgE antibodies are never found without IgG antibodies to the same allergen, and that the quantities of these two classes are correlated (Figure 19.8);

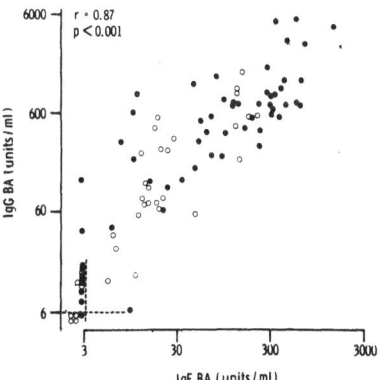

Figure 19.8 Correlation between IgG antibody and IgE antibody in sera from allergic patients who have not received desensitizing injections. Antibodies expressed as binding activity – BA – were measured by antigen-binding assay using radiolabelled mite allergen. The minimum level of sensitivity of each assay is indicated (----). The patients who were all skin-test-positive to *D. pteronyssinus* came from Hong Kong (●) and London (○) (from ref. 34 by permission of *Int. Arch. Allergy Appl. Immunol.*)

(2) that the antibodies in nasal secretions are locally produced while IgG and IgE antibodies found in serum are probably derived predominantly from local lymph nodes;

(3) that most non-allergic, i.e. skin test negative, individuals do not have detectable antibodies to allergens of any class either in their serum or nasal secretions[5, 33, 36].

These results led to the tentative conclusion that the individuals who develop hay fever are those with sufficiently good local immunity to recognize and respond to inhaled allergens.

MEASUREMENT OF TOTAL IgE

As soon as purified IgE was available it became possible to develop a double-antibody inhibition RIA for IgE[37, 38]. This assay is similar to the inhibition assays used for hormones. In general, immunoglobulins are easy to radiolabel and it is not difficult to raise good antisera to IgE in rabbits. Antisera to myeloma proteins include antibodies against the variable region (anti-idiotype antibodies). Anti-idiotype antibodies can create problems because they cannot be inhibited by normal IgE (Figure 19.9). This problem can be overcome either by obtaining sera directed only against the heavy-chain determinants of IgE, or by using two different IgE myeloma proteins. The inhibition RIA for IgE is suitable for measuring IgE in secretions and can be modified to measure concentrations of IgE down to 0.2 ng/ml (i.e. ~ 0.1 IU/ml; one international unit of IgE $= 2.4$ ng)[39]. As with all RIA it is necessary to separate bound radiolabelled protein from free. This is normally

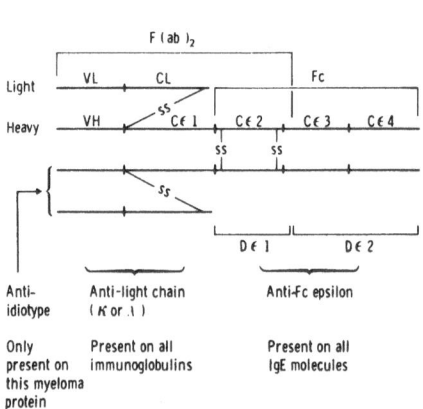

Figure 19.9 Antisera to IgE. Heavy and light chain variable (V) and constant (C) region domains of IgE are shown with only the interchain disulphide bridges indicated. The fragments that can be obtained by papain (Fc), or pepsin (Fab'₂), digestion are shown. The main antigenic sites include the variable region (idiotypic determinants), the light chains (both IgE ND and IgE PS have light chains) and the Fc portion of the heavy chain. The heavy chain antigenic determinants have been divided into two groups: De1 and De2; antisera to these two groups can be obtained separately

done with goat, donkey or sheep anti-rabbit IgG. With other classes of Ig there are often problems because the antisera against rabbit IgG cross-react with human Ig; this is not a problem with IgE. In many laboratories the RIA for IgE is used for routine measurements of serum IgE. Because of the work involved in maintaining reagents and in washing precipitates, two solid-phase techniques for total IgE have been developed and are commercially available.

Solid-phase assays for IgE involve the use of anti-IgE linked covalently to a particle or disc (an immunosorbent). As with RAST assays a major practical advantage of these systems is in the ease of washing a cellulose disc. This requires about one-fifth of the time required for washing precipitates, and does not require a centrifuge because the discs settle by gravity. By contrast assays using solid-phase Sepharose are difficult to wash because they have to be centrifuged and sucked off. Washing fluid can be tipped off a precipitate; but Sepharose beads will pour and the fluid can only successfully be removed by suction. There are two different approaches to determining how much IgE has bound to anti-IgE on the particle. The first technique involves direct inhibition; radiolabelled IgE is added to determine how much anti-IgE had been blocked (the radioimmunosorbent technique or RIST)[40] (Figure 19.10).

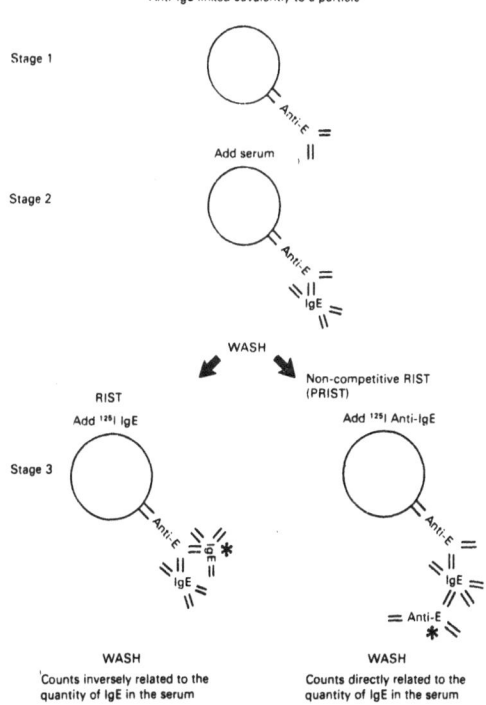

Figure 19.10 Comparison of two solid-phase assays for measuring IgE. In the RIST assay, any non-specific factor that 'blocks' anti-IgE on the surface of the solid phase will reduce the amount of radiolabelled IgE bound. This reduction is likely to be interpreted as indicating the presence of IgE. By contrast, in the non-competitive RIST assay, or paper RIST (PRIST), blocking some of the anti-IgE will have very little effect provided there is sufficient anti-IgE on the solid phase

This assay is very prone to non-specific inhibition and has caused considerable confusion because non-specific inhibition has been interpreted as implying the presence of IgE. The second approach is to use radiolabelled anti-IgE to determine how much IgE is present on the surface of the particle (the non-competitive RIST or Paper RIST (PRIST)[41] (Figure 19.10). The non-competitive RIST is an elegant assay which can be modified to become very sensitive, can be used for assaying IgE in secretions and does not appear to suffer from the problems of RIST. However, as with all solid-phase assays there remains the possibility that the radiolabel will bind (or fail to bind) to the particle for reasons that are not immediately obvious. Thus the inhibition RIA should be the reference technique for measuring total IgE, and in any new situation, e.g. *in vitro* cultures, the results obtained with a solid-phase technique should be checked by RIA.

The problems with RIST are interesting because they illustrate how difficult it can be to identify a problem with an assay even when it is severe. Because the assay depends on identifying anti-IgE which has not been blocked (Figure 19.10), any substance which can bind to the anti-IgE would appear to be IgE. If there were no other technique for detecting IgE then there would be no way of distinguishing between mucus bound to the anti-IgE and IgE bound to the anti-IgE. The reason for believing that the RIA is an accurate measurement of IgE is that the results correlate so well with other techniques. Erroneous results with RIST have predominantly been obtained in fluids other than serum. Thus high levels of IgE have been reported in milk, urine, and nasal secretions which turned out to be absent or much lower than had been reported[33, 42, 43]. However, RIST also tends to over-estimate low IgE levels in serum. This appears to be because concentrated serum contains substances which can bind non-specifically[18, 44, 45]. Using RIST normal levels of IgE were found in sera from patients with hypogammaglobulinaemia[46]. This result is clearly erroneous since these sera contain no IgE by RIA, or non-competitive RIST, and furthermore these patients show no evidence of IgE antibodies in their sera or in the skin by skin testing with allergens or anti-IgE. Thus while it may be very difficult to prove whether inhibition of RIST is caused by IgE or is non-specific, evidence from several sources is available to suggest that inhibition of RIST can occur due to factors other than IgE.

The role of IgE measurements in clinical practice is still not clearly established. Curiously total IgE measurements are often used to give a guide as to whether a patient is allergic or not, i.e. whether they have IgE antibodies. Measurements of total IgG, IgA or IgM in serum are never used in this way. This is because a total IgG value can give no guidance about whether a patient has made IgG antibodies to any specific antigen. However, IgG levels are very constant when compared with IgE (see Table 19.1). The IgG levels in normal sera vary from 6 to 12 mg/ml in 'western' populations, values below 4 mg/ml usually indicate immunodeficiency and values above 14 mg/ml usually indicate some chronic inflammatory disease. By comparison normal adult IgE

Table 19.1 Immunoglobulin classes and the antibody response to inhalant allergens

	IgE	IgG	IgA	IgM
*Total**				
Serum concentration	0.001–10 μg	6–12 mg	0.2–3.0 mg	0.2–2 mg
Nasal secretions	< 1.0–10 ng	~ 45 μg	~ 74 μg	< 1 μg
Specific Antibodies to Grass pollen allergen – Rye I †				
Serum units/ml	200	800	50	< 10
(~ ng/ml)	(100)	(400)	(25)	< 5
Antibody to Rye I as a percentage of total	1–50	0.01	0.005	< 0.002
Nasal secretions, units/ml	3–5	20	26	< 1
(~ ng/ml)	(2)	(10)	(13)	(< 1)
Antibody to Rye I as a percentage of total	30	0.2	0.1	–

* Serum IgG, IgA and IgM measured by radial immunodiffusion. Serum IgE and all classes in secretions measured by radioimmunoassay.

† Mean values for 45 patients with grass pollen hay fever, antibodies measured by antigen binding radioimmunoassay[16,33].

levels range from 2 to 200 IU/ml. Asymptomatic individuals may be found who have total serum IgE levels < 1 IU/ml or greater than 1000 IU/ml. In patients with hypogammaglobulinaemia values < 0.2 IU/ml are common while patients with helminthiasis or severe atopic eczema often have total IgE levels > 10 000 IU/ml. In routine allergy practice, measurement of serum IgE levels on patients with hay fever or perennial allergic rhinitis may not be very useful. This is because almost 50% of uncomplicated cases will have IgE levels in the normal range. In asthma and eczema IgE levels are of considerable value in considering whether the disease has an allergic basis. Values < 50 IU/ml are rare in extrinsic asthma and very rare in atopic eczema. Total serum IgE levels may also be useful in assessing patients who have a variety of syndromes which might be related to allergy, e.g. staphylococcal infection of the skin, gastrointestinal symptoms, migraine etc.[47,48].

IMMUNOASSAYS FOR ALLERGENS

There are two reasons for wanting to measure allergen concentrations; firstly to quantitate *in vivo* exposure to allergens, and secondly to standardize allergen extracts for skin testing or desensitization treatment. Traditionally allergen extracts have been assessed by their protein content or their skin reactivity. The protein content of pollen extracts may give a reasonable guide to their allergen content; however only a minority of the protein in these extracts is allergen. It is possible for allergen content to vary from < 1% to 25%. In keeping with this Baer *et al.*[49,50] found that the skin reactivity of ragweed and grass pollen extracts was only very poorly related to their p.n.u. values (p.n.u. = protein nitrogen unit = 0.01 μg protein N). For the most important allergens it would be possible to find sufficient, selectively sensitive patients who could be used for skin testing[51]. However, skin testing does carry some hazards and for many less important allergens it would be difficult to identify patients for repeated skin testing. There is therefore a great need for a reliable, simple technique to assess the allergen content of extracts *in vitro*.

The allergens involved in immediate hypersensitivity are defined by the fact that patients have IgE antibodies specific for them. Consequently the most satisfactory techniques for quantitating allergens use human IgE antibodies to detect the allergens. In almost all cases human antibodies to inhalant or food allergens will not make precipitates *in vitro*, so that immunodiffusion techniques cannot be used. Human IgE antibodies will bind to allergens which are fixed either in a precipitate or on an allergosorbent. This binding can be used to assess allergens, either by linking a variety of allergens to beads (direct RAST), or by using a standard extract on the bead and using a variety of extracts to inhibit the binding (RAST inhibition) (Figure 19.11). RAST

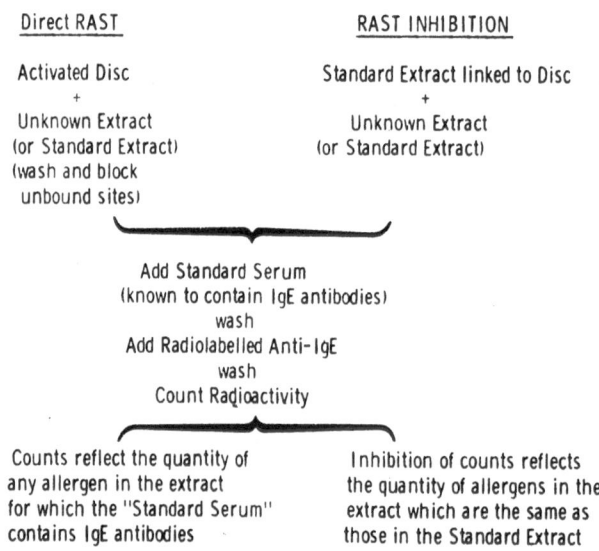

Solid Phase Techniques for Assessing Allergen Extracts

Direct RAST   RAST INHIBITION

Activated Disc   Standard Extract linked to Disc
+   +
Unknown Extract   Unknown Extract
(or Standard Extract)   (or Standard Extract)
(wash and block
unbound sites)

Add Standard Serum
(known to contain IgE antibodies)
wash
Add Radiolabelled Anti-IgE
wash
Count Radioactivity

Counts reflect the quantity of   Inhibition of counts reflects
any allergen in the extract   the quantity of allergens in the
for which the "Standard Serum"   extract which are the same as
contains IgE antibodies   those in the Standard Extract

Figure 19.11   RAST inhibition is potentially an important technique in allergen standardization, since an 'unknown' extract can be directly compared with a standard extract. The direct RAST technique is more difficult to carry out, and may give positive results because the standard serum contains antibodies against an allergen which is present in the unknown extract but is not present in the standard allergen extract. Thus direct RAST is not so suitable for allergen standardization but may be very useful for investigating an allergen suspected of being responsible for symptoms or IgE antibody formation

inhibition is the most practical technique for assessing allergen extracts *in vitro*[52-55]. The advantages are that:

(1) large batches of discs can be made and the same discs can be used for detecting IgE antibodies by RAST;

(2) a large pool of allergic sera can be stored indefinitely, either frozen or lyophylized; and

(3) the radiolabelled anti-IgE is the same as that used for RAST and the non-competitive RIST.

Although the technique of RAST inhibition is simple to carry out, the inhibition is often very complicated because the allergen extracts contain many different proteins, and a 'standard serum' often contains IgE (and IgG) antibodies against a variety of different allergens. It has been suggested that the slope of inhibition curves can give useful information about the composition of an extract, but for routine use results are given as the quantity of extract (in μl) necessary to cause 50% inhibition[55,56].

An alternative approach to standardizing allergens is to use rabbit antisera raised against allergen extracts. These antisera will produce easily visible precipitin lines against many different proteins in an extract[57,58]. However, demonstrating multiple proteins is of no use unless it is possible to identify which proteins are the important allergens. If a major allergen has been identified it is possible to measure it with antisera against the allergen and a quantitative immunodiffusion technique, e.g. radial immunodiffusion or rocket electrophoresis. Løwenstein and his colleagues[58] have developed a beautiful technique for identifying which of the bands seen on Laurell electrophoresis of an allergen extract are allergens. This technique is called crossed radioimmunoelectrophoresis (CRIE); it involves layering allergic sera over the immunodiffusion, followed by radiolabelled anti-IgE. The bands that contain allergens can then be visualized by autoradiography. This technique can also be modified to measure the quantities of allergens in an extract. The problem with CRIE is that it is technically difficult to carry out and it is also difficult to compare results between laboratories. This technique might be a good method for a central laboratory to compare allergen extracts from different manufacturers. It is certainly possible to identify multiple different allergens in each extract and to quantitate them approximately. However, the work involved in carrying out and assessing CRIE on a wide range of allergen extracts would be formidable.

An important feature of the proof that pollen grains cause hay fever was the correlation between pollen counts and symptoms. Even today pollen counts are the best available method for assessing exposure to airborne allergens. It is also fairly simple to examine pollen to ensure purity of the source material used for preparing allergen extracts. Similarly it is possible to define with reasonable accuracy the source material used for preparing animal dander extracts. Indeed the purity of source material is the only practical way in which the presence of irrelevant allergens can be avoided in an extract. Theoretically either RAST inhibition or CRIE could be used to screen extracts for contamination with irrelevant allergens. However, these techniques would probably not be sufficiently sensitive to detect a minor contamination of grass pollen in another pollen extract which might be clinically very confusing. Isoelectric focusing is a useful technique for identifying multiple proteins in an extract. However, at present there is no simple way of identifying which of the multiple bands seen are allergens; many allergens may be present in different isoelectric forms[17,59]. At present there seems no basis on which isoelectric focusing could be used to standardize allergen extracts.

Standardization of house dust extracts poses special problems. Here the source material includes many different substances and there is no way of comparing different source materials. It is possible to assess house dust extracts by skin testing on a range of patients, but the information might not be relevant to patients in other areas. Alternatively one can use extracts of each of the constituents of house dust and try to standardize each separately. Some authors believe that crude 'house dust' extract should never be used. In Europe, Australia, Africa and the Far East house dust mites have been shown to be responsible for much of the allergenicity of house dust[60]. Either house dust extracts or extracts of mite cultures can be assessed by RAST inhibition[55,61] (Figure 19.12). Recently we[17,27] have purified a major allergen

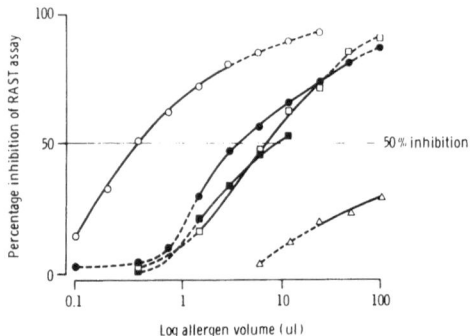

Figure 19.12 Assay of mite allergen content in five extracts of house dust mite culture, using RAST inhibition. The allergen content can be compared on the basis of the volume of extract necessary to give 50% inhibition. In this experiment the points joined by solid lines were used to calculate the slope. Differences in slope suggest that the composition of the extract may be different (from ref. 55 by permission of *Clin. Allergy*)

from cultures of *Dermatophagoides pteronyssinus* – antigen P_1. Using this antigen it has been possible to develop a RIA for an important allergen in house dust or dust mite cultures[62] (Figure 19.13). More importantly this assay has made it possible to identify the distribution of this allergen in dust mite cultures. These studies have demonstrated unequivocally that the most important source of allergen is the faecal particles produced by the mites.

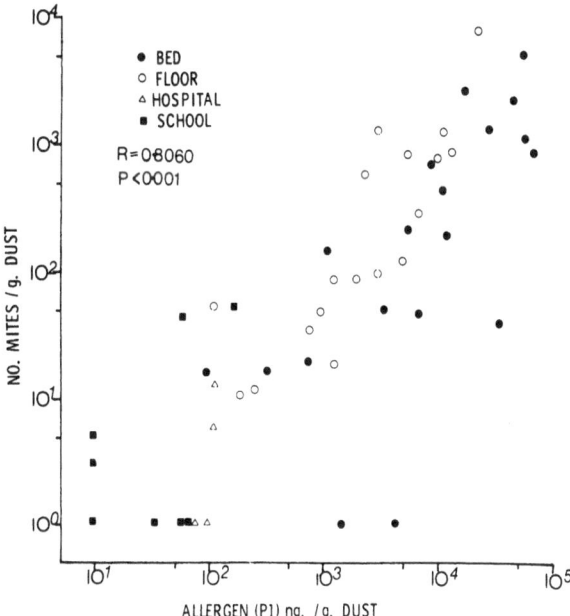

Figure 19.13 Dust samples were sieved and the fine dust was either examined for mites microscopically or extracted with saline. The content of dust mite allergen P_1 was determined by double-antibody inhibition RIA. More detailed assessment of the dust, and of dust mite cultures, suggests that the number of mites is relevant only as a guide to the quantity of accumulated mite faeces in the dust sample[62, 64]

These particles account for most of the antigen P_1 content of cultures (> 90%) and in addition the allergen on the faecal particles elutes very rapidly in aqueous solution. The presence of a protein which can elute rapidly from the surface of a particle is very similar to the situation with pollen wall proteins[59, 63]. The size of faecal particles (10–40 μm) is similar to that of pollen grains. Preliminary evidence suggests that faecal particles have similar aerodynamic properties to pollen grains. In order to assess allergen exposure it is necessary to know the allergen content of the air and the size of particles with which the allergen is associated. It is possible that a count of mite faecal particles in the air (comparable to a pollen count) would give more information than accurate measurements of allergen content in floor dust. Meanwhile, assessment of floor dust allergen content, either by RAST inhibition or by measuring mite allergens by RIA, is the best available technique for comparing different houses[61, 64]. During our studies of house dust mite allergens it appeared that antigen P_1 represented a large proportion (up to 20%) of the protein in an aqueous extract of dust mite culture. A similar conclusion has been reached about ragweed pollen where antigen E appears to be the 'most abundant' protein in aqueous extracts of ragweed pollen[65]. The dust mite allergen (antigen P_1) has a molecular weight on SDS polyacrylamide

L

gel electrophoresis of 24000 daltons. This is very similar to all the major pollen allergens which range from 10 000 to 40 000 daltons. This size would appear to be defined by the size of molecule which can penetrate the nasal mucosa and which is nonetheless a good immunogen. Thus a major allergen is a protein which is present as a high proportion of the rapidly soluble proteins of the correct size, and is associated with a particle which can become airborne and will be deposited on the nasal mucosa. If assays of *in vivo* allergen exposure are to have meaning they will have to reflect these properties. At present no immunoassay of pollen allergens can give more information than the traditional pollen count. Ideally we need a comparable assessment of airborne allergens for dust and animal dander allergens.

CONCLUSIONS

Having briefly (and highly selectively) reviewed the state of the art in immunoassays for allergy, it is worth returning to the reasons why the RAST assay for IgE antibodies has been so successful. These reasons explain why in general this type of assay is not suitable for measuring antibodies to other types of antigens or for measuring other classes of antibody:

(1) important allergens often represent a large proportion (10–20%) of the protein in an aqueous allergen extract;
(2) although the antibody response to inhalant allergens includes IgG antibodies, the serum IgG antibodies are usually only 2–6-fold greater than the IgE antibody response – therefore the IgG antibodies generally do not block the allergen on RAST beads;
(3) compared with other classes of immunoglobulin, total serum IgE levels are very low and IgE antibody responses to a single allergen often represent a large proportion (2–50%) of the total – this reflects the fact that most antibody responses (e.g. to bacteria, diphtheria toxoid, viruses, etc.) do not usually include IgE antibodies.

Thus a RAST bead can be coated with crude allergen extract and the quantity of specific IgE antibody bound will be significant relative to both IgG antibodies and non-specific binding of IgE. Despite the fact that RAST is able to measure IgE antibodies to many different allergens, it is not clear that it has an important role in routine diagnosis. The reason for this is that prick testing usually gives as much information as any of the *in vitro* tests. Skin testing has the advantage that further tests can be carried out rapidly and the results are immediately clear to the patient. There may be an important role for *in vitro* measurements of IgE antibodies in conditions where skin testing is difficult or unreliable, e.g. infants or atopic eczema. In sera from patients with atopic eczema total IgE is often very high, i.e. > 5000 IU/ml so that RAST becomes unreliable and antigen-binding assays may be more suitable. At present there is considerable confusion about the role of allergens in atopic eczema, but preliminary studies in which allergen avoidance has been based on the results of antigen-binding assays for IgE antibody suggests that this approach might be successful. For clinical purposes, establishing that a patient has IgE antibodies either by skin testing or by an *in vitro* technique is often adequate. In research studies it is usually necessary to know total serum IgE and IgG antibody levels as well. In these situations antigen-binding assays have great advantages because the quantities of different classes can be directly compared.

A wide range of RIAs have been developed for the investigation of allergy. It is not yet clear whether these assays have an important role in clinical allergy. Measurements of total serum IgE play an important role in academic medicine. Measurements of IgE antibodies *in vitro* may have an important role in penicillin allergy and bee venom allergy[66, 67]. The present uncritical use of RAST on a semi-quantitative basis without total IgE measurements is probably not justified. In the assessment of allergen extracts immunodiffusion techniques are being used to assess the antigen E content of ragweed pollen extracts. It should be possible to extend similar assays of major allergen content to a few more extracts, e.g. grass pollen and dust mite. In Denmark CRIE is used routinely to assess many allergen extracts; it seems unlikely that it will prove acceptable to many countries which are less sophisticated immunochemically. Despite some progress, in most countries allergen extracts are still only assessed by protein content. It would seem sensible to insist on RAST inhibition as a minimum assessment for the important extracts and certainly for any extracts which are used for 'desensitizing' injections. The demand for accurate allergy diagnosis stems from three requirements: to reassure and inform the patient; to guide attempts at desensitization; and to guide allergen avoidance. The first requirement is best satisfied by skin testing. Desensitizing injections remain hazardous and unpredictable in their results, and are probably not justified either for asthma or hay fever. Certainly there is little evidence that desensitization is more effective today than it was in 1920, while pharmacological management of immediate hypersensitivity has progressed enormously over the last 40 years. It has been suggested that measurements of IgG (or 'blocking') antibodies can help in assessing the results of desensitizing injections. This may be true for bee venom allergy[28, 67, 68], but there is very little evidence that measurements of IgG antibody production can be used to control or predict the results of desensitization for inhalant allergens[34, 69]. Allergen avoidance is likely to remain an important part of the management of allergic disease. During the 1980s it should be possible to apply presently available assays to rational allergen avoidance. In particular it should be possible to use assays to guide clinical advice or research on the control of household dust antigens.

References

1. Taylor, G. and Walker, J. (1973). Charles Harrison Blackley 1820–1900. *Clin. Allergy*, **3**, 103
2. Prausnitz, C. and Küstner, H. (1921). Studien veger die verbering findlichkeit. *Zentralbl. Bakteriol., Parasitenkd, Infectionskr. Hyg. Abt.* 1, Orig. *86*, 160
3. Ishizaka, K., Ishizaka, T. and Hornbrook, M. M. (1967). Allergen binding activity of γE, γG and γA, antibodies in sera from atopic patients: *in vitro* measurements of reaginic antibody. *J. Immunol.*, **98**, 490
4. Ishizaka, K. and Ishizaka, T. (1975). Biology of immunoglobulin E. Molecular basis of reaginic hypersensitivity. *Progr. Allergy*, **19**, 60
5. Bennich, H. and Johansson, S. G. O. (1971). Structure and function of human immunoglobulin E. *Adv. Immunol.*, **13**, 1
6. Klinman, N. R. and Taylor, R. B. (1969). General methods for the study of cells and serum during the immune response: the response to dinitrophenyl in mice. *Clin. Exp. Immunol.*, **4**, 473
7. Wide, L., Bennich, H. and Johansson, S. G. O. (1967). Diagnosis of allergy by an *in vitro* test for allergen antibodies. *Lancet*, **2**, 1105
8. Ceska, M., Eriksson, R. and Varga, J. M. (1972). Radioimmunosorbent assay of allergens. *J. Allergy Clin. Immunol.*, **49**, 1
9. Wide, L. (1973). Clinical significance of measurement of reaginic (IgE) antibody by RAST. *Clin. Allergy*, **3**, suppl. 583
10. Pepys, J., Roth, J. and Carroll, K. B. (1975). RAST, skin and nasal tests and the history in grass pollen allergy. *Clin. Allergy*, **5**, 431
11. Berg, T., Bennich, H. and Johansson, S. G. O. (1971). *In vitro* diagnosis of atopic allergy. I. A comparison between provocation tests and the radioallergosorbent test. *Int. Arch. Allergy*, **40**, 770
12. Aas, K. (1978). The diagnosis of hypersensitivity to ingested foods: reliability of skin prick testing and the radioallergosorbent test with different materials. *Clin. Allergy*, **8**, 39
13. Delespesse, G., Debisschop, M. J. and Flament, J. (1979). Measurement of IgG antibodies to house dust mite and grass pollen by a solid-phase radioimmunoassay. *Clin. Allergy*, **9**, 503
14. Gleich, G. J. and Jacob, G. L. (1975). Immunoglobulin E antibodies to pollen allergens account for high percentages of total immunoglobulin E protein. *Science*, **190**, 1106
15. Schellenberg, R. R. and Adkinson, N. F. (1975). Measurement of absolute amounts of antigen-specific human IgE by a radioallergosorbent test (RAST) elution technique. *J. Immunol.*, **115**, 1577
16. Platts-Mills, T. A. E., Snajdr, M. J., Ishizaka, K. and Frankland, A. W. (1978). Measurement of IgE antibody by an antigen binding assay: correlation with P-K activity and IgG and IgA antibodies to allergens. *J. Immunol.*, **120**, 1201
17. Chapman, M. D. and Platts-Mills, T. A. E. (1980). Purification and characterization of the major allergen from *Dermatophagoides pteronyssinus* – Antigen P_1. *J. Immunol.*, **125**, 587
18. Aalberse, R. C. (1974). *Immunoglobulin E, Allergens and their Interaction.* (Amsterdam: Rudopi NV)
19. Gleich, G. J. and Jones, R. T. (1975). Measurement of IgE antibodies by the radioallergosorbent test. *J. Allergy Clin. Immunol.*, **55**, 334
20. Johansson, S. G. O., Bennich, H. and Bert, T. (1971). *In vitro* diagnosis of atopic allergy. III. Quantitative estimation of circulating IgE antibodies by the radioallergosorbent test. *Int. Arch. Allergy Appl. Immunol.*, **41**, 443
21. Lidd, D. and Farr, R. S. (1962). Primary interaction between I^{131} labelled ragweed pollen and antibodies in the sera of humans and rabbits. *J. Allergy*, **33**, 45
22. Osler, A. G., Mulligan, J. J. and Rodriguez, I. (1966). Weight estimates of rabbit anti-human serum albumin based on antigen-binding and precipitin analyses: specific haemagglutinating activities of 7S and 19S components. *J. Immunol.*, **96**, 334

23. Newcomb, R. W., Ishizaka, K. and de Vald, B. L. (1969). Human IgG and IgA diphtheria antitoxins in serum, nasal fluids and saliva. *J. Immunol.*, **103**, 215

24. Yunginger, J. W. and Gleich, G. J. (1973). Seasonal changes in IgE antibodies and their relationship to IgG antibodies during immunotherapy for ragweed hay fever. *J. Clin. Invest.*, **52**, 1268

25. Lichtenstein, L. M., Ishizaka, K., Norman, P. S., Sobotka, A. K. and Hill, B. M. (1973). IgE measurements in ragweed hay fever. Relationship to clinical severity and the results of immunotherapy. *J. Clin. Invest.*, **52**, 472

26. Platts-Mills, T. A. E., von Maur, R. K., Ishizaka, K., Norman, P. S. and Lichtenstein, L. M. (1976). IgA and IgG anti-ragweed antibodies in nasal secretions. Quantitative measurements of antibodies and correlation with inhibition of histamine release. *J. Clin. Invest.*, **57**, 1041

27. Chapman, M. D. and Platts-Mills, T. A. E. (1978). Measurement of IgG, IgA and IgE antibodies to *Dermatophagoides pteronyssinus* by antigen-binding assay, using a partially purified fraction of mite extract (F_4P_1). *Clin. Exp. Immunol.*, **34**, 126

28. Sobotka, A. K., Valentine, M. D., Ishizaka, K. and Lichtenstein, L. M. (1976). Measurement of IgG-blocking antibodies: development and application of a radioimmunoassay. *J. Immunol.*, **117**, 84

29. Zeiss, C. R., Pruzansky, J. J., Patterson, R. and Roberts, M. (1973). A solid phase radioimmunoassay for the quantitation of human reaginic antibody against ragweed antigen E. *J. Immunol.*, **110**, 414

30. Sano, Y. and Ito, K. (1978). Correlation between the antigen binding activity and the relative concentration of IgE antibodies to mite. *Ann. Allergy*, **40**, 124

31. Paull, B. R., Jacob, G. L., Yunginger, J. W. and Gleich, G. L. (1978). Comparison of binding of IgE and IgG antibodies to honey bee venom phospholipase-A. *J. Immunol.*, **120**, 1917

32. Zeiss, C. R., Pruzansky, J. J., Levitz, D. and Wang, J. (1978). The quantitation of IgE antibody specific for ragweed antigen E (AgE) from the basophil surface in patients with ragweed pollenosis. *Immunology*, **35**, 237

33. Platts-Mills, T. A. E. (1979). Local production of IgG, IgA and IgE antibodies in grass pollen hay fever. *J. Immunol.*, **122**, 2218

34. Chapman, M. D., Platts-Mills, T. A. E., Gabriel, M., Ng, H. K., Allan, W. G. L., Hill, L. E. and Nunn, A. J. (1980). Antibody response following prolonged hyposensitization with Dermatophagoides pteronyssinus extract. *Int. Arch. Allergy Appl. Immunol.*, **61**, 431

35. Chapman, M. D., Fuenmajor, M., Champion, R. H., Pope, M. and Platts-Mills, T. A. E. (1981). IgE and IgG antibodies to inhalant allergens in patients with atopic eczema: measurement by antigen binding assay. (In preparation)

36. Tse, K. S., Wicher, K. and Arbesman, C. E. (1973). Effect of immunotherapy on the appearance of antibodies to ragweed in external secretions. *J. Allergy Clin. Immunol.*, **51**, 208

37. Ishizaka, K., Tomioka, H. and Ishizaka, T. (1970). Mechanisms of passive sensitization. Presence of IgE and IgG molecules on human leucocytes. *J. Immunol.*, **105**, 1459

38. Gleich, G. J., Averback, A. K. and Svedlund, H. A. (1971). Measurement of IgE in normal and allergic serum by radioimmunoassay. *J. Lab. Clin. Med.*, **77**, 690

39. Nakajima, S., Gillespie, D. N. and Gleich, G. J. (1975). Differences between IgA and IgE as secretory proteins. *Clin. Exp. Immunol.*, **21**, 306

40. Wide, L. (1971). Solid-phase antigen–antibody systems. In Kirkham, K. E. and Hunter, W. M. (eds.) *Radioimmunoassay Methods*. (Edinburgh: E. and S. Livingstone)

41. Ceska, M. and Lundquist, U. (1972). A new and simple radioimmunoassay method for the determination of IgE. *Immunochemistry*, **9**, 1021

42. Underdown, B. J., Knight, A. and Papsin, F. R. (1976). The relative paucity of IgE in human milk. *J. Immunol.*, **116**, 1435

43. Turner, M. W., McClelland, D. B. L., Medlen, A. R. and Stokes, C. R. (1977). IgE in human urine and milk. *Scand. J. Immunol.*, **6**, 343

44. Johansson, S. G. O., Berglund, A. and Kjellman, N. I. M. (1976). Comparison of IgE values

as determined by different solid phase radioimmunoassay methods. *Clin. Allergy*, **6**, 91

45. Nye, L., Merrett, T. G., Landon, J. and White, R. J. (1975). A detailed investigation of circulating IgE levels in a normal population. *Clin. Allergy*, **5**, 13

46. McLaughlan, P., Stanworth, D. R., Webster, A. D. B. and Asherson, G. L. (1974). Serum IgE in immune deficiency disorders. *Clin. Exp. Immunol.*, **16**, 374

47. Lichtenstein, L. M. and Hamburger, R. N. (1978). IgE and atopic disease. In Samter, M. (ed.) *Immunological Diseases*, 3rd edn. (Boston: Little Brown & Co.)

48 Platts-Mills, T. A. E. (1981). Hay fever and perennial allergic rhinitis. In Lachmann, P. and Peters, D. K. (eds.) *Clinical Aspects of Immunology*, 4th edn. (In press)

49. Baer, H., Godfrey, H., Maloney, C. J., Norman, P. S. and Lichtenstein, L. M. (1970). The potency and antigen E content of commercially prepared ragweed extracts. *J. Allergy*, **45**, 347

50. Baer, H., Maloney, C. J., Norman, P. S. and Marsh, D. G. (1974). The potency and group I antigen content of six commercially prepared grass pollen extracts. *J. Allergy Clin. Immunol.*, **54**, 157

51. Aas, K. and Belin, L. (1972). Standardization of diagnostic work in allergy. *Acta Allergol.* (K6L), **27**, 439

52. Foucard, T., Johansson, S. G. O., Bennich, H. and Berg, T. (1972). *In vitro* estimation of allergens by a radioimmune antiglobulin technique using human IgE antibodies. *Int. Arch. Allergy. Appl. Immunol.*, **43**, 360

53. Gleich, G. J., Larson, J. B., Jones, R. T. and Baer, H. (1974). Measurement of the potency of allergen extracts by their inhibitory capacities in the radioallergosorbent test. *J. Allergy Clin. Immunol.*, **53**, 158

54. Yman, L., Ponterius, G. and Brandt, R. (1975). RAST based allergen assay methods. *Dev. Biol. Standard.*, **29**, 151

55. Tovey, E. and Vandenberg, R. (1979). Mite allergen content in commercial extracts and bed dust determined by radioallergosorbent tests. *Clin. Allergy*, **9**, 253

56. Gleich, G. J. and Yunginger, J. W. (1976). Standardization of allergens. In Rose, N. R. and Friedman, H. (eds.) *Manual of Clinical Immunology.* (American Society for Microbiology)

57. Augustin, R. and Hayward, B. J. (1962). Grass pollen allergens. IV. The isolation of some of the principal allergens of *Phleum pratense* and *Dactylis glomerata* and their sensitivity spectra in patients. *Immunology*, **5**, 424

58. Løwenstein, H. (1978). Quantitative immunoelectrophoretic methods as a tool for the analysis and isolation of allergens. *Progr. Allergy*, **25**, 1

59. Marsh, D. G. (1975). Allergens and the genetics of allergy. In Sela, M. (ed.) *The Antigens*, Vol. III. (New York: Academic Press)

60. Spieksma, F. Th. M. and Voorhorst, R. (1969). Comparison of skin reactions to extracts of house dust, mites and human skin scales. *Acta Allergol.*, **24**, 124

61. Burr, M. L., Dean, B. V., Merrett, T. G., Neale, E., St. Leger, A. S. and Verrier-Jones, E. R. (1980). The effects of anti-mite measures on children with mite sensitive asthma. A controlled trial. *Thorax*, **35**, 506

62. Tovey, E., Chapman, M. D. and Platts-Mills, T. A. E. (1980). Production of allergens in cultures of *Dermatophagoides pteronyssinus*. Mite faecal particles are a major source of allergen P_1. (In preparation)

63. Knox, R. B., Willing, R. R. and Ashford, A. E. (1972). Role of pollen-wall proteins as recognition substances in interspecific incompatibility in poplars. *Nature (London)*, **237**, 381

64. Tovey, E., Chapman, M. D. and Platts-Mills, T. A. E. (1981). The quantities and distribution of mite aeroallergens. (In preparation)

65. King, T. P. (1979). Immunochemical properties of some atopic allergens. *J. Allergy Clin. Immunol.*, **64**, 159

66. Kraft, D., Roth, A., Mischer, P., Pichler, H. and Ebner, H. (1977). Specific and total serum IgE measurements in the diagnosis of penicillin allergy. A long-term follow-up study. *Clin. Allergy*, **7**, 21

67. Hunt, K. J., Valentine, M. D., Sobotka, A. K. and Lichtenstein, L. M. (1976). Diagnosis of allergy to stinging insects by skin testing with hymenoptera venoms. *Ann. Intern. Med.*, **85**, 56

68. Lessof, M. N., Sobotka, A. K. and Lichtenstein, L. M. (1977). Protection against anaphylaxis in hymenoptera-sensitive patients by passive immunization. *Monogr. Allergy*, Vol. 12. (Basel: Karger)

69. Norman, P. S. (1980). An overview of immunotherapy: implications for the future. *J. Allergy Clin. Immunol.*, **65**, 87

20
Immonuassay Screening for Open Neural-tube Defects: Practical Aspects

N. J. WALD

INTRODUCTION

During the second half of the 1970s we have seen the widespread introduction of the immunoassay for α-fetoprotein (AFP) in maternal serum as a method of general population screening for open neural-tube defects. With the further extension of AFP screening during the 1980s, both in the UK and overseas, it is timely to consider certain practical aspects such as the influence of assay performance on the results of screening, the organization of screening and its monitoring.

SCREENING FOR OPEN NEURAL-TUBE DEFECTS

When to screen

The best time to perform the maternal serum AFP screening test is between 16 and 18 weeks of pregnancy. The detection efficiency of the test for anencephaly increases during pregnancy up to about 16–20 weeks, and for open spina bifida increases up to about 16–18 weeks. In the UK Collaborative AFP Study[1], at 16–18 weeks of pregnancy, 86% (44/51) of pregnancies with anencephaly and 76% (25/33) of those with open spina bifida had maternal serum AFP levels equal to or greater than the 97th percentile for unaffected singleton pregnancies.

Units

The concentration of AFP in maternal serum is usually determined in ng/ml or IU/ml, the latter being increasingly adopted. With the more general use of the WHO AFP Standard (72/225) or the British Standard (72/227), systematic differences between laboratories in the measurement of maternal serum AFP will decrease. Much of the inter-laboratory variation can also be reduced by expressing an AFP result as a multiple of the laboratory's own median level at the relevant gestational time. The use of 'multiple of the median' (MoM) has been increasingly adopted for AFP screening because it is simple to derive and use, it is robust (for example the median is hardly influenced at all by occasional outlying values), and while the absolute concentration of AFP increases during the second trimester of pregnancy, expressing results in terms of multiples of the median at a given gestational age automatically takes account of this increase. For example, a value of 2 MoM at 16 weeks of gestation will, in absolute units, be lower than 2 MoM at 18 weeks, but both will be associated with a similar risk of a neural-tube defect.

Distribution of serum AFP levels

Figure 20.1 shows the distribution of maternal serum AFP in unaffected pregnancies, open spina bifida pregnancies and anencephalic pregnancies (all

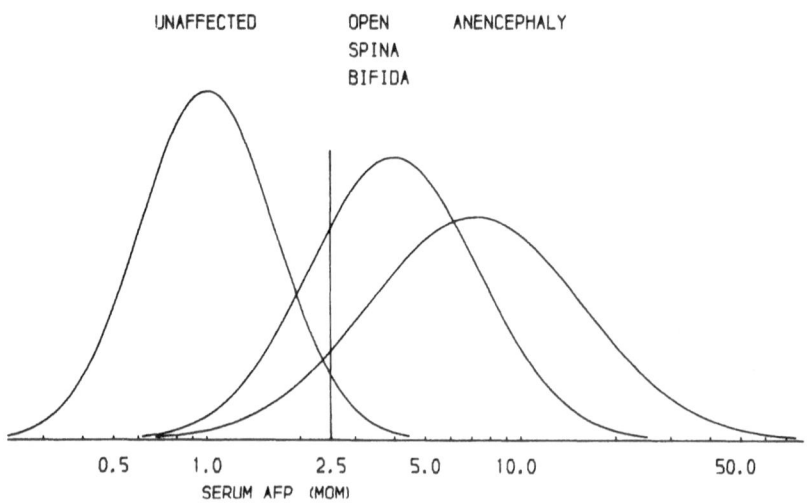

Figure 20.1 Distribution of maternal serum AFP at 16–18 weeks of gestation in singleton pregnancies (from the Report of the UK Collaborative Study on Alpha-fetoprotein in Relation to Neural-Tube Defects[1])

singleton) from 16 to 18 weeks' gestation. The three distributions overlap so there is no obvious level of serum AFP that will separate affected from unaffected pregnancies. Most centres in the UK use a cut-off level of about 2.5 times the median, where about 90% of anencephalic pregnancies and 80% of open spina bifida can be expected to be detected, and where about 3% of unaffected pregnancies will be found to have raised levels, representing the screening false-positive rate.

After the serum AFP test

After a woman has been identified as having a raised serum AFP level several courses of action can be taken. An ultrasound scan can next be performed, to identify multiple pregnancy (itself associated with raised serum AFP levels), to check on gestational age by measuring the biparietal diameter of the fetal skull and to identify anencephaly or possibly spina bifida. Alternatively, a repeat serum AFP test can be done either before or at the same time as the scan. Each policy will have a different consequence and some of these are discussed elsewhere[2]. Figure 20.2 shows the outcome of pregnancy among women with high maternal serum AFP levels who had an ultrasound scan, based on screening in Oxford when it was normal practice to perform only one serum AFP estimation[3]. About half were found to have elevated AFP levels on account of the under-estimation of gestational age ('wrong dates'), or a

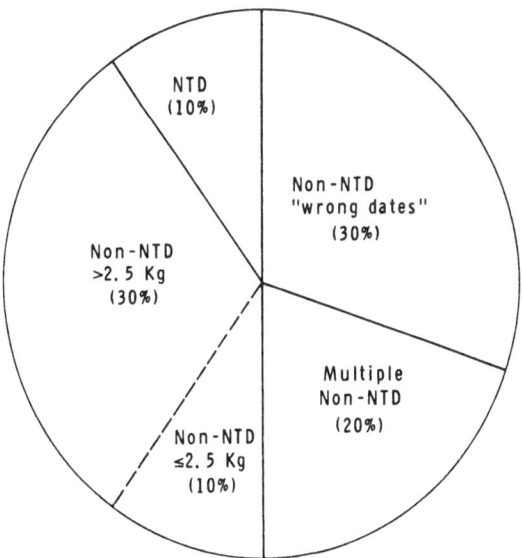

Figure 20.2 Outcome of pregnancy among 101 women with high serum AFP levels who had an ultrasound scan in connection with screening (NTD = neural-tube defect) (from Wald *et al.*[3])

multiple pregnancy. About 10% had neural-tube defects and the remaining false-positives included a high proportion associated with low birth weight, an observation described in greater detail separately[4].

A policy of repeat AFP testing will result in a decrease in the false-positive rate, but there will also be a reduction in the detection rate, which can be largely avoided by either retesting women with AFP values just below the cut-off level, or using a lower cut-off level for the second test.

Knowledge of the local birth prevalence of open neural tube defects is important in the interpretation of a serum AFP result. Table 20.1 shows the approximate probability of having a single fetus with spina bifida, given a serum AFP level equal to or greater than 2.5 MoM, according to the birth prevalence of open spina bifida in the community. In the UK, where the birth prevalence is approximately 2/1000, the probability of having open spina bifida is about 10% using a cut-off level of 2.5 MoM.

Table 20.1 Serum AFP at 16–18 weeks' gestation: approximate probability of having a singleton fetus with open spina bifida given a serum AFP level $\geqslant 2.5$ MoM*

Birth prevalence (per 1000) of open spina bifida	Probability of having open spina bifida (%)
0.5	3
1.0	5
2.0	10

* It is assumed that ultrasound scanning reduces the proportion of unaffected pregnancies with raised serum AFP levels by about one-third, and that repeat testing results in a further one-third reduction.

The amniotic fluid AFP test

The Second UK Collaborative AFP Study Report[5] deals with amniotic fluid AFP measurement as a method of diagnosing open neural-tube defects. At 16–18 weeks of gestation the detection rate for either open spina bifida or anencephaly is 98% and the false-positive rate 0.4% if a single amniotic fluid AFP estimation is performed. If a second amniocentesis is performed on patients yielding amniotic fluid which is bloodstained or on those with borderline results, the false-positive rate can be reduced to 0.2% or less. Table 20.2 shows the probability of having a single fetus with open spina bifida according to the amniotic fluid AFP cut-off level and the reason for amniocentesis. The probabilities shown assume a prevalence of open spina bifida at birth of 2/1000 and a 10-fold increase in risk associated with previously having had an affected child. They are also based on a single amniotic fluid AFP estimation. The risk of having an affected fetus given a positive result is highest among women with positive screening tests, lower for those who have previously had an infant with a neural-tube defect, and much lower for other

Table 20.2   Amniotic fluid AFP at 16–18 weeks' gestation: probability of having a singleton fetus with open spina bifida expressed as a percentage according to cut-off level and reason for amniocentesis (if prevalence of open spina bifida is 2 per 1000)

	Amniotic fluid AFP cut-off level (MoM)	
Reason for aminiocentesis	*3.0(%)*	*4.0(%)*
Single serum AFP >2.5 × median and ultrasound to correct 'dates'	95	97
Previous infant with a neural-tube defect	83	90
Other	33	50

Data from UK Collaborative AFP Study 1979[5]

women where the probability is only about 33% using an amniotic fluid AFP cut-off level of 3 times the median – that is, only one out of three positive results would be associated with open spina bifida. To avoid the high risk of error among women in the third group (those not at special risk of having a fetus with a neural-tube defect) a serum AFP determination should be done on blood taken before the amniocentesis. Then both a high serum and amniotic fluid AFP level would mean that the probability of having an affected fetus is similar to that applicable to screened women.

The future

The discovery that amniotic fluid acetylcholinesterase (AChE) measurement can be used to diagnose open neural-tube defects[6] holds promise that in the future the termination of normal pregnancies on account of false-positive AFP results will be very rare. The most effective assay is the one based on polyacrylamide gel electrophoresis employing the specific AChE inhibitor BW 284C51 dibromide. The test has been evaluated on amniotic fluid samples from several hundred patients including a disproportionately high number incorrectly classified on the basis of AFP results as having normal fetuses (false-negative) or neural-tube defect fetuses (false-positive). To date the only viable pregnancies other than those with an open neural-tube defect which yielded positive results were those associated with exomphalos. Research undertaken during the 1980s will probably determine whether amniotic fluid AChE measurement is a better diagnostic test for open neural-tube defects than amniotic fluid AFP measurement.

THE ROLE OF ASSAY PERFORMANCE

Accuracy

Since the screening detection rate for open spina bifida can be estimated reliably in terms of multiples of the median, it is possible for an AFP assay to be effective provided it can accurately measure *relative* differences in AFP concentration. This type of accuracy has been termed 'relative accuracy' in contrast to the ability to obtain the 'true' concentration (absolute accuracy) which is, from a practical screening point of view, unnecessary[7]. If a laboratory cannot accurately measure relative differences in maternal serum AFP concentration the detection rate for open neural-tube defects and the proportion of unaffected pregnancies with high AFP levels at a given cut-off level will differ from those expected from the distributions shown in Figure 20.1. For example, consider an assay which is inaccurate in the way characterized by Figure 20.3 (the plot of observed AFP values expressed in

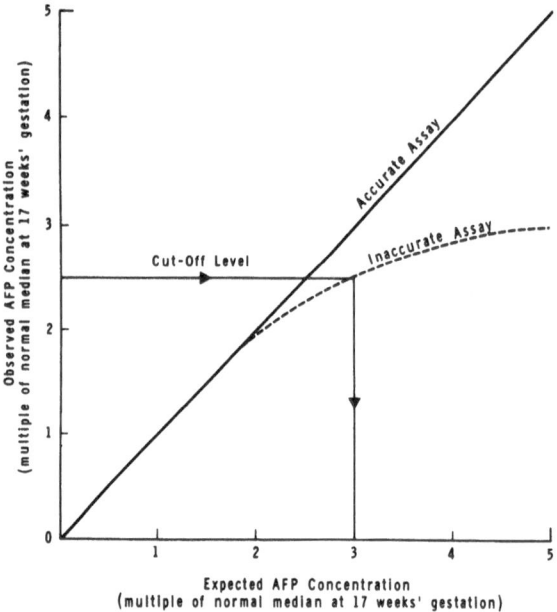

Figure 20.3 The observed and expected AFP concentrations of samples of a serum specimen diluted by known amounts using an accurate assay (in a continuous line) and an inaccurate one (dotted line). The serum specimen has an AFP concentration of 5 multiples of the normal median for 17 weeks' gestation (from Wald and Cuckle[7])

multiples of the median against known relative (or expected) AFP values for a serum specimen diluted by known amounts). Using this assay a cut-off level thought to be at 2.5 times the median would in fact be at 3 times the median; the detection rate for open spina bifida would then be 70% instead of 79%; and the proportion of unaffected pregnancies with high AFP levels would be 1.4%

instead of 3.3%. A 'dilution curve' such as that shown in the figure can readily be plotted and used to indicate the extent of relative inaccuracy of an assay and its effect on screening. The actual AFP value of a cut-off level will be the known (or expected) AFP level corresponding to the observed cut-off level, and the results on the detection rate and false-positive rate can then be determined by reference to Table IX in the First UK Collaborative AFP Study Report[1]. It will be noted that inaccuracy will lead either to a decrease in the detection rate and a decrease in the false-positive rate (as in the example cited) or to an increase in both the detection rate and the false-positive rate, but not an increase in one and a decrease in the other.

Precision

In the course of the UK Collaborative AFP Study the assay imprecision (the random error of AFP measurement when a serum specimen is assayed repeatedly in many analytical batches) was estimated by distributing many specimens drawn from a few maternal serum pools to each participating laboratory where they were assayed as if they were routine specimens. It was then possible to estimate the proportion of the variance of the logarithm of serum AFP concentration in a 1-week gestational period among women with singleton unaffected pregnancies (the normal within-week AFP variance) which was due to the imprecision of AFP measurement. This proportion, the relative assay imprecision, was found to be only about 15% of the normal within-week AFP variance. The remaining 85% of the within-week AFP variance was due to within-person differences in AFP, errors in estimating gestational age, and biological differences between different individuals in the population.

The fact that the assay accounts for only 15% of the AFP variation among different women suggests that differences in AFP assay performances are unlikely to make a substantial impact on the practical results of AFP screening. This can be seen by the examples shown in Figure 20.4 based on data collected by the UK Collaborative AFP Study. The figure shows how a relatively imprecise assay with an across-batch coefficient of variation* of about 30% (dotted line) is associated with a wider AFP distribution than a more precise assay with an across-batch coefficient of variation of about 5% (continuous line). At a cut-off level of 2.5 times the median the proportion of unaffected pregnancies with high AFP levels associated with the imprecise assay is double that associated with the precise one (4% compared with 2%). However, the proportion of open spina bifida pregnancies with high levels is only slightly higher (80% compared with 78%).

---

* The term 'across-batch' (rather than the more usual 'between-batch') coefficient of variation is used because it represents a combination of within-batch and between-batch random assay errors. In the examples that follow it was estimated by assaying a serum specimen once in each of about 50 batches.

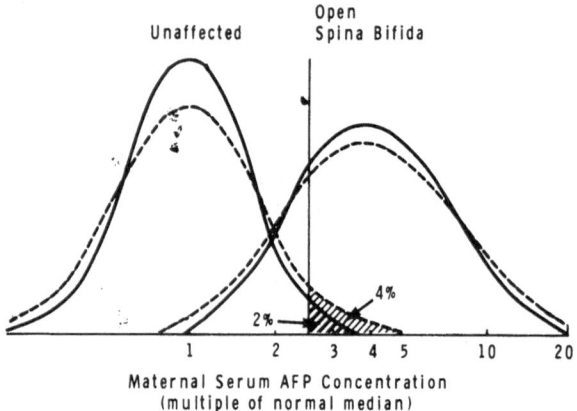

Figure 20.4 The distribution of AFP values from unaffected and open spina bifida pregnancies at 16–18 weeks of pregnancy using a precise assay (straight line) and an imprecise one (dotted line). The shaded areas show the proportion of unaffected pregnancies with AFP levels above 2.5 times the median using each assay (from Wald and Cuckle[7])

An across-batch coefficient of variation of 30% is considerably higher than that generally associated with maternal serum AFP measurement, while one of 5% represents above-average performance. These extremes of assay performance can thus alter the false-positive rate by a factor of two and have only a very small effect on the detection rate.

MONITORING

Assay quality assessment

The most immediate form of monitoring is quality assessment of the AFP assay, although it is an indirect and incomplete measure of screening performance. In Oxford the across-batch coefficient of variation at AFP levels close to the cut-off level is regularly checked; at the end of 1979 it was about 4%. The accuracy of the assay is periodically reviewed by performing dilution and recovery experiments and ensuring that the ratio of the observed AFP to the expected AFP concentration always lies between 0.9 and 1.1. Reference preparations of maternal serum and amniotic fluid are regularly assayed to check for intra- and inter-assay drift.

Short-term epidemiological monitoring

Short-term epidemiological monitoring, involving the collection and reviewing of data approximately every 3 months, can be a very effective method of determining whether screening performance is satisfactory. Table 20.3 shows

Table 20.3 Short-term epidemiological monitoring of AFP screening (Oxford data)

	Gestation (completed weeks)		
	16	17	18
Number of women screened	274	221	172
Screening medians (previously defined) IU/ml	32	37	44
Current medians IU/ml	32	38	45
Ratio of 90th percentile/median	1.7	1.6	1.5
Proportion of women with serum AFP values ⩾ cut-off level		2.1%	

the information that is routinely collected in Oxford and, as an example, the figures obtained under each heading over a recent 3-month period. The 'screening medians' indicated in the table are defined on the basis of data collected during one period of time and then used in screening at a future period. The 'current medians' indicated in the table are those observed during the latter period, and if the assay remained stable the medians in both periods should be very close, say within about 2 IU/ml if there are more than 100 women tested in each week of gestation. If the discrepancy is greater the cause should be determined; it is likely to be due either to assay drift or to some systematic change in the way gestational age is estimated.

The ratio of the 90th percentile of serum AFP to the median in a specified week of gestation gives an indication of the dispersion of values, a large ratio indicating a wide distribution and a small ratio indicating a narrow one. This ratio makes no assumptions about the *shape* of the distribution and, unlike the standard deviation, is hardly influenced by occasional outlying values which can arise in the collection of biochemical results. Using information given in the UK Collaborative AFP Study[1] the ratio can be used as a guide to the proportion of unaffected pregnancies with serum AFP levels equal to or greater than a specified cut-off level such as 2.5 MoM; for example, at 16–18 weeks' gestation this proportion was 1.5%, 2.8% and 5.7% among centres at which the ratio was about 1.7, 1.8–1.9 and 2.0 or more respectively. The ratio will be influenced not only by the precision of measuring AFP but also by the precision with which gestational age is measured, so that if the ratio were found to increase over time the cause would need to be investigated. With greater numbers the false-positive rate can be estimated directly by recording the proportion of women with serum AFP values equal to or greater than a specified cut-off level. It will provide a reasonable estimate as long as the ratio of NTD to non-NTD pregnancies with positive screening tests is reasonably small (say 1:5 or less) as it will be if cut-off levels less than about 3 MoM are used.

Long-term epidemiological monitoring

Long-term epidemiological monitoring in Oxford includes the collection of information specified in Table 20.4. The table also shows actual data relating

Table 20.4 Long-term epidemiological monitoring of AFP screening (Oxford data, 1975–9)

Proportion of women having amniocentesis	1.4%
Number of open neural-tube defects screened	36
Number of neural-tube defects detected	33 (92%)
Pregnancies terminated – affected : unaffected	15 : 1

to AFP screening in Oxford in the period 1975–9. The ratio of the number of affected to unaffected pregnancies terminated is an important statistic; the ratio of 15:1 for Oxford excludes a fetus terminated with biochemical evidence of congenital nephrosis (but without electronmicroscopic evidence) and also excludes a fetus with a skin abnormality extending from the occiput to the lower thoracic region.

Costs

It is useful to monitor the costs of screening – a difficult task if one attempts to determine the full costs including those connected with alterations to antenatal clinic practice, changes in doctor/patient consultation, and procedures such as amniocentesis often performed by existing staff. The figures shown in Table 20.5 represent the costs of additional staff, reagents and equipment needed to undertake AFP screening in Oxford without which a service would not have been available. In 1979 it amounted to about £2500 per neural tube defect detected.

Table 20.5 Monitoring costs of AFP screening (Oxford data, 1979)

	£
Cost per woman screened	3.50
Cost per neural-tube defect detected	2500
Cost per open spina bifida detected	4000

ORGANIZATION OF SCREENING

AFP screening is an example of a medical investigation which does not arise from a patient's request for advice in connection with a specific complaint. Because the investigation is initiated by doctors there is a responsibility to ensure that the overall result of screening and the consequences that follow from it result in a net benefit, and do not use limited resources that could be better utilized in other medical areas. This broad responsibility suggests that the organization of AFP screening should lie within the remit of community medicine or the Public Health Service.

The actual AFP test is a straightforward biochemical test which can be supervised by a biochemist or a doctor with some laboratory experience. What is more difficult is establishing a system of defining cut-off levels in accordance with certain targets agreed in the light of information on the prevalence of the defect in the population, the risks of subsequent investigations such as amniocentesis, and the resources available. All these variables need to be assimilated into a coherent policy, and simple data collection systems set up in order to monitor the results of the policy.

In AFP screening, arrangements need to be made to obtain maternal blood samples at the appropriate gestational age and offer counselling and special tests to women who have raised AFP levels within no more than 1 or 2 weeks. Although not widely adopted there is merit in reporting only results relating to women with high AFP levels. The opportunity for clerical error is thus substantially reduced and the cost of handling, communicating and filing in patients' notes, say 100 instead of three results a week is saved. Confirmation of the safe receipt of samples in the laboratory can be provided at little cost and virtually no chance of error if a self-addressed envelope is enclosed with each specimen.

As I have indicated, AFP assay imprecision is a relatively minor source of AFP variation, and random errors in the estimation of gestational age appear to have a greater effect. The person in charge of an AFP screening programme needs to determine what improvements in the estimation of gestational age are practical, say, by ultrasound scanning, and to what extent these will improve the results of screening. Many patients have an ultrasound scan regardless of AFP screening, and in such an event the linking of the results of the ultrasound scan to the AFP results will avoid an unnecessary second ultrasound scan.

It is unwise to recommend any single protocol for AFP screening. For example, there is no sound basis in adopting rigid guidelines on whether a serum AFP test should always be repeated or whether an ultrasound scan should be carried out before or after a serum AFP test. It is preferable if those responsible for organizing a screening programme are familiar with the practical problems and have an understanding of how varying the different components of screening will influence the final results.

Acknowledgments

I thank my colleagues Dr H. S. Cuckle, Dr Jillian Boreham and Mr R. D. Barlow for their help in providing information presented here.

The Oxford AFP Screening Programme is supported by the Department of Health and Social Security and the Oxfordshire Area Health Authority

(Teaching). Financial support was also provided by the R. J. Harris Trusts, and Dr Jillian Boreham is the holder of a Laing Fellowship in Preventive Medicine.

References

1. Report of UK Collaborative Study on Alpha-fetoprotein in Relation to Neural-tube Defects (1977). Maternal serum alpha-fetoprotein measurement in antenatal screening for anencephaly and spina bifida in early pregnancy. *Lancet*, **1**, 1323
2. Wald, N. J. and Cuckle, H. S. (1980). Alpha-fetoprotein in the antenatal diagnosis of open neural-tube defects. *Br. J. Hosp. Med.*, **23**, 473
3. Wald, N. J., Cuckle, H. S., Boreham, J., Brett, R., Stirrat, G. M., Bennett, M. J., Turnbull, A. C., Solymar, M., Jones, N., Bobrow, M. and Evans, C. J. (1979). Antenatal screening in Oxford for fetal neural-tube defects. *Br. J. Obstet. Gynaecol.*, **86**, 91
4. Wald, N., Cuckle, H., Stirrat, G. M., Bennett, M. J. and Turnbull, A. C. (1977). Maternal serum alpha-fetoprotein and low birth weight. *Lancet*, **2**, 268
5. Second Report of the UK Collaborative Study on Alpha-fetoprotein in Relation to Neural-tube Defects (1979). Amniotic fluid alpha-fetoprotein measurement in antenatal diagnosis of anencephaly and open spina bifida in early pregnancy. *Lancet*, **2**, 651
6. Smith, A. D., Wald, N. J., Cuckle, H. S., Stirrat, G. M., Bobrow, M. and Lagercrantz, H. (1979). Amniotic fluid acetylcholinesterase as a possible diagnostic test for neural-tube defects in early pregnancy. *Lancet*, **1**, 685
7. Wald, N. J. and Cuckle, H. S. (1980). The quality control of alpha-fetoprotein reagents and assay for the antenatal screening and diagnosis of open neural-tube defects: the report of a workshop sponsored by the National Institute of Child Health and Human Development, USA. *Clin. Chim. Acta*, **105**, 9.

21
Immunoassays in Haematology

G. S. CHALLAND

INTRODUCTION

Saturation analysis techniques were first applied to haematology in 1961 by Ekins and co-workers[1] in their pioneering work on the assay of vitamin B_{12}. Subsequent development was slow, but since the subject was reviewed in 1974[2] there have been many developments of research interest and of clinical importance. The major areas of clinical interest at present are the haematinics, vitamin B_{12} and folate; ferritin; and coagulation and lytic factors. The first three are now of established clinical value, but despite a considerable research effort on the latter, there is as yet no immunoassay for the reliable detection of thrombosis or the prethrombotic state.

VITAMIN B_{12} AND FOLATES

The interrelationship of folate and cobalamins has been reviewed by Chanarin[3] and the clinical usefulness of their measurement is unquestioned.

Vitamin B_{12}

The history of assays for cobalamin (vitamin B_{12}) has been reviewed by Mollin *et al.*[4]. Binding assays depend on the addition of cyanide, and a shift of pH and boiling to release the vitamin from its protein-bound complex. Subsequently, a tracer amount of (^{57}Co) cyanocobalamin and a vitamin B_{12}-binding protein are added. Many different binding proteins have been used such as human serum[1], intrinsic factor[5], and chicken serum[6].

Although such binding assays are sensitive, and more precise than microbiological assays, the majority give numerical results which are higher than microbiological assays[6] and it has become apparent that some patients with pernicious anaemia have normal B_{12} results by binding assays[7]. The reason for this discrepancy was established by Kolhouse and co-workers[8]. Most binding agents contain both proteins which specifically bind B_{12} and proteins of the so-called R type which bind a wide range of cobalamins and cobalamin-like materials. Serum contains a mixture of different cobalamins, all of which are detected when an impure binding agent is used, but only the biologically active cobalamins are detected by a microbiological assay. It is therefore necessary to modify the binding agent, either by selective purification or by blocking the R proteins with cobamide[8,9], to achieve a binding assay of clinical validity.

It may be of value to develop radioimmunoassays (RIAs) specific for methyl cobalamin, the major plasma component, or adenosyl cobalamin, the major tissue component. Attempts to do this have so far been unsuccessful.

Folates

The standard binding assay for folates uses a binding protein present in the β-lactoglobulin fraction of milk[10-12]. At pH 9.3, this reacts equally both with 5-methyl-tetrahydrofolate, the major serum folate, and with the minor component, tetrahydrofolate. The number of glutamate residues present on the folate does not appear to affect binding. These assays therefore measure total serum folates, and correlation with microbiological assays is adequate[13,14].

RIAs have been described for folates[15] but numerical results have not been in good agreement with other assay methods. This may be caused by antisera to folates differentiating between the different numbers of glutamate residues attached to the folate molecule, and thus failing to recognize all folates.

Combined assays

Recently, combined binding assays have appeared which measure both vitamin B_{12} and folates simultaneously, utilizing a ^{57}Co tracer for B_{12} and a ^{125}I-tagged tracer for folates[16]. These have some advantages of convenience over the separate performance of conventional binding assays, but there are technical disadvantages and the appropriate choice of experimental conditions is critical to their validity[17].

BINDING PROTEINS

Ferritin

Ferritin is the principal tissue iron-storage protein in the reticuloendothelial systems of liver, spleen, and bone marrow. Its concentration in serum is thought to be closely related to total body iron stores[18,19]. The early development of ferritin RIAs was hindered by difficulty in preparing a suitable tracer[20] and the first method with adequate sensitivity for clinical use was an immunoradiometric assay[21]. Since then, improved radioiodination methods have made possible the development of sufficiently sensitive RIAs[22-24].

The ferritins in different tissues which may contain one or more different types of subunits are known as isoferritins. Although their electrophoretic mobility differs, antisera raised against one type cross-react in general equally with ferritins of other types. Whether it is of clinical importance to measure a single isoferritin rather than all circulating ferritins is at present unknown.

Although ferritin is primarily implicated in iron storage, evidence is accumulating that it may have other roles. In the gastric mucosal cell and in the placenta[25], ferritin appears to be implicated in the transport of iron. Significant concentrations of ferritin are found in urine; these are not related to proteinurea (McLean and Challand, unpublished observations).

The traditional method of assessing iron stores by chemical means is to measure iron and iron-binding capacity. These methods have been frequently criticized and do not correlate well with ferritin measurements[23]. It would be unwise at present to replace them by ferritin RIAs, particularly as ferritin is an acute phase reactant, but it is now certain that measurement of ferritin will be commonly requested in clinical practice. Much more work will need to be done on this interesting protein.

Transferrin

Transferrin concentrations are normally assessed chemically by determination of the total iron-binding capacity of serum. A less direct binding method has been described in which the transferrin–iron complex is dissociated and the free transferrin is then used as a binding agent[26]. This method offers no advantages over chemical methodology. RIAs for transferrin have been developed, but do not as yet appear to be of clinical value.

COAGULATION AND LYSIS

Haemostasis, the arrest of bleeding at a site of injury, is of intense research interest. Thrombosis, haemostasis in the wrong place, is a major clinical problem, and considerable efforts have been made to produce a reliable diagnostic test. Both have been recently reviewed[27,28].

The mechanism of haemostasis is a complex series of reactions which are summarized in Table 21.1. These are: first, a group of platelet reactions; second, the activation of the coagulation cascade of enzyme reactions; third, the formation of a fibrin clot; fourth, the lysis of fibrin and subsequent dissolution of the clot.

Table 21.1   The sequence of reactions involved in haemostasis

(1) Damage to blood vessel wall.
(2) Platelet adhesion to damaged endothelium.
(3) Platelet aggregation and release of platelet factors.
(4) Activation of the coagulation cascade, leading to the formation of thrombin.
(5) Conversion, by thrombin, of fibrinogen to fibrin monomer.
(6) Polymerization of fibrin monomer to form fibrin chains through the platelet mass which stabilize the clot.
(7) Lysis of fibrin chains by plasmin to dissolve the clot.

Platelet factors

After damage to the vessel wall, platelets adhere to the damaged site by either of two mechanisms; adhesion to exposed subendothelial structures such as collagen[29], or by a complex series of prostaglandin reactions[30]. In the intact vessel wall, prostacyclin is synthesized from endoperoxides produced in part by the platelet. This stimulates adenylate cyclase in platelets, which inhibits platelet aggregation through the production of cyclic AMP. When vessel wall cells are damaged, prostacyclin synthesis falls, and endoperoxides are metabolized primarily to thromboxane A2 in the platelet. This inhibits adenylate cyclase, the production of cyclic AMP falls and of ADP rises, which stimulates platelet aggregation. Platelet adhesion depends on the relative concentration of prostacyclin and thromboxane A2 around the vessel wall. Both of these are short-lived products, but both are metabolized to relatively long-lived products which should be measurable by RIA. If binding assays are developed for these products, it may be possible to monitor the earliest stages of haemostasis and thrombosis.

When platelets aggregate, they release a variety of products, which can be measured to assess platelet aggregation.

Platelet factor 4

RIAs have been developed for measurement of platelet factor 4, a protein with heparin-neutralizing activity released by platelets on aggregation. High levels in plasma are associated with thrombotic events[31]. However, levels in patients with thrombi overlap the normal range, so the test is not suitable for diagnosis.

β-Thromboglobulin

β-Thromboglobulin is a platelet-specific protein of unknown function which is released when platelets aggregate[32]. The measurement of plasma concentrations by RIA was initially promising for the diagnosis of deep vein thrombosis[33]. These early results were not substantiated, and a large overlap was found between controls and patients with deep vein thrombosis.

The main problem in developing a biochemical test to detect thrombus formation is that the taking of a blood sample initiates haemostasis. Extreme care is therefore needed during phlebotomy, and a complex group of inhibitors must be added to the blood sample to prevent coagulation. Any carelessness in sampling leads to a false-positive result. An alternative approach is to measure factors released in thrombus formation found in urine rather than blood, since this avoids the sampling difficulty. Initial results with β-thromboglobulin in urine are promising[34].

Factors of the coagulation cascade

The biochemistry of the coagulation cascade has been recently reviewed[35]. It is traditionally divided into the intrinsic pathway, which starts with the activation of Factor XII initiated by blood contact with a foreign surface; the extrinsic pathway, probably the most important initiation pathway *in vivo*; and the common pathway, which starts at the activation of Factor X and finishes with the formation of thrombin and ultimate polymerization of fibrin. Individual factors are usually measured by bioassay but immunological methods, including RIAs, are being increasingly employed.

Factor VIII, antihaemophilic factor

Haemagglutination inhibition, immunoelectrophoresis, RIA[36] and an immunoradiometric assay[37] for Factor VIII have all been described. Factor VIII has three distinct properties: clot-promoting activity; antigenic activity; and an activity which is deficient in Von Willebrand's disease. These may be on separate subunits of the molecule[38]. For diagnostic purposes, it is usually necessary to measure both antigenic and biological activity. Thus, carriers of haemophilia A could be detected by comparing antigenic and biological activities[39]. However, the abnormality of Factor VIII in Von Willebrand's disease was suggested to be associated with the antigenic site, since a lack of parallelism was found in an immunoradiometric assay[37].

Other coagulation factors

A RIA for plasminogen and plasmin has been described[40], and it proved possible to distinguish the two by appropriate choice of experimental conditions[41]. As with Factor VIII, there is a difference between biological and immunological activity.

RIA, or other immunological assays, have been described for several other factors important in the coagulation cascade, for example, prothrombin[42]. The diagnostic usefulness of these is yet to be established.

It is now apparent that the traditional view of the coagulation pathway described above is oversimplified. Precursors can be activated by many different proteolytic enzymes, and the whole system is unlikely to be a strict linear pathway[35]. Some factors are now considered to be regulatory proteins rather than proteolytic enzymes, and the whole system is kept in check by an elaborate network of inhibitors, activators and feedback loops.

For any factor, there are likely to be precursor molecules, active and inactive fragments which may be bound to inhibitor molecules, all circulating *in vivo*. This, coupled with the complexity of the cascade, suggests that the development of RIAs for isolated factors is unlikely to yield valuable diagnostic information. Such RIAs are, however, of research interest and may provide information on inherited deficiencies of isolated factors.

Fibrinogen, fibrin and their degradation fragments

The last steps in the haemostatic mechanism are the conversion of fibrinogen to fibrin monomer with the release of fibrinopeptides, the polymerization of fibrin and its cross-linking and the subsequent digestion by plasmin to give degradation fragments.

RIAs have been developed for the fibrinopeptides A and B[43, 44] and applied clinically[45]. Elevated levels were found in patients with venous thrombosis or pulmonary embolism; however, this proved of limited diagnostic usefulness.

As early as 1968, a RIA was described for fibrinogen and fibrin[46]. Because of cross-reaction between fibrinogen and degradation fragments of fibrinogen and fibrin, this assay has not been applied clinically. Subsequent efforts have been devoted to developing RIAs for degradation fragments in which fibrinogen does not cross-react. Assays for Fragments D and E were described[47] although some cross-reaction with fibrinogen was experienced. As with fibrinopeptides, patients with deep vein thrombosis and pulmonary embolism had elevated levels, but there was no clear distinction from normals[48, 49]. Subsequent efforts have been directed towards producing antisera specific to neoantigenic determinants on the fragments[50] or the only unique fibrin degradation fragment, D-dimer[51]. These have been largely unsuccessful.

CONCLUSIONS

The last 5 years have seen some solid advances in the application of saturation assays to haematology. Thus, a binding assay for folate, a modified binding assay for vitamin B_{12}, and a RIA for ferritin are now of proven clinical validity. In other areas of haematology the situation is less clear. Despite a considerable research effort, the development of RIAs for coagulation and lytic factors has not resulted in a reliable test for thrombosis. Although it is apparent that several molecules are candidates for measurement, technical difficulties in their RIA, sampling problems, and the complexity of the system have hindered progress. A single test to detect the presence of a thrombus – or, better, to detect those patients at risk of a thrombus prior to surgery – remains a dream.

The most obvious other area of haematological interest in which immunoassays could be applied is in the study and classification of blood groups. Although it should be possible to develop rapid techniques which can readily be automated in place of the present labour-intensive methods, little progress on this has yet been made.

References

1. Barakat, R. M. and Ekins, R. P. (1961). Assay of Vitamin B12 in blood. *Lancet*, **2**, 25
2. Newmark, P. A. and Gordon, Y. B. (1974). Haematology. *Br. Med. Bull.*, **30**, 86
3. Chanarin, I. (1977). Folates, cobalamins and their interrelationship in man. In Marks, V. and Hales, C. N. (eds.) *Essays in Medical Biochemistry*, Vol. 3, pp. 1–24. (London: The Biochemical Society and the Association of Clinical Biochemists)
4. Mollin, D. L., Anderson, B. B. and Burman, J. F. (1976). The serum vitamin B12 level: its assay and significance. *Clin. Haematol.*, **5**, 521
5. Lau, K. S., Gottlieb, C., Wasserman, L. R. and Herbert, V. (1965). Measurement of serum Vitamin B12 level using radioisotopic dilution and coated charcoal. *Blood*, **26**, 202
6. Newmark, P., Green, R., Musso, A. and Mollin, D. L. M. (1972). Radioisotopic assay of serum Vitamin B12 levels using chicken serum as the binding protein. *Scand. J. Clin. Lab. Invest.* Suppl. no. 126, 6.11 (Abstract)
7. Cooper, B. A. and Whitehead, V. M. (1978). Evidence that some patients with pernicious anaemia are not recognised by radiodilution assay for cobalamin in serum. *N. Engl. J. Med.*, **299**, 816
8. Kolhouse, J. F., Kondo, H., Allen, N. C., Podell, E. and Allen, R. H. (1978). Cobalamin analogues are present in human plasma and can mask cobalamin deficiency because current radioisotope dilution assays are not specific for true cobalamin. *N. Engl. J. Med.*, **299**, 785
9. Allen, R. H., Seetharam, B., Allen, N. C., Podell, E. R. and Alpers, D. H. (1978). Correction of cobalamin malabsorption in pancreatic insufficiency with a cobalamin analogue that binds with high affinity to R. protein but not to intrinsic factor. *J. Clin. Invest.*, **61**, 1628
10. Ford, J. E., Salter, D. N. and Scott, K. J. (1969). The folate binding protein in milk. *J. Dairy Res.*, **36**, 435
11. Waxman, S., Schreiber, C. and Herbert, V. (1971). Radioisotopic assay for measurement of serum folate levels. *Blood*, **38**, 210
12. Rothenberg, S. P., da Costa, M. and Rosenberg, Z. (1972). A radioassay for serum folate: use of a two-phase sequential incubation ligand binding system. *N. Engl. J. Med.*, **286**, 1335
13. Hill, P. W. and Dawson, D. W. (1977). Evaluation of a commercial radioisotopic kit for folate assays. *J. Clin. Pathol.*, **30**, 449
14. Waxman, S., Schreiber, S., Rose, M., Johnson, I., Sheppard, R., Sumbler, K., Keen, A. and Guilford, H. (1977). Measurement of serum folate by ^{75}Se-selenofolate radioassay. *Am. J. Clin. Pathol.*, **70**, 359
15. Da Costa, M. and Rothenberg, S. P. (1971). Identification of an immunoreactive folate in serum extracts by radioimmunoassay. *Br. J. Haematol.*, **21**, 121
16. Gutcho, S. and Mansbach, L. (1977). Simultaneous radioassay of serum Vitamin B12 and folic acid. *Clin. Chem.*, **23**, 1609
17. Lee-Own, V., Bolton, A. E. and Carr, P. J. (1979). Formation of a Vitamin B12 serum complex on heating at alkaline pH. *Clin. Chim. Acta*, **93**, 239
18. Walter, G. O., Miller, F. M. and Worwood, M. (1973). Serum ferritin concentrations and iron stores in normal subjects. *J. Clin. Pathol.*, **26**, 770

19. Lipschitz, D. A., Cook, J. D. and Finch, C. A. (1974). A clinical evaluation of serum ferritin as an index of iron stores. *N. Engl. J. Med.*, **290**, 1213

20. Reller, H. (1971). Radioimmunologischer nachweis von ferritin mit der solid-phase methode. *Pathol. Microbiol.*, **37**, 201

21. Addison, G. M., Beamish, M. R., Hales, C. N., Hodgkins, M., Jacobs, A. and Llewellin, P. (1972). An immunoradiometric assay for ferritin in the serum of normal subjects and patients with iron deficiency and iron overload. *J. Clin. Pathol.*, **25**, 326

22. Bolton, A. E., Lee-Own, V., McLean, R. K. and Challand, G. S. (1979). Three different radioiodination methods for human spleen ferritin compared. *Clin. Chem.*, **25**, 1826

23. Goldie, D. J. and Thomas, M. J. (1978). Measurement of serum ferritin by radioimmunoassay. *Ann. Clin. Biochem.*, **15**, 102

24. Wide, L. and Birgegard, G. (1977). A solid-phase radioimmunoassay for ferritin in serum using ^{125}I-labelled ferritin. *Uppsala J. Med. Sci.*, **82**, 15

25. McLean, R. K., Jones, H. M., Challand, G. S. and Chard, T. (1980). Ferritin levels in fetal and maternal compartments in late pregnancy. (In preparation)

26. Herbert, V., Gottlieb, C. W., Lau, K. S., Gevirtz, N. R., Sharney, L. and Wasserman, L. (1967). Coated charcoal assay of plasma iron binding capacity and iron using radioisotope dilution and hemoglobin-coated charcoal. *J. Nucl. Med.*, **8**, 529

27. Haemostasis (whole issue). *Br. Med. Bull.*, **33**, No. 3 (1977).

28. Thrombosis (whole issue). *Br. Med. Bull.*, **34**, No. 3 (1978).

29. Baumgartner, H. R., Muggli, R., Tschopp, T. B. and Turitto, V. T. (1976). Platelet adhesion, release and aggregation in flowing blood: effects of surface properties and platelet function. *Thromb. Haemost.*, **35**, 124

30. Moncada, S. and Vane, J. R. (1978). Unstable metabolites of arachidonic acid and their role in haemostasis and thrombosis. *Br. Med. Bull.*, **34**, 129

31. Bolton, A. E., Ludlam, C. A., Pepper, D. S., Moore, S. and Cash, J. D. (1976). A radioimmunoassay for platelet factor 4. *Thromb. Res.*, **8**, 51

32. Moore, S., Pepper, D. S. and Cash, J. D. (1975). The isolation and characterisation of a platelet-specific β-globulin (β-thromboglobulin) and the detection of antiurokinase and antiplasmin released from thrombin-aggregated washed human platelets. *Biochim. Biophys. Acta*, **379**, 360

33. Ludlam, C. A., Moore, S., Bolton, A. E. and Cash, J. D. (1975). New rapid method for diagnosis of deep venous thrombosis. *Lancet*, **2**, 259

34. Bolton, A. E., Cooke, E. D., Lekhwani, C. P. and Bowcock, S. A. (1980). Urinary β-thromboglobulin levels as a diagnostic marker for post-operative deep vein thrombosis. (In preparation)

35. Esnouf, M. P. (1977). Biochemistry of blood coagulation. *Br. Med. Bull.*, **33**, 213

36. Hoyer, L. W. (1972). Immunologic studies of anti-hemophilic factor (AHF, factor VIII). IV. Radioimmunoassay of AHF antigen. *J. Lab. Clin. Med.*, **80**, 822

37. Peake, I. R. and Bloom, A. L. (1977). The use of an immunoradiometric assay for Factor VIII related antigen in the study of atypical Von Willebrand's disease. *Thromb. Res.*, **10**, 27

38. Bloom, A. L. and Peake, I. R. (1977). Factor VIII and its inherited disorders. *Br. Med. Bull.*, **33**, 219

39. Zimmerman, T. S., Ratnoff, O. D. and Littell, A. S. (1971). Detection of carriers of classic hemophilia using an immunologic assay for antihemophilic factor (Factor VIII). *J. Clin. Invest.*, **50**, 255

40. Rabiner, S. F., Goldfine, I. D., Hart, A., Summaria, L. and Robbins, K. C. (1969). Radioimmunoassay of human plasminogen and plasmin. *J. Lab. Clin. Med.*, **74**, 265

41. Hart, A., Robbins, K. C., Summaria, L. and Rabiner, S. F. (1971). Differentiation of plasminogen from plasmin by radioimmunoassay. *Fed. Proc.*, **30**, 367 (Abstract)

42. Johnston, M. F. M., Kipfer, R. K. and Olson, R. E. (1972). Studies of prothrombin biosynthesis in cell-free systems. I. Comparison of coagulation and immunochemical assays. *J. Biol. Chem.*, **247**, 3987

43. Nossel, H. L., Younger, L. R., Wilner, G. D., Procupez, T., Canfield, R. E. and Butler, V. P. (1971). Radioimmunoassay of human fibrinopeptide A. *Proc. Natl. Acad. Sci. USA*, **68**, 2350

44. Nossel, H. L., Chatpar, R., Butler, V. P. and Canfield, R. E. (1972). Radioimmunoassay of fibrinopeptide B. *Blood*, **40**, 955 (Abstract)

45. Nossel, H. L., Yudelman, I., Canfield, R. E., Butler, V. P., Spanondis, K., Wilner, G. D. and Qureshi, G. D. (1974). Measurement of fibrinopeptide A in human blood. *J. Clin. Invest.*, **54**, 43

46. Catt, K. J., Hirsh, J., Castelan, D. J., Niall, H. D. and Tregear, G. W. (1968). Radioimmunoassay of fibrinogen and its proteolysis products. *Thromb. Diath. Haemorrh.*, **20**, 1

47. Gordon, Y. B., Martin, M. J., Landon, J. and Chard, T. (1975). The development of radioimmunoassays for Fibrin(ogen) degradation products: Fragments D and E. *Br. J. Haematol.*, **29**, 109

48. Cooke, E. D., Bowcock, S. A., Pilcher, M. F., Ibbotson, R. M., Gordon, Y. B., Sola, C. M., Chard, T. and Ainsworth, M. E. (1975). Serum fibrin(ogen) degradation products in diagnosis of deep-vein thrombosis and pulmonary embolism after hip surgery. *Lancet*, **2**, 51

49. Butler, M. J., Gordon, Y. B., Irving, M. H., Sola, C. M. and Chard, T. (1976). Serum levels of fibrin(ogen) degradation fragment E antigen in the diagnosis of deep vein thrombosis after abdominal and inguinal surgery. *Thromb. Res.*, **8**, 167

50. Gordon, Y. B., Martin, M. J., McNeilly, A. S., Rees, L. H. and Chard, T. (1975). Observations on radioimmunoassays for neoantigenic sites. In Pasternak, C. A. (ed.) *Radioimmunoassay in Clinical Biochemistry*, pp. 263–8. (London: Heyden)

51. Ferguson, E. W., Fratto, L. J. and McKee, P. A. (1975). A re-examination of the cleavage of fibrinogen and fibrin by plasmin. *J. Biol. Chem.*, **250**, 7210

22
Immunoassays in Tissue Typing

C. C. ENTWISTLE

Transplantation can be likened to the mixing of tissues from different creatures, and the more different they are, the more likely is the outcome to be rejection of transplanted tissue. In transplantation, the host's immune system recognizes the graft by different sets of characteristics present on the cells of the graft. The identification *in vitro* of those cellular characteristics is what tissue typing is all about.

We know that the inheritance of many of these characteristics so far recognized is genetically determined, by genes at a number of loci carried at what is called the 'major histocompatibility complex' (MHC), situated in man on the short arm of the sixth autosomal chromosome. Similar MHCs have also been discovered in all laboratory and domestic animals so far studied.

In each MHC there are a number of separate loci, which in man are now known as the HLA loci: A, C and B being defined serologically, D defined by cellular interaction only. In addition there are other characteristics called DR (HLA-D related) antigens which for practical purposes are only carried on B lymphocytes and macrophages. These are also recognized serologically, and are very closely related though not identical to the HLA-D determinants mentioned above. Let us consider some of the assays available to study the products of each of these gene loci, starting with the cellular determinants.

The simplest technique is the 'mixed lymphocyte culture' or MLC, which has been with us for about 16 years. Basically it is very simple: mix cells from two individuals in a suitable culture situation for a few days and see whether either recognizes the other as 'foreign'. If it does, it will undergo blast-cell transformation which is usually measured by the incorporation of radio-labelled (tritiated) thymidine, while absence of such a reaction should indicate that the two cells share the same HLA-D determinants. Unfortunately, the

MLC test system is not so simple as that. It requires a very large number of both 'stimulator' as well as 'responder' cells, strictly sterile and highly standardized technique, many replicates to allow for test variability, expensive β-radiation counters, and a complicated data analysis methodology; worst of all, the whole test takes several days to complete which takes it largely out of the realm of practicality for transplant compatibility testing, apart from the live donor situation.

One attempt to short-circuit this problem is the 'primed lymphocyte test' or PLT. In this, an MLC test is allowed to proceed for about 10 days, when all the responding cells are either harvested for use immediately, or are frozen down for future use. On rechallenge, these cells will behave differently according to whether they are exposed to the same determinant they met before, which precipitates an accelerated or secondary type of response in 36 h, or any totally new determinant, in which case a normal MLC response peaking in 3–6 days will take place. Primed lymphocyte tests are undoubtedly quicker, and have generated a lot of most useful information. However, even these take a couple of days to conclude, and our surgical colleagues cannot usually wait that long to decide what to do with a cadaver kidney. For this reason, most of the laboratory work concerned with attempts to find the most suitable recipients for a given graft have so far been based on serological tests which take only a few hours. Let us consider some of these.

Leukocyte agglutination is the oldest and perhaps the simplest. It stems from the fact that while we should ideally be testing kidney tissues to match up kidney grafts, such tissues are not available for laboratory work and we are therefore dependent upon what tissues we can readily get – blood – which we hope will give us near enough the same answers. In fact, we know that blood, and white blood cells in particular, do share histocompatibility antigens with most tissues of the body and hence tests done with leukocytes should give us good clues to graft acceptability. Whole leukocyte preparations are of course very crude, unstandardized (having variable mixtures of lymphocytes, granulocytes, platelets etc.), have to be fresh, and carry antigens which form part of many different systems (HLA, granulocyte and platelet-specific, etc). Nonetheless, such tests gave us an early insight into compatibility testing, and even now still find occasional usefulness in the investigation of transfusion reactions.

Platelet complement fixation has the advantage of using, as substrate, platelets which are fixed in azide and oxalate and can be stored at room temperature for many months. Conveniently, the tests are also macroscopic. However, platelet complement fixation tests are relatively insensitive, there are *very* few good sera available, and there is also the problem of variable extent of antigen expression on the surface of platelets according to the antigens concerned. Other techniques were soon devised and, without doubt, most of our present-day knowledge of tissue typing has come from one form or another of complement-dependent lymphocyte toxicity test.

Several variations have been devised of such 'lymphocytotoxicity' tests, the two best known being the one-stage Kissmeyer–Nielsen technique, wherein the test cells, suspended in rabbit/human complement-containing serum, are allowed to react with test serum at 37 °C, then assessed for degree of cell death produced. This technique has the advantage of requiring only 1 h incubation, but is undoubtedly less sensitive than the now more or less standard two-stage, so-called 'NIH' technique. In this, cells suspended in suitable buffer are allowed to react with test serum for 30 min at 22 °C, then rabbit serum (standardized complement) is added for a further 60 min before degree of cell death is assessed. The latter can be done by one of various methods: simple-phase contrast microscopy, exclusion of supravital dyes (trypan blue or eosin) or the fluorochrome ethidium bromide; or loss of another fluórochrome fluoresceine diacetate or of a radiolabel ^{51}Cr from live cells. Both these last two methods can lend themselves to automation, but neither is very practical for routine purposes in most laboratories.

The NIH test has many technical pitfalls for the unwary. Cell concentration, background viability, purity, must all be acceptable; the complement *must* be well-standardized and of proven potency; the timing of the reactions is fairly critical, and the temperature *must* be standardized between 20 and 24 °C – 'room temperature' is *not* enough (too variable).

One of the biggest problems comes not so much with the execution of the tests as with interpretation. Throughout tissue typing, considerable confusion arises out of the phenomenon of antigenic cross-reactivity. This is manifest by the frequent observation of apparently 'pure' sera reacting with cells carrying other antigens related to the one supposed to be specific to that serum; this happens particularly where those cells are carrying a double dose, or are homozygous, for the related antigen. We are only now beginning to understand the possible mechanism of such cross-reactivity. Recent sequencing studies have demonstrated, for instance, that the closely related antigens A2 and A28 share not less than 61 of the 64 known amino acids in their basic structure, so it is perhaps not surprising that there are very few sera which will react with A28 cells and do not have at least some reactivity with A2-positive cells (especially homozygous A2-positive cells). A corollary to this problem is the serum availability situation. Thus, while there are adequate supplies of operationally monospecific antisera for many of the established specificities, for many others there are *very few sera in the world*, and this despite very intensive efforts by large numbers of laboratories to improve the situation.

To illustrate this point, in the UKTS laboratory in Bristol, we annually screen up to about 10 000 antenatal sera for possible use as typing reagents. From these, only about 1000 (in round figures) have any sort of recognizable HLA activity and are studied again with a more comprehensive system. A mere couple of hundred turn out to be worthy of further consideration and we make efforts to try to secure a reasonable-sized serum donation from those ladies. Inevitably it takes a while to obtain such donations and in many

M

instances the antibody reactivity is then perhaps not as useful as we first thought, being either too weak or too broadly reactive. Only about 100 sera a year are anywhere near good enough for possible reagent use, but of these only the best 20 or so end up being offered to other laboratories for kidney donor and recipient typing, and a mere handful are of sufficient quality to be offered for international exchanges. All in all, there is thus a very small return for a lot of screening, and this is the sort of pattern seen in all laboratories. Also, it should be remembered that although there are a limited number of specificities and perhaps many sera for defining any one of them, nonetheless no two sera behave in exactly the same way. The end-result of this is that there are *no perfect standard reference reagents* for tissue typing such as there are for many other immunoassays. The best we have available are alloantisera which have been studied through international exchanges and tested against comprehensive panels of cells.

When we turn to the serological identification of the HLA-D related or DR antigens, we are confronted by additional problems. DR antigens are present on a minor subpopulation of lymphocytes. One way to identify that subpopulation within a mixture of peripheral blood lymphocytes is to use two-colour fluorescence. In this, the B-cells which carry surface immunoglobulin can be labelled with one fluorochrome (FDA) conjugated to anti-IgG, while dead cells are identified by another fluorochrome of a different colour, such as ethidium bromide. Alternatively, and currently more commonly, the B cells (and some macrophages) can be 'enriched' by eliminating most of the T cells by their incorporation in EA rosettes with enzyme-treated (papain, AET or neuraminidase) sheep cells.

Other ways of 'purifying' B cells depend on different principles. If a whole lymphocyte suspension is passed through a nylon-wool column, the B cells are sticky and adhere to the wool while the T and null cells tend to pass on through. The adherent cells can later be dislodged to give a reasonably pure suspension without damaging the cells too much. Other columns containing extracts of *Helix pomatia* bound to sepharose similarly bind the B cells which again can be recovered after other cells have been washed out. More recently a technique has been described whereby sepharose beads complexed to monoclonal anti-DR antibody (non-cytotoxic) can be used. These bind loosely to the B cells and after separation from remaining cells the bead/B cell adhesion can be disrupted – again leaving the cells in a viable state suitable for toxicity tests. Following purification or enrichment of B cells, the serological tests for DR detection all take longer to perform than conventional HLA tests, and require a better quality of complement. There are as yet relatively few DR antigens to define, and all are thought to belong to a single locus. There are hints that there may be another locus but this awaits proof. There are only nine established antigens, but at present the number of sera to define them, and the volumes of these sera available, are still abysmally small although progress in this direction is being made all the time.

Why do we do all this, how far has it got us, and where do we go from here?

Ideally, what we are aiming to achieve is a graft success rate using unrelated donors similar to that seen in identical-twin transplants. So far this seems something of a Utopian dream. What we do know is that transplants performed between family members who are apparently identical for the tissue type factors so far identified undoubtedly do better than those who are mismatched. Even the latter seem to do better than so-called 'matched' unrelated grafts, presumably because of the many other factors which have so far defied laboratory recognition and yet which are of biological importance to transplantation. Indeed, it is now becoming patently obvious that graft success or failure is dependent upon a multitude of factors; some definable, many not. Clinical factors such as patient selection, history of transfusion, previous disease, previous sensitization from pregnancy, grafts etc., are every bit if not more important than tissue factors, though the latter cannot be ignored. So how much does their recognition help?

Almost all studies, both from individual centres and from multicentre analyses, have agreed that in cadaver transplantation, grafts well-matched for HLA A and B locus antigens will on *average* do statistically rather better than those which are mismatched. The advantage is in the order of 15–20% better graft survival overall after 1 and after 2 years. There is also a further advantage for recipients of well-matched grafts that, should the latter fail, such patients are in general less troubled by sensitization from that first graft, and it may be rather easier to find a suitable subsequent graft for them.

If that is all the advantage from HLA-A and B locus matching, what about HLA-DR? There is still rather limited information on this subject, but it does appear that grafts which are DR identical put into non-sensitized recipients do much better than DR mismatched grafts; also, there is some evidence that DR matching may overcome any disadvantage accruing from recipients lacking a previous blood transfusion. However, more information is needed to confirm or refute these early reports.

What improvements can we expect in tissue typing? Mechanically, the work-load can be made much easier by plate-oiling machines, serum dispensing machines and other semi-automatic innovations. Fully automatic microscope stages are being developed and in time these must lead to automatic recording of results, computerized data entry and analyses.

Other likely changes in the 80s must include further development of monoclonal antibodies, though it will probably be some time before these exotic (and rather expensive) refinements become freely available for general use and replace alloantisera. Meanwhile, standardized cell-lines may help in screening programmes of pregnancy-associated and other human sera. Further clarification will I am sure emerge for the reactions we currently observe. Many can be explained on the basis of HLA, but there is a lot more to it than that. We are only just beginning to recognize reactions due to autoantibodies, better definition of granulocyte and platelet-specific antibodies will follow, the newly recognized monocyte-specific and associated vascular endothelial antigens will be better defined, and it is likely that there may well be further specificities peculiar to T cell subpopulations. All of these will be elucidated in time and will give us a greater understanding of what is going on.

On the cellular front, a new microversion of MLC type tests has already been developed, which will greatly facilitate wider use of these techniques so badly hampered by the large number of cells needed in conventional tests. Again, automation and computerization will simplify the interpretation of such tests performed on a larger scale.

On the disease-association front, a considerable volume of work has already been done, and a number of statistically valid associations have been described with antigens of all loci. However, the associations are rather tenuous, and must be regarded as being of very limited real clinical value. Indeed there are relatively few situations where the establishment of the presence or otherwise of a particular HLA antigen materially alters the clinical management of a given patient. In the future, however, perhaps even closer associations may be recognized which may be of more practical use.

Finally, when a few more clouds of ignorance have been swept away – perhaps in the 1980s – then possibly we may understand how it is that seemingly 'well-matched' grafts may fail, while others which on the face of things are hopelessly unsuitable sometimes defy all the odds and support life in a state of happy symbiosis.

23
Immunoassays for Acute Phase Proteins

M. B. PEPYS

THE ACUTE PHASE RESPONSE

The acute phase response consists of increased synthesis and raised circulating concentrations of a number of plasma proteins, the so-called acute phase reactants[1,2]. It is initiated by most forms of tissue injury, infection or inflammation and high levels of some acute phase proteins persist in chronic active inflammation and malignancy[3,4]. Acute phase responses occur in all mammals and birds which have been studied and proteins homologous with C-reactive protein (CRP), the classical acute phase reactant, are apparently present in all vertebrates[5,6]. The general nature of the response and the evolutionary conservation of these molecules suggests that they probably have beneficial functions. Functions for many acute phase proteins are known or suspected and their possible role in processes of resolution and repair is obvious (Table 23.1). However there is also evidence that in some circumstances acute phase proteins may exacerbate tissue damage during inflammation[7,8].

The underlying mechanism of the acute phase response, and the functions and control of metabolism of specific acute phase proteins, are poorly understood. Most of these proteins are glycoproteins and many are produced in the liver[1,9,10] where their rates of synthesis and secretion are increased apparently under the influence of humoral mediators derived directly or indirectly from sites of tissue damage or inflammation[11-14]. Although the liver is clearly important it is not necessarily the only site of acute phase protein synthesis. For example a number of complement components which are acute phase reactants, including C3, can be synthesized by macrophages[15]. Increased levels of such biologically important proteins could thus be produced locally at the site of an inflammatory lesion with 'spill-over' into the plasma as a secondary phenomenon[16].

Table 23.1 Plasma protein profile in the acute phase response

Proteins	Increased	Decreased
Coagulation proteins	fibrinogen prothrombin factor VIII plasminogen	
Protease inhibitors	α_1-antitrypsin α_1-antichymotrypsin	inter-α-antitrypsin
Transport proteins	haptoglobin haemopexin caeruloplasmin	transferrin
Complement proteins	C1s, C1INH C2, factor B C3, C4, C5 C$\overline{56}$	properdin
Miscellaneous	C-reactive protein (CRP) α_1-acid glycoprotein Gc globulin cold-insoluble globulin serum amyloid A-related protein (SAA)	albumin prealbumin α_1-lipoprotein β-lipoprotein

The peak serum concentration of particular acute phase proteins may correlate with the extent of tissue damage or the intensity of stimulation, but not necessarily so; it may therefore be impossible to compare the effects of qualitatively different stimuli[3]. The precise profile of timing and relative levels of different proteins in the response to different stimuli or in different individuals have been examined in the past but without consistent result, and much of the early clinical work on CRP was with semi-quantitative assays. Although this yielded useful information, the application of precise, specific and sensitive immunochemical assay methods in sera from carefully clinically categorized individuals can be more valuable. This chapter will deal with the assay of C-reactive protein and related proteins in man and animals, and illustrate the role of such measurements in routine clinical management.

C-REACTIVE PROTEIN AND SERUM AMYLOID P-COMPONENT

C-reactive protein (CRP) and serum amyloid P-component (SAP) are closely related plasma proteins in man. They share about 60% homology of amino acid sequence[17, 18], have a similar molecular configuration[5, 17] and both show calcium-dependent ligand binding properties[19, 20]. The CRP molecule consists of five identical subunits non-covalently associated in a disc-like configuration with cyclic pentameric symmetry[17]. SAP is composed of two such pentameric discs interacting face-to-face[19]. In the presence of calcium ions CRP binds to free phosphoryl choline with an affinity constant of $1-2 \times 10^{-7}$ mol, a value comparable to that of many antigen–antibody interactions[21]. As a result of this affinity CRP binds to the many diverse molecules which contain phosphoryl choline residues, including phospholipids[22,23] and the so-called C-polysaccharides (or peptidopolysaccharides) of bacterial, fungal, parasite and plant origin[24,25]. CRP also reacts with polycations and polyanion–polycation complexes[26]. Once complexed with these ligands CRP activates the classical complement pathway as efficiently as IgG antibody[27].

SAP does not bind phosphoryl choline but in the presence of calcium it reacts with certain polysaccharides (agarose[19], other galactans[28], zymosan[29]), and with isolated amyloid fibrils[29]. SAP is not required for complement activation[30] but it is not known whether it can itself activate the complement system. SAP is also not a necessary procoagulant[31]. A protein which is immunochemically indistinguishable from circulating SAP is present in human vascular basement membrane, localized to the lamina rara interna of the glomerular basement membrane[32,33].

Knowledge of the calcium-dependent ligand binding properties of CRP and SAP has greatly facilitated their isolation from serum and other fluids by affinity chromatography techniques[19,20]. Using the same procedures as in man, proteins closely resembling human CRP and SAP have been isolated from a wide range of vertebrate species[5]. All have the pentameric disc configuration with one or two such discs in each molecule. In the marine teleost *Pleuronectes platessa* L. (the plaice) partial amino-terminal amino acid sequencing of CRP and SAP has formally established homology with human CRP and SAP[6].

ASSAY METHODS FOR CRP AND SAP

Availability of isolated CRP and SAP from man and other animals has permitted production of specific antisera for use in immunoassays and a variety of different techniques has been used. In addition CRP, by virtue of its binding to pneumococcal C-polysaccharide (CPS) has been assayed by precipitation with CPS[34] and by the capsular swelling reaction it causes when it reacts with whole intact CPS-bearing pneumococci[35]. Although used in much of the early clinical work on CRP[36,37] these methods are now only of historical interest. The semi-quantitative capillary tube immunoprecipitation assay using anti-CRP antiserum[38,39] is still in use, as are passive agglutination assays with anti-CRP-coated latex particles. However these techniques, by virtue of their relatively low sensitivity and non-quantitative results, yield less valuable information than the more modern precise immunochemical methods such as radial immunodiffusion and electroimmunoassay[40]. We routinely use the latter because of its superior sensitivity, excellent precision and reproducibility and greater speed than radial immunodiffusion. In addition various radiometric[41, 42] and fluorimetric[43] assays have been designed but are only necessary for measurement of CRP levels in normal sera when they are below 1 μg/ml, or in the mouse, for example[44], in which even acute phase CRP levels do not exceed 1–2 μg/ml.

A novel radiometric assay for CRP has recently been developed (de Beer, F. C., Shine, B., Forrest, G. C. and Pepys, M. B. unpublished observations), which utilizes the binding affinity of CRP for CPS. CPS is covalently coupled to a solid phase and CRP in serum is estimated by its competitive displacement of radioiodinated pure CRP tracer from the solid phase. This approach has the advantage that it measures 'functional' CRP, or at least CRP molecules with available binding sites. A discrepancy between results in this assay and measurements made of CRP as an antigen would suggest that some of the circulating CRP molecules are in complexed form and, whilst still reactive with anti-CRP, are not available to compete against labelled tracer for CPS. There is some preliminary evidence for the existence of such complexed CRP which may have pathogenetic significance in terms of complement activation and inflammatory activity.

BEHAVIOUR OF CRP AND SAP AS ACUTE PHASE REACTANTS IN DIFFERENT SPECIES

Acute phase proteins which cross-react immunochemically with human CRP and also have calcium-dependent binding specificity for CPS have been described in the rabbit, monkey, dog, mouse and chicken[44–51]. In the marine teleosts, the plaice (*Pleuronectes platessa* L.)[52] and the lumpsucker (*Cyclopterus lumpus* L.)[53], CRP is present in appreciable amounts in the sera of all the putatively normal fish and does not increase during inflammation. CRP has recently been isolated and characterized for the first time in rats and, even in specific pathogen-free animals, there are very high normal levels of CRP which increase only relatively modestly following acute phase stimuli[54]. SAP also shows considerable inter-species differences in terms of normal levels and acute phase behaviour (Table 23.2). For example, in man and the rat normal levels are about 20–60 μg/ml and change little after an acute stimulus, although in patients with chronic active inflammatory disease SAP levels do rise significantly[6, 54, 55]. In contrast mouse SAP is a major acute phase reactant, and furthermore different inbred strains of mice have marked differences in their normal SAP levels, in the ranges 1–10 μg/ml in C57Bl to 40–60 μg/ml in CBA and over 80 μg/ml in DBA/2 mice[56]. These differences between strains and species (Table 2) provide valuable experimental models

for investigation of the pathophysiology of the acute phase response in general
and the specific function of CRP and SAP in particular.

Table 23.2 Comparison of CRP and SAP levels in different species

	Normal	*Acute phase*
Human CRP	< 1 μg/ml	up to 500 μg/ml
Human SAP	20–50 μg/ml	no change with acute stimuli up to 90 μg/ml in chronic active disease
Mouse CRP	about 50 ng/ml	about 500 ng/ml
Mouse SAP	2–100 μg/ml in different strains	up to 600 μg/ml
Rat CRP	400–600 μg/ml	up to 900 μg/ml
Rat SAP	20–40 μg/ml	no change with acute stimuli
Plaice CRP*	40–60 μg/ml	fall by up to 30%
Plaice SAP*	180–250 μg/ml	fall by up to 50%

* Fletcher, T. C., White, A. and Pepys, M. B., unpublished observations

Table 23.3 Clinical applications of CRP assays

Infections
Post-operative
Septicaemia and bacterial meningitis in neonates and infants
Symptomatic urinary tract infection in childhood
Intercurrent infection in systemic lupus erythematosus
Intercurrent infection in leukaemia

Inflammatory/allergic/autoallergic disorders
Rheumatic fever
Rheumatoid arthritis
Still's disease
Ankylosing spondylitis
Psoriatic arthritis
Polymyalgia rheumatica
Systemic vasculitis
Crohn's disease
Ulcerative colitis
Familial Mediterranean fever

Miscellaneous
Thromboembolic disease
Threatened abortion
Malignant neoplasia

CLINICAL APPLICATIONS OF CRP ASSAYS

Although widely used in the past, testing for serum CRP fell out of favour in
clinical practice because the semi-quantitative results were non-specific and
often provided no information of significance for patient management. More

recently, however, it has been established that precise quantitative measurements can be useful and in some situations provide valuable information which would not otherwise be available.

Infections

Serum CRP levels increase rapidly in response to infection although they may reach higher levels in bacterial than in viral disease[3]. In patients after surgery or myocardial infarction failure of the CRP to return to normal following the rise initiated by the initial insult is a sensitive index of intercurrent infection, for example in the wound or the respiratory tract[57]. Secondary rises in CRP may also herald venous thromboembolic phenomena[57]. In neonates, including premature babies, and in infants elevation of the serum CRP caused by bacteraemia or septicaemia and bacterial meningitis is as sensitive an index as culture techniques in assessing response to chemotherapy or possible relapse after cessation of therapy[58, 59]. In children with symptomatic urinary tract infection, a raised CRP level is one of the best signs that the process involves the kidney and not just the lower outflow tract[60]. In some chronic inflammatory diseases, including systemic lupus erythematosus[61,62] and dermatomyositis[63], CRP levels are not greatly elevated in response to the disease process. In such conditions intercurrent microbial infections do, however, cause the CRP to rise and this provides a most important aid to differential diagnosis[61,62] (see below). In leukaemia, in which intercurrent infection is a common diagnostic and therapeutic problem, CRP levels are significantly higher in infected than in non-infected patients[64]. In all these situations the speed and ease with which results can be obtained enhances the value of this test.

Inflammatory and immunological disorders

In many inflammatory disorders of unknown aetiology, often with immunological abnormalities, the serum CRP concentration is raised when the disease process is active, and correlates well with the overall level of disease activity. For example, CRP measurements provide a useful objective index of disease activity and response to therapy in rheumatic fever[65], rheumatoid arthritis[66], Still's disease (Ansell, B. and Pepys, M. B., unpublished observations), psoriatic arthritis (Hughes, G. R. V. and Pepys, M. B., unpublished observations), ankylosing spondylitis[67], polymyalgia rheumatica, many forms of systemic vasculitis (Peters, D. K., Pusey, C. and Pepys, M. B., unpublished observations), familial Mediterranean fever[68] and Crohn's disease[69,70]. In these disorders the assay of CRP is superior to the assay of other acute phase proteins which have been tested because its normal level is lower, its incremental range is greater and the rate at which the concentration rises and falls in response to – respectively – increased or diminished disease activity is more rapid. It is also more useful as a prospective measurement than the erythrocyte sedimentation rate because it responds more promptly and precisely in most situations, is less affected by other variables such as haematocrit and feeding, and it covers an extended incremental range. CRP measurements have particular value in the clinical management of Crohn's disease in which the affected organ may be relatively inaccessible for examination and objective assessment is difficult[70]. For example, in seriously ill patients, in whom the choice of treatment may lie between persisting with medical measures or resorting to surgery, an objective criterion of day-to-day progress, such as is provided by the serum CRP level, may be invaluable. Another application is in the conduct of therapeutic trials in which objective assessment of response is essential.

In marked contrast there are certain inflammatory conditions in which the CRP response is relatively modest even in patients with severe active disease. For example in both ulcerative colitis[69, 70] and systemic lupus erythematosus (SLE)[61, 62] the serum CRP is usually only slightly increased above normal. Although it tends to be higher in groups of patients with active rather than inactive disease[62] there are frequent individual exceptions. Measurement of serum CRP is thus of little use in monitoring these disorders but it may have differential diagnostic value between Crohn's disease and ulcerative colitis[69, 70] and between SLE and rheumatoid arthritis[71] respectively. A further application of CRP measurements is in the differential diagnosis of pyrexia in SLE, which usually lies between an exacerbation of the underlying disease and an intercurrent microbial infection, especially in patients on immunosuppressive and anti-inflammatory therapy. SLE patients with documented microbial infection – bacterial, fungal or viral – have significantly higher CRP levels than patients with active SLE alone[61, 62]. Patients with active lupus and no infection often have no significant elevation of CRP despite having high fever, leukocytosis and sedimentation rate greater than 100 mm in the first hour. Although this has been disputed by one group of workers[72], a careful analysis of their own results reveals that they conform closely with those of other groups in showing that the great majority of patients with SLE have only modest levels of CRP and that markedly elevated CRP levels in the absence of infection are very rare. They may occur, particularly, in our experience, when the disease is manifest as a fulminating systemic vasculitis with multi-organ involvement, but it is always essential to exclude infection, by thorough culture studies (for viruses and fungi as well as bacteria) and repeated serological tests, before ascribing the CRP response to SLE alone.

Miscellaneous

Raised CRP levels are much more commonly seen in patients with malignant neoplasms than in those with benign tumours[73] and in Hodgkin's disease, for example, there is a good positive correlation between the serum CRP concentration and the extent and secondary effects of the tumour[55, 74]. Precise prospective correlative studies of CRP in malignancy have not yet been conducted, although in both man and animals CRP (or SAP respectively) have been mistakenly identified as specific tumour markers. There are, however, some grounds for supposing that CRP measurements might be useful under certain circumstances in suggesting metastatic disease or in the early detection or prediction of relapse following apparently successful primary therapy.

The CRP level may help to distinguish between those patients with threatened abortion who will miscarry and those in whom the pregnancy is retained[75].

CONCLUSIONS

The acute phase response to injury is a general phenomenon among homoeothermic animals and the CRP/SAP family of plasma proteins, which are such characteristic acute phase reactants, have been conserved throughout vertebrate evolution. They probably have important biological functions and their isolation, characterization and assay in various animal species will facilitate elucidation of the mechanisms and significance of the acute phase response in general as well as their specific functions. In the practice of clinical medicine precise immunoassay of serum CRP provides valuable information in a variety of different settings:

(1) as a screening test, since raised CRP is unequivocal evidence of organic disease;
(2) as an objective index of disease activity and response to therapy in those disorders in which CRP becomes markedly elevated;
(3) as a sign of microbial infection, particularly when the usual clinical indicators are obscured by an intercurrent disease or standard investigative methods are technically difficult.

With more general awareness and rapid availability of results, serum CRP measurement should find a place as a routine procedure in the screening, investigation and management of a wide range of conditions.

References

1. Koj, J. (1974). Acute phase reactants. In Allison, A. C. (ed.) *Structure and Function of Plasma Proteins*, pp. 73–125. (London: Plenum Press)
2. Gordon, A. H. (1976). The acute phase plasma proteins. In Bianchi, R., Mariani, G. and MacFarlane, A. S. (eds.). *Plasma Protein Turnover*, pp. 381–94. (London: Macmillan)
3. Kindmark, C.O. (1976). Sequential changes in plasma proteins in various acute diseases. In

Bianchi, R., Mariani, G. and MacFarlane, A. S. (eds.) *Plasma Protein Turnover*, pp. 395–402. (London: Macmillan)

4. Pepys, M. B. (1979). Acute phase phenomena. In Cohen, A. S. (ed.) *The Science and Practice of Clinical Medicine: Rheumatology and Immunology*, pp. 85–8. (New York: Grune & Stratton)

5. Pepys, M. B., Dash, A. C., Fletcher, T. C., Richardson, N., Munn, E. A. and Feinstein, A. (1978). Analogues in other mammals and in fish of human plasma proteins, C-reactive protein and amyloid P-component. *Nature (London)*, **273**, 168

6. Pepys, M. B., Baltz, M. L., Dyck, R. F., de Beer, F. C., Evans, D. J., Feinstein, A., Milstein, C. P., Munn, E. A., Richardson, N., March, J., Fletcher, T. C., Davies, A. J. S., Gomer, K., Cohen, A. S., Skinner, M. and Klaus, G. G. B. (1980). Studies of serum amyloid P-component (SAP) in man and animals. In Glenner, G. G., Pinho e Costa, P. and de Freitas, F. (eds.). *Amyloid and Amyloidosis*, pp. 373–383. (Amsterdam: Excerpta Medica)

7. Parish, W. E. (1976). Studies in vasculitis. VII. C-reactive protein as a substance perpetuating chronic vasculitis. Occurrence in lesions and concentrations in sera. *Clin. Allergy*, **6**, 543

8. Parish, W. E. (1977). Features of human spontaneous vasculitis reproduced experimentally in animals. Effects of antiglobulins, C-reactive protein and fibrin. In *Bayer-Symposium VI, Experimental Models of Chronic Inflammatory Diseases*, pp. 117–51. (Berlin: Springer-Verlag)

9. Hurlimann, J., Thorbecke, G. and Hochwald, G. (1966). The liver as the site of C-reactive protein formation. *J. Exp. Med.*, **123**, 365

10. Kushner, I. and Feldmann, G. (1978). Control of the acute phase response. Demonstration of C-reactive protein synthesis and secretion by hepatocytes during acute inflammation in the rabbit. *J. Exp. Med.*, **148**, 466

11. Darcy, D. A. (1968). Liver cell fractions which stimulate increase of an acute phase protein in the rat. *Br. J. Exp. Pathol.*, **49**, 614

12. Darcy, D. A. (1968). Polymorphonuclear cell fractions which stimulate increase of an acute phase protein in the rat. *Br. J. Exp. Pathol.*, **49**, 525

13. Wannemacher, R. W., Jr., Pekarek, R. S., Thompson, W. L., Curnow, R. T., Beall, F. A., Zenser, T. V., De Rubertis, F. R. and Beisel, W. R. (1975). A protein from poly-morphonuclear leukocytes (LEM) which affects the rate of hepatic amino acid transport and synthesis of acute-phase globulins. *Endocrinology*, **96**, 651

14. Merriman, C. R., Pullian, L. A. and Kampschmidt, R. F. (1975). Effect of leukocytic endogenous mediator on C-reactive protein in rabbits. *Proc. Soc. Exp. Biol. Med.*, **149**, 782

15. Colten, H. R. and Einstein, L. P. (1976). Complement metabolism: cellular and humoral regulation. *Transplant. Rev.*, **32**, 3

16. Pepys, M. B., Baltz, M. L., Musallam, R. and Doenhoff, M. J. (1980). Serum protein concentrations during *Schistosoma mansoni* infection in intact and T-cell deprived mice. I. The acute phase proteins, C3 and serum amyloid P-component (SAP). *Immunology*, **39**, 249

17. Osmand, A. P., Friedenson, B., Gewurz, H., Painter, R. H., Hofmann, T. and Shelton, E. (1977). Characterization of C-reactive protein and the complement subcomponent C1t as homologous proteins displaying cyclic pentameric symmetry (pentraxins), *Proc. Natl. Acad. Sci. USA*, **74**, 739

18. Skinner, M., Pepys, M. B., Cohen, A. S., Keller, L. M. and Lian, J. B. (1980). Studies of amyloid protein AP. In Glenner, G. G., Pinho e Costa, P. and de Freitas, F. (eds.). *Amyloid and Amyloidosis*, pp. 384–391. (Amsterdam: Excerpta Medica)

19. Pepys, M. B., Dash, A. C., Munn, E. A., Feinstein, A., Skinner, M., Cohen, A. S., Gewurz, H., Osmand, A. P. and Painter, R. H. (1977). Isolation of amyloid P-component (protein AP) from normal serum as a calcium-dependent binding protein. *Lancet*, **1**, 1029

20. Pepys, M. B., Dash, A. C. and Ashley, J. (1977). Isolation of C-reactive protein by affinity chromatography. *Clin. Exp. Immunol.*, **30**, 32

21. Anderson, J. K., Stroud, R. M. and Volanakis, J. E. (1978). Studies of the binding specificity

of human C-reactive protein for phosphoryl choline. *Fed. Proc.*, **37**, 1495

22. Hokama, Y., Tam, R., Hirano, W. and Kumura, L. (1974). Significance of C-reactive protein binding by lecithin; a simplified procedure for CRP isolation. *Clin. Chim. Acta*, **50**, 53

23. Kaplan, M. H. and Volanakis, J. E. (1974). Interaction of C-reactive protein complexes with the complement system. I. Consumption of human complement associated with the reaction of C-reactive protein with pneumococcal C-polysaccharide and with the choline phosphatides, lecithin and sphingomyelin. *J. Immunol.*, **112**, 2135

24. Pepys, J. and Longbottom, J. L. (1971). C-substance activities of related glycopeptides from fungal, parasitic and vegetable sources. *Int. Arch. Allergy Appl. Immunol.*, **41**, 219

25. Baldo, B. A., Fletcher, T. C. and Pepys, J. (1977). Isolation of peptido-polysaccharide from the dermatophyte *Epidermophyton floccosum* and a study of its reaction with human C-reactive protein and a mouse anti-phosphoryl choline myeloma serum. *Immunology*, **32**, 831

26. Claus, D. R., Siegel, J., Petras, K., Skor, D., Osmand, A. P. and Gewurz, H. (1977). Complement activation of interaction of polyanions and polycations. III. Complement activation by interaction of multiple polyanions and polycations in the presence of C-reactive protein. *J. Immunol.*, **118**, 83

27. Claus, D. R., Siegel, J., Petras, K., Osmand, A. P. and Gewurz, H. (1977). Interactions of C-reactive protein with the first component of human complement. *J. Immunol.*, **119**, 187

28. Uhlenbruck, G., Karduck, D., Haupt, M. and Schwick, H. G. (1979). C-reactive protein (CRP), $9.5S\alpha_1$ glycoprotein and C1q: serum proteins with lectin properties. *Z. Immunol. Forsch.*, **155**, 262

29. Pepys, M. B., Dyck, G. F., de Beer, F. C., Skinner, M. and Cohen, A. S. (1979). Binding or serum amyloid P-component (SAP) by amyloid fibrils. *Clin. Exp. Immunol.*, **38**, 284

30. Painter, R. H. (1977). Evidence that C1t (amyloid P-component) is not a subcomponent of the first component of complement (C1). *J. Immunol.*, **119**, 2203

31. Pepys, M. B., Becker, G. J., Dyck, R. F., McCraw, A., Hilgard, P., Merton, R. E. and Thomas, D. P. (1980). Studies of human serum amyloid P-component (SAP) in relation to coagulation. *Clin. Chim. Acta*, **105**, 83

32. Dyck, R. F., Kershaw, M., McHugh, N. and Pepys, M. B. (1980). Immunohistochemical staining of normal, and pathological human tissues with antibody to serum amyloid P-component (SAP). In Glenner, G. G., Pinho e Costa, P. and de Freitas, F. (eds.). *Amyloid and Amyloidosis*, pp. 50–54. (Amsterdam: Excerpta Medica)

33. Dyck, R. F., Kershaw, H., McHugh, N., Lockwood, C. M., Duance, V. Baltz, M. L. and Pepys, M. B. (1980). Amyloid P-component is a constituent of normal human glomerular basement membrane. *J. Exp. Med.* (In press)

34. Tillet, W. S. and Francis, T. (1930). Serological reactions in pneumonia with a non-protein somatic fraction of pneumococcus. *J. Exp. Med.*, **52**, 561

35. Löfström, G. (1944). Comparison between the reactions of acute phase serum with pneumococcus C-polysaccharide and with pneumococcus type 27. *Br. J. Exp. Pathol.*, **25**, 21

36. Hedlund, P. (1947). The appearance of acute phase protein in various diseases. *Acta Med. Scand.*, **128**, (Suppl. 196). 579

37. Hedlund, P. (1961). Clinical and experimental studies on C-reactive protein (acute phase protein). *Acta Med. Scand.*, **169** (Suppl. 361), 1

38. Roantree, R. J. and Rantz, L. A. (1955). Clinical experience with the C-reactive protein test. *Arch. Intern. Med.*, **96**, 674

39. Yocum, R. S. and Doerner, A. A. (1957). A clinical evaluation of the C-reactive protein test. *Arch. Intern. Med.*, **99**, 74

40. Kindmark, C. O. (1969). Quantitative measurement of C-reactive protein in serum. *Clin. Chim. Acta*, **26**, 95

41. Kindmark, C. O. and Thorell, J. I. (1972). Quantitative determination of individual serum proteins by radio-electroimmuno assay and use of ^{125}I-labelled antibodies (application to C-reactive protein). *Scand. J. Clin. Lab. Invest.*, **29** (Suppl. 124), 49

42. Claus, D. R., Osmand, A. P. and Gewurz, H. (1976). Radioimmunoassay of human C-reactive protein and levels in normal sera. *J. Lab. Clin. Med.*, **87**, 120

43. Siboo, R. and Kulisek, E. (1978). A fluorescent immunoassay for quantification of C-reactive protein. *J. Immunol. Methods*, **23**, 59

44. Pepys, M. B. (1979). Isolation of serum amyloid P-component (protein SAP) in the mouse. *Immunology*, **37**, 637

45. Löfström, G. (1947). Acute phase protein in rabbits. I. The capacity of pneumococcus strains which react with antipneumococcus type 16 serum to cause non-specific capsular swelling with acute phase serum from rabbits. *Acta Med. Scand.* (Suppl. 196), 575

46. Anderson, H. D. and McCarthy, M. (1951). The occurrence in the rabbit of an acute phase protein analogous to human C-reactive protein. *J. Exp. Med.*, **93**, 25

47. Gotschlich, E. and Stetson, C. A. (1960). Immunologic cross-reactions among mammalian acute phase proteins. *J. Exp. Med.*, **111**, 441

48. Patterson, L. T. and Mora, E. C. (1964). Occurrence of a substance analogous to C-reactive protein in the blood of the domestic fowl. *Texas Rep. Biol. Med.*, **22**, 716

49. Dillman, R. C. and Coles, E. H. (1966). A canine serum fraction analogous to human C-reactive protein. *Am. J. Vet. Res.*, **27**, 1769

50. Riley, R. F. and Coleman, M. K. (1970). Isolation of C-reactive proteins of man, monkey, rabbit and dog by affinity chromatography on phosphorylated cellulose. *Clin. Chim. Acta*, **30**, 483

51. Bodmer, B. and Siboo, R. (1977). Isolation of mouse C-reactive protein from liver and serum. *J. Immunol.*, **118**, 1086

52. Baldo, B. A. and Fletcher, T. C. (1973). C-reactive protein-like precipitins in plaice. *Nature (London)*, **246**, 145

53. Fletcher, T. C., White, A. and Baldo, B. (1977). C-reactive protein-like precipitin and lysozyme in the lumpsucker *Cyclopterus lumpus* L. during the breeding season. *Comp. Biochem. Physiol.*, **57B**, 353

54. de Beer, F. C., Baltz, M. L., Munn, E. A., Feinstein, A. and Pepys, M. B. (1980). Isolation and characterisation of C-reactive protein (CRP) and serum amyloid P-component (SAP) in the rat. (Submitted for publication)

55. Pepys, M. B., Dash, A. C., Markham, R. E., Thomas, H. C., Williams, B. D. and Petrie, A. (1977). Comparative clinical study of protein SAP amyloid P-component and C-reactive protein in serum. *Clin. Exp. Immunol.*, **32**, 119

56. Pepys, M. B., Baltz, M. L., Gomer, K., Davies, A. J. S. and Doenhoff, M. (1979). Serum amyloid P-component is an acute phase reactant in the mouse. *Nature (London)*, **278**, 259

57. Fischer, C. L., Gill, C., Forrester, M. G. and Nakamura, R. (1976). Quantitation of 'acute-phase proteins' postoperatively. *Am. J. Clin. Pathol.*, **66**, 840

58. Sabel, K. G. and Hanson, L. A. (1974). The clinical usefulness of C-reactive protein (CRP) determinations in bacterial meningitis and septicemia in infancy. *Acta Paediatr. Scand.*, **63**, 381

59. Sabel, K. G. and Wadsworth, Ch. (1979). C-reactive protein (CRP) in early diagnosis of neonatal septicaemia. *Acta Paediatr. Scand.*, **68**, 825

60. Jodal, U., Lindberg, U. and Lincoln, K. (1975). Level diagnosis of symptomatic urinary tract infections in childhood. *Acta Paediatr. Scand.*, **64**, 201

61. Honig, S., Gorevic, P. and Weissmann, G. (1977). C-reactive protein in systemic lupus erythematosus. *Arthritis Rheum.*, **20**, 1065

62. Becker, G. J., Waldburger, M., Hughes, G. R. V. and Pepys, M. B. (1980). Value of serum C-reactive protein measurement in the investigation of fever in systemic lupus erythematosus. *Ann. Rheum. Dis.*, **39**, 50

63. Haas, R. H., Dyck, R. F., Pepys, M. B. and Dubowitz, V. (1980). C-reactive protein in childhood dermatomyositis. (Submitted for publication)

64. Mackie, P. H., Crockson, R. A. and Stuart, J. (1979). C-reactive protein for rapid diagnosis of

infection in leukaemia. *J. Clin. Pathol.*, **32**, 1253

65. Anderson, H. C. and McCarthy, M. (1950). Determination of C-reactive protein in the blood as a measure of the activity of the disease process in acute rheumatic fever. *Am. J. Med.*, **8**, 445

66. Amos, R. S., Constable, T. J., Crockson, R. A., Crockson, A. P. and McConkey, B. (1977). Rheumatoid arthritis. Relation of serum C-reactive protein and erythrocyte sedimentation rates to radiographic changes. *Br. Med. J.*, **1**, 195

67. Cowling, P., Ebringer, R., Cawdell, D., Ishii, M. and Ebringer, A. (1980). C-reactive protein, ESR and *Klebsiella* in ankylosing spondylitis. *Ann. Rheum. Dis.*, **39**, 45

68. Frensdorff, A., Shibolet, S., Lamprecht, S. and Sohar, E. (1964). Plasma proteins in familial Mediterranean fever. *Clin. Chim. Acta*, **10**, 106

69. Pepys, M. B., Druguet, M., Klauss, H. J., Dash, A. C., Mirjah, D. D. and Petrie, A. (1977). Immunological studies in inflammatory bowel disease. In Porter, R. R. and Knight, J. (eds.) *Immunology of the Gut: Ciba Foundation Symposium 46* (new series), pp. 283–304. (Amsterdam: Elsevier/Excerpta Medica/North Holland)

70. Fagan, E. A., Dyck, R. F., Hodgson, H. J. F., Chadwick, V. S. and Pepys, M. B. (1980). Serum levels of C-reactive protein in Crohn's disease and ulcerative colitis. (Submitted for publication)

71. Pereira da Silva, J. A., Elkon, K. B., Hughes, G. R. V., Dyck, R. F. and Pepys, M. B. (1980). C-reactive protein levels in systemic lupus erythematosus; a classification criterion? *Arthritis Rheum.*, **23**, 770

72. Zein, N., Ganuza, C. and Kushner, I. (1979). Significance of serum C-reactive protein elevation in patients with systemic lupus erythematosus. *Arthritis Rheum.*, **22**, 7

73. Baruah, B. D. and Gogoi, B. C. (1975). C-reactive protein in malignant tumours. *Ind. J. Cancer*, **12**, 39

74. Wood, H. F., Diamond, H. D., Craver, L. F., Pader, E. and Elster, S. K. (1958). Determination of C-reactive protein in blood of patients with Hodgkin's disease. *Ann. Intern. Med.*, **48**, 823

75. Jones, W. R. (1970). Serum C-reactive protein in pregnancy, labour and the puerperium. *Aust. N.Z. J. Obstet. Gynaecol.*, **10**, 221

24
Rapid Virus Diagnosis

P. S. GARDNER

Rapid virus diagnosis means a diagnosis during the acute stage of the illness when the diagnosis within 2–3 h of admission may influence the management of the patient. This will usually mean detection of antigen in the patient or possibly the detection of specific IgM in his blood[1].

The techniques in use for rapid virus diagnosis are many and depend on three factors:

(1) The site of lesion in which the virus is to be detected and its accessibility.

(2) The concentration of virus at that site; for example, hepatitis is relatively easy to diagnose by use of serum as there are masses of hepatitis B surface antigen present in the blood and various techniques are suitable for its detection. On the other hand, though many other viruses have a viraemic phase, such as measles, rubella, cytomegalovirus, the chances of detecting these agents in the bloodstream by a test is almost nil because their concentration is well below the threshold of normal methods of detectability. In the respiratory tract the problems are different: if antigen can be visualized in shed respiratory tract cells by immunofluorescence then, with a smaller concentration of virus, a specific diagnosis can be made even with a single positive cell. There is probably too little antigen to be detectable by other rapid diagnostic techniques[2]. One of the most fruitful sites of all for diagnosing virus infections is the faeces. Concentrations of virus here may run to titres as high as 10^{10} on occasions, and the detectable level by electronmicroscopy in good hands can be about 10^6. Because of this high concentration, a large number of tests can be used for the detection of rotaviruses in faeces[3]. Another site loaded with heavy virus concentration is skin warts.

(3) The expertise of the virologist and the equipment available in the department.

The various techniques which are available, and which will be the subject of this chapter, are illustrated in Table 24.1. They are all, except electronmicroscopy (EM), based on the use of antisera, but radioimmunoassay

Table 24.1   Techniques

(1) Electronmicrosopy (EM) and immunoelectronmicroscopy (IEM)
(2) Fluorescent antibody techniques (FAT)
(3) Enzyme-linked immunoassays (ELISA)
(4) Radioimmunoassays (RIA)
(5) Solid-phase aggregation of coupled erythrocytes (SPACE)

(RIA), the fluorescent antibody technique (FAT), solid-phase aggregation of coupled erythrocytes (SPACE) and enzyme-linked immunoassay (ELISA) all have the same principal of being dependent on an antigen–antibody reaction on a solid phase. The main difference in these techniques is that the detecting system in each has been altered. RIA has a large essential part to play in diagnostic virology; it has an enormous sensitivity but has been used mainly for detection of hepatitis antigen in situations where it is vital that all potential carriers of the antigen are found; for example, in the screening of blood transfusion donors. Its other main use has been for the detection of various viral antibodies and except when specific IgM is sought, cannot be considered as rapid diagnosis. Therefore its uses will be covered elsewhere in this volume. Figure 24.1 compares the three solid-phase techniques with which this paper is

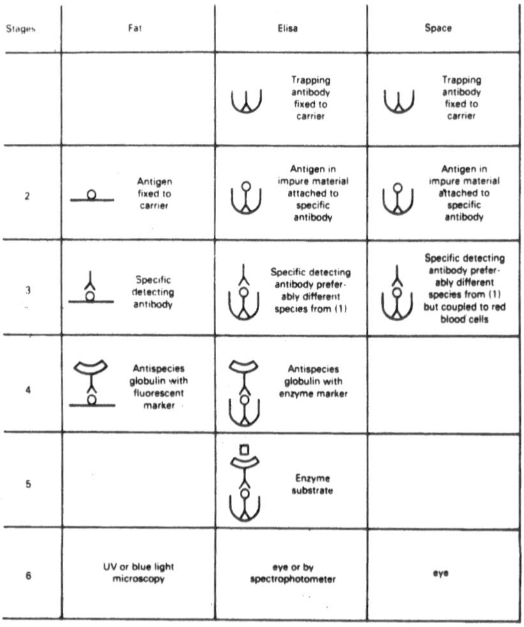

Figure 24.1   Solid-phase techniques compared

mainly concerned. SPACE[3] and ELISA[4] depend on a capture antibody in order to semi-purify the virus usually from dirty material, such as faeces. FAT does not require this stage as one is actually seeing the antigen. All three techniques need a carrier system and all three depend on the trapped antigen reacting with a highly specific antibody; in the case of SPACE the specific antibody and the detecting system, the red blood cell, are combined. In the other two systems conjugated antispecies antibodies are required; the enzyme system requires the additional stage of a substrate. Figure 24.1 has been designed to illustrate the indirect technique in both FAT and ELISA. Although there is no reason why a direct test cannot be used in these two systems (that is labelling the detecting specific antiserum) the indirect test is to be encouraged because in diagnostic work many viral agents are sought at the same time, and it would be impractical and uneconomic to label all the detecting antisera. This would not only be laborious but greatly decrease the titres of valuable specific antisera and also commit their use to one system only. This means that only one common reagent needs to be labelled, provided that a single species has been used for the production of the antisera.

Again outside the terms of reference of this chapter is the question of the quality of the reagents used, and therefore the assumption will be made that all reagents which are being used have been not only standardized and found to be of good potency, but have also been tested against clinical material to make sure they are of good quality and of specific reaction. All these tests depend on the highest quality of the reagents; therefore the need for effective quality control cannot be emphasized too much.

Table 24.2 lists the sites from which viruses in clinical material may be

Table 24.2 Clinical materials used for rapid virus diagnosis

(1) Secretions of the respiratory tract
(2) Skin scraping or skin biopsy
(3) Eye scrapings
(4) Central nervous system
(5) Faeces
(6) Post-mortem and biopsy material
(7) Urine

obtained for rapid virus diagnosis, and each of the sites in turn will be examined, with discussion as to which is the most effective method of diagnosing the viral cause of the lesion. The methods used for detecting respiratory viruses are FAT and possibly ELISA. There is no doubt that the method of choice at present is FAT. For reasons already given, other techniques are not sensitive enough to detect the small amount of antigen present, and it is only seeing the occasional presence of antigen within intact cells that makes this technique as sensitive as the time-consuming isolation of the virus on tissue culture. The immunofluorescence in cells shed from the respiratory tract should show the following characteristics for a specific diagnosis to be made: the fluorescence must be intracellular; the colour should be apple green if fluorescein is in the labelled conjugate; the virus should show the typical pattern that is normally associated with it; and it should be in cells in which one is accustomed to seeing the virus. RSV in respiratory tract cells from a child with bronchiolitis would show virus in ciliated cells, the distribution being cytoplasmic with particulate fluorescence as well as large inclusion bodies. In contrast, in influenza A, the intracellular fluorescence would be mainly intranuclear but still in ciliated cells[2]. (If in any of these examples the fluorescence had been in squamous cells then one would have had grave doubts about the diagnosis.)

There is no point in recommending a technique unless it has been carefully evaluated against the most sensitive current techniques used, and in the case of respiratory syncytial virus a careful comparison with standard isolation procedures has been made (Table 24.3). Of the last 618 isolations only seven

Table 24.3 Comparison of results by two techniques (immunofluorescence and virus isolation) for respiratory syncytial virus, influenza A and parainfluenza viruses types 1, 2 and 3

Virus	Virus isolated		Virus not isolated		Co-positivity (%)	Co-negativity (%)	Overall agreement (%)
	FA+	FA−	FA+	FA−			
Respiratory syncytial virus	611	7	41	1387	98.9	97.1	97.7
Influenza A	274	10	17	2261	96.5	99.3	98.9
Parainfluenza type 1	120	10	11	4918	92.3	99.8	99.6
Parainfluenza type 2	57	3	11	1554	95.0	99.3	99.1
Parainfluenza type 3	211	11	34	5508	95.1	99.4	99.2

were not diagnosed on admission by FAT. These seven cases were entirely due to poor preparation with insufficient material and cells in the secretions. There were 41 secretions which showed positive fluorescence in shed cells from which respiratory syncytial virus was not isolated. It must be asked whether the fluorescence was real or was it non-specific? All 41 had a history of illness of more than 5 days; some as long as 14 days, and the fluorescent appearance of all the shed cells was dull and hazy. It has now been proved conclusively, by using a double-staining technique which stained virus and antibody with different colours, that these infected cells were coated with specific antibody produced by the patient. This led to difficulty in culturing the virus *in vitro*, but in real life this is probably a factor which leads to loss of infectivity of the patient and also assists in his recovery[5].

Similar surveys with similar results have been obtained with influenza A diagnosed by immunofluorescence on cells shed by the respiratory tract and also for the parainfluenza viruses (Table 24.3).

McIntosh in the United States has used ELISA with secretions, to diagnose RS virus infection. He has reported that he obtained 23 positive results out of 29 specimens from which the virus was isolated. He also obtained one positive among 35 culture negative specimens[6]. This work has yet to be confirmed. It is the author's opinion that it is unlikely that there would be sufficient antigen there to be detected in this way and that it is probable that fluorescence will prove, for some time to come, the most reliable and sensitive technique.

The techniques which may be used to detect viruses, particularly those causing lesions of the skin and also in the conjunctivae, are EM and FAT. ELISA may prove successful where much antigen is present but is as yet untested. EM comes into its own here as the method of choice in rapidly diagnosing (and differentiation by morphology) the viruses in the lesion of a possible pox infection from that of a herpes virus. Skin scrapings and conjunctival scrapings too can be diagnosed by immunofluorescence[7]. Skin lesions tend to crust, and once this has occurred it is more difficult to diagnose specific skin lesions from non-specific staining, except with long experience. If one could confine oneself to the examination of the earlier vesicular lesions there would be no problems, as these show little or no non-specific staining (Table 24.4). In contrast to skin, Table 24.5 demonstrates that the conjunctival

Table 24.4 Correlation of immunofluorescence and virus isolation with scrapings of skin lesions

$FA+$ isolation$+$	$FA+$ isolation$-$	$FA-$ isolation$-$	$FA-$ isolation$+$
55	3	97	7

Table 24.5 Relationship of isolation of herpesvirus to direct fluorescent antibody (FA) technique (conjunctival specimens)

$FA+$ isolation$+$	$FA+$ isolation$-$	$FA-$ isolation$-$	$FA-$ isolation$+$	Total
45	10	72	0	127

scrapings present no non-specific problems because the amount of material is limited, the majority of the scraping is used for FAT, and the little left on the scalpel blade may be too small for isolation of virus.

The two main tests which can be used on brain biopsy material are EM and FAT. The diagnosis does not depend solely on the ability of the virologist or the technique employed, but also on the skill of the surgeon who must put his needle into the correct site. If either of these techniques fails to show a positive biopsy, material can be cultured which, after a few hours on sensitive cells – e.g. human diploid cells – can be shown to contain the presence of the growing virus by FAT. In viral emergency situations such as the diagnosis of herpes encephalitis when antiviral therapy can influence the course of the illness, one is often tempted to attempt a diagnosis by staining cells in the cerebrospinal fluid by FAT. Though this has been described by many workers its success as a technique, despite these claims, remains unproven. White cells are notoriously bad for producing non-specific staining, and many of the so-called successes reported have been non-specific reactions. Viruses have rarely been isolated from the cerebrospinal fluid to support these claims. Other workers have put very high concentrations of herpes virus into the cerebrospinal fluid of rabbits and have had difficulty in detecting positive cells there[8].

Many techniques, e.g. EM, IEM, ELISA, SPACE, FAT, can be success-fully employed for the detection of rotavirus in faeces, mainly because of their abundance there. EM is an efficient technique in the diagnosis of human and animal rotaviruses, though cannot be used on a large scale. Diagnosis is usually by straight observation – not by IEM, which takes a little longer although it does increase the sensitivity of the technique. All the methods that have been listed for use in rotavirus detection are approximately of equal sensitivity, i.e. ELISA, FAT, SPACE and EM.

FAT can be used for diagnosis of a rotavirus infection[9]. Human rotaviruses cannot be propagated in tissue culture but if a 10% suspension of faeces is placed on to a continuous monkey-kidney cell line such as LLCMK2 and grown overnight, the first abortive cycle of the virus can be stained the next day.

At the moment the smaller viruses which occur in faeces, such as astroviruses and the non-cultivated adenoviruses, are best detected by EM. These techniques should be applicable to the other faecal viruses causing diarrhoea, and in due course should achieve success.

Rapid virus techniques can be used to investigate post-mortem material and are invaluable in assessing the amount of virus present and also the cause of death[10]. Virus infectivity rapidly declines in post-mortem material but antigen can be still detected and FAT has an important role to play. Sudden deaths, especially in infants, can be caused by a number of viruses, often RS virus, where little virus appears sufficient to produce this fatal result. Sudden deaths are always reported to the coroner and a rapid virus diagnosis can rapidly clear suspicion and help to relieve the anguish of bereaved parents.

Urine will not be emphasized because looking for a virus in urine is like looking for the proverbial 'needle in a haystack'. Cytomegalovirus is relatively easy to grow from urine but extremely difficult to diagnose rapidly in the cells of urine deposits; probably the best method is FAT, but even that has a low success rate.

Finally, immunosuppression often allows a large amount of virus to grow in patients of an older age group than one is accustomed to finding it[11]. Measles giant cells occur in the secretions of normal children up to about the third day, but in leukaemia examples of much longer excretion can be found; as long as 21 days has been recorded, with a rash lasting as long. Respiratory syncytial virus may also show long excretion under these conditions. In a child of 4, with a very severe bronchitis which lasted eventually for 60-odd days, this was found to be caused by RS virus not normally seen producing illness of this severity in this age group. However in leukaemia and other immunosuppressed conditions local antibody is not found coating the infected cells and this may be why the virus goes on being excreted.

The précis of the potential immunological methods that can be used in rapid virus diagnosis must leave all unsatisfied because of what still needs to be achieved. Rapid virus diagnosis could be self-destructive by pricing itself out of routine use and certainly for use in developing countries. RIA needs expensive labelling material, reagents are unstable and expensive counting apparatus is required. ELISA is better in this respect, the reagents being more stable; but for large-scale use the reagents are relatively expensive and one also needs reading apparatus. With FAT, one needs expensive microscopes, expensive reagents and with all these techniques, as well as SPACE, one needs a high standard of purity of reagents which must add to the cost. New and more effective methods of antisera production are needed and techniques need to be made as simple as possible which is an exciting thought to leave you with. Professor Coombs advocates the increased use of red cells as markers and the question must therefore be asked whether relatively simple techniques, shown to be sufficiently sensitive for antigen detection in various clinical material, can be developed further for routine work. We could be returning to unsophisticated cheap methods of universal applicability where even the relatively unsophisticated laboratories of developing countries could make use of them.

References

1. Gardner, P. S. (1977). Rapid virus diagnosis. *J. Gen. Virol.*, **36**, 1
2. Gardner, P. S. and McQuillin, J. (1978). In *Rapid Virus Diagnosis, Application of Immunofluorescence*, 2nd Edn. (London: Butterworth)
3. Bradbourne, A. F., Almeida, J. D., Gardner, P. S., Moosai, R. B., Nash, A. A. and Coombs, R. R. A. (1979). A solid phase system (SPACE) for the detection and quantitation of rotavirus in faeces. *J. Gen. Virol.*, **44**, 615
4. Yolken, R. H., Barbour, B., Wyatt, R. G., Kalica, A. R., Kapikian, A. Z. and Chanock, R. M. (1978). Enzyme-linked immunosorbent assay for identification of rotaviruses from different animal species. *Science*, **201**, 259
5. Gardner, P. S. and McQuillin, J. (1978). The coating of RS virus infected cells in the respiratory tract by immunoglobulins. *J. Med. Virol.*, **2**, 77
6. McIntosh, K., Chao, R. and Fishaut, J. M. (1978). An enzyme-linked immunosorbent assay (ELISA) for detection of RS virus in nasal secretions. Abstracts of the IVth International Congress. *Int. Virol.*, **4**, 634

7. Gardner, P. S., McQuillin. J., Black, M. M. and Richardson, J. (1968). Rapid diagnosis of Herpesvirus hominus infections in superficial lesions by immunofluorescent antibody techniques. *Br. Med. J.*, **4**, 89

8. Grumbach, K., Baringer, R. J. and Klassen, T. (1977). Herpes simplex antigen in rabbit CSF. *Lancet*, **1**, 149

9. Moosai, R. B., Gardner, P. S., Almeida, J. D. and Greenaway, M. A. (1979). A simple immunofluorescent technique for the detection of human rotavirus. *J. Med. Virol.*, **3**, No. 3, 189

10. Downham, M. A. P. S., Gardner, P. S., McQuillin, J. and Ferris, J. A. J. (1975). The role of respiratory viruses in childhood mortality. *Br. Med. J.*, **1**, 235

11. Craft, A. W., Reid, M. M., Gardner, P. S., Jackson, E., Kernahan, J., McQuillin, J., Noble, T. C. and Walker, W. (1979). Virus infections in children with acute lymphoblastic leukaemia. *Arch. Dis. Childh.*, **54**, 755

25
Viral Hepatitis with special Reference to Hepatitis B

A. J. ZUCKERMAN

INTRODUCTION

Viral hepatitis has emerged as a major public health problem occurring endemically in all parts of the world. The general term viral hepatitis refers to infections caused by at least three different viruses, hepatitis A (infectious or epidemic hepatitis), hepatitis B (serum hepatitis) and the more recently identified form of hepatitis, non-A, non-B hepatitis which is most probably caused by more than one virus.

Acute viral hepatitis is a generalized or systemic infection with particular emphasis on inflammation of the liver. The clinical picture of the infection ranges in its presentation from inapparent or subclinical infection, slight malaise, mild gastrointestinal symptoms and the anicteric form of the disease, acute icteric illness, severe prolonged jaundice to acute fulminant hepatitis. The incidence of individual symptoms and signs varies, therefore, both in different outbreaks and in sporadic cases. In addition, hepatitis B and non-A, non-B hepatitis may progress to chronic liver disease, which may be severe, and there is substantial evidence of a close association between hepatitis B virus and primary liver cancer.

Hepatitis A and hepatitis B can now be differentiated by specific laboratory tests for antigens and antibodies associated with these infections[1,2]. Laboratory tests for non-A, non-B hepatitis are under development. This chapter reviews the more sensitive immunoassays which are available for hepatitis type B.

HEPATITIS B

Serological markers of infection

Infection with hepatitis B virus leads to the appearance in the plasma during the incubation period of a specific antigen, hepatitis B surface antigen (originally referred to as Australia antigen) some 2–8 weeks before bio-chemical evidence of liver damage or the onset of jaundice. The antigen persists during the acute illness and it is usually cleared from the circulation during convalescence. Next to appear in the circulation is DNA polymerase associated with the core or nucleocapsid of the virus and *e* antigen, again preceding serum aminotransferase elevations. The *e* antigen is a distinct soluble antigen which is specifically associated with hepatitis B and is located within the core of the virus particle. Antibody to the core is found in the serum 2–4 weeks after the appearance of the surface antigen and is usually detectable during the early phase of the illness persisting after recovery. The next antibody to appear in the circulation is directed against the *e* antigen. Antibody to the surface antigen component is the last to appear, late during convalescence. More recently, precipitating antibodies reacting with specificities on the complete virus particle have been described[3]. These antibodies may be relevant to the clearance of circulating hepatitis B virions and the termination of acute infection, and their absence in all but one of the patients with chronic active hepatitis examined might explain why the infection persists in such patients. In addition to the complex serological events which take place during the course of uncomplicated infection, cell-mediated immune responses to hepatitis B antigens have been described[4].

The serological markers (Table 25.1), which can now be detected by

Table 25.1 Simplified guide for the interpretation of serological markers of hepatitis B

Surface antigen	e antigen	Anti-e	DNA polymerase	Core antibody	Surface antibody	Clinical interpretation
+	+	−	+	−	−	incubation period or early acute hepatitis
+	+	−	+	+	−	(1) acute hepatitis B (2) persistent carrier state
−	−	+	−	+	+	convalescence from acute hepatitis B
+	−	+	−	+	−	persistent carrier state
−	−	−	−	+	+	past infection
−	−	−	−	+	−	infection with hepatitis B virus without detectable (excess) surface antigen
−	−	−	−	−	+	immunization without infection; repeated exposure to surface antigen without infection

Reproduced with permission from the *British Medical Journal* (1979), **2**, 84

sensitive techniques such as radioimmunoassay (RIA) and enzyme immunoassay, have proved extremely useful for unravelling the epidemiology of hepatitis B, established the global dissemination and public health importance of this infection, led to the routine screening of blood donors for the surface antigen and resulted in remarkable advances in the knowledge of the virology and pathogenesis of hepatitis B and its associated chronic liver disorders.

A carrier state of hepatitis B virus, which may be lifelong, becomes established in some patients. Such a carrier state may be associated with liver damage ranging from minor changes in the nucleus of the hepatocyte to chronic active hepatitis and cirrhosis. A number of factors have been identified which increase the risk of developing the carrier state. The carrier state is commoner in males, more likely to follow infection acquired in childhood and more likely to occur in patients with natural or acquired immune deficiencies[5]. Seroepidemiological surveys reveal that there is a large reservoir of persistent carriers of hepatitis B virus in the world estimated to number more than 176 million. The carrier state is characterized serologically by persistence of hepatitis B surface antigen and absence of free surface antibody. Core antibody is present often in high titre and there are reports that core antibody of the IgM class remains detectable. In some carriers hepatitis B DNA polymerase activity remains elevated, not infrequently fluctuating in titre, and e antigen persists, whereas in others hepatitis B DNA polymerase is not detectable and anti-e is found. Hepatitis B e antigen has been reported to be commoner in young than in adult carriers, while the prevalence of anti-e appears to increase with age.

Hepatitis B virus

There is substantial evidence that the 42 nm particle is the hepatitis B virus. The core has a subunit structure organized according to the principles of icosahedral symmetry and has an endogenous core antigen-associated DNA-dependent DNA polymerase in close association with a DNA template. Double-stranded DNA has been isolated from circulating virus particles and also from cores extracted from the nuclei of infected hepatocytes. The DNA consists of circular nucleic acid molecules with a mean contour length of 0.79 ± 0.09 μm, with a molecular weight of about 2.3×10^6. The DNA has been characterized by gel electrophoresis and restriction enzyme cleavage as approximately 3600 nucleotides in length containing a single-stranded gap of 600–2100 nucleotides. The endogenous DNA polymerase reaction appears to repair the gap, but the relevance of the gapped circular DNA to the mode of replication of the virus is not clear.

Hepatitis B surface antigen carries a common group determinant, termed a, and a number of major subdeterminants, d, y, w and r in various combinations, which are coded by the virus genome. The major subtypes have differing geographical distribution. For example, in northern Europe, the

Americas and Australia subtype *adw* predominates. Subtype *ayw* occurs in a broad zone which includes northern and western Africa, the eastern Mediterranean, eastern Europe, northern and central Asia and the Indian subcontinent. Both *adw* and *adr* are found in Malaysia, Thailand, Indonesia and Papua New Guinea, while the *adr* subtype predominates in other parts of south-east Asia including China, Japan and the Pacific.

Laboratory tests for hepatitis B surface antigen and antibody

Many laboratory methods of varying sensitivity and specificity are now available for detecting the surface antigen and its antibody[2, 5-7]. The two-dimensional micro-Ouchterlony immunodiffusion test, which was the first method employed, allows direct comparisons to be made between precipitin lines and is the simplest technique for detecting the surface antigen and the surface antibody, but it is also the least sensitive. Somewhat more sensitive techniques include counterimmunoelectrophoresis, rheophoresis, complement-fixation, passive haemagglutination inhibition (for antigen), and immunofluorescence microscopy. Greater sensitivity for detection of antigen has been achieved by reverse passive haemagglutination, immune adherence haemagglutination, reverse passive latex agglutination and immunoelectron-microscopy. The technique of passive haemagglutination for the assay of surface antibody is sensitive. The most sensitive methods for detection of surface antigen and surface antibody are RIAs, including solid-phase RIA, and radioimmunoprecipitation. More recently enzyme-linked immunosor-bent assay (ELISA or enzyme assay) has been adapted for detection of surface antigen and surface antibody. This technique has been shown to have a sensitivity similar to that of RIA. Reactions obtained with the highly sensitive techniques must be confirmed as specific by means of neutralization or blocking with unlabelled surface antibody or surface antigen as appropriate.

Passive haemagglutination and haemagglutination-inhibition

Red cells coated with purified antigen, using chromic chloride as a coupling agent, are agglutinated by very small amounts of antibody, and the results may be read within 2 h. This technique of passive haemagglutination is very sensitive, being as much as 10 000 times more sensitive than the immunodiffu-sion technique. However, the precipitation of suitable antigen-coated red cells with chromic chloride is difficult, and different batches of cells vary considerably in their sensitivity. Non-specific agglutination is frequently found with low dilutions of sera and control erythrocytes must be used. Non-specific agglutinins can be absorbed with control erythrocytes before retesting and by heat inactivation. False-negative results may be obtained with low dilutions of high titre antibody because of the formation of prozones and sera should, therefore, be tested at several dilutions.

Inhibition of haemagglutination by sera under test as a result of neutralization by known antibody preparations may be used for the detection of the surface antigen. The sensitivity of haemagglutination-inhibition is about the same as complement-fixation.

Human blood group O, Rh-negative erythrocytes have been tanned and sensitized with purified hepatitis B surface antigen. The sensitized cells were used for the detection of antigen by two-stage haemagglutination-inhibition, and the technique has been reported to be very sensitive. A direct haemagglutination test was applied for the detection of hepatitis B surface antibody and the order of sensitivity, based on titration, was high.

Surface antigen has also been purified by adsorption to and elution from glass particles. The antigen was subsequently stabilized with dextran and adsorbed to the surface of freshly washed erythrocytes. The test can be modified for antigen detection by inhibition or by coating red cells with surface antibody.

Reverse passive haemagglutination (RPHA)

RPHA for detection of hepatitis B surface antigen was first described in 1969 using purified surface antibody attached to formalin-fixed erythrocytes. Since then red cells of various species have been coated by several techniques with purified surface antibody of human or animal origin and used for the detection of surface antigen. This method, which has the obvious attraction of simplicity and rapidity, does not attain the sensitivity of RIA or ELISA, although increase in sensitivity has recently been described[8].

A number of non-specific false-positive results on screening are inherent in the method due to species-specific red cell agglutinins. Confirmatory tests are therefore required and appropriate reagents are available. RPHA has generally been considered to be a practical compromise between the highly sensitive but technically more complex RIA and ELISA and other simple but less sensitive techniques.

Radioimmunoassay (RIA)

RIA, which combines the specificity of antigen–antibody reaction with the sensitivity of radioisotope detection, has provided extremely sensitive assays for the minute amounts of many of the peptide hormones present in plasma. All RIA techniques depend upon the quantitation of non-antibody-bound antigen, non-antigen-bound antibody or the extent of antigen–antibody reaction. The most frequently used procedure has been the introduction of an isotope of iodine, ^{131}I or ^{125}I, into the tyrosine residues of the peptides. Iodination with ^{125}I is more convenient because of its longer half-life and lower energy radiation, with consequent increased ease of handling.

The various RIA procedures differ mainly according to the method of separation. The aim of separation is to resolve a reaction mixture into two portions containing free and bound reactants respectively at the end of the incubation period. Numerous techniques of separation are now available based on the ability of paper, charcoal, talc and so on to adsorb small amounts of antigens more readily than the larger antibody molecules. Some methods utilize the size, charge and differences in solubility between antigen and antibody, and there are also methods in which the antibody is fixed to sephadex or to polystyrene by chemical or physical bonding.

The first RIA technique for the detection of hepatitis B surface antigen and antibody by the use of the surface antigen labelled with ^{125}I was described in 1970. An RIA adaptation of a double-antibody precipitation method to a microtitre system for detecting the surface antibody was described subsequently. This technique combines specificity with high sensitivity, and furthermore the procedure is relatively easy and rapid. The method can also be used for assaying the antigen by the competitive blocking of the reaction of ^{125}I-labelled antigen and antibody by the addition of unlabelled antigen. A two-step direct, non-competitive radioimmune technique[9] uses polypropylene tubes or polystyrene beads coated with hepatitis B surface antibody raised in animals and specific hepatitis B immunoglobulin labelled with [125]I. The sandwich-type RIA technique has also been adapted for subtyping of the surface antigen using subtype-specific antisera. The technique has also been adapted for the detection of surface antibody by coating the solid phase with surface antigen. Radiolabelled antigen is used for the assay of bound antibody.

An important development has been the use of the protein A of *Staphylococcus aureus* for the separation of bound antigen from free antigen. Radioimmunocompetition is used for testing. Antibody is measured by direct binding of radiolabelled hepatitis B surface antigen. The principle of the technique is as follows: protein A combines specifically with the Fc part of IgG, types 1, 2 and 4, which in normal sera comprises more than 90% of the total IgG. The reaction between protein A and the combining site on the IgG molecule is very rapid and there seems to be no difference in the combining properties to protein A between free and antigen-bound IgG. Radiolabelled antigen which reacted with its specific antibody develops, after attachment to protein A fixed to the staphylococcus, into a solid phase which is readily precipitated by light centrifugation. The pellet can be counted directly without washing, once the supernatant containing the unbound radiolabelled antigen has been removed. The sensitivity for detection of the antigen is similar to that of the sandwich-type RIA technique, and the sensitivity for measurement of antibody is at least that of passive haemagglutination[10].

A number of other RIA procedures have also been described, including micro-solid-phase techniques and double-antibody methods. All these methods differ primarily in the technique of separation of the antigen–antibody complex and the placing of the label on purified antigen or purified antibody. The purity of the labelled preparation is, of course, the essential component of the specificity of the technique.

Enzyme immunoassay

The use of radioisotopes for labelling reactants in immunoassays obviated the need for monospecific antisera, enhanced sensitivity and permitted the assay of haptens as well as proteins. Enzyme labelling provides a feasible alternative to RIA and such assays provide objective results and are extremely sensitive[11]. Although the amplification made possible by the use of enzymes to attain sensitivity will also magnify any error, advantages include the availability and relative cheapness of many enzymes and of manual and automated systems for their assay, the long shelf life of the labelled reagent, and the lack of hazards during labelling and subsequent handling of the reagents. The potential of ELISA was also discussed by Kato et al.[12] in which the point was made that while RIA is routinely used to measure femtomole (10^{-15} mol) amounts of hormones, ELISA has been used to detect 30 attomoles (1 attomole $= 10^{-18}$ mol) of ornithine aminotransferase.

The assay for hepatitis B surface antigen is based on a non-competitive solid-phase procedure using disposable polystyrene microhaemagglutination plates containing sheep (or other species) antibody to the surface antigen immobilized on the inner surface of each well. Bound antigen is subsequently detected by a further reaction with the γ-globulin fraction of purified hepatitis B surface antibody conjugated with horseradish peroxidase. The presence of the bound antigen is detected after the addition of a colourless enzyme substrate as a result of hydrolysis by the enzyme yielding a coloured reaction product which is visible to the naked eye or can be read with a spectrophotometer[13]. Various laboratories have reported that ELISA and RIA for hepatitis B surface antigen have a similar order of sensitivity and specificity[14-18]. Specific confirmation of positive reactions is based on in-situ blocking by surface antigen bound to the solid-phase antibody. A technique for detection of surface antibody has also been described[19,20]. The subject has been reviewed by Waart et al.[21], outlining the techniques for detection of hepatitis B surface antigen and antibody, e antigen and anti-e and hepatitis A virus and its antibody.

Laboratory tests for hepatitis B core antigen and antibody

Hepatitis B core antibody is a useful and consistent marker of infection with hepatitis B virus, and persisting high titres suggest continuing viral replication, although this antibody remains detectable long after the cessation of viral replication. Various techniques are available for demonstrating core antibody ranging from immunofluorescence to RIA. Core antibody may be found in serum in the absence of other markers of hepatitis B virus, and the possibility that under some circumstances blood from such individuals may contain infective virus in the absence of excess production of surface antigen is under investigation. Reference has been made to the possible value of the assay of IgM core antibody. Free core antigen has not been detected in the circulation.

Fluorescent antibody techniques and thin-section EM demonstrate clearly the core antigen in the nuclei of hepatocytes. Core antibody is readily shown in the serum by indirect immunofluorescence using as a substrate, cryostat sections of liver obtained at autopsy from patients with hepatocytes containing a large number of core antigen particles. This technique is widely used. Immune adherence haemagglutination for the assay of core antibody is used in some countries[2].

A micro-solid-phase RIA technique for the detection of core antigen and core antibody was described several years ago. The wells of polyvinyl microtitre plates formed the solid phase to which was adsorbed a diluted human convalescent serum to hepatitis B. Core antigen was prepared by the treatment of circulating hepatitis B virus particles with Nonidet P40, a nonionic detergent found previously to be more efficient than Tween 80 for complete removal of the outer surface antigen envelope. The detection of core antibody by its ability to inhibit the binding of radiolabelled core antibody to core antigen provided a means of measuring this antibody in sera with concomitant surface antibody.

The direct radiolabelling of core antigen by activation of the endogenous DNA polymerase activity offers an alternative radioimmune procedure.

A radioimmune precipitation technique has also been described whereby antigen–antibody complexes were separated from unbound labelled antigen by precipitation with antiglobulin. A similar procedure utilizing staphylococcal protein A for the removal of immune complexes has shown that a chimpanzee serum at a dilution of 1 : 500 000 was found to precipitate 50% of added core antigen in comparison to a titre of 1 : 256–1 : 1024 obtained by complement-fixation. For optimal sensitivity radiolabelled core antigen is separated from both unlabelled core antigen and incompletely disrupted virus particles by equilibrium centrifugation in caesium chloride. It is often necessary to adjust the amount of radiolabelled core antigen used when different batches of antigen are employed as the specific activity of each preparation varied according to the source of plasma.

Another technique[22] utilizes core antigen obtained from the sera of persistent carriers of hepatitis B virus by centrifugation and treatment with Nonidet P40 and 2-mercaptoethanol. The separated core is labelled with ^{125}I and employed in a RIA procedure of high sensitivity for the detection of core antibody. Vyas and Roberts[23] described a technique for the detection of core antigen and core antibody whereby the core antigen isolated from complete virus particles in plasma of a carrier and the autologous IgG labelled with ^{125}I can be used in a solid-phase RIA. The inherent advantages of this technique also include the use of empty cores, autologous core antibody and cores as reagents virtually eliminating non-specific reactions. The inhibition of binding of cores to the solid phase obviates the need for neutralization tests. Foreseeable developments for the detection of core antibody include ELISA and methods for the measurement of core antibody of the IgM class.

Tests for detection of hepatitis B *e* antigen and anti-*e*

The presence of *e* antigen in the serum appears to correlate with the replication of hepatitis B virus in the host. There is a highly significant correlation between *e* antigen, DNA polymerase activity and circulating complete virus particles and therefore infectivity. Anti-*e*, on the other hand, signifies reduced or relatively low infectivity, but virus production has been reported in the presence of antibody to *e* antigen in some carriers[24, 25].

Several serological methods are now available for detection of *e* antigen and its antibody. In order of increasing sensitivity these include immunodiffusion, rheophoresis, immune adherence haemagglutination, passive haemagglutination and more recently ELISA and solid-phase RIA[7, 20, 26].

Hepatitis B virion (Dane particle) antibody

Alberti *et al.*[3] labelled the complete hepatitis B virus with [³H]thymidine using the endogenous DNA polymerase. After incubation with the serum under test, antibody-coated virus was precipitated by anti-immunoglobulin and the loss of radioactivity from the supernatant was measured. The antibody reacting with specificities on the complete virion did not correlate with anti-*e*, although it was considered possible that only one of the various determinants of *e* antigen was involved. This precipitating antibody appeared to be relevant to the clearance of circulating hepatitis B virus and the termination of acute infection, and the absence of this antibody in all but one of the patients with chronic active hepatitis might explain why the infection persists in such patients. Further studies are in progress.

The delta antigen–antibody system

During the examination by immunofluorescence of liver biopsies of patients with hepatitis B surface antigenaemia, it was observed that a serum containing core antibody stained core antigen, demonstrable by EM, and also nuclei which did not contain core antigen particles[27]. It was found that some anti-core sera reacted with either one or other liver substrates associated with hepatitis B virus infection. The reacting antigen is distinct from the surface antigen, the core antigen and *e* antigen and was named the delta antigen. Delta antigen was detected by direct immunofluorescence in the liver cell nuclei of patients with chronic liver disease associated with hepatitis B infection. The delta and core antigen determinants in the hepatocyte nuclei appear to be mutually exclusive. Delta antibodies may be present or absent in sera containing core antibody. Delta antibody is found in the serum of persistent carriers of the surface antigen, with a higher prevalence in patients with liver damage. An immunofluorescence blocking test allows the detection of anti-delta in serum by specific inhibition of the fluorescence produced by delta antisera conjugated with fluorescein. More recently delta antibody has been detected by a microtitre solid-phase blocking RIA[28]. The nature of delta antigen and the significance of its association with chronic hepatitis B surface antigen liver disease are unknown.

NON-A, NON-B HEPATITIS

The specific laboratory diagnosis of hepatitis A and hepatitis B has revealed a previously unrecognized form of hepatitis which is clearly unrelated to either type and which is referred to as non-A, non-B hepatitis. It is now the most common form of hepatitis occurring after blood transfusion and the infusion of certain plasma derivatives in some areas of the world[5]. The infection has also been transmitted experimentally to chimpanzees. Although specific laboratory tests for identifying this new type of hepatitis are not available, and the diagnosis can only be made by exclusion, there is considerable information about the epidemiology of this infection. Non-A, non-B hepatitis has been found in every country in which it has been sought, and it has a number of features in common with hepatitis B. This form of hepatitis has been most commonly recognized as a complication of blood transfusion[29], and in countries where all blood donations are screened for hepatitis B surface antigen by very sensitive techniques non-A, non-B hepatitis may account for up to 90% of all cases of post-transfusion hepatitis. Outbreaks of non-A, non-B hepatitis have also been reported after the administration of blood clotting Factors VIII[30,31] and IX[32]. Non-A, non-B hepatitis has occurred in haemodialysis[33] and other specialized units[34] and among drug addicts[35]. In several countries a significant number of cases are not associated with transfusion and such sporadic cases of non-A, non-B hepatitis have been found to account for 10–20% of all adult patients with recognized viral hepatitis. In general, the illness is mild and often subclinical or anicteric. However, there is evidence that the infection may be followed by prolonged viraemia and the development of a persistent carrier state. Several recent studies of the histopathological sequelae[36] of acute non-A, non-B infection indicate that chronic hepatitis may occur in as many as 40–50% of the patients.

Clinical, epidemiological and experimental studies in a number of laboratories suggest that non-A, non-B hepatitis may be caused by two or more infectious agents. Clinical evidence is based on the observation of multiple attacks of hepatitis in individual patients. Epidemiologically, short-incubation and long-incubation forms of non-A, non-B hepatitis have been described, although it is possible that differences in the incubation period represent differences in the infective dose. Experimental evidence for the existence of at least two distinct non-A, non-B hepatitis viruses has been obtained from recent cross-challenge transmission studies in chimpanzees[31, 37]. The initial finding of two different types of ultrastructural cytoplasmic and nuclear changes in the hepatocytes of infected chimpanzees appear to represent different phases of structural changes and are not mutually exclusive[38].

Serological procedures for antigens and antibodies which are specifically associated with this recently recognized form of viral hepatitis are being sought.

Acknowledgments

The work on hepatitis in progress at the London School of Hygiene and Tropical Medicine is generously supported by grants from the Medical Research Council, the Department of Health and Social Security, the Wellcome Trust and the World Health Organization.

References

1. Zuckerman, A. J. (1979). Specific serological diagnosis of viral hepatitis. *Br. Med. J.*, **2**, 84
2. Zuckerman, A. J. and Howard, C. R. (1979). *Hepatitis Viruses of Man.* (London and New York: Academic Press)
3. Alberti, A., Diana, S., Scullard, G. H., Eddleston, A. L. W. F. and Williams, R. (1978). Detection of a new antibody system reacting with Dane particles in hepatitis B virus infection. *Br. Med. J.*, **2**, 1056
4. Lee, W. M., Reed, W. D., Osman, C. G., Vahrman, J., Zuckerman, A. J., Eddleston, A. L. W. F. and Williams, R. (1977). Immune responses to hepatitis B surface antigen and liver specific lipoprotein in acute type B hepatitis. *Gut*, **18**, 250
5. World Health Organization (1977). *Advances in Viral Hepatitis.* Report of the WHO Expert Committee on Viral Hepatitis. *Techn. Rep. Ser.*, No. 602 (Geneva)
6. Zuckerman, A. J. (1975) *Human Viral Hepatitis*, 2nd Edn. (Amsterdam: North-Holland/American Elsevier)
7. *Diagnostic Methods in Viral Hepatitis* (1978). Proceedings of a Symposium held in London, January 1978, organized by the European Group for Rapid Virus Diagnosis. *J. Med. Virol.*, **3**, 1
8. Barbara, J. A. J., Harrison, P. J., Howell, D. R., Briggs, M. and Cameron, C. H. (1979). A sensitive single reverse passive haemagglutination test for detecting both HBsAg and anti-HBs. *J. Clin. Pathol.*, **32**, 1180
9. Ling, C. M. and Overby, L. R. (1972). Prevalence of hepatitis B virus antigen as revealed by direct radioimmune assay with ^{125}I-antibody. *J. Immunol.*, **109**, 834
10. Figenschau, K. J. and Ulstrup. J. C. (1974). Staphylococcal radioimmunoassay for hepatitis B antigen and antibody. *Acta Pathol. Microbiol. Scand.*, **82**, 422
11. Landon, J. (1977). Enzymeimmunoassay: techniques and uses. *Nature (London)*, **268**, 483
12. Kato, K., Hamaguchi, Y., Okawa, S., Ishikawa, E., Kobayashi, K. and Katunuma, N. (1977). Enzyme immunoassay in rapid progress. *Lancet*, **1**, 40
13. Wolters, G., Kuijpers, L., Kacaki, J. and Schuurs, A. (1976). Solid-phase enzyme

immunoassay for detection of hepatitis B surface antigen. *J. Clin. Pathol.*, **29**, 873

14. Ukkonen, P., Koistinen, V. and Penttinen, K. (1977). Enzyme immunoassay in the detection of hepatitis B surface antigen. *J. Immunol. Methods*, **15**, 343

15. Kacaki, J., Wolters, G., Kuijpers, L. and Stulemeyer, S. (1978). Results of a multicentre clinical trial of the solid-phase enzyme immunoassay for hepatitis B surface antigen. *Vox Sang.*, **35**, 65

16. Vandervelde, E. M., Cohen, B. J. and Cossart, Y. E. (1977). An enzyme linked immunosorbent assay test for hepatitis B surface antigen. *J. Clin. Pathol.*, **30**, 714

17. Babes, V. T. and Aderca, I. (1978). HBsAg detection by micro-ELISA. *Rev. Roum. Med. Virol.*, **29**, 161

18. Crovari, P., Rivano, R., Bennicelli, C., Zanacchi, P. and de Flora, S. (1978). Comparative study of an enzyme immunoassay and of a radioimmunoassay for the detection of hepatitis B surface antigen. *Boll. Ist. Sieroter. Milan*, **57**, 434

19. Spano, C., Patti, S. and Palazzo, U. (1978). Detection of anti-HBs antibody by means of an indirect micro-ELISA method. *Bull. WHO*, **56**, 653

20. Wolters, G., Kuijpers, L. and Schuurs, A. (1979). Detection of human antibodies to hepatitis B surface antigen (HBsAg) by an enzyme immunoassay for HBsAg. *J. Clin. Pathol.*, **32**, 1264

21. Waart, M. v. d., Swelting, A., Cichy, J., Wolters, G. and Schuurs, A. (1978). Enzyme immunoassay in the diagnosis of hepatitis with emphasis on the detection of 'e' antigen (HBeAg). *J. Med. Virol.*, **3**, 43

22. Howard, C. R. and Zuckerman, A. J. (1977). Core antigen and circulating anti-core antibody in hepatitis B infection. *J. Immunol. Methods*, **14**, 391

23. Vyas, G. N. and Roberts, I. M. (1977). Radioimmunoassay of hepatitis B core antigen and antibody with autologous reagents. *Vox Sang.*, **33**, 369

24. Howard, C. R., Zanetti, A. R., Thal, S. and Zuckerman, A. J. (1978). Viral antigens and antibodies in hepatitis B infection. *J. Clin. Pathol.*, **31**, 681

25. Howard, C. R. and Zuckerman, A. J. (1979). The separation and analysis of hepatitis B *e* antigen. *J. Med. Virol.*, **4**, 303

26. Bonino, F., Recchia, S., Ponzetto, A., Filippone, B., Palla, M., Zanetti, A. R. and Ferroni, P. (1980). A solid-phase enzyme immunoassay (EIA) for detection of HBeAg and anti-HBe. *J. Immunol. Methods*, **33**, 195

27. Rizzetto, M., Canese, M. G., Arico, S., Crivelli, O., Trepo, C., Bonino, F. and Verme, G. (1977). Immunofluorescence detection of a new antigen–antibody system (δ/anti-δ) associated with the hepatitis B virus in the liver and in the serum of HBsAg carriers. *Gut*, **18**, 997

28. Rizzetto, M., Shih, J. W.-K., Gocke, D. J., Purcell, R. H., Verme, G. and Gerin, J. L. (1979). Incidence and significance of antibodies to delta antigen in hepatitis B virus infection. *Lancet*, **2**, 986

29. Tabor, E. and Gerety, R. J. (1979). Non-A, non-B hepatitis: new findings and prospects for prevention. *Transfusion*, **19**, 669

30. Bradley, D. W., Cook, E. H., Maynard, J. E., McCaustland, K. A., Ebert, J. W., Dolana, G. H., Petzel, R. A., Kantor, R. J., Heilbrunn, A., Fields, H. A. and Murphy, B. L. (1979). Experimental infection of chimpanzees with antihemophilic (Factor VIII) materials: recovery of virus-like particles associated with non-A, non-B hepatitis. *J. Med. Virol.*, **3**, 253

31. Tsiquaye, K. N. and Zuckerman, A. J. (1979). New human hepatitis virus. *Lancet*, **1**, 1135

32. Wyke, R. J., Tsiquaye, K. N., Thornton, A., White, Y., Portmann, B., Das, P. K., Zuckerman, A. J. and Williams, R. (1979). Transmission of non-A, non-B hepatitis to chimpanzees by factor IX concentrates after fatal complications in patients with chronic liver disease. *Lancet*, **1**, 520

33. Galbraith, R. M., Dienstag, J. L., Purcell, R. H., Gower, R. H., Zuckerman, A. J. and Williams, R. (1979). Non-A, non-B hepatitis associated with chronic liver disease in a haemodialysis unit. *Lancet*, **1**, 951

34. Meyers, J. D., Dienstag, J. L., Purcell, R. H., Thomas, E. D. and Holmes, K. K. (1977).

Parenterally transmitted non-A, non-B hepatitis. An epidemic reassessed. *Ann. Intern. Med.*, **87**, 57

35. Mosley, J. W., Redeker, A. G., Feinstone, S. M. and Purcell, R. H. (1977). Multiple hepatitis viruses in multiple attacks of acute viral hepatitis. *N. Engl. J. Med.*, **296**, 75

36. Berman, M., Alter, H. J., Ishak, K. G., Purcell, R. H. and Jones, E. A. (1979). The chronic sequelae of non-A, non-B hepatitis. *Ann. Intern. Med.*, **91**, 1

37. Tsiquaye, K. N., Bird, R. G., Tovey, G., Wyke, R. J., Williams, R. and Zuckerman, A. J. (1980). Further evidence of cellular changes associated with non-A, non-B hepatitis. *J. Med. Virol.*, **5**, 63

38. Tsiquaye, K. N., Amini, S., Kessler, H., Bird, R. G., Tovey, G. and Zuckerman, A. J. (1980). Ultrastructural changes in the liver in experimental non-A, non-B hepatitis. (Submitted for publication)

26
Immunoassays for Hepatitis A

L. R. MATHIESEN

INTRODUCTION

Immunoassay for hepatitis A is a field where the development has been very rapid during the last 7 years and today test methods for hepatitis A are among the best for a rapid diagnosis in viral diseases. This is despite the fact that hepatitis A virus (HAV) until recently could not be cultured *in vitro*[1].

Development began in the late 1960s with a demonstration of the marmoset monkey as a susceptible animal for hepatitis A infection[2]. It was thus possible to measure HAV by infectivity studies, and a neutralization test was also developed for detection of antibody to HAV (anti-HAV)[3] but the practical application of these tests was very limited.

IMMUNOELECTRONMICROSCOPY

The first immunoassay for hepatitis A became available in 1973 when Feinstone *et al.*[4] reported the discovery by immunoelectronmicroscopy (IEM) of HAV in stool collected during the acute phase of experimental hepatitis A infection. Mixing a 2% suspension of an acute phase stool with dilution of a convalescent serum they were able to precipitate and, with the electronmicroscope, visualize complexes of 27 nm particles coated with antibody.

Presence of anti-HAV in serum can be tested using a known positive stool sample, and presence of HAV in stool using a known anti-HAV-positive serum. The amount of anti-HAV can be measured semi-quantitatively on a scale of 0–4+, and rises in anti-HAV levels can be detected during hepatitis A infection.

The IEM technique is very specific and sensitive for detection of both HAV and anti-HAV and has been widely accepted as a basic reference technique[5-8]. The test is, however, quite cumbersome, requires special equipment and also takes considerable expertise before reliable results can be obtained.

COMPLEMENT-FIXATION AND IMMUNE ADHERENCE HAEMAGGLUTINATION ASSAYS

Much more convenient for detection of anti-HAV are the complement-fixation assay (CF) and the immune adherence haemagglutination assay (IAHA) developed by Provost et al.[9] and Miller et al. in 1975[10].

IAHA proved to be superior to CF for detection of anti-HAV due to its greater sensitivity and because sera taken during acute hepatitis are frequently anti-complementary. Both assays utilize HAV from livers of marmosets infected with HAV but marmosets are now an endangered species and are no longer generally available as a laboratory animal. To resolve this problem Moritsugu et al.[11] purified HAV from human stool collected during the acute phase of hepatitis A infection. By combining gradient and zonal centrifugation it was possible to purify HAV to an extent that it gave only specific reaction in IAHA.

The IAHA is a very easy test to perform once the antigen has been purified. It is based on the observation that antigen–antibody–complement complexes can bind to complement C3 receptors on erythrocytes, thereby forming a haemagglutination pattern easily visible in a microtitre plate.

This principle is widely used in Japan for detection of hepatitis B surface antigen (HBsAg)[12] and has a sensitivity comparable with other third-generation assays.

Normally a buffer control is incorporated in the test but as there is no means of using blocking experiments the specificity for anti-HAV depends entirely on the purification of the antigen utilized in the test; specific detection of HAV in stool suspensions is not possible because monospecific anti-HAV is not available.

With purified HAV the test is easy to perform and it is now possible to perform large serological surveys for anti-HAV in different populations around the world[13, 14]. Development of anti-HAV as detected by IAHA is delayed 2–6 weeks as compared with IEM, solid-phase radioimmunoassay (SPRIA) and enzyme-linked immunosorbent assay (ELISA) where anti-HAV can be demonstrated from the onset of acute illness during hepatitis A infection (Figure 27.9)[11, 15-19]. This has the practical advantages that seroconversion for anti-HAV can be demonstrated by IAHA during hepatitis A infection; using IEM, SPRIA and ELISA it can be difficult to show a fourfold titre rise because the anti-HAV titre by these methods can be fairly high within a few days of onset of acute illness. A negative result for anti-HAV by IAHA, combined with a positive result by one of the other methods in an acute phase serum, is presumptive evidence for acute hepatitis A infection[18-23].

SOLID-PHASE RADIOIMMUNOASSAY

Shortly after IAHA was described, Purcell *et al.*[24] and Hollinger *et al.*[25] simultaneously described a SPRIA for detection of HAV based on the principle used in similar tests for HBsAg[26] and hepatitis B core antigen (HBcAg)[27]. The test is performed in microtitre plates precoated with human serum containing anti-HAV. The material to be tested is added, and if HAV is present it is adsorbed to the anti-HAV-treated plates. After washing, radiolabelled IgG prepared from human anti-HAV serum is added and binding of radioactivity discloses the presence of HAV (Figure 26.1).

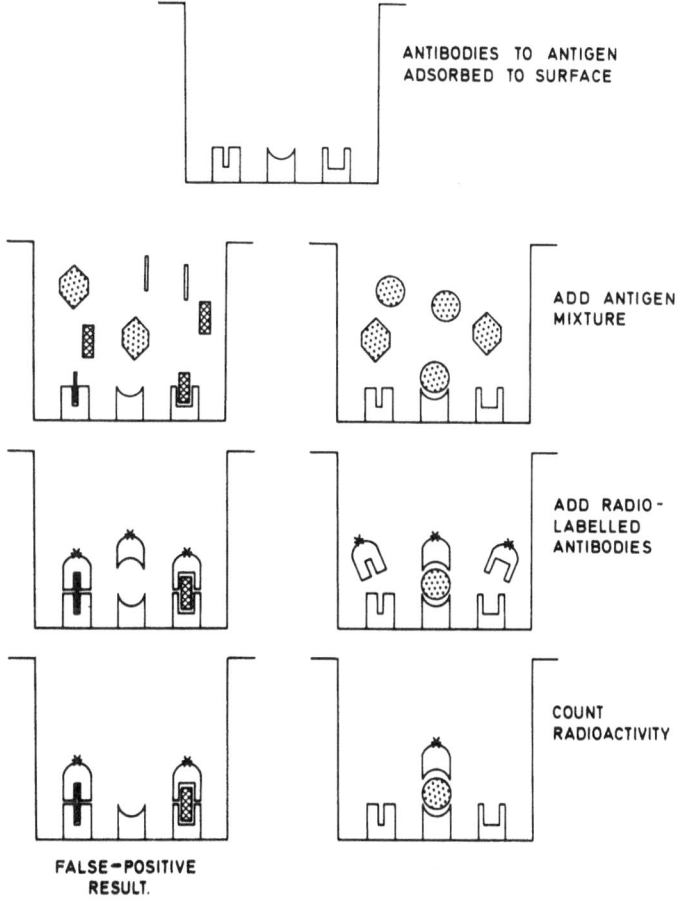

Figure 26.1   Solid-phase radioimmunoassay for detection of antigen

The test proved to be useful for monitoring HAV during the purification step but as monospecific anti-HAV is not available, non-specific results were often obtained when stool suspensions were tested[24].

Using purified HAV as antigen it is also possible to detect anti-HAV by SPRIA. Purcell *et al.*[24] used a blocking procedure where the serum to be tested is added before the conjugate, and if anti-HAV is present in serum it will bind to the adsorbed HAV and block the binding of the conjugate to the plates (Figure 26.2). Usually a 50% reduction in activity bound to the plates

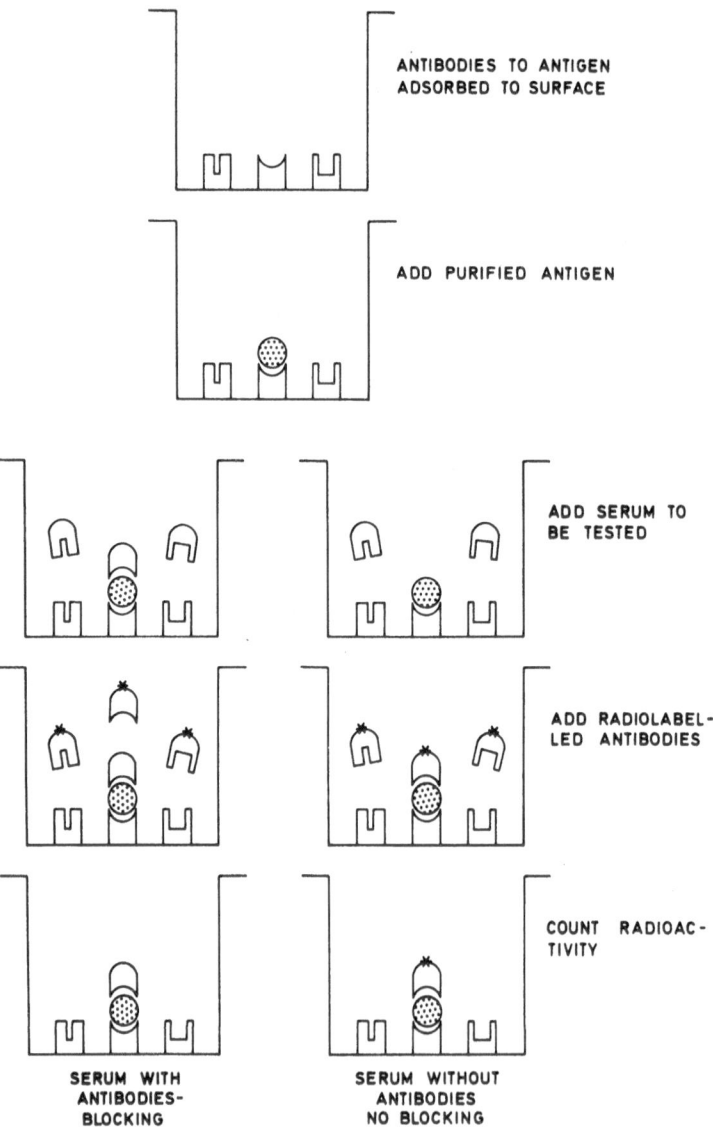

ANTIBODIES TO ANTIGEN
ADSORBED TO SURFACE

ADD PURIFIED ANTIGEN

ADD SERUM TO
BE TESTED

ADD RADIOLABEL-
LED ANTIBODIES

COUNT RADIOAC-
TIVITY

SERUM WITH
ANTIBODIES-
BLOCKING

SERUM WITHOUT
ANTIBODIES
NO BLOCKING

Figure 26.2 Blocking solid-phase radioimmunoassay for detection of antibodies

compared with a negative control is considered positive for anti-HAV. Normally the serum is diluted ten-fold and an exact titre can then be calculated by interpolation, either by plotting the results in a semilog graph or, more easily, by calculation on a programmable calculator using the data of the two dilutions around the 50% reduction in activity (Figure 26.3).

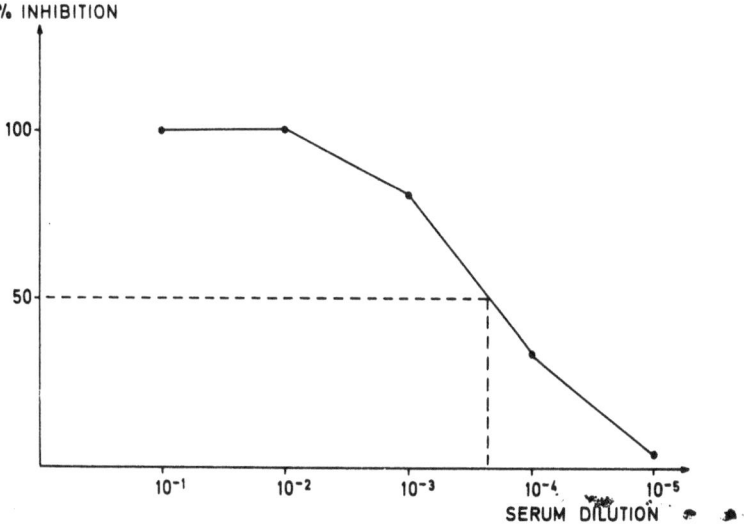

Figure 26.3 Calculation of exact titre corresponding to 50% inhibition after testing ten-fold dilutions of serum in solid-phase radioimmunoassay

Hollinger *et al.*[26] used the serum to be tested as a precoating agent, and if the serum contained anti-HAV activity the subsequent addition of HAV and anti-HAV conjugate will result in binding of radioactivity to the plates and give a positive response. No activity will bind if the serum is devoid of anti-HAV. This can also be used quantitatively by testing dilutions of sera.

ENZYME-LINKED IMMUNOSORBENT ASSAY (ELISA)

ELISA has been widely used since the original observation by Engvall and Perlmann[28] and Van Weemen and Schuurs[29] that an enzyme conjugate can be used instead of a radioactive-labelled conjugate.

ELISA and SPRIA are normally equally sensitive and there is no difference in their specificity, but ELISA has three advantages over SPRIA:

(1) there is no radiation safety hazard in ELISA;
(2) the enzyme conjugates are stable for months to years compared with only 2–4 weeks for most ^{125}I-conjugates;
(3) no expensive equipment is necessary for detection of activity in ELISA as

Table 26.1 Methods for detection of HAV and anti-HAV

Method	Sensitivity	Specificity	Comments (references)
Marmoset inoculation	good for HAV	not without serological testing	very laborious and expensive, not in use any more[2,3]
Immune electron-microscopy (IEM)	comparable to SPRIA and ELISA	with proper experience and controls	requires expensive equipment and great experience; time-consuming[4,8]
Complement-fixation (CF)	lower than IAHA	with purified HAV and proper controls	sera from patients with acute viral hepatitis are frequently anti-complementary, not in use[9]
Immune adherence haemagglutination assay (IAHA)	comparable to SPRIA and ELISA	with purified HAV and proper controls	does not detect anti-HAV until 2–4 weeks after onset of type A hepatitis, requires purified HAV[10,11,13,23]
Solid-phase radioimmunoassay (SPRIA)	comparable to IEM, IAHA and ELISA	with proper controls	radioactive health hazard; shelf life only 2–4 weeks of conjugate, difficult to detect rise in anti-HAV titre during type A hepatitis[24,25,32,33]
Enzyme-linked immunosorbent assay (ELISA)	comparable to IEM, IAHA and SPRIA	with proper controls	same principle as SPRIA but no radiation health hazard and shelf life of conjugate months to years, difficult to detect rise in anti-HAV titre during type A hepatitis[6,19,30,31]
Immunofluorescence (IF)	better than IEM, SPRIA and ELISA	with proper controls	usually necessary for detection of HAV in tissue culture, primary research tool[53,55,57]
Immunoperoxidase (IP)	less than IF	with proper controls	can label HAV for EM localization[57]
Tissue culture	not evaluated	depends on test for detection of HAV after culture	takes several weeks before growth can be detected, laborious[1,62]

it can be read by eye or, if more exact quantitation is needed, by a simple spectrophotometer.

In 1978 Mathiesen et al.[6], Duermeyer et al.[30] and Locarnini et al.[31] independently developed an ELISA using the same principle described for SPRIA but substituting the ^{125}I-conjugate with peroxidase-labelled IgG with anti-HAV activity. Mathiesen et al.[6] demonstrated that ELISA and SPRIA were equally sensitive for detection of HAV and anti-HAV when the same anti-HAV-containing sera were used for precoat and conjugate (Table 26.1).

As ELISA and SPRIA use the same principle, except for the difference in conjugate, false-positive results are also a frequent problem in ELISA when

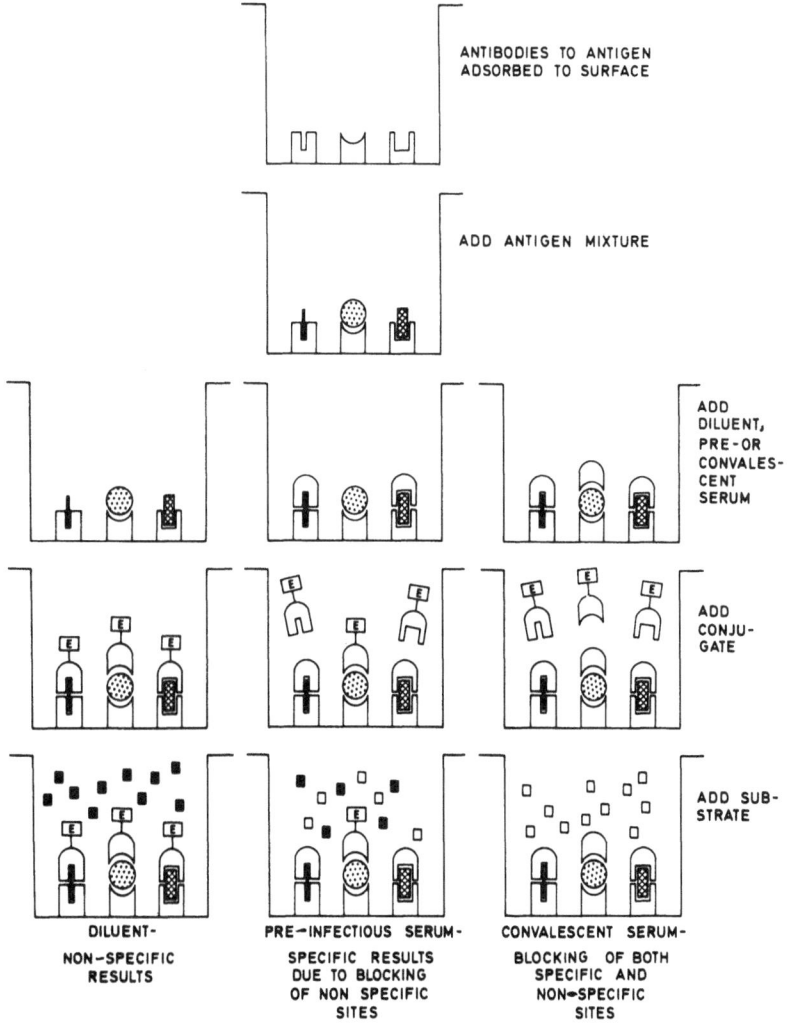

Figure 26.4   Test for antigen specificity in eynzme linked immunosorbent assay by blocking with preinoculation and convalescent sera

stool suspensions are tested for HAV[6]. Initially this problem was solved by parallel blocking with preinoculation and convalescent sera from a chimpanzee experimentally infected with hepatitis A (Figure 26.4). Non-specific activity was then blocked by the preinoculation serum without anti-HAV, whereas activity due to HAV in stool was only blocked by the convalescent serum. This system with parallel blocking was very useful but required three parallel tests, and Mathiesen *et al.*[19] in later experiments routinely avoided non-specific results by diluting the enzyme conjugate in 50% normal pooled human sera negative for anti-HAV (Figure 26.5). In this way unlabelled antibodies are in great excess except for anti-HAV, and it is only if HAV is present in the stool that the enzyme conjugate can bind to the plates. In the absence of available monospecific antibodies this competition with great excess of unlabelled antibodies to all possible antigens that might give false-positive results, is one of the great advantages in the sandwich method. This also means that purified HAV is not necessary for detection of anti-HAV by

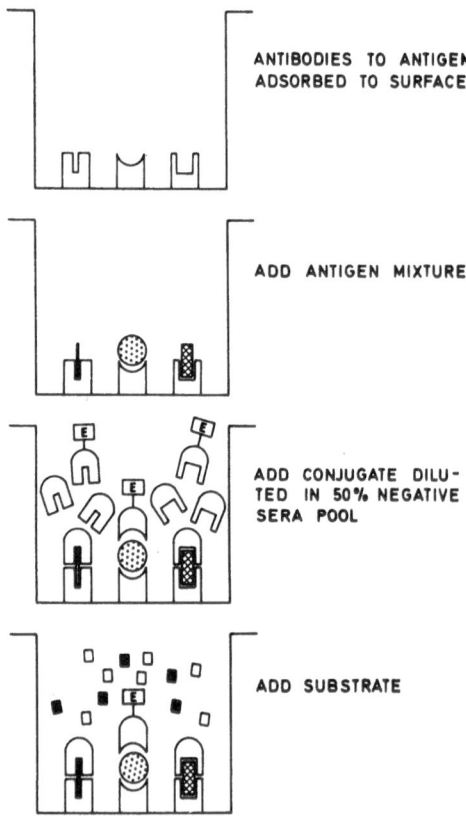

ANTIBODIES TO ANTIGEN ADSORBED TO SURFACE

ADD ANTIGEN MIXTURE

ADD CONJUGATE DILUTED IN 50% NEGATIVE SERA POOL

ADD SUBSTRATE

Figure 26.5 Specific detection of antigen in mixture by enzyme-linked immunosorbent assay diluting the conjugate in excess of unlabelled sera pool lacking the specificity to be tested for

the blocking ELISA, but a HAV-containing stool suspension can be used directly[19].

With IAHA seroconversion for anti-HAV can be demonstrated during hepatitis A infection but by blocking SPRIA or ELISA anti-HAV can always be demonstrated from the onset of acute illness during hepatitis A infection. The titre rises rather abruptly; it reaches a maximum about 3 months after the onset of acute illness and can be demonstrated for years, probably throughout life, protecting the individual from reinfection (Figure 26.9).

Thus detection of anti-HAV in a single serum only means that the individual has been exposed to HAV at some time earlier in life and as this is a fairly common event[13] the diagnostic significance of detectable anti-HAV in serum is very limited for making an aetiological diagnosis during acute hepatitis.

As in other viral infections a four-fold rise in anti-HAV titre has been used for making a diagnosis of acute hepatitis A infection, but this can be difficult to demonstrate by the blocking SPRIA and ELISA[19,32,33].

Mathiesen et al.[19] have compared the blocking and the competition ELISA for detection of anti-HAV during acute hepatitis A infection. The blocking ELISA is performed by adding the serum dilution to the HAV-coated plates before the conjugate, whereas the competition ELISA is performed by mixing the serum dilutions with the conjugate and then adding the mixture to the HAV-coated plates.

They found that blocking ELISA was not useful for detection of rise in anti-HAV titre during hepatitis A infection as an almost equal number of patients demonstrated a two-fold rise in titre and a two-fold fall in titre when an acute phase and an early convalescent phase serum were tested. This was due to a fairly high anti-HAV titre already found in the acute phase serum. Using the competition ELISA a lower titre was usually found in the acute phase serum and detection of a four-fold titre rise was possible in more than half of the patients with hepatitis A infection. For diagnostic purposes this is still not satisfactory and an alternative approach has been the demonstration of IgM anti-HAV.

DETECTION OF IgM ANTI-HAV

As in other self-limiting viral infections, the first antibodies detectable after HAV exposure are of IgM class, but during convalescence IgM antibodies fall to undetectable levels and only IgG antibodies can be demonstrated. Locarnini et al.[34] were the first to describe IgM-like structures in immune complexes formed when acute phase hepatitis A sera reacted with HAV-containing stools. Later several laboratories have separated IgM and IgG by sucrose gradient centrifugation and found anti-HAV in the IgM fractions in the acute phase sera but not in convalescent sera (Table 26.2)[35-37].

Table 26.2 Methods for detection of IgM anti-HAV

Method	Sensitivity	Specificity	Comments (references)
IEM	low	low	laborious[34]
Sucrose gradient centrifugation	medium	good	very laborious[35,37]
Staphylococcal protein A absorption	low	variable	does not absorb all IgG, results depend on local experience[39,40]
Mercaptoethanol destruction of IgM	low	variable	results depend on local experience[41,43]
Precoating SPRIA	low	variable	requires end-point titration and very good controls, not in general use[38]
ELISA with catching antibodies	medium	good	only very small difference between a positive and a negative result, not in general use[44]
Reverse ELISA or SPRIA with anti-IgM precoating	high	good	easy to perform, high diagnostic accuracy, rheumatoid factor generally not a problem, routinely used in several laboratories[8,19,45,51]

Sucrose gradient centrifugation is rather time consuming and Bradley *et al.*[38] therefore modified their SPRIA, so that IgM anti-HAV could be determined. They used the serum to be tested as a precoating agent and if the serum was able to bind HAV and thus the conjugate, the serum contained anti-HAV activity. If the binding of HAV could be abolished by an extra incubation step with anti-IgM, the anti-HAV was of IgM class. This principle required titration of the serum, and their initial results have not been confirmed by others.

Absorption of the sera with staphylococcal protein A, which binds to IgG but not to IgM, before testing the sera in a competition SPRIA for anti-HAV has been described[3]. In order to get reliable results using this technique, it seems necessary to re-evaluate the conditions for each new batch of SPRIA kit, as well as individually to determine the dilution of sera to be used[39], otherwise false-positive results can be obtained[40].

Testing for anti-HAV before and after destruction of IgM antibodies by mercaptoethanol has also been used by some with some success[41,42] whereas others have not found it useful[43].

Another approach has recently been described by Locarnini *et al.*[44]. They determined IgM anti-HAV as being present in sera by applying the sera to HAV-coated solid-phase and adding enzyme-conjugated anti-IgM as the top layer in a sandwich test (Figure 26.6). Using this approach they could usually detect IgM anti-HAV up to 6 weeks after onset of dark urine and no patients were positive longer than 115 days. Their method, however, did not discriminate very well between sera positive and negative for IgM anti-HAV, as the highest positive/negative ratio in their test was only about 2 times their cut-off level of 1.6. This means that only a slight variation in the procedure might invalidate the results.

Recently a new principle for detection of IgM anti-HAV has been described by Duermeyer *et al.*[8,45,46] and techniques using this approach have been further evaluated by Møller *et al.*[47] and Mathiesen *et al.*[19,48] using ELISA, and Flehmig *et al.*[49], Roggendorf *et al.*[50], Papaevangelou *et al.*[51] and Hanson *et al.* (personal communication) using SPRIA (Table 26.2).

In contrast to the usual approach for detecting IgM antibodies in virology by SPRIA or ELISA (Figure 27.2), Duermeyer *et al.* coated solid-phase with anti-IgM and added test sera for binding of antibodies of IgM class to the phase. Thereafter they tested the bound IgM for anti-HAV specificity by adding HAV followed by anti-HAV conjugate (Figure 26.7).

Using this approach there is no competition between IgM and IgG antibodies of the same specificities but only between IgM antibodies of different specificities, Møller and Mathiesen[47] have shown that an ELISA using this approach is very specific and sensitive for detection of IgM anti-HAV, detecting IgM anti-HAV from onset of clinical illness during HAV infections and the following 2–4 months but not thereafter (Figures 26.8 and 26.9). No false-positive results due to rheumatoid factor in IgG anti-HAV

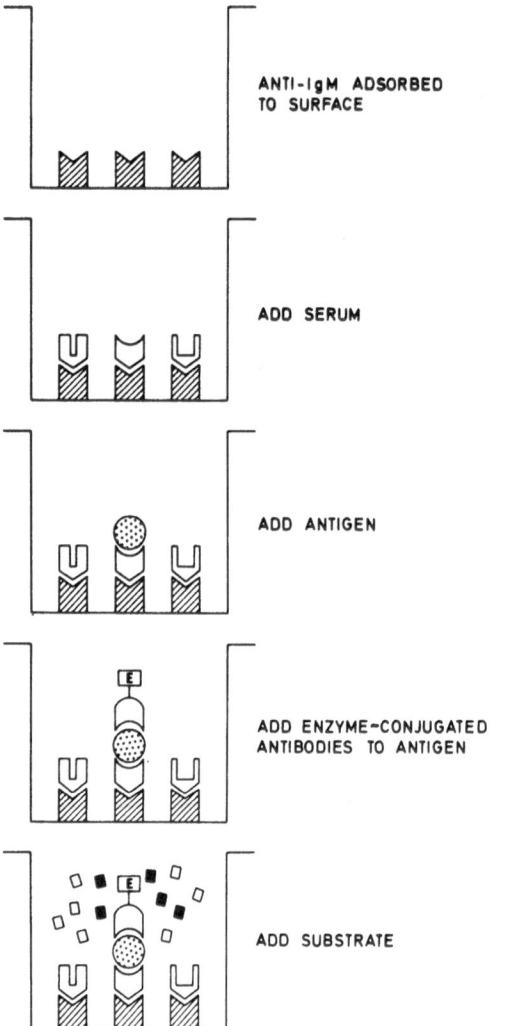

ANTI-IgM ADSORBED
TO SURFACE

ADD SERUM

ADD ANTIGEN

ADD ENZYME-CONJUGATED
ANTIBODIES TO ANTIGEN

ADD SUBSTRATE

Figure 26.6 Enzyme-linked immunosorbent assay for detection of IgM antibodies using catching antibodies and anti-IgM conjugate

containing sera were observed, and a high accuracy for both a positive and negative result was obtained when testing a group of patients with acute hepatitis serologically confirmed as type A, B or non-A, non-B.

Using other dilutions and conditions for precoating and incubation Flehmig et al.[35] could detect IgM anti-HAV in serum taken up to 12 months after the acute infection with HAV. Duermeyer et al.[46] could, under extreme conditions, by mixing a high-titred IgG anti-HAV serum with a sera containing a high titre of rheumatoid factor, produce false-positive results even when a F(ab) conjugate was used; this was not observed by others using 1% aggregated IgG[35] or fetal sera[47] for dilution of the sera to be tested and

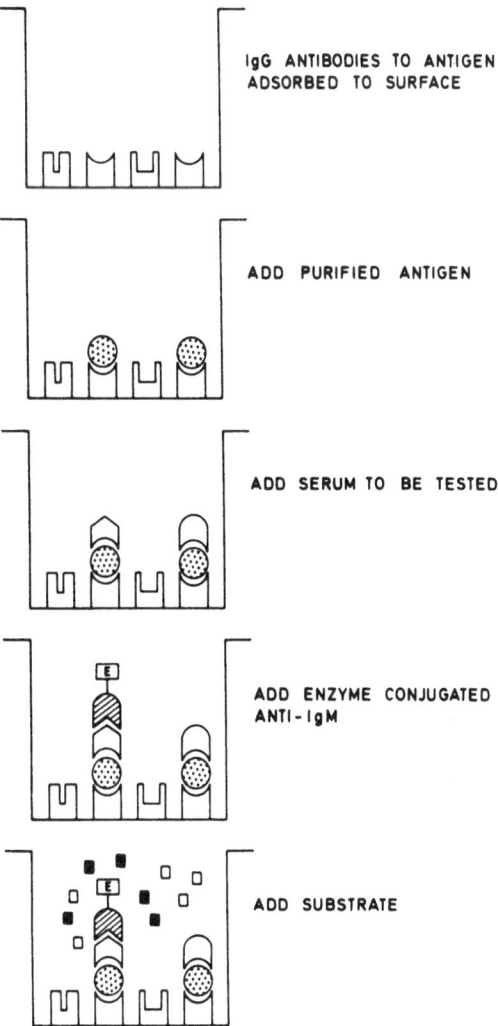

IgG ANTIBODIES TO ANTIGEN
ADSORBED TO SURFACE

ADD PURIFIED ANTIGEN

ADD SERUM TO BE TESTED

ADD ENZYME CONJUGATED
ANTI-IgM

ADD SUBSTRATE

Figure 26.7 Reverse enzyme-linked immunosorbent assay for detection of IgM antibodies using anti-IgM precoat (reproduced by permission from reference 47)

50% normal human sera for dilution of the conjugate.

The test is easy to perform and allows a great number of sera to be tested daily by one technician.

The principle of extraction of IgM to anti-IgM pre-coated plates followed by testing for specificities of the antibody has great potential also in other viral diseases where detection of specific IgM antibodies is of diagnostic value. So far a similar test has been described for detection of IgM antibodies to HBcAg[52], but work is in progress using the same principle for detection of IgM antibodies to rubella (Duermeyer et al., personal communication).

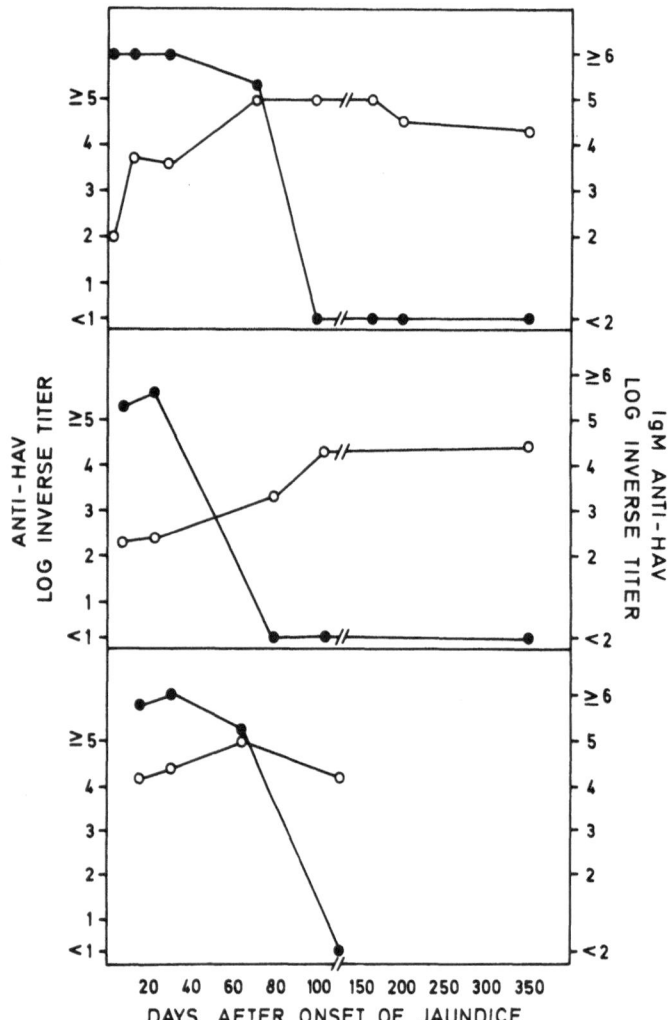

Figure 26.8 Serial determination of anti-HAV (○) by competition ELISA and IgM anti-HAV (●) by reverse ELISA in three patients with acute hepatitis type A (reproduced by permission from reference 47)

IMMUNOFLUORESCENCE AND IMMUNOPEROXIDASE METHODS

In 1977 Mathiesen *et al.*[53] reported the detection of HAV by immunofluores-cence (IF) in the cytoplasm of hepatocytes and Kupffer cells using snap-frozen liver biopsies taken during the acute stage of experimental HAV infections in chimpanzees. The appearance was very fine granules concentrated in the cytoplasm of hepatocytes scattered throughout the tissue (Figure 26.10).

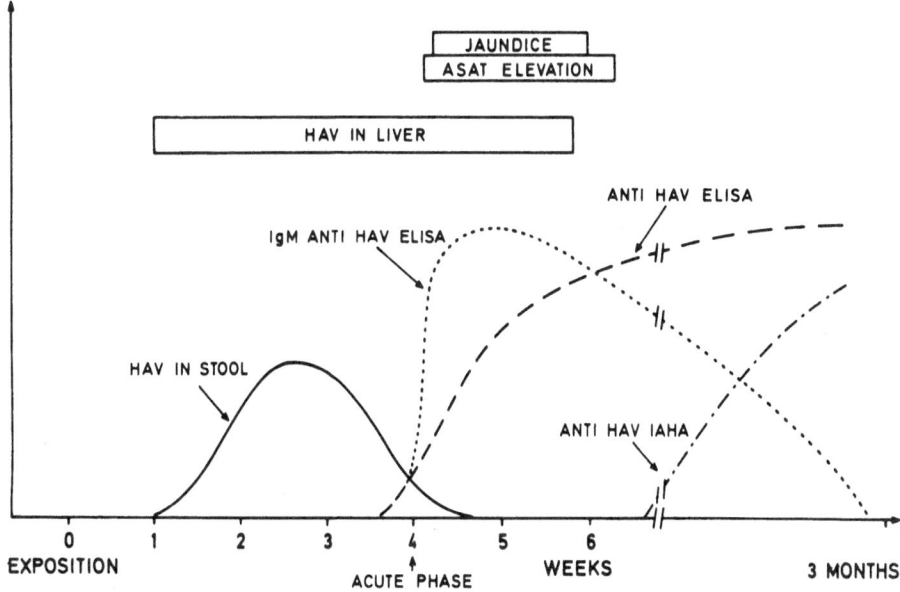

Figure 26.9 Idealized course of the different serological findings during the typical HAV infection

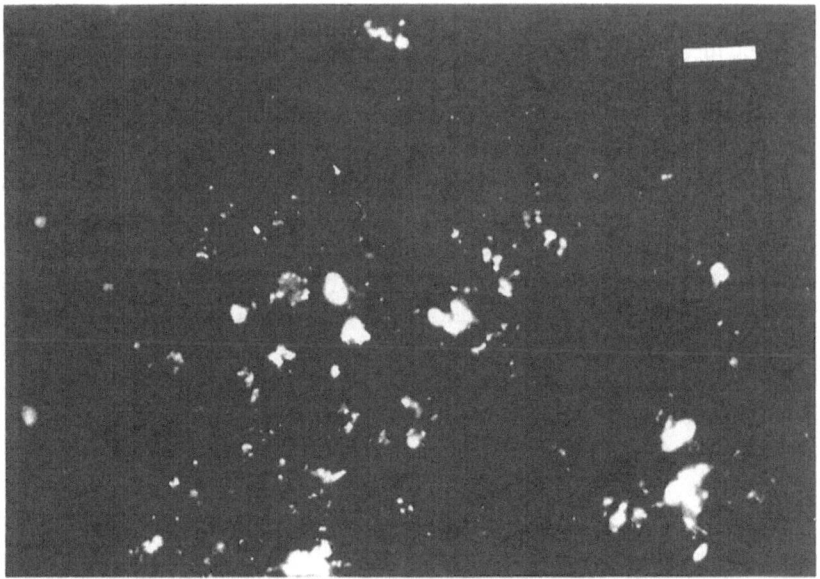

Figure 26.10 Hepatitis A virus demonstrated by direct immunofluorescence in a liver biopsy from a patient with acute type A hepatitis. Bar = 20 μm. (reproduced from reference 18)

The same principle, previously found to be successful in detection of HBsAg and HBcAg in liver biopsies, was used[54]. IgG from a serum with a high anti-HAV titre was isolated and conjugated to fluorescein isothiocyanate (FITC) and used in a direct immunofluorescence technique. In order to visualize HAV in the biopsies it was necessary to change the microscope to vertical illumination and diminish the autofluorescence using a combination of a LP 455 and a KP 490 as excitation filters. This only allows light between 455 and 490 nm to reach the tissue, and it is in this interval that FITC has absorption maximum. Finally it was also necessary to use an objective with a high aperture in order to get the brightest fluorescence possible. In later experiments a 75 W xenon bulb was preferred to a HBO 200 W/2 mercury bulb for FITC fluorescence because the emission from the xenon bulb is better in the wavelength where FITC has absorption maximum (unpublished observation).

The specificity of the fluorescence was easily shown by blocking with preinoculation and convalescent sera from humans and chimpanzees experimentally infected with HAV. The IF technique proved to be very sensitive for detection of HAV in tissue and Mathiesen et al.[53] were able to demonstrate HAV in serial liver biopsies, before faecal shedding of HAV was demonstrated and extending about 3 weeks beyond detectable shedding of HAV in stools. These results have been confirmed by Murphy et al.[55], and in a subsequent experiment Mathiesen et al.[56] made a direct comparison between IF, IEM and ELISA on marmoset liver tissue and demonstrated that IF was superior for detection of HAV in tissue. It was even possible by IF to detect HAV deposited in glomeruli lymph nodes and spleen during the acute phase of HAV infections in marmosets inoculated intravenously with HAV. The high sensitivity for detection of HAV in tissue was also demonstrated when liver biopsies from patients with acute hepatitis A infection were tested for HAV; 11 out of 17 patients studied demonstrated HAV in the liver by IF, where normally less than one-third has detectable HAV in stool by ELISA or SPRIA when presenting to a physician[18].

The IF has been very valuable in the study of the pathogenesis of HAV infections and the subsequent development of an immunoperoxidase method also enabled the study of the ultrastructural localization of HAV in membrane-bound cytoplasmic vesicles[57]. For normal routine diagnostic work the detection of anti-HAV and IgM anti-HAV in serum is much easier and more accurate for making a diagnosis of acute hepatitis A infection[18,47].

TISSUE CULTURE

During the last 30 years numerous investigators have tried to grow HAV in tissue culture[58] and several reports with promising results have been published[59], however, on each occasion it was shown to be some other virus, or the results could not be confirmed by others[60,61].

It was not until well-characterized HAV was generated in marmosets[2] and the very sensitive immunofluorescence method was developed for detection of HAV in tissue[58] that the propagation of HAV in tissue culture was demonstrated by Provost et al.[1]. The observation has subsequently been confirmed by Frösner et al.[62], Purcell et al. and Gust et al. (unpublished observations) and they have also shown that HAV obtained directly from human stool, without passage in marmoset, also grows in tissue culture.

So far, HAV has not been shown to produce cytopathic changes in tissue culture and the demonstration of growth therefore depends on secondary demonstration of HAV by IF, SPRIA or ELISA. Propagation of HAV in tissue culture might prove to be a very sensitive way to detect HAV in stool and tissue, but it takes several weeks before HAV can be detected, even by IF, and the procedure is very laborious compared to other methods.

The culture of HAV allows generation of large amounts of HAV necessary as antigen in the different methods for detection of anti-HAV. A more complete study of the biochemical and biophysical properties of HAV isolated from different outbreaks is also possible now. The ultimate aim with the cultivation of HAV is development of a vaccine. So far, HAV has only been cultured in primary cells or cell lines not suitable for vaccine production, but further progress will hopefully make the development of a killed or attenuated vaccine possible. It has already been shown in marmosets that a crude vaccine prepared from marmoset livers containing HAV, and inactivated by heat and formalin, induces an anti-HAV response and protects the animals from HAV infections when they are rechallenged[63].

CONCLUSION

For detection of HAV in stool and liver homogenates IEM is suitable, but ELISA or SPRIA are easier to perform and are specific if appropriate controls are used. By these methods HAV can in general only be detected in stool suspension from about one-third of the patients with acute hepatitis A.

For detection of HAV in tissue or tissue culture IF is the method of choice. By IF it is possible to detect HAV in liver biopsies in about two-thirds of the patients with hepatitis A infection if the biopsies are taken during the acute stage. It is possible that HAV can be detected in stool and tissue with greater sensitivity by propagation in tissue culture followed by detection by an immunoassay.

The IEM, IAHA, CF, SPRIA and ELISA methods are all suitable for detecting anti-HAV, but the tests vary in sensitivity, specificity and ease of performance. IAHA is the simplest, if purified HAV is available, and has been widely used for seroepidemiologic studies. Although it is at least as sensitive as the other tests available, IAHA does not detect anti-HAV until 2–6 weeks after the onset of illness, and seroconversion for anti-HAV can therefore be demonstrated by IAHA during acute hepatitis A infection.

This is not possible with the now commonly used SPRIA and ELISA. These methods are very useful for seroepidemiologic studies and demonstration of immunity, but as anti-HAV by SPRIA and ELISA is present from the onset of acute illness and can be detected for years, probably throughout life, demonstration of a significant rise in anti-HAV titre is necessary for making a diagnosis of acute hepatitis A infection. The competition ELISA for detection of anti-HAV has been found superior to the blocking ELISA for detection of rise in anti-HAV titre during acute hepatitis A infection. However, demonstration of four-fold rise in anti-HAV titre by competition SPRIA or ELISA is normally only possible in about half of the patients with acute hepatitis A infection.

Detection of IgM anti-HAV in acute phase serum is therefore today the method of choice in making a diagnosis of acute hepatitis A infection. Here the reverse SPRIA or ELISA with absorption of IgM to anti-IgM precoated solid-phase, followed by testing for anti-HAV specificity by adding HAV and anti-HAV conjugate, are the best methods available. These methods are very sensitive and specific and are able to detect IgM anti-HAV in all patients with hepatitis A infection for up to 3–12 months after onset of illness but not thereafter. It is thus possible to demonstrate acute or recent hepatitis A infection testing a single serum for IgM anti-HAV.

The described immunoassays for hepatitis A have made possible a rapid increase in our knowledge of the hepatitis A infection and have led to the successful propagation of HAV in tissue culture which will hopefully result in development of a vaccine in the near future.

References

1. Provost, P. J. and Hilleman, M. R. (1979). Propagation of human hepatitis A virus in cell culture in vitro. *Proc. Soc. Exp. Biol.*, **160**, 213
2. Holmes, A. W., Wolfe, L., Rosenblate, H. and Deinhardt, F. (1969). Hepatitis in marmosets: induction of disease with coded specimens from a human volunteer study. *Science*, **165**, 816
3. Provost, P. J., Ittensohn, L., Villarejos, V. M., Arguedas, J. A. and Hilleman, M. R. (1973). Etiologic relationship of marmoset-propagated CR326 hepatitis A virus to hepatitis in man. *Proc. Soc. Exp. Biol.*, **142**, 1257
4. Feinstone, S. M., Kapikian, A. Z. and Purcell, R. H. (1973). Hepatitis A: detection by immune electron microscopy of a viruslike antigen associated with acute illness. *Science*, **182**, 1026
5. Locarnini, S. A., Gust, I. D., Ferris, A. A., Stott, A. C. and Wong, M. L. (1976). A prospective study of acute viral hepatitis with particular reference to hepatitis A. *Bull. WHO*, **54**, 199
6. Mathiesen, L. R., Feinstone, S. M., Wong, D. C., Skinhoej, P. and Purcell, R. H. (1978). Enzyme-linked immunosorbent assay for detection of hepatitis A antigen in stool and antibody to hepatitis A. Antigen in sera: comparison with solid-phase radioimmunoassay,

immune electron microscopy, and immune adherence hemagglutination assay. *J. Clin. Microbiol.*, **7**, 184

7. Rakela, J. and Mosley, J. W. (1977). Fecal excretion of hepatitis A virus in humans. *J. Infect. Dis.*, **135**, 933

8. Tufvesson, B., van der Veen, J., Duermeyer, W., Niklasson, P. M. and Johnsson, T. (1979). An outbreak of hepatitis A investigated by immune electron microscopy and enzyme-linked immunosorbent assay. *Scand. J. Infect. Dis.*, **11**, 97

9. Provost, P. J., Ittensohn, O. L., Villarejos, V. M. and Hilleman, M. R. (1975). A specific complement-fixation test for human hepatitis A employing CR326 virus antigen. Diagnosis and epidemiology. *Proc. Soc. Exp. Biol.*, **148**, 962

10. Miller, W. J., Provost, P. J., McAleer, W. J., Ittensohn, C. L., Villarejos, V. M. and Hilleman, M. R. (1975). Specific immune adherence assay for human hepatitis A antibody. Application to diagnostic and epidemiologic investigations. *Proc. Soc. Exp. Biol.*, **149**, 254

11. Moritsugu, Y., Dienstag, J. L., Valdesuso, J., Wong, D. C., Wagner, J., Routenberg, J. A. and Purcell, R. H. (1976). Purification of hepatitis A antigen from faeces and detection of antigen and antibody by immune adherence hemagglutination. *Infect. Immun.*, **13**, 898

12. Mayumia, M., Okochi, K. and Nichioka, K. (1971). Detection of Australia antigen by means of immune adherence hemagglutination test. *Vox Sang.*, **20**, 178

13. Dienstag, J. L., Szmuness, W., Stevens, C. E. and Purcell, R. H. (1978). Hepatitis A virus infection: new insights from seroepidemiologic studies. *J. Infect. Dis.*, **137**, 328

14. Szmuness, W., Dienstag, J. L., Purcell, R. H., Stevens, C. E., Wong, D. C., Ikram, H., Har-Shany, S., Beasley, P., Desmyter, J. and Gaon, J. A. (1977). The prevalence of antibody to hepatitis A antigen in various parts of the world: a pilot study. *Am. J. Epidemiol*, **106**, 392

15. Dienstag, J. L., Alaama, A., Mosley, J. W., Redeker, A. G. and Purcell, R. H. (1977). Etiology of sporadic hepatitis B surface antigen-negative hepatitis. *Ann. Intern. Med.*, **87**, 1

16. Dienstag, J. L., Mathiesen, L. R. and Purcell, R. H. (1978). Test methods and animal models for HAV infection. In Vyas, C. N., Cohen, S. M. and Schmid, R. (eds.) *Viral Hepatitis*, pp. 13–21. (Philadelphia: The Franklin Institute)

17. Gust, I. D., Dienstag, J. L., Purcell, R. H. and Lucas, C. R. (1977). Non-B hepatitis in Melbourne: a serological study of hepatitis A virus infection. *Br. Med. J.*, **1**, 193

18. Mathiesen, L. R., Fauerholdt, L., Møller, A. M., Aldershvíle, J., Dietrichson, O., Hardt, F., Nielsen, J. O., Skinhøj, P. and CHAP (1979). Immunofluorescence studies for hepatitis A virus and hepatitis B surface and core antigen in liver biopsies from patients with acute viral hepatitis. *Gastroenterology*, **77**, 623

19. Mathiesen, L. R., Skinhøj, P., Hardt, F., Nielsen, J. O., Sloth, K., Zoffmann, H., Møller, A. M., Wong, D., Purcell, R. H. and CHAP (1979). Epidemiology and clinical characteristics of acute hepatitis types A, B, and non-A non-B. *Scand. J. Gastroenterol.*, **14**, 849

20. Mathiesen, L. R., Papaevangelou, G., Purcell, R. H., Grammatikopoulos, D., Contoyannis, P. and Wong, D. (1980). Etiologic characterization of HBsAg-negative hepatitis among adult patients in Athens, Greece. *J. Clin. Microbiol.*, **11**, 297

21. Mathiesen, L. R., Skinhøj, P., Nielsen, J. O., Purcell, R. H., Wong, D. and Ranek, L. (1980). Hepatitis type A, B and non-A non-B in fulminant hepatitis. *Gut*, **21**, 72

22. Rakela, J., Redeker, A. G., Edwards, V. M., Decker, R., Overby, L. R. and Mosley, J. W. (1978). Hepatitis A virus infection in fulminant hepatitis and chronic active hepatitis. *Gastroenterology*, **74**, 879

23. Rakela, J., Stevenson, D., Edvards, V. M., Gordon, I. and Mosley, J. W. (1977). Antibodies to hepatitis A virus: patterns by two procedures. *J. Clin. Microbiol.*, **5**, 110

24. Purcell, R. J., Wong, D. C., Moritsugu, Y., Dienstag, J. L., Routenberg, J. A. and Boggs, J. D. (1976). A microtiter solid-phase radioimmunoassay for hepatitis A antigen and antibody. *J. Immunol.*, **116**, 349

25. Hollinger, P. B., Bradley, D. W., Maynard, J. E., Dreesman, G. R. and Melnick, J. L. (1975). Detection of hepatitis A viral antigen by radioimmunoassay. *J. Immunol.*, **115**, 1464

26. Purcell, R. H., Wong, D. C., Alter, H. J. and Holland, P. V. (1973). Microtiter solid-phase radio immunoassay for hepatitis B antigen. *Appl. Microbiol.*, **26**, 478

27. Purcell, R. H., Gerin, J. L., Almeida, J. D. and Holland, P. V. (1973). Radio immuno assay for the detection of the core of the Dane particle and antibody to it. *Intervirology*, **2**, 231

28. Engvall, E. and Perlmann, P. (1971). Enzyme-linked immunosorbent assay (ELISA). Quantitative assay of immunoglobulin. *Immunochemistry*, **8**, 871

29. Van Weemen, B. K. and Schuurs, A. H. W. M. (1971). Immuno assay using antigen enzyme conjugates. *FEBS Letters*, **15**, 232

30. Duermeyer, W., Veen, van der, J. and Koster, B. (1978). ELISA in hepatitis A. *Lancet*, **1**, 823

31. Locarnini, S. A., Garland, S. M., Lehmann, N. I., Pringle, R. C. and Gust, I. D. (1978). Solid-phase enzymelinked immunosorbent assay for detection of hepatitis A virus. *J. Clin. Microbiol.*, **8**, 277

32. Müller, R., Willers, H., Frösner, G. G., Gerlich, W., Knocke, K. W., Sipos, S., Deicher, H. and Höpken, W. (1978). The seroepidemiological pattern of acute viral hepatitis. *Infect.* **6**, 65

33. Norkrans, G., Frösner, G., Hermodsson, S., Nenonen, N. and Iwarson, S. (1978). The epidemiological pattern of hepatitis A, B and non-A, non-B in Sweden. *Scand. J. Gastroenterol.*, **13**, 873

34. Locarnini, S. A., Ferris, A. A., Stott, A. and Gust, I. D. (1974). The antibody response following hepatitis A infection. *Intervirology*, **4**, 110

35. Flehmig, B., Ranke, M., Frank, H. and Gerth, H.-J. (1978). Application of a solid-phase radio immuno assay and immune electron microscopy for hepatitis A in diagnosis and research. *Med. Microbiol. Immunol.*, **166**, 187

36. Frösner, G. G., Scheid, R., Wolf, H. and Deinhardt, F. (1979). Immunoglobulin M anti-hepatitis A virus determination by reorienting gradient centrifugation for diagnosis of acute hepatitis A. *J. Clin. Microbiol.*, **9**, 476

37. Locarnini, S. A., Ferris, A. A., Lehmann, N. I. and Gust, I. D. (1977). The relationship between a 27 nm virus-like particle and hepatitis A as demonstrated by immune electron microscopy. *Intervirology*, **8**, 309

38. Bradley, D. W., Maynard, J. E., Hindman, S. H., Hornbeck, C. L., Fields, H. A., McFaustland, K. A. and Cook, E. H. (1977). Serodiagnosis of viral hepatitis A: detection of acute-phase immunoglobulin M anti-hepatitis A virus by radio immunoassay. *J. Clin Microbiol.*, **5**, 521

39. Bradley, D. W., Fields, H. A., McMaustland, K. A., Maynard, J. E., Decker, R. H., Whittington, R. and Overby, L. R. (1979). Serodiagnosis of viral hepatitis A by a modified competitive binding radioimmunoassay for immunoglobulin M anti-hepatitis A virus. *J. Clin. Microbiol.*, **9**, 120

40. Williams, W. L., Roudreaux, V., Gohd, R., Cornway, C. T. and McFarland, L. (1979). Pseudo outbreak of hepatitis A – Louisiana. *Morbidity and Mortality Weekly Report*, **28**, 473

41. Girardet, C., Peitrequin, R. and Frei, P. C. (1979). Radioimmunoassay diagnosis of hepatitis type A. *Lancet*, **1**, 876

42. Pastore, G., Angarano, G., Dentico, P. and Schiraldi, O. (1979). Radio immuno assay diagnosis of hepatitis type A. *Lancet*, **1**, 876

43. Berg, J. V. R., Bergdahl, S., Lindh, G., Lundberg, P., Sjöblom, R., Weiland, O. and Flehmig, B. (1979). Limitations of commercial test for antibody to hepatitis A virus. *Lancet*, **1**, 212

44. Locarnini, S. A., Coulepis, A. G., Stratton, A. M., Kaldor, J. and Gust, I. D. (1979). Solid phase enzyme-linked immunosorbent assay for detection of hepatitis A-specific immunoglobulin M. *J. Clin. Microbiol.*, **9**, 459

45. Duermeyer, W. and Veen, van der, J. (1978). Specific detection of IgM-antibodies by ELISA, applied in hepatitis A. *Lancet*, **2**, 684

46. Duermeyer, W., Wielaard, F. and Veen, van der, J. (1979). A new principle for the detection of specific IgM antibodies applied in an ELISA for hepatitis A. *J. Med. Virol.*, **4**, 25

47. Møller, A. M. and Mathiesen, L. R. (1979). Detection of IgM antibodies to hepatitis A virus. *Clin. Microbiol.*, **10**, 628

48. Mathiesen, L. R., Hardt, F., Dietrichson, O., Purcell, R. H., Wong, D., Skinhøj, P., Nielsen, J. O., Zoffmann, H., Iversen, K. and CHAP. (1978). The role of acute hepatitis type A, B, and non-A non-B in the development of chronic active liver disease. *Scand. J. Gastroenterol.*, **15**, 49

49. Flehmig, B., Ranke, M., Berthold, H. and Gerth, H.-J. (1979). A solid-phase radio immuno assay for detection of IgM antibodies to hepatitis A virus. *J. Infect. Dis.*, **140**, 169

50. Roggendorf, M., Frösner, G., Deinhardt, F., Rodt, H. and Scheid, R. (1978). Comparison of solid phase enzyme immunoassay (ELISA), solid phase radio immuno assay (RIA) and density gradient centrifugation for demonstration of anti-HAV of the IgM-class. *Gastroenterology*, **76**, 1298

51. Papaevangelou, G., Decker, R., Contoyannis, P. and Overby, L. (1979). Differential serodiagnosis of sporadic acute viral hepatitis. *Proc. Soc. Exp. Biol.*, **161**, 322

52. Gerlich, W. H. and Lüer, W. (1979). Selective detection of IgM-antibody against core antigen of the hepatitis B virus by a modified enzyme immuno assay. *J. Med. Virol.*, **4**, 227

53. Mathiesen, L. R., Feinstone, S. M., Purcell, R. H. and Wagner, J. A. (1977). Detection of hepatitis A antigen by immunofluorescence. *Infect. Immunol.*, **18**, 524

54. Murphy, B. L., Peterson, J. M., Ebert, J. W., Bergquist, K. K., Maynard, J. E. and Purcell, R. H. (1975/76). Immunofluorescent localization of hepatitis B antigens in chimpanzee tissue. *Intervirology*, **6**, 207

55. Murphy, B. L., Maynard, J. E., Bradley, D. W., Ebert, J. W., Mathiesen, L. R. and Purcell, R. H. (1978). Immunofluorescence of hepatitis A virus antigen in chimpanzees. *Infect. Immunol.*, **21**, 663

56. Mathiesen, L. R., Drucker, J., Lorenz, D., Wagner, J., Gerety, R. J. and Purcell, R. H. (1978). Localization of hepatitis A antigen in marmoset organs during acute infection with hepatitis A virus. *J. Infect. Dis.*, **138**, 369

57. Shimizu, Y. K., Mathiesen, L. R., Lorenz, D., Drucker, J., Feinstone, S. M., Wagner, J. A. and Purcell, R. H. (1978). Localization of hepatitis A antigen in liver tissue by peroxidase-conjugated antibody method: light and electron microscopic studies. *J. Immunol.*, **121**, 1671

58. Taylor, A. R., Rightsel, W. A., Boggs, J. D. and McLean, I. W. (1962). Tissue culture of hepatitis virus. *Am. J. Med.*, **32**, 679

59. Boggs, J. D., Melnick, J. L., Conrad, M. E. and Felsher, F. (1970). Viral hepatitis. Clinical and tissue culture studies. *J. Am. Med. Assoc.*, **214**, 1040

60. World Health Organization Expert Committee on viral hepatitis (1977). Advances in viral hepatitis. Technical report series 602

61. Zuckerman, A. J. (1970). In *Virus Diseases of the Liver*, Chap. 8 (London: Butterworths)

62. Frösner, G. G., Deinhardt, F., Scheid, R., Gauss-Müller, V., Holmes, N., Messelberger, V., Siegl, G. and Alexander, J. J. (1979). Propagation of human hepatitis A virus in hepatoma cell line. *Infection*, **7**, 303

63. Provost, P. J. and Hilleman, M. R. (1978). An inactivated hepatitis A virus vaccine prepared from infected marmoset liver. *Proc. Soc. Exp. Biol.*, **159**, 201

27
Immunoassays for the TORCH programme

M. VEJTORP

INTRODUCTION

Toxoplasma, rubellavirus, cytomegalovirus (CMV) and herpes simplex virus (HSV) infections constitute the TORCH group of infectious diseases[1]. These can cause malformation or devastating disease of the newborn infant following an often symptomless or mild infection of the mother during pregnancy. Severe damage due to the congenital infection may also arise in children without symptoms or recognized disease at birth.

The clinical manifestations of the TORCH diseases may be characteristic for the causative agent; however, laboratory tests are normally essential for establishment of the diagnosis. The infections induce changes in the cell-mediated immune response, but at present the immunoassays for *in vitro* measurement of this response are mainly research tools, and their potential usefulness for diagnosis of the TORCH diseases has not yet been evaluated. Isolation and identification of the infecting agent is commonly necessary for routine diagnosis of CMV and HSV infections and occasionally for the diagnosis of toxoplasmosis. However, these techniques require propagation of the agent in tissue cultures or laboratory animals and accordingly, they exclude an early diagnosis.

During recent years immunoassays for diagnosis of pre- and postnatally acquired TORCH infections by detection of specific antibodies and antigens have been improved considerably. These methods, being rapid, specific and sensitive, will probably during the 1980s completely replace present diagnostic techniques.

PATHOGENESIS OF THE TORCH DISEASES

The most important route of the intrauterine infections caused by the agents of the TORCH group is a haematogenous transplacental dissemination from the mother to the fetus. Antibodies acquired by a previous infection of the mother generally protect the fetus. Intrauterine CMV infections in consecutive pregnancies and in previously immune pregnant women have, however, been reported, but the congenital infections were asymptomatic[2-4]. Postnatal transmission of CMV to newborn infants has not been associated with damage.

Transplacental transmission of HSV to the fetus in early gestation probably as a rule results in spontaneous abortion[5] and only a few cases of congenital damages due to prenatal infections are known[6]. The neonatal HSV infections are usually transmitted to the fetus during the passage through an infected birth canal or by an ascending infection of the genital tract of the mother following rupture of the membranes[7]. Another source of infection may be a non-genital HSV infection of the mother, or others nursing the infant.

An HSV type 1 is primarily associated with non-genital and an HSV type 2 primarily with genital infections[8]. Either of the types may be transmitted to the newborn infant. Prenatally transferred maternal antibodies may not be relied on to protect the newborn infant.

IMMUNE RESPONSE TO POSTNATAL TORCH INFECTIONS

The humoral immune responses to the TORCH diseases have been elucidated during the last decade by assays, which separately detect specific antibodies belonging to different immunoglobulin classes.

The specific IgM class antibodies appear in serum early after the primary infection and disappear usually within 1–3 months. The specific IgG antibodies can commonly be demonstrated a few days after appearance of the IgM antibodies. The concentration of the IgG globulins increases to reach a plateau level after several weeks. A minor decline may then be observed, but detectable specific IgG antibodies probably persist for lifetime. The specific IgA antibodies constitute the main part of the immunoglobulins in secretions. They also appear in the serum early after an infection, but the time of persistence may be variable.

Reinfections normally cause an increase only in the concentration of the specific IgG antibodies. Reinfections or reactivations of CMV and HSV may, however, occasionally also initiate a synthesis of specific IgM antibodies. Consequently the serodiagnosis of a recent infection may be based on a demonstration of a significant increase in the level of specific IgG antibodies in paired sera or on detection of specific IgM antibodies. The latter is the method of choice, when acute phase sera are lacking or when a rapid diagnosis based on testing only one blood specimen is required. Demonstration of specific IgG antibodies is indicative of past infection.

IMMUNE RESPONSE TO PRENATAL TORCH INFECTIONS

The immunoglobulin synthesis in the human fetus is initiated during the end of the first trimester[9]. The fetally produced immunoglobulins are mainly of IgM class. Almost all of the IgG in the fetal circulation is transferred from the mother through placenta by an active transport mechanism, whereas the IgM antibodies are normally not transferred to the fetus[10]. The level of serum IgG in the fetus at birth is equivalent to that of the mother. The concentration of the transferred antibodies declines thereafter, corresponding to a half-life of 20–30 days.

An intrauterine infection elicits a fetal synthesis of the specific IgM class antibodies. After birth the production of the specific immunoglobulins gradually changes from specific IgM to IgG antibodies.

Due to the high frequency of specific IgG antibodies to the agents of the TORCH group found in sera from normal pregnant women, the early serodiagnosis of the respective congenital infections is based on assays which detect the specific IgM class antibodies. The diagnosis may alternatively be established by a demonstration of the persistence of the specific IgG antibodies after disappearance of the maternal antibodies.

IMMUNOASSAYS FOR DETECTION OF ANTIBODIES

Several methods are available for serodiagnosis of the TORCH diseases. These include the neutralization test (NT), dye test (DT), complement-fixation (CF) test, agglutination tests, haemagglutination inhibition (HI) test, haemolysis-in-gel (HIG) test, fluorescent antibody (FA) test, radioimmunoassay (RIA) and enzyme-linked immunosorbent assay (ELISA).

Neutralization test

The NT depends on the ability of the specific antibodies to neutralize the infectivity of the corresponding virus. The infectivity is demonstrated in cell cultures either by a direct cytopathic effect or by interference with a challenge virus. The NT is time-consuming, laborious, technically difficult and only occasionally used for routine laboratory diagnosis. The NT has, however, been valuable as a sensitive reference method during the development of later assays.

The NT for detection of CMV antibodies has revealed antigenically different strains[11]. An antigenically broadly reactive laboratory strain AD 169 is commonly employed in assays for anti-CMV immunoglobulins. However, specific antibodies not detected by the AD 169 may occasionally be demonstrated by other strains.

The NT has been established for determination of type-specific HSV antibodies[12], but difficulties may be encountered in detection of type 2 antibodies, when type 1 antibodies also are present in the serum[13].

Dye test

The DT, developed in 1948 by Sabin and Feldman[14] for detection of toxoplasma antibodies, is based on the observation of changes, in the presence of complement, in living toxoplasma organisms after exposure to human serum. In serum without specific antibodies the parasites swell and are stained by Methylene Blue. If specific antibodies are present in the serum, the parasites will be distorted and remain unstained. The titre is the serum dilution in which half of the protozoa are stained or distorted.

About 1–3 weeks following acute toxoplasmosis, the DT becomes positive and maximum titres are reached after 1–2 months. The titres normally decrease a few months later, but high titres may persist for many years. The DT may be employed for the diagnosis of congenital toxoplasmosis by demonstration of persisting antibodies[15].

A disadvantage of the test is the requirement for living *Toxoplasma gondii* and for microscopic reading of the result. However, the assay is widely used for routine diagnosis due to the high precision, sensitivity and specificity. The method has been employed for the detection of IgM class toxoplasma antibodies in serum fractionated by rate zonal ultracentrifugation[16].

Complement-fixation test

The CF test utilizes the fixation of added complement to complexes of antigen and antibody. The reaction is visualized by red cells sensitized by a haemolysin. If the complement has been attached to the antigen–antibody complexes, none will be available for lysis of the sensitized red cells. The antigen can be supplied commercially or from a central national source, and micromodification of the technique is relatively easy to perform.

The CF test for toxoplasma antibodies may measure antibodies to a soluble antigen or to a cell wall antigen[17–19]. The CF antibodies to the soluble antigen develop later than the antibodies measured by the DT; the test may become negative a few years after an infection or remain positive for at least 10 years[20].

Rubella-specific CF antibodies appear from a few days up to 2–3 weeks after a rubella infection and disappear again a few years later[21]. The method is relatively insensitive and cannot be used as the only test for diagnosis of postnatal rubella. It may, however, be utilized as a supplement to the HI test for detection of increases in titre of paired samples obtained at a time when the HI antibodies have reached their maximal level[22]. The assay detects only antibodies of IgG class[23,24] and is consequently unsuited for the early diagnosis of congenital rubella. The limited time of persistence precludes application for screening for past infection.

The CF antibodies to CMV commonly appear approximately 2 weeks after the infection[25] and significant increases have been observed after primary as well as secondary infections[26]. Following an infection the maximal titre does not exceed those found in sera from blood donors[27], and the titres may later decline to undetectable levels[28]. Differences of CMV CF titres should probably be regarded with some reservation, as large fluctuations have been observed in a longitudinal study of plasma donors[29].

The CF test may be applied for diagnosis of postnatal HSV infections, but the method is relatively insensitive and unable to differentiate between antibodies to HSV types 1 and 2.

Agglutination and haemagglutination inhibition tests

The agglutination tests are based on the ability of specific antibodies to agglutinate particles which carry antigen on their surface. A titre is given as the highest dilution of the test serum which is able to agglutinate the particles.

In the Fulton direct agglutination test formalin-treated toxoplasma parasites are agglutinated by specific antibodies[30]. Non-specific agglutinators may occasionally cause false-positive results[31].

Tanned erythrocytes coated with antigen have been applied for the detection of antibodies to toxoplasma[32], rubellavirus[33], CMV[34] and HSV types 1 and 2[35].

The platelet aggregation test is applied for detection of antibodies by observation of the sedimentation patterns of platelets in a chequerboard of dilutions of test sera and CMV[36] or rubellavirus[24] antigens.

Rubellavirus and HSV antigens are able to agglutinate red blood cells. An inhibition of the agglutination by binding of specific antibodies to the antigens is utilized in the HI tests. Non-specific inhibitors and agglutinins which interfere in the reaction must be removed before the test by absorption to kaolin, heparin–$MnCl_2$ or dextran. Simultaneous absorption of specific antibodies or incomplete absorption of the non-specific inhibitors may cause false-negative or positive results[37]. The test is, however, generally considered reliable and sensitive and is widely applied as a routine method for determination of rubella antibodies.

The HI antibody titres increase very rapidly after an infection. This is a serious disadvantage, as significant increases cannot be determined if the first serum specimen has been obtained only a few days after appearance of the symptoms.

o

The tests detect immunoglobulins of all classes. A selective detection of IgM class-specific antibodies therefore requires a previous separation of the immunoglobulins in each sample. Rate zonal ultracentrifugation and separate testing of serum fractions containing the IgM antibodies by the HI test is widely applied for the detection of rubella-specific IgM antibodies[38]. The method is, however, laborious and the number of samples which can be tested is limited by the capacity of the ultracentrifuge. Gel filtration[39] and affinity chromatography[40] have also been applied for the separation of the IgM antibodies from the other immunoglobulins, but these procedures may be too inconvenient for large-scale use.

Contamination of the IgM containing fractions with minute amounts of IgG may cause false-positive results, particularly if the titre of the specific IgG antibodies is high. The separation of the immunoglobulins must therefore be controlled, e.g. by single radial immunodiffusion. Low levels of IgG antibodies – which could be responsible for false results – may, however, escape detection. Other methods have utilized a significant decrease of the IgM fractions after reduction by 2-mercaptoethanol for confirmation of positive results[41, 42].

In a recent modification of the HI test anti-IgM on a solid phase consisting of microtitration trays was employed for immunoabsorption of IgM antibodies in the test serum. Rubella-specific IgM antibodies attached to the solid phase were subsequently detected by a conventional HI test performed on the microtitration tray[43].

Haemolysis-in-gel test

The HIG test is based on the diffusion of antibodies in a gel plate containing antigen-coated erythrocytes. The test sera are added to prepunched wells in the gel, and the erythrocytes will be lysed in the presence of antibodies and complement. The diameters of the haemolytic zones, which are recorded after an overnight incubation, are proportional to the concentration of the specific antibodies. The results of the test adapted for determination of rubella antibodies[44] correlate well with those obtained by the HI test[45]. Specific IgM antibodies are not detected by the HIG test. The increase of the antibodies after a rubella infection is therefore delayed in relation to the HI test and diagnostic differences may be detected between samples obtained at a time when a constant level of the HI titres has been reached[45]. The performance of the test is technically very simple and special equipment is not required. The test has therefore been recommended as a suitable method for screening for rubella antibodies[46]. The shelf-life of the gel plates, which are commercially available, is restricted to a few weeks.

Fluorescent antibody test

In the FA test, infected tissue cultures grown on glass slides or in the bottom of microtitration trays are incubated with serial dilutions of the test sera. Specific antibodies in the serum samples bind to the antigen. Unbound serum constituents are removed by a washing procedure, and the cells are incubated with a solution of fluorescein-labelled anti-human immunoglobulin, which may be heavy chain specific. After repeated washing the slides are examined under a dark field microscope in ultraviolet light[47]. The presence of specific antibodies in the test serum will produce a yellow-green fluorescence of the infected cells. The method enables selective detection of antibodies of different classes without previous separation of the immunoglobulins.

Shortly after the development of the FA test it was realized that IgM RF might cause false-positive results of assays for detection of specific IgM antibodies. Further this interference is seen as a serious source of error in the RIA[48] and the ELISA[49], which also utilizes labelled anti-human IgM for detection of specific IgM antibodies. The false-positive results have been explained by a secondary binding of IgM RF to complexes of antigen and specific IgG[50].

Concentrations of IgM RF higher than approximately 3.5 IU/ml have been sufficient to produce false-positive results of an ELISA for rubella IgM antibodies[51]. Such concentrations were found in the sera from approximately 5% of healthy individuals. The conventional agglutination tests for measurement of RF are not sensitive enough to reveal all sera with a level of RF, which might cause false-positive results. Sensitive RIAs[52] or ELISA[53] may be utilized for this purpose.

The false-positive results can be avoided by removal of IgM RF or of IgG from the sample prior to the assay. The rate zonal ultracentrifugation may be applied for separation of IgG and IgM antibodies. Alternatively IgG can be absorbed by anti-γFc[54] or by protein A[49], which removes approximately 95% of the IgG antibodies, but also 30–40% of the IgM antibodies[55]. The removal of IgM RF can be accomplished by absorption to heat-aggregated human IgG[50] or by heat-aggregated IgG bound to latex particles[51, 52].

Antinuclear factors, which are IgG and IgM class antibodies to DNA[56] and other nuclear antigens may cause false-positive results if nuclear material is incorporated in the antigen. This has been reported in an FA test for toxoplasma antibodies[57] and in an ELISA for CMV antibodies[58]. Control antigens from non-infected cell cultures may disclose the false results of the CMV assays.

The antigen applied in FA tests for toxoplasma antibodies is a preparation of killed toxoplasma organisms. As the antigen can be stored, a continuous production of living parasites is not needed. The FA test and the DT measure antibodies against cell wall antigens and a close agreement between the results obtained by the two methods has been reported[59]. However, Remington and Desmonts[60] hold the opinion that the DT offers a more precise quantitation of the specific antibodies.

The IgM class toxoplasma antibodies detected by the FA test appear in the serum early during the disease, and disappear usually within 3–4 months, but may occasionally persist for longer periods[60]. These antibodies have been detected in sera from only 25% of infants with congenital toxoplasmosis[15]. In the absence of the specific IgM antibodies the serological diagnosis of the congenital infection depends on a demonstration of persisting IgG class antibodies measured, for example, by the IgG FA test or the DT.

In rubella serology the FA test has mainly been employed for detection of specific IgM class antibodies. The sensitivity is relatively low, when unseparated sera are tested[61] due to a competition between the specific IgM and IgG for the same antigenic sites. Removal of IgG prior to the test, e.g. by rate zonal ultracentrifugation, increases the sensitivity[62]. Specific IgM antibodies detected by this method persist usually for 1–3 months after the postnatal infection.

In studies of sera from infants with congenital rubella, specific IgM was detected in the majority of cases at an age of 6 months and in a few cases up to 2 years after birth[62].

The FA technique for measurement of IgG, IgA and IgM class CMV antibodies is applied without preceding separation of the immunoglobulins. The method detects antibodies to antigens situated in the nuclei of infected cell cultures. Sera from patients with varicella zoster or Epstein–Barr virus infections may cross-react in this assay[63].

Serum CMV IgM antibodies appear early in the postnatal infection[64] and persist usually for several months. The synthesis of the specific IgM immunoglobulins is not limited to primary infections, but has also been demonstrated after reinfections or reactivated disease[65].

For the diagnosis of congenital CMV infection the test for CMV-specific IgM antibodies is less sensitive than the demonstration of cytomegaloviruria. It is, however, assumed that the CMV macroglobulin-negative infants with CMV in the urine are most commonly unaffected by the congenital infection[66]. Newborn infants with symptoms due to a congenital CMV infection usually produce CMV IgM for months after birth[66].

An FA technique has been utilized for the detection of antibodies against the two HSV types. The antigens consisted of cell cultures infected with HSV type 1 and 2, respectively. The method was more sensitive than the CF test, but cross-reactions between antibodies against the HSV types were observed[67]. The detection of HSV IgM antibodies by the FA test has encountered problems possibly related to competition between specific IgG and IgM in the test and to interaction of IgM RF[68]. The HSV IgM antibodies may appear in sera from infected newborn infants 2–3 weeks after birth and persist during the first year of life[69].

Radioimmunoassay

The first RIAs for detection of antibodies were carried out in a liquid phase.

The radiolabelled antigen was incubated with the diluted test sera, the antigen–antibody complexes were precipitated by anti-immunoglobulins and the radioactivity in the precipitate determined. The liquid-phase RIA is a rather cumbersome method, due to the requirement for centrifugation or other methods for isolation of the antigen–antibody complexes and the need for an individual labelling of each antigen.

In the solid-phase RIAs for detection of specific antibodies the antigens used initially consisted of infected cell cultures on coverslides. However, a decrease of the background radioactivity and an increase of the sensitivity and specificity of the assay was obtained by the application of purified antigens from cell lysates or from the supernatants of infected cell cultures. The antigens can subsequently be non-specifically adsorbed to a solid phase, which may consist of the surface of polystyrene tubes, polystyrene or polyvinyl chloride microtitration trays or polystyrene beads. Alternatively, the antigens can be bound immunologically to specific antibodies attached to the solid phase.

After an incubation of the diluted serum specimens with the solid-phase antigen, specific antibodies are detected by ^{125}I-labelled anti-immunoglobulins. Labelled heavy chain specific anti-immunoglobulins can be applied for separate detection of specific antibodies belonging to different immunoglobulin classes, and the same labelled anti-immunoglobulins can be used for the detection of antibodies to different agents.

The solid-phase RIAs are generally sensitive and precise. The procedures can readily be automated and are thus suited for laboratories receiving large numbers of samples. The equipment is, however, expensive, the reagents unstable and a radiation hazard inherent.

A RIA developed for the detection of rubella IgG antibodies was more sensitive than the HI test[70]. Antibodies measured by this method appeared rapidly after rubella infections and usually reached the maximum level after 1 week[71]. As the IgM antibodies contribute to the HI test, but not to the IgG RIA, a significant increase in the titres in paired sera could occasionally be detected by the RIA at a time when the HI titre in the first sample had reached the maximum level[72].

The RIAs for measurement of rubella IgM antibodies have been applied without previous separation of the immunoglobulins. The method was more sensitive than the FA test[73] and the HI test after separation of the immunoglobulins by rate zonal ultracentrifugation[74] or by gel filtration[55]. Following postnatal rubella, the RIA IgM antibodies appeared within the first 4 days after the rash and persisted usually for 40–80 days[71].

The RIA has been used for an evaluation of the incidence of rubella IgM antibodies in the sera from infants born after maternal rubella during pregnancy[73]. The highest detection rate was observed after infections in early pregnancy and during the last months before delivery. The low frequency of rubella IgM detected in the sera from children born after maternal rubella 2–3 months prior to the birth, might be explained by a IgM antibody response in late pregnancy, which may resemble the postnatal response. The rubella IgM antibodies persisted in the sera from infants with congenital malformations or neonatal disease due to rubella from a few months until more than 2 years after birth[73]. These results indicate that the RIA may be a sensitive method for screening for congenital rubella.

In a RIA for detection of CMV-specific IgG and IgM antibodies, the antigen applied was a sonicate of CMV-infected cell cultures dried onto the surface of the wells in microtitration plates. The competition between specific IgG and IgM in the assay for CMV IgM was avoided by protein A absorption of IgG, and IgM RF was absorbed to IgG polymerized by glutaraldehyde[75].

An early RIA, for type-specific detection of HSV antibodies, utilized cell cultures in glass vials after infection with HSV type 1 or 2, respectively. Type-specific HSV antibodies were detected after absorption of the type-heterologous antibodies to infected cell cultures[76]. Kalimo et al.[77] applied a semi-purified HSV antigen on polystyrene beads and ^{125}I-labelled anti-human-γ or anti-human-ρ for detection of immunoglobulin class-specific HSV antibodies. The IgG RIA was more sensitive than the CF test. Severe reinfections elicited increases of both specific IgG and IgM antibodies. The method was suited also for the detection of antibodies in the cerebrospinal fluid[78].

Enzyme-linked immunosorbent assay

In ELISA, which was developed simultaneously by Engvall and Perlmann[79] and by van Weemen and Schuurs[80], labelled antibodies and antigens are applied in techniques which are analogous to the RIA. The radioactive isotope label has, however, been replaced by an enzyme. The results of an ELISA can thus be measured by a simple colorimeter or by an observation of the change of colour of an added substrate. As the assay is sensitive, inexpensive and rather easy to perform, it has attracted attention as a possible future screening method for the TORCH diseases.

In ELISAs for serodiagnosis of toxoplasmosis, the antigens applied have been either a crude supernatant or an extract from the supernatants obtained after centrifugation of a suspension of disrupted Toxoplasma gondii[81, 82]. The specific antibodies were detected by anti-human-immunoglobulin[82, 83] or by anti-IgG conjugates[81, 84]. The sensitivity of an ELISA was equal to that of the haemagglutination test, the FA technique and the DT, and an acceptable correlation between ELISAs and reference methods has been reported[81, 82, 84]. The lack of complete correlation may be explained by the complexity of the toxoplasma antigens and differences in the time of appearance of antibodies against the different antigens used in the assays. The ELISA can probably be developed for detection of antibodies against purified selected antigens and for determination of the IgM class-specific antibodies[84].

The detection of antibodies to rubella by the ELISA was described in 1975 by Voller and Bidwell[85]. The antigen employed in this assay has most commonly been the supernatants of infected cell cultures after purification by rate zonal ultracentrifugation[86,87] or by membrane and ultrafiltration[88]. Cellular antigens caused a high non-specific binding of immunoglobulins even after purification[89]. A control antigen from non-infected cell cultures was essential for identification of non-specific reactions in an ELISA for rubella IgM antibodies[90], but has not been mandatory in assays for rubella IgG antibodies (Vejtorp, unpublished).

The level of rubella antibodies has been given as a titre obtained by visual reading after the testing of serial dilutions of the serum specimens[86]. A measurement of the absorbence by spectrophotometry allows, however, a fully quantitative determination of the antibody level by examination of a single serum dilution. The absorbance can be related to a standard curve and the result given as IU or μg/ml[87].

Following postnatal rubella specific IgM antibodies were detected by an ELISA in serum samples obtained during the first 2 days after the rash. The appearance of the IgM antibodies commonly preceded the development of the specific IgG antibodies. The peak concentration was reached after approximately 1 week, and the specific IgM antibodies disappeared generally after 2–12 weeks[90].

The results of the rubella IgG ELISA correlated well with those of the HI and the HIG tests, the HI test, however, being the least sensitive[85,88,91]. The specific IgG antibodies in serial serum samples from patients with rubella were detected by ELISA approximately 4 days after the rash, and a plateau was reached after 50–120 days. The antibodies persisted for at least 10 years, although a minor decline of the concentration was observed[90]. The rather slow increase in antibody level indicates that a significant difference may be detected in paired sera, even when the first sample has been obtained with a delay of 10–20 days after the rash.

An ELISA for determination of CMV antibodies developed by Voller and Bidwell[92] has later been modified for selective measurement of specific IgG[28,93] and IgM antibodies[28,58]. Cappel et al.[28] employed a commercial antigen, whereas Schmitz et al.[58] reported non-specific reactions using two commercial antigens and preferred a purified nuclear antigen from CMV-infected cells. The results of a direct haemagglutination test[93] and a CF test[28] agreed with those of the ELISA for specific IgG antibodies, although higher titres were generally obtained by the ELISA. A close correlation was also found between the results of the CMV IgM ELISA and of the FA test for specific IgM antibodies[58].

Only little information is yet available on the potentials of the CMV IgM antibody ELISA for diagnosis of congenital CMV infections. However, Cappel et al.[28], have tested sera collected from 150 apparently healthy infants 1–2 days after birth and detected CMV IgM antibodies in only the two infants who excreted CMV in the urine.

During primary CMV infections in renal transplant patients[28,94] the development of the specific IgG and IgM antibodies was studied by an ELISA. The IgM antibodies persisted for 2–3 months in the sera from six of the ten patients and disappeared within 11 months in the remaining four patients. Reinfection or reactivation was commonly associated with the development of specific IgM antibodies and cytomegaloviuria.

Crude HSV type 1 and 2 antigens have been employed in the ELISA for the detection of type-specific HSV IgG antibodies. The antigens were bound immunologically to the solid phase and type-common antigenic sites blocked by type-heterologous rabbit antibodies[94]. Alternatively, purified HSV type 1 and type 2 antigens have been used in type-specific assays[95,96].

IMMUNOASSAYS FOR DETECTION OF ANTIGENS

Immunoassays for detection of antigens have been utilized only to a very limited extent for diagnosis of the TORCH diseases. Since infants with congenital CMV infections shed CMV in the urine at birth, and viruria also follows the postnatal infections, such methods could presumably be valuable for the diagnosis.

A type-specific detection of HSV antigens was accomplished by a FA technique developed by Nahmias et al. [97]. Cells from suspected lesions were fixed on coverslides and incubated with type-specific antibodies, which were fluorescein-labelled. In an analogous RIA, the fluorescein label was replaced by ^{125}I[98].

A double-sandwich ELISA developed by Miranda et al. [99] for detection of HSV type 1 antigen was less sensitive than the virus isolation technique. Vestergaard[100] has modified the assay by application of rabbit antibodies to HSV type 1 or type 2 antigens as 'catching' and 'detecting' antibodies on a solid phase consisting of microtitration trays. The assay was type-specific and more sensitive than the virus isolation method. By this test as little as 1 ng HSV antigen on a swab from a lesion could be detected within 3 h.

SCREENING FOR THE TORCH DISEASES

Screening is defined as the identification of unrecognized disease or defect by a rapidly applied test or examination[101]. Before the initiation of a screening procedure it has been advocated that a list of criteria should be satisfied[102]. The disease should constitute an important health problem either due to the severity or high prevalence. The test should be inexpensive and the predictive values of positive and negative results high. The possibilities for amelioration or cure should be better than if the disease was diagnosed at a stage at which symptoms had appeared.

Screening for the TORCH diseases has not been generally recommended, apart from the antibody testing prior to rubella vaccination, probably due to the lack of easy and reliable diagnostic methods and hence the necessary epidemiological information. Furthermore, specific therapy has not been available except for toxoplasmosis.

The incidence of congenital toxoplasmosis varies from area to area and detection rates between 1 in 1000 and 1 in 5000 have been reported[60, 103]. Early diagnosis and specific chemotherapy could presumably reduce the damage due to the congenital infection. A reliable screening method, however, is not yet available, since sera from only approximately 25% of infected newborn infants contain specific IgM antibodies detectable by the FA test. Identification of seronegative women, and abortion or specific therapy after seroconversion during pregnancy, constitutes another possible method for prevention, but it is unknown whether the costs of this approach are balanced in relation to the benefits.

Screening of women of child-bearing age for rubella antibodies, and vaccination of susceptibles, form an integrated part of established vaccination programmes. Since approximately 80–90% of adult women are immune to rubella due to previous infection, an antibody screening reduces the number of vaccinees and thus the risk of inadvertent vaccination of pregnant women. Vaccination programmes have in the USA significantly diminished the incidence of congenital rubella[104] and in the UK increased the proportion of young women who are immune to rubella[105].

The impact of congenital CMV infections varies widely, and incidences between 3 and 12 per 1000 infants have been published[106, 107]. A prospective study of an urban population in the USA has showed a high risk of intellectual impairment and of hearing loss among children who were prenatally infected, but without symptoms at birth. Prospective studies from Scandinavia have, however, detected very low incidences of congenital CMV and no neurological damage[108, 109].

Vaccines against CMV have been developed, but problems related to safety and effectivity remain to be solved[110]. The birth of some of the infected infants may be prevented by termination of the pregnancy upon demonstration of seroconversion during early pregnancy, but a more detailed knowledge of the effectiveness of this approach is needed before a screening programme is initiated. A screening for congenital CMV infections in selected population groups by detection of CMV IgM in cord blood may prove valuable, if a therapy capable of improving the prognosis of the infected children becomes available.

The incidence of the neonatal HSV infection has been estimated at 1 per 3500–30 000 deliveries[7]. Some of the infections could possibly be prevented by screening pregnant women for genital HSV infections, followed by Caesarean section or local treatment of the lesions in the infected women. However, precise information is not available on the incidence of the neonatal HSV infection, the risk for this infection in the presence of herpetic lesions of the mother and on the effectiveness of Caesarean section in the prevention of the neonatal disease. An ELISA for detection of HSV antigens would presumably constitute the most suitable screening procedure.

CONCLUSIONS

Reliable, easily performed and inexpensive immunoassays are needed for epidemiological surveys, which should be conducted for estimation of the requirements for prophylactic measures. Such assay could also be employed for testing of specimens from pregnant women or infants, who clinically are suspect of a TORCH disease.

The utilization of a single technique and common equipment would presumably be advantageous. Several of the necessary tests are available as RIAs and ELISAs, and both techniques seem suited for large-scale epidemiological surveys. However, the reagents and the equipment for an ELISA are less expensive, and an accelerating development of instruments for automation will facilitate the large-scale use of this technique. For testing small numbers of samples, ELISA is preferable due to the stability of the reagents, the need for only simple equipment and to the availability of an increasing range of commercial kits.

References

1. Nahmias, A. J., Walls, K. W., Steward, J. A., Herrmann, K. L. and Flynt, J. Jr. (1971). The TORCH complex – perinatal infections associated with toxoplasma and rubella, cytomegol- and herpes simplex viruses. *Pediatr. Res.*, **5**, 405

2. Embil, J. A., Ozere, R. L. and Haldane, E. V. (1970). Congenital cytomegalovirus infection in two siblings from consecutive pregnancies. *J. Pediatr.*, **77**, 417

3. Krech, U., Konjajev, Z. and Jung, M. (1971). Congenital cytomegalovirus infection in siblings from consecutive pregnancies. *Helv. Paediat. Acta*, **26**, 355

4. Stagno, S., Reynolds, D. W., Huang, E., Thames, S. D., Smith, R. J. and Alford, C. A. Jr. (1977). *Congenital cytomegalovirus infection*. Occurrence in an immune population. *N. Engl. J. Med.*, **296**, 1254

5. Nahmias, A., Josey, W., Naib, Z., Freeman, M., Fernandez, R. and Wheeler, J. (1971). Perinatal risk associated with maternal genital herpes simplex infection. *Am. J. Obstet. Gynecol.*, **110**, 825

6. Florman, A. L., Gershon, A. A., Blackett, P. R. and Nahmias, A. J. (1973). Intrauterine infection with herpes simplex virus: resultant congenital malformations. *J. Am. Med. Assoc.*, **225**, 129

7. Nahmias, A. J. and Visintine, A. M. (1976). Herpes simplex. In Remington, J. S. and Klein, J. O. (eds.) *Infectious Diseases of the Fetus and Newborn Infant*, pp. 156–90. (Philadelphia: W. B. Saunders Co.)

8. Nahmias, A. J. and Roizman, B. (1973). Herpes simplex viruses. *N. Engl. J. Med.*, **289**, 667

9. Gitlin, D. and Biasucci, A. (1969). Development of gamma G, gamma M, beta I_C, beta I_A, C′1 esterase inhibitor, ceruloplasmin, transferrin, hemopexin, haptoglobin, fibrinogen,

plasminogen, alpha-l-antitrypsin, orosomucoid, beta-lipoprotein, alpha-2-macroglobulin and pre-albumin in the human conceptus. *J. Clin. Invest.*, **48**, 1433

10. Gitlin, D., Kumate, J., Urrusti, J. and Morales, C. (1964). The selectivity of the human placenta in the transfer of plasma proteins from mother to fetus. *J. Clin. Invest.*, **43**, 1938

11. Andersen, H. K. (1972). Studies of human cytomegalovirus strain variations by kinetic neutralization tests. *Arch. Ges. Virusforsch.*, **38**, 297

12. Nahmias, A. J., Josey, W. E., Naib, Z. M., Luce, C. F. and Duffey, A. (1970). Antibodies to herpesvirus hominis type 1 and 2 in humans. *Am. J. Epidemiol.*, **91**, 539

13. Skinner, G. R. B., Thouless, M. E. and Jordan, J. A. (1971). Antibodies to type 1 and type 2 herpesvirus in women with abnormal cervical cytology. *J. Obstet. Gynaecol. Br. Commonw.*, **78**, 1031

14. Sabin, A. B. and Feldman, H. A. (1948). Dyes as microchemical indicators of a new immunity phenomenon affecting a protozoon parasite (toxoplasma). *Science*, **108**, 660

15. Desmonts, G. and Couvreur, J. (1975). Toxoplasmosis: epidemiologic and serologic aspect of perinatal infection. In Krugman, S. and Gershon, A. A. (eds.) *Infections of the Fetus and the Newborn Infant. Progress in Clinical and Biological Research*, Vol. 3, pp. 115–32. (New York: Alan R. Liss, Inc.)

16. Remington, J. S., Miller, M. J. and Brownlee, I. (1968). IgM antibodies in toxoplasmosis. I: Diagnostic significance in congenital cases and a method for their rapid demonstration. *Pediatrics*, **41**, 1068

17. Warren, J. and Sabin, A. (1942). The complement fixation in toxoplasmic infection. *Proc. Soc. Exp. Biol. Med.*, **51**, 11

18. Fleck, D. G. and Payne, R. A. (1963). Tests for toxoplasma antibody. *Mon. Bull. Minist. Health and Public Health Lab. Serv.*, **22**, 97

19. Karim, K. A. and Ludlam, B. (1975). The relationship and significance of antibody titres as determined by various serological methods in glandular and ocular toxoplasmosis. *J. Clin. Pathol.*, **28**, 42

20. Feldman, H. A. (1958). Toxoplasmosis. *Pediatrics*, **22**, 559

21. Vesikari, T., Kauppinen, M. A. and Vaheri, A. (1970). A two-year follow-up of rubella antibodies in a female population with special reference to reinfections. *Scand. J. Infect. Dis.*, **2**, 81

22. Banatvala, J. E., Best, J. M., Bertrand, J., Bowern, N. A. and Hudson, S. M. (1970). Serological assessment of rubella during pregnancy. *Br. Med. J.*, **3**, 247

23. Best, J. M., Banatvala, J. E. and Watson, D. (1969). Serum IgM and IgG responses in postnatally acquired rubella. *Lancet*, **2**, 65

24. Vesikari, T., Vaheri, A. and Leinikki, P. (1971). Antibody response to rubella virion (V) and soluble (S) antigens in rubella infection and following vaccination with live attenuated rubella virus. *Arch. Ges. Virusforsch.*, **35**, 25

25. Andersen, H. K. (1974). Cytomegalovirus infektion. *Thesis*. Aarhus.

26. Weller, T. H. (1971). The cytomegaloviruses: ubiquitous agents with protean clinical manifestations. *N. Engl. J. Med.*, **285**, 267

27. Mirkovic, R., Werch, J., South, M. A. and Benyesh-Melnick, M. (1971). Incidence of cytomegaloviremia in blood-bank donors and in infants with congenital cytomegalic inclusion disease. *Infect. Immunol.*, **3**, 45

28. Cappel, R., de Cuyper, F. and de Braekeleer, J. (1978). Rapid detection of IgG and IgM antibodies for cytomegalovirus by the enzyme-linked immunosorbent assay (ELISA). *Arch. Virol.*, **58**, 253

29. Waner, J. L., Weller, T. H. and Kevy, S. V. (1973). Patterns of cytomegaloviral complement-fixing antibody activity: a longitudinal study of blood donors. *J. Infect. Dis.*, **127**, 538

30. Fulton, J. D. and Turk, J. L. (1959). Direct agglutination test for *Toxoplasma gondii*. *Lancet*, **2**, 1068

31. Desmonts, G., Baufine, Ducrocq, H., Couqineau, P. and Peloux, Y. (1974). Anticorps

toxoplasmiques naturels. *Nouv. Presse Med.*, **3**, 1547

32. Jacobs, L. and Lunde, M. N. (1957). A hemagglutination test for toxoplasmosis. *J. Parasitol.*, **43**, 308

33. Safford, J. W. and Whittington, R. (1976). A passive hemagglutination assay for detecting rubella antibody. *Fed. Proc.*, **35**, 813

34. Fucillo, D. A., Moder, F. L., Traub, R. G., Hensen, S. and Sever, J. L. (1971). Micro indirect hemagglutination test for cytomegalovirus. *Appl. Microbiol.*, **21**, 104

35. Fucillo, D. A., Moder, F. L., Catalano, L. W. Jr., Vincent, M. M. and Sever, J. L. (1970). Herpesvirus hominis types I and II: a specific microindirect hemagglutination test. *Proc. Soc. Exp. Biol. Med.*, **133**, 735

36. Penttinen, K., Kääriäinen, L. and Myllylä, G. (1970). Cytomegalovirus antibody assay by platelet aggregation. *Arch. Ges. Virusforsch.*, **29**, 189

37. Schmidt, N. J. and Lennette, E. H. (1970). Variables of the rubella hemagglutination-inhibition test and their effect on antigen and antibody titres. *Appl. Microbiol.*, **19**, 491

38. Vesikari, T. and Vaheri, A. (1968). Rubella: a method for rapid diagnosis of a recent infection by demonstration of the IgM antibodies. *Br. Med. J.*, **1**, 221

39. Pattison, J. R., Dane, D. S. and Mace, J. E. (1975). Persistence of specific IgM after natural infection with rubella virus. *Lancet*, **1**, 185

40. Barros, M. F. and Lebon, P. (1975). Séparation des anticorps IgM anti-rubéole par chromatographie d'affinité. *Biomed. Express (Paris)*, **23**, 184

41. Newman, S., Horta-Barbosa, L. and Sever, J. L. (1969). Serological test for rubella. *Lancet*, **2**, 432

42. Field, P. R. and Murphy, A. M. (1972). The role of specific IgM globulin estimates in the diagnosis of acquired rubella. *Med. J. Austr.*, **2**, 1244

43. Krech, U. and Wilhelm, J. A. (1979). A solid-phase immunosorbent technique for the rapid detection of rubella IgM by haemagglutination inhibition. *J. Gen. Virol.*, **44**, 281

44. Strannegård, Ö., Grillner, L. and Lindberg, I. (1975). Hemolysis-in-gel test for the demonstration of antibodies to rubella virus. *J. Clin. Microbiol.*, **1**, 491

45. Väänänen, P. and Vaheri, A. (1979). Hemolysis-in-gel test in immunity surveys and diagnosis of rubella. *J. Med. Virol.*, **3**, 245

46. Vaheri, A., Saksela, O. and Väänänen, P. (1979). Rubella screening by haemolysis-in-gel test. *Lancet*, **2**, 644

47. Fraser, K. B., Shirodaria, P. V. and Stanford, C. F. (1971). Fluorescent staining and human IgM. *Br. Med. J.*, **3**, 707

48. Meurman, O. H. and Ziola, B. R. (1978). IgM class rheumatoid factor interference in the solid-phase radioimmunoassay of rubella-specific IgM antibodies. *J. Clin. Pathol.*, **31**, 483

49. Leinikki, P. O., Shekarchi, I., Dorsett, P. and Sever, J. L. (1978). Determination of virus-specific IgM antibodies by using ELISA: elimination of false-positive results with protein A-Sepharose absorption and subsequent IgM antibody assay. *J. Lab. Clin. Med.*, **92**, 849

50. Shirodaria, P. V., Fraser, K. B. and Stanford, F. (1973). Secondary fluorescent staining of virus antigens by rheumatoid factor and fluorescein-conjugated anti-IgM. *Ann. Rheum. Dis.*, **32**, 53

51. Vejtorp, M. (1980). The interference of IgM rheumatoid factor in enzyme-linked immunosorbent assays of rubella IgM and IgG antibodies. *J. Virol, Methods*, **1**, 1

52. Ziola, B., Meurman, O., Matikainen, M., Salmi, A. and Kalliomäki, J. L. (1978). Determination of human immunoglobulin M rheumatoid factor by a solid-phase radioimmunoassay which uses human immunoglobulin G in antigen–antibody complexes. *J. Clin. Microbiol.*, **8**, 134

53. Vejtorp, M., Høier-Madsen, M. and Halberg, P. (1979). Enzyme-linked immunosorbent assay for determination of IgM rheumatoid factor. *Scand. J. Rheumatol.*, **8**, 65

54. Gispen, R., Nagel, J., Brand-Saathof, B. and de Graaf, S. (1975). Immunofluorescence test for IgM rubella antibodies in whole serum after absorption with anti-γFc. *Clin. Exp. Immunol.*, **22**, 431

55. Kangro, H. O., Pattison, J. R. and Heath, R. B. (1978). The detection of rubella-specific IgM antibodies by radioimmunoassay. *Br. J. Exp. Pathol.*, **59**, 577

56. Aotsuka, S., Okawa, M., Ikebe, K. and Yokohari, R. (1979). Measurement of anti-double-stranded DNA antibodies in major immunoglobulin classes. *J. Immunol. Methods*, **28**, 149

57. Araujo, F. G., Barnett, E. V., Gentry, L. O. and Remington, J. S. (1971). False-positive anti-toxoplasma fluorescent-antibody tests in patients with antinuclear antibodies. *Appl. Microbiol.*, **22**, 270

58. Schmitz, H., Doerr, H.-W., Kampa, D. and Vogt, A. (1977). Solid-phase enzyme immunoassay for immunoglobulin M antibodies to cytomegalovirus. *J. Clin. Microbiol.*, **5**, 629

59. Walton, B. C., Benchoff, B. M. and Brooks, W. H. (1966). Comparison of the indirect fluorescent antibody test and methylene blue dye test for detection of antibodies to toxoplasma gondii. *Am. J. Trop. Med. Hyg.*, **15**, 149

60. Remington, J. S. and Desmonts, G. (1976). Toxoplasmosis. In Remington, J. S. and Klein, J. O. (eds.) *Infectious Diseases of the Fetus and Newborn Infants*, pp. 191–332. (Philadelphia: W. B. Saunders Co.)

61. Baublis, J. V. and Brown, G. C. (1968). Specific responses of the immunoglobulins to rubella infection. *Proc. Soc. Exp. Biol. Med.*, **128**, 206

62. Cradock-Watson, J. E., Ridehalgh, M. K. S. and Chantler, S. (1976). Specific immunoglobulins in infants with the congenital rubella syndrome. *J. Hyg. Camb.*, **76**, 109

63. Hanshaw, J. B., Niederman, J. C. and Chessin, L. N. (1972). Cytomegalovirus macroglobulin in cell-association herpesvirus infections. *J. Infect. Dis.*, **125**, 304

64. Lang, D. L. and Hanshaw, J. B. (1969). Cytomegalovirus infection and the postperfusion syndrome. *N. Engl. J. Med.*, **280**, 1145

65. Schmitz, H., Kampa, D., Doerr, H. W., Luthardt, T., Hillemanns, H. G. and Würtele, A. (1977). IgM antibodies to cytomegalovirus during pregnancy. *Arch. Virol.*, **53**, 177

66. Hanshaw, J. B. (1969). Congenital cytomegalovirus infection: laboratory methods of detection. *Pediatrics*, **75**, 1179

67. Leinikki, P. (1971). Immunofluorescent assay of herpesvirus type 1 and type 2 antibodies in rabbit and human sera. *Arch. Ges. Virusforsch.*, **35**, 349

68. Nahmias, A. J., Visintine, A. M., Reimer, C. B., Buono, I. D., Shore, S. L. and Starr, S. E. (1975). Herpes simplex virus infection of the fetus and newborn. In Krugman, S. and Gershon, A. A. (eds.) *Infections of the Fetus and the Newborn Infant. Progress in Clinical and Biological Research*, Vol. 3, pp. 63–77. (New York: Alan R. Liss, Inc.)

69. Nahmias, A. J., Dowdle, W. R., Josey, W. E., Naib, Z. M., Painter, L. M. and Luce, C. (1969). Newborn infection with herpesvirus hominis type 1 and 2. *Pediatrics*, **75**, 1194

70. Sugishita, C., O'Shea, S., Best, J. M. and Banatvala, J. E. (1978). Rubella serology by solid-phase radioimmunoassay: its potential for screening programmes. *Clin. Exp. Immunol.*, **31**, 50

71. Meurman, O. H. (1978). Persistence of immunoglobulin G and immunoglobulin M antibodies after postnatal rubella infection determined by solid-phase radioimmunoassay. *J. Clin. Microbiol.*, **7**, 34

72. Meurman, O. and Granfors, K. (1977). Completion of hemagglutination inhibition test by solid-phase radioimmunoassay test in routine diagnostic rubella serology. *Med. Biol.*, **55**, 241

73. Pattison, J. R., Anderson, M. J., Cradock-Watson, J. E., Ridehalgh, M. K. S. and Kangro, H. O. (1979). Comparison of immunofluorescence and radioimmunoassay for detecting IgM antibody in infants with the congenital rubella syndrome. Presented at the Meeting of European Association against Virus Diseases, 5–7 September, Munich

74. Meurman, O. H., Viljanen, M. K. and Granfors, K. (1977). Solid-phase radioimmunoassay of rubella virus immunoglobulin M antibodies: comparison with sucrose density gradient centrifugation test. *J. Clin. Microbiol.*, **5**, 257

75. Knez, V., Steward, J. A. and Ziegler, D. W. (1976). Cytomegalovirus specific IgM and IgG

response in humans studied by radioimmunoassay. *J. Immunol.*, **117**, 2006

76. Forghani, B., Schmidt, N. J. and Lennette, E. H. (1975). Solid phase radioimmunoassay for typing herpes simplex viral antibodies in human sera. *J. Clin. Microbiol.*, **2**, 410

77. Kalimo, K. O. K., Ziola, B. R., Viljanen, M. K., Granfors, K. and Toivanen, P. (1977). Solid-phase radioimmunoassay of herpes simplex virus IgG and IgM antibodies. *J. Immunol. Methods*, **14**, 183

78. Kalimo, K. O. K., Marttila, R. J., Ziola, B. R., Matikainen, M.-T. and Panelius, M. (1977). Radioimmunoassay of herpes-simplex and measles virus antibodies in serum and cerebrospinal fluid of patients without infections or demyelinating diseases of the central nervous system. *J. Med. Microbiol.*, **10**, 431

79. Engvall, E. and Perlmann, P. (1971). Enzyme-linked immunosorbent assay (ELISA). Quantitative assay of immunoglobulin G. *Immunochemistry*, **8**, 871

80. Van Weemen, B. K. and Schuurs, A. H. W. M. (1971). Immunoassay using antigen-enzyme conjugates. *FEBS Lett.*, **15**, 232

81. Walls, K. W., Bullock, S. L. and English, D. K. (1977). Use of the enzyme-linked immunosorbent assay (ELISA) and its microadaptation for the serodiagnosis of toxoplasmosis. *J. Clin. Microbiol.*, **5**, 273

82. Voller, A., Bidwell, D. E., Bartlett, A., Fleck, D. G., Perkins, M. and Oladehin, B. (1976). A microplate enzyme-immunoassay for toxoplasma antibody. *J. Clin. Pathol.*, **29**, 150

83. Denmark, J. R. and Chessum, B. S. (1978). Standardization of enzyme-linked immunosorbent assay (ELISA) and the detection of toxoplasma antibody. *Med. Lab. Science*, **35**, 227

84. Boniolo, A., Dovis, M., Petruzzelli, E., Rolleri, E., Zannino, M. and Malvano, R. (1979). In Malvano, R. (ed.) *The Immunoenzymatic Assay*. Proc. Europ. Workshop, Tirrenia, Pisa, 23–27 April. (The Hague: Martinus Nijhoff)

85. Voller, A. and Bidwell, D. E. (1975). A simple method for detecting antibodies to rubella. *Br. J. Exp. Pathol.*, **56**, 338

86. Gravell, M., Dorsett, P. H., Gutenson, O. and Ley, A. C. (1977). Detection of antibody to rubella virus by enzyme-linked immunosorbent assay. *J. Infect. Dis.* (Suppl.), **136**, 300

87. Leinikki, P. O., Shekarchi, I., Dorsett, P. and Sever, J. L. (1978). Enzyme-linked immunosorbent assay determination of specific rubella antibody levels in micrograms of immunoglobulin G per milliliter of serum in clinical samples. *J. Clin. Microbiol.*, **8**, 419

88. Vejtorp, M. (1978). Enzyme-linked immunosorbent assay for determination of rubella IgG antibodies. *Acta Path. Microbiol. Scand.*, *B*, **86**, 387

89. Forghani, B. and Schmidt, N. J. (1979). Antigen requirements, sensitivity and specificity of enzyme immunoassays for measles and rubella viral antibodies. *J. Clin. Microbiol.*, **9**, 657

90. Vejtorp, M., Fanøe, E. and Leerhoy, J. (1979). Diagnosis of postnatal rubella by the enzyme-linked immunosorbent assay for rubella IgM and IgG antibodies. *Acta Path. Microbiol. Scand.*, *B*, **87**, 155

91. Morgan-Capner, P., Pullen, H. J. M., Pattison, J. R., Bidwell, D. E., Bartlett, A. and Voller, A. (1979). A. comparison of three tests for rubella antibody screening. *J. Clin. Pathol.*, **32**, 542

92. Voller, A. and Bidwell, D. E. (1976). Enzyme-immunoassays for antibodies in measles, cytomegalovirus infections and after rubella vaccination. *Br. J. Exp. Pathol.*, **57**, 243

93. Castellano, G. A., Hazzard, G. T., Madden, D. L. and Sever, J. L. (1977). Comparison of the enzyme-linked immunosorbent assay and the indirect hemagglutination test for detection of antibody to cytomegalovirus. *J. Infect. Dis.* (Suppl.), **136**, 337

94. Vestergaard, B. F. and Grauballe, P. C. (1979). ELISA for herpes simplex virus type-specific antibodies in human sera using HSV type 1 and type 2 polyspecific antigens blocked with type-heterologous rabbit antibodies. *Acta Path. Microbiol. Scand.*, *B*, **87**, 261

95. Vestergaard, B. and Grauballe, P. C. (1979). Isolation of the major herpes simplex virus type 1-specific glycoprotein by hydroxylapatite chromatography and its use in ELISA for titration of human type 1-specific antibodies. *J. Clin. Microbiol.*, **10**, 772

96. Grauballe, P. C. and Vestergaard, B. F. (1977). ELISA for herpes simplex virus type 2 antibodies. *Lancet*, **2**, 1038

97. Nahmias, A. J., Buono, I. del, Pipkin, J., Hutton, R. and Wickliffe, C. (1971). Rapid identification and typing of herpes simplex virus types 1 and 2 by a direct immunofluorescence technique. *Appl. Microbiol.*, **22**, 455

98. Forghani, B., Schmidt, N. J. and Lennette, E. H. (1974). Solid phase radioimmunoassay for identification of herpesvirus hominis types 1 and 2 from clinical materials. *Appl. Microbiol.*, **28**, 661

99. Miranda, Q. R., Bailey, G. D., Fraser, A. S. and Tenoso, H. J. (1977). Solid-phase enzyme immunoassay for herpes simplex virus. *J. Infect. Dis.* (Suppl.), **136**, 304

100. Vestergaard, B. F. (1980). Diagnosis and typing of herpes simplex virus in clinical samples by the enzyme-linked immunosorbent assay. Presented at the International Conference on Human Herpesviruses, 17–21 March, Atlanta.

101. Commission on Chronic Illness (1957). *Chronic Illness in the United States*, Vol. 1. (Cambridge, Mass.: Harvard University Press)

102. Wilson, J. M. G. and Jungner, G. (1968). *Principles and Practice of Screening for Disease.* (Geneva: World Health Organization)

103. Fleck, D. G. (1979). Toxoplasmosis. *J. Antimicrob. Chemother.* (Suppl. A), **5**, 78

104. Preblud, S. T., Brandling-Bennett, A. D. and Hinman, A. R. (1979). An update on measles, mumps and rubella. Presented at the 14th Immunization Conference, 12–15 March, St. Louis, Missouri.

105. Clarke, M., Schild, G. C., Boustred, J., Seagroatt, V., Pollock, T. M., Finlay, S. E. and Barbara, J. A. J. (1979). Effect of rubella vaccination programme on serologic status of young adults in United Kingdom. *Lancet*, **1**, 1224

106. Ahlfors, K., Ivarsson, S.-A., Johnsson, T. and Svanberg, L. (1979). Preliminary report: a prospective study on congenital and acquired cytomegalovirus infections in infants. *Scand. J. Infect. Dis.*, **11**, 177

107. Starr, J. G., Bart, R. D. and Gold, E. (1970). Inapparent congenital cytomegalovirus infection. Clinical and epidemiological characteristics in early infancy. *N. Engl. J. Med.*, **282**, 1075

108. Hanshaw, J. B., Scheiner, A. P., Moxley, A. W., Gaev, L., Abel, V. and Scheiner, B. (1976). School failure and deafness after 'silent' congenital cytomegalovirus infection. *N. Engl. J. Med.*, **295**, 468

109. Andersen, H. K., Brostrøm, K., Hansen, K. B., Leerhoy, J., Pedersen, M., Østerballe, O., Felsager, U. and Mogensen, S. (1979). *Acta Paedatr. Scand.*, **68**, 329

110. Dudgeon, J. A. (1973). Future developments in prophylaxis. In *Intrauterine Infections*. Ciba Foundation Symposium 10 (new series), p. 179. (Amsterdam: Associated Scientific Publishers)

28
Current Status of Specific IgM Antibody Assays

SHIREEN CHANTLER and J. A. DIMENT

The presence of specific IgM antibody in neonatal and adult sera is usually indicative of active or recent infection[1-14]. Reliable methods of detecting low levels of IgM class antibody are of considerable clinical value for the early detection of infections and parasitic diseases.

Radioimmunoelectrophoresis, described by Miller and Owen in 1960, was the first method of determining the immunoglobulin class of antibody bound to a particular antigen[15]. Modifications of the original method have been described using immunodiffusion to immobilize each class of test antibody prior to flooding the gel with radiolabelled antigen[16]. Several sera can be examined by this technique but the procedure is lengthy, requires radio-labelled antigen and the results are qualitative. Nonetheless, the system does provide a useful 'at a glance' assessment of the class of reactive antibody and the method is still used, particularly in the field of allergy. The red cell linked antigen : antiglobulin test has also been used to detect specific IgA, IgG, IgE and IgM antibody by Coombs and his colleagues[17,18]. In this method antigen-coupled red blood cells (RBCs) are reacted with sub-agglutinating levels of test serum followed by exposure to immunoglobulin class-specific antibody which gives rise to visible agglutination if the appropriate immunoglobulin is bound at the first stage. Attempts to overcome the difficulties of binding antigen to RBCs and eliminating the interference of the major classes of antibody in the detection of the minor immunoglobulin classes include the use of mixed agglutination and indicator RBCs coupled with class-specific antisera[19]. This approach has been less widely exploited than that using labelled class-specific reagents.

DETECTION OF SPECIFIC IgM BY LABELLED DETECTOR ANTIBODY TECHNIQUES

These assays utilize antigen physically or chemically bound to a solid phase or present in microscopical slide preparations to bind antibody from the test serum. The presence of bound antibody is detected by the use of labelled antibody immunospecific for the immunoglobulin class under test (Figure 28.1). The principle of this type of assay is analogous irrespective of whether

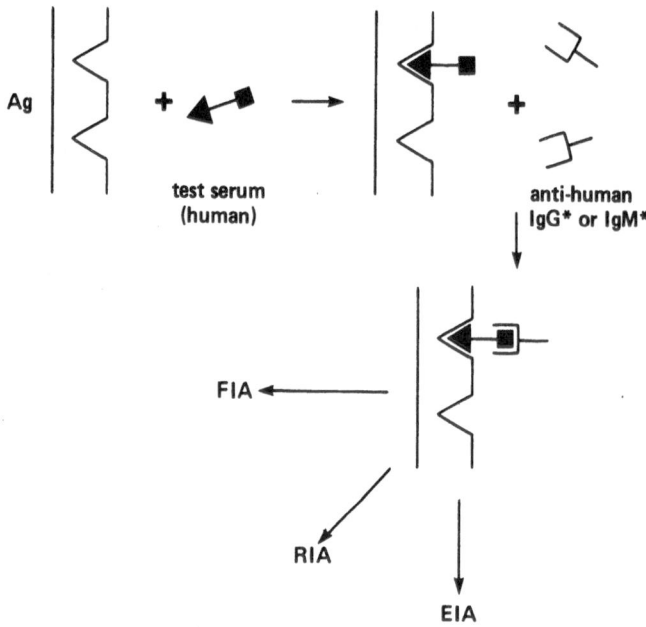

Figure 28.1 Schematic diagram of labelled detector antibody method. ■—▸ , antibody; ⊐— labelled antihuman IgM

the label is a radioisotope, a fluorescent dye, an enzyme or RBC. The only difference between these procedures is the method used for measuring or visualizing the presence of bound marker.

Immunofluorescent tests using fluorochrome-labelled anti-human IgM conjugates were extensively used in the late 1960s to demonstrate IgM antibody against viruses[3, 4, 10], bacteria[6, 9, 14] and parasites[5, 13] and were followed by the application of less subjective radioimmunoassays[20-28]. Concurrent with this was the development of enzyme-linked immunosorbent assays (ELISA) by Engvall and Perlmann[29, 30] which were later modified to detect specific IgM antibody[31]. The use of antigen adsorbed to individual spheres[27, 32] and microtitre plates[33, 34] in preference to the antigen-containing slide preparations used in immunofluorescence has considerable practical advantages which, coupled with the ease of qualitative and quantitative assessment of the soluble coloured reaction products obtained with enzyme labels, has resulted in the increased use of ELISA assays for the detection of specific IgM antibody[35-46].

Labelled detector antibody procedures are extensively used for the demonstration of specific IgM in test samples but many studies clearly indicate several limitations to this approach. These include the use of conjugates of uncertain immunospecificity[47,48], the failure to detect low levels of specific IgM in the presence of proportionally high levels of IgG antibody as a result of competitive inhibition between IgG and IgM antibodies for the same antigenic sites[11,49-54] and the interference by IgM class anti-immunoglobulin in the test sample reacting with IgG antibody which has combined with antigen so giving a false-positive IgM reaction[51,52,55-62]. A schematic illustration of these technical limitations is shown in Figure 28.2.

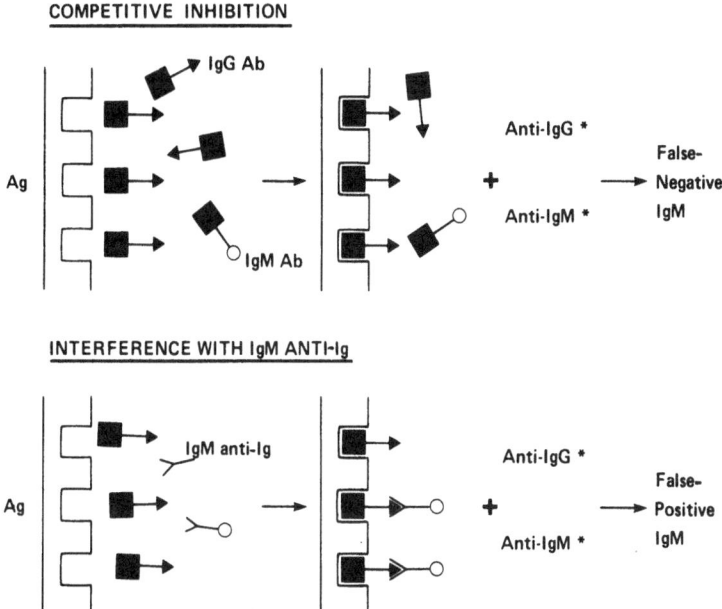

Figure 28.2 Schematic illustration of factors affecting interpretation of IgM status in labelled detector antibody method. ▮→ , IgG antibody; ▮—○, IgM antibody; ⊃—○ , IgM anti-Ig

The use of defined systems of comparable sensitivity to that used in the test procedure for evaluation of immunospecificity of conjugates[48,52,63] has eliminated problems relating to dubious specificity of reagents. An analysis of the contribution of competitive inhibition in labelled detector antibody procedures raises some intriguing anomalies. Competitive inhibition clearly participates in immunofluorescent tests for rubella-specific IgM[28,49,52] but does not appear to be a problem if radiolabelled[25,26,28] or enzyme-labelled[41,42,46] detector antibody is used. Differences in the nature, quantity and spatial distribution of the substrate antigen may account for these divergent results. The interference by IgM class anti-immunoglobulin has been observed to participate in most of these assays[25,26,28,42,46].

Considerable effort has been directed towards eliminating the inherent problems of competitive inhibition and interference by IgM anti-Ig. The methods commonly involve pretreatment of the test sample prior to assessing class-specific or total antibody activity in conventional immunoassays. The major procedures adopted are summarized in Table 28.1.

Table 28.1   Serum pretreatment procedures used in specific IgM antibody assays

Category	Procedure	Immunoassay
Separation of IgG and IgM	chromatography	IF, HA, HAI, RIA
	density gradient centrifugation	IF, HA, HAI, RIA
Removal IgM anti-Ig	aggregated IgG or latex IgG	IF, RIA, ELISA
Removal IgG	protein A	IF, HAI, ELISA
	anti-IgG	IF
Removal IgM	2ME	IF, HA, HAI
Removal IgG + IgM anti-Ig	protein A + latex IgG or aggregated IgG	IF

IF: Immunofluorescence
HA: Haemagglutination
HAI: Haemagglutination inhibition
RIA: Radioimmunoassay
ELISA: Enzyme-linked immunosorbent assay

PHYSICAL SEPARATION METHODS

On theoretical grounds methods which enable complete separation of IgG and IgM should eliminate the above limitations. Physical separation by filtration chromatography using dextran[63-65], agarose[66,67] or controlled pore size glass[68] and sucrose density gradient centrifugation[7,8,52,69-74] may achieve this objective. These procedures are time-consuming and certainly impractical if large numbers of samples are to be handled, give rise to dilution of the test sample which may result in decreased sensitivity, and can result in incomplete separation of IgG and IgM[71,75], so that some method of monitoring fractions in test runs to ensure the use of fractions showing total separation of immunoglobulin classes is mandatory. The monitoring system must have an equivalent sensitivity to the immunoassay used in the second step to avoid erroneous results due to contamination of samples[63,74,76]. Separation procedures reliant upon differences in molecular size are also subjected to the possibility that IgM anti-Ig : specific IgG complexes eluted in the high molecular weight fraction (i.e. IgM fraction) may give false-positive reactions in haemagglutination (HA) or haemagglutination inhibition (HAI) tests which do not discriminate between different classes of antibody. Several groups using fractionation in combination with HAI have reported ambiguous results, and postulate that polymers of IgG present in the high molecular weight fraction could account for these findings[67,71]. On the other hand, other workers have found sucrose density gradient fractionation of sera prior to evaluation in HAI or in class discriminatory assays to provide a reliable test for specific IgM[8,52].

Despite the limitations separation of immunoglobulin class does minimize the possibility of false-negative IgM by decreasing the possibility of competitive inhibition, as recently shown by Pyndiah et al.[53].

SELECTIVE REMOVAL OF IgM ANTI-IMMUNOGLOBULIN (IgM ANTI-Ig)

Several workers have used aggregated IgG or IgG coupled to latex particles as a means of eliminating false-positive IgM reactions due to IgM anti-Ig[56,57,60-62]. Although these procedures are effective in the majority of cases they are not invariably so, presumably due to the differing avidity of IgM anti-Ig. The data in Table 28.2 illustrate the problems encountered in the

Table 28.2 Detection of toxoplasma-specific IgM by immunofluorescence in serum samples absorbed with latex IgG

Samples with defined specific IgM*		Presence of IgM after absorption with latex IgG	
+	−	+	−
16		14	2
	11	2	9

* Specific IgM defined as IgM activity after sequential absorption with protein A-positive *Staphylococcus aureus* and latex IgG

demonstration of toxoplasma IgM antibody in serum samples absorbed with latex IgG where two of the 11 known IgM-negative sera gave false-positive IgM staining despite absorption. The major disadvantage of this simple absorption procedure lies in its failure to eliminate competitive inhibition by specific IgG antibody. This is seen in Table 28.2 where two of the 16 known IgM-positive samples were not detected. The practical significance of competition between IgG and IgM antibodies in diagnostic systems is likely to vary but cannot be ignored in specific IgM assays.

SELECTIVE REMOVAL OF IgG

It is well established that protein A present on the cell wall of certain strains of *Staphylococcus aureus* combines with the Fc region of human IgG[77-80]. This preferential removal of IgG forms the basis of specific IgM assays utilizing protein A-positive organisms or protein A Sepharose adsorbents[42,61,81-84]. These methods are easy and rapid to perform allowing a large number of samples to be processed, avoid dilution of the test sample, and minimize competitive inhibition, but opinion is divided on the efficacy of indisputable IgM detection.

Although extensive early work claimed that IgM was not removed by protein A[78-80] subsequent reports have shown that some IgM can be adsorbed and the amount varies with different test samples, as seen in Table 28.3[54,61,83,85,86]. This may influence the ease of detecting low levels of

Table 28.3 Percentage removal of total IgG and IgM from human sera following absorption with protein A-positive *Staphylococcus aureus*

No. of samples	Percentage removal of:	
	IgG	IgM
33	94.5 ± 4.9	
27		46.5 ± 21

specific IgM and should be considered in any assay. However, a single dilution drop in titre would not be regarded as significant in any assay utilizing titration by serial-doubling dilution. Protein A absorption fails to remove IgA, hence any residual specific IgA even at low levels could give rise to reactivity wrongly attributed to IgM in assays measuring total antibody activity. Protein A absorbents remove a substantial amount, but not all, of IgG. The failure to completely remove IgG can result in reactivity in subsequent total antibody assays or give false-positive IgM reactivity due to interaction with IgM anti-Ig in antibody class discriminatory assays. Some investigators claim that false-positive IgM reactivity is removed by protein A absorbents[42] but the data shown in Table 28.4, and that reported by other groups[61,62,83,84], indicate that this does not always occur. Five of 17 toxoplasma IgM-negative samples listed in the table gave false-positive IgM staining following absorption with *Staphylococcus aureus* alone. Additional absorption with aggregated IgG or latex IgG to remove IgM anti-Ig[61,82] or 2ME treatment to confirm IgM participation[54,74] has been advocated as a means of overcoming this problem.

Alternative procedures for removing IgG by the addition of anti-human IgG have been reported[59,87] but the use of liquid antiserum is not to be recommended because of the likelihood of specific IgG: anti-IgG-soluble

Table 28.4 Detection of specific IgM by immunofluorescence in serum samples absorbed with protein A containing *Staphylococcus aureus*

Samples with defined specific IgM*		Presence of IgM after absorption with Staph. aureus	
+	−	+	−
23		23	0
	17	5	12

* As for Table 28.2

complex formation which could interfere in subsequent immunoassay. The use of solid-phase anti-IgG absorbents would be preferable, but in practice we have found these to lack the capacity to effectively remove all IgG when used in rapid tube centrifugation methods.

SELECTIVE REMOVAL OF IgM

Many serological tests for specific IgM rely upon the selective chemical denaturation of IgM by 2-mercaptoethanol pretreatment of test serum. A significant decrease in the end-point titre in subsequent immunoassay compared with the untreated sample is indicative of the presence of specific IgM antibody in the original sample[1,2,88-90]. This test has produced some useful data but has been found to be unreliable in rubella[8,71,89] and toxoplasma[69,90]. We have observed a fall in titre in sera from patients with toxoplasma indicating IgM antibody participation in the absence of specific IgM and conversely no decreased response in samples with defined IgM activity (Table 28.5). In the presence of low levels of specific IgM and high levels of specific IgG antibody, denaturation of IgM will fail to have a significant effect on the total antibody titre. In conjunction with class discriminatory assays, 2ME treatment will not differentiate between IgM

Table 28.5 Effect of chemical denaturation of IgM on the haemagglutination activity (HA) obtained with sera from patients with toxoplasmosis

Samples with defined specific IgM*		HA titre after 2ME	
+	−	Change †	No change
7		3	4
	6	3	3

* As for Table 28.2
† Minimum four-fold decrease in titre

reactivity due to specific antibody and that due to interaction between specific IgG and IgM anti-Ig.

It is clear that all procedures adopted so far for the detection of specific IgM suffer from some kind of limitation. There is indisputable evidence that IgM anti-Ig can affect most assays; the practical significance of competitive inhibition is less certain as recent data suggest that the extent of its participation may be related to the nature and spatial distribution of the antigen substrate employed. A critical analysis of the extensive work done in this area indicates that at the present time the most reliable results are obtained by sequential absorption of the sample with both protein A and IgG absorbents, or the use of monitored fractions obtained by physical separation followed by class-specific detection methods for both IgG and IgM.

ANTIBODY CLASS CAPTURE ASSAYS (ACCA) FOR DETECTION OF SPECIFIC IgM ANTIBODY

The principle of antibody class capture assays reverses the conventional approach of selecting antibody from test serum on the basis of its specificity for antigen[91-95]. In this approach, shown schematically in Figure 28.3, IgM is

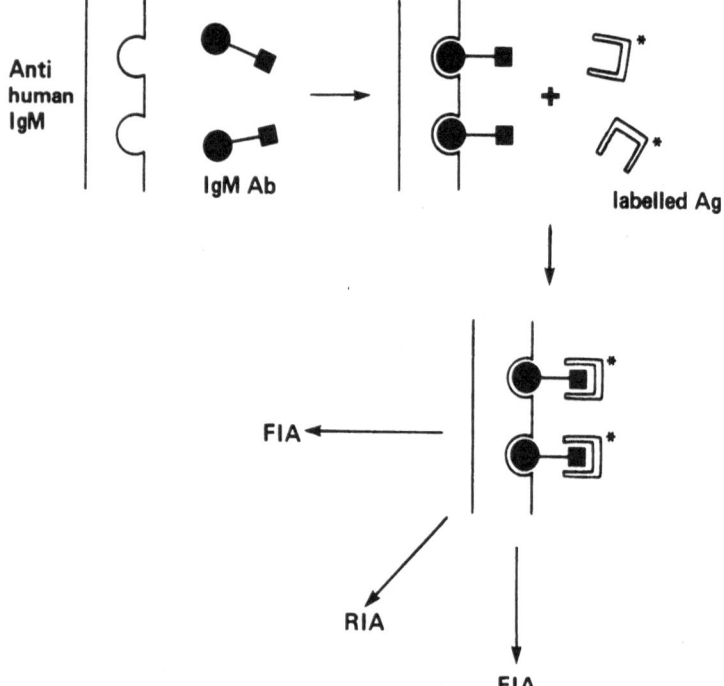

Figure 28.3 Schematic diagram of antibody class capture assay (ACCA). ■—●, IgM antibody; ⊐, labelled antigen

selectively removed from the test sample by anti-IgM antiserum physically adsorbed or chemically coupled to a solid phase. The immunoreactivity of bound IgM for a particular antigen is determined by the use of labelled antigen[91–93,96] or alternatively unlabelled antigen and labelled antibody directed against the test antigen[94,95,97,98]. The potential technical and diagnostic value of this method has stimulated its use for the detection of IgM antibody against hepatitis A[94,95,100], hepatitis B[98], Sendai virus[97], rubella[99] and *Mycoplasma pneumoniae*[96] as shown in Table 28.6. The extended application of these assays will depend upon the specificity and sensitivity achieved in practice.

Table 28.6   Antibody class capture assays (ACCA)

Ig class	Solid phase	Antigen	Detection system	Reference
IgE	cellulose	β-lactoglobulin	[^{125}I]β-lactoglobulin	91
IgG	Sepharose	subtilisin	[^{125}I]subtilisin	92
IgG/IgM	Sepharose	pigeon IgG	[^{125}I]pigeon IgG	93
IgM	PVC	hepatitis A	HRP–F(ab')$_2$ anti-HAV	94, 95
IgM	PVC	Sendai virus	HRP–Sendai virus	97
IgM	PS	hepatitis B	HRP–IgG anti-HBc	98
IgM	PVC	hepatitis A	HRP–IgG anti-HAV	100
IgM	PS	rubella	haemagglutination inhibition	99
IgM	PVC	*Mycoplasma pneumoniae*	[^{3}H]*M. pneumoniae*	96

PVC: Polyvinyl chloride microtitre plates
PS: Polystyrene microtitre plates
HRP: Horseradish peroxidase

Recent studies employ physical adsorption of the capture antibody to microtitre plates which offers the practical advantage of handling large numbers of test samples. The capacity of this capture antibody : solid phase is limited by the surface area of the microtitre well and the quality of the coating antibody used. it is essential that a high proportion of IgM from the test sample is adsorbed. In the absence of this the result will be influenced by the total IgM levels in individual samples and it is likely that test sera with low specific IgM and high total IgM will present the greatest problems. Stringent selection of coating antibody with high capacity is likely to be of paramount importance in achieving the desired level of sensitivity.

There are insufficient data on the relative sensitivity of ACCA assays and other conventional assays. Although Ertl *et al.* find an IgM class capture assay to be substantially more sensitive than an IgM ELISA no detailed comparisons have been made[97]. The criteria used to discriminate between positive and negative samples in these assays vary considerably between different workers. The 'cut-off' value, commonly greater than twice the negative control value, is somewhat arbitrary and it is likely that the greatest problem will be in interpreting the IgM status of borderline values. The data in Table 28.7 illustrate the interpretative problems encountered in an ACCA system for rubella IgM. Samples with significant levels of IgM antibody present no problem, but some sera with low levels of IgM antibody give only marginally higher values than control samples which, on the basis of conventional assays, are IgM-negative.

Table 28.7   Detection of rubella-specific IgM in ACCA using ^{125}I-labelled antibody

Serum	IgM status*	Binding ratio †
1	−	0.67
2	−	0.8
3	weak +	1.2
4	+	1.65
5	+	3.41
6	+	5.47
7	+	7.0

* Presence of IgM determined by conventional assay

† Expressed as ratio of counts by test/negative +3 SD

The specificity of the capture antibody solid phase, and an awareness of the factors which can affect this, are important. The specificity of the test can be influenced by non-immunological binding of IgG antibody or immunological binding of IgG antibody as a result of cross-reactivity present in the coating anti-IgM or subsequent to the adsorption of IgM anti-IgG on the solid phase, as shown schematically in Figure 28.4. High binding ratios have been observed with occasional sera which are not reduced by 2ME treatment, indicating that IgG antibody is bound to the solid phase[96]. Whether this is due to poor specificity of the anti-IgM coating antibody, or non-immunological binding of specific IgG, is uncertain; but other workers do not find cross-reactivity of coating antibody to be a problem with different antisera on the solid phase[95]. The absorption of IgM anti-Ig to the solid phase may lead to erroneous results, either by binding IgG antibody which in turn reacts with the test antigen, or alternatively by binding the labelled antibody conjugate used in the final step. IgM anti-Ig in test samples has been shown to interfere in these assays[95,98]; pre-absorption of samples with aggregated IgG[98,99], and the use of F(ab')$_2$ conjugates[95] have been found to abolish this interference.

The theoretical advantages of the ACCA principle for the determination of

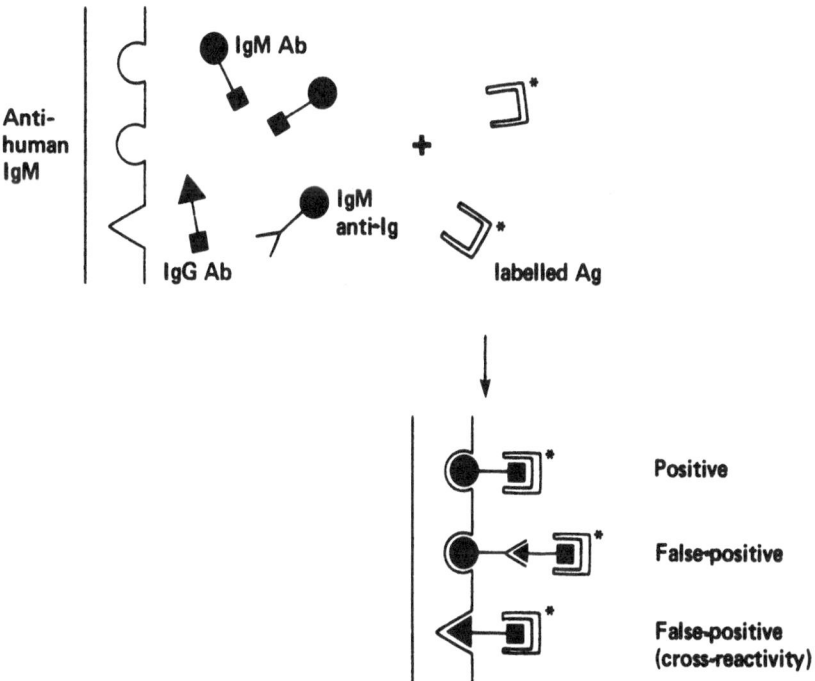

Figure 28.4 Schematic illustration of factors affecting specificity of ACCA. ■—●, IgM antibody; >—●, IgM anti-Ig; ■—▶, IgG antibody

specific IgM antibody are considerable. Since IgM is selectively attached to the solid phase immunoadsorbent during the first incubation competitive inhibition, which is an inherent problem in conventional immunoassays for IgM, is eliminated. The difficulties of obtaining antigens in a purified form suitable for conventional assays or attaching them physically or chemically to a solid phase without loss of antigenicity are eliminated, as the antibody absorbed from the test sample effectively immunopurifies the antigen '*in situ*'. The assay also offers considerable flexibility in enabling the choice of using labelled antigen or antibody for the detection of IgM antibodies against a variety of different antigens by radioimmunoassay[91-93], enzyme immuno-assay[93,95,98,100] and agglutination systems[99]. The use of antibody class capture assays for the detection of specific IgM is in its infancy. A considerable effort is required to determine the specificity and sensitivity of the assay in comparison with methods currently in use, and to eliminate the possibility of false-positive and false-negative results which bedevil current assays. If these requirements can be met, IgM class capture assays are likely to be the method of choice for the detection of specific IgM antibody.

References

1. Schluederberg, A. (1965). *Nature*, **205**, 1232
2. Banatvala, J. E., Best, J. M., Kennedy, E. A., Smith, E. E. and Spence, M. E. (1967). *Br. Med. J.* **3**, 285
3. Baublis, J. V. and Brown, G. C. (1968). *Proc. Soc. Exp. Biol. (N.Y.)*, **128**, 206
4. Cohen, S. M., Ducharme, C. P., Carpenter, C. A. and Deibel R. (1968). *J. Lab. Clin. Med.*, **72**, 760
5. Remington, J. S., Miller, M. J. and Brownlee, I. (1968). *J. Lab. Clin. Med.*, **71**, 855
6. Scotti, A. T. and Logan, L. (1968). *J. Pediatr.*, **73**, 242
7. Vesikari, T. and Vaheri, A. (1968). *Br. Med. J.*, **1**, 221
8. Best, J. M., Banatvala, J. E. and Watson, D. (1969). *Lancet*, **2**, 65
9. Julian, A. J., Logan, L. C. and Norins, L. C. (1969). *J. Immunol.*, **102**, 1250
10. Haire, M. and Hadden, D. S. M. (1970). *Br. Med. J.*, **3**, 130
11. Cradock-Watson, J. E., Bourne, M. S. and Vandervelde, E. M. (1972). *J. Hyg.*, **70**, 473
12. Haire, M. and Hadden, D. S. M. (1972). *J. Med. Microbiol.*, **5**, 237
13. Matossian, R. M., Kane, G. J., Chantler, S. M., Batty, I. and Sarhadian H. (1972). *Immunology*, **22**, 423
14. O'Neill, P. and Nicol, C. S. (1972). *Br. J. Venereol. Dis.*, **48**, 460
15. Miller, H. and Owen, G. (1960). *Nature*, **188**, 67
16. Zavagal, V. and Stagner, A. (1970). *Acta Allergol.*, **25**, 1
17. Coombs, R. A. R., Jonas, W. E., Lachmann, P. J. and Feinstein, A. (1965). *Int. Arch. Allergy*, **27**, 321
18. Coombs, R. A. R., Hunter, A., Jonas, W. E., Bennich, H., Johansson, S. G. O., and Danzani, R. (1968). *Lancet*, **2**, 1115
19. Sanderson, C. J. (1971). *Immunology*, **21**, 719
20. Daugharty, H., Warfield, D. T., Hemingway, W. D. and Casey, H. L. (1973). *Infect. Immun.*, **7**, 380
21. Charlton, D. and Blanford, G. (1975). *J. Immunol. Methods*, **8**, 319
22. Nassau, E., Parsons, E. R. and Johnson, G. D. (1975). *J. Immunol. Methods*, **6**, 261
23. Kalimo, K. O. K., Meurman, O. H., Halonen, P. E., Ziola, B. R., Viljanen, M. K., Granfors, K. and Toivanen, P. (1976). *J. Clin. Microbiol.*, **4**, 117
24. Knez, V., Stewart, J. A. and Zeigler, D. W. (1976). *J. Immunol.*, **117**, 2006
25. Meurman, O. H., Viljanen, M. K. and Granfors, K. (1977). *J. Clin. Microbiol.*, **5**, 257
26. Kangro, H. O., Pattison, J. R. and Heath R. B. (1978). *Br. J. Exp. Pathol.*, **59**, 577
27. Kalimo, K. O. K., Ziola, B. R., Viljanen, M. K., Granfors, K. and Tiovanen, P. (1977). *J. Immunol. Meth.*, **14**, 183
28. Cradock-Watson, J. E., Ridehalgh, M. K. S., Pattison, J. R., Anderson, M. J. and Kangro, H. O. (1979). *J. Hyg., Camb.*, **83**, 413
29. Engvall, E. and Perlmann, P. (1971). *Immunochemistry*, **8**, 871
30. Engvall, E. and Perlmann, P. (1972). *J. Immunol.*, **109**, 129
31. Voller, A. and Bidwell, D. E. (1976). *Br. J. Exp. Pathol.*, **57**, 243
32. Pattison, J. R. and Smith, K. O. (1975). *J. Clin. Microbiol.*, **2**, 130
33. Rosenthal, J. D., Hayashi, K. and Notkins, A. L. (1973). *Appl. Microbiol.*, **25**, 567
34. Voller, A., Bidwell, D. E., Huldt, G. and Engvall, E. (1974). *Bull. WHO*, **51**, 209
35. Carlsson, H. E., Lindberg, A. A. and Hammerstrom, S. (1972). *Infect. Immun.*, **6**, 703
36. Prevot, J. and Guesdon, J. L. (1977). *Ann. Microbiol.* (Inst. Pasteur), **128B**, 531
37. Schmitz, H., Doerr, H. W., Kampa, D. and Vogt, A. (1977). *J. Clin. Microbiol.*, **5**, 629
38. Atanasiu, P., Savy, V. and Gibert, C. (1978). *Med. Microbiol. Immunol.*, **166**, 201
39. Cappel, R., de Cuyper, F. and de Brackeleer, J. (1978). *Arch. Virol.*, **58**, 253
40. Camargo, M. E., Ferreira, A. W., Mineo, J. R., Takigati, C. K. and Nakahara, O. S. (1978). *Infect. Immun.*, **21**, 55

41. Leinikki, P., Shekarchi, I., Dorsett, P. and Sever, J. (1978). *J. Clin. Microbiol.*, **8**, 419
42. Leinikki, P., Shekarchi, I., Dorsett, P. and Sever, J. (1978). *J. Lab. Clin. Med.*, **92**, 849
43. Luckins, A. G. and Mehlitz, D. (1978). *Trop. Anim. Health Prod.*, **10**, 149
44. Matthiesen, L. R., Feinstone, S. M., Wong, D. C., Skinhoej, J. P. and Purcell, R. M. (1978). *J. Clin. Microbiol.*, **7**, 184
45. Yolken, R. H., Wyatt, R. G., Kim, H. W., Kapikian, A. Z. and Chanock, R. M. (1978). *Infect. Immun.*, **19**, 540
46. Vejtorp, M. Fanøe, E. and Leerhoy, J. (1979). *Acta Pathol. Microbiol. Scand. Sect. B.*, **87**, 155
47. Remington, J. S. and Desmonts, G. (1973). *J. Pediatr.*, **83**, 27
48. Chantler, S. M. and Haire, M. (1972). *Immunology.*, **23**, 7
49. Cohen, I. R., Norins, L. C. and Julian, A. J. (1967). *J. Immunol.*, **98**, 143
50. Juchau, S., Linscott, W. D., Schachter, J. and Jawetz, E. (1972). *J. Immunol.*, **108**, 1563
51. Reimer, C. B., Black, C. M., Phillips, D. J., Logan, L. C., Hunter, E. F., Pender, B. J. and McGrew, B. E. (1975). *Ann. N.Y. Acad. Sci.*, **254**, 77
52. Cradock-Watson, J. E., Ridehalgh, M. K. S. and Chantler, S. (1976). *J. Hyg. Camb.*, **76**, 109
53. Pyndiah, N., Krech, U., Price, P. and Wilhelm J. (1979). *J. Clin. Microbiol.*, **9**, 170
54. Field, P. R., Shanker, S. and Murphy, A. M. (1980). *J. Immunol. Methods.*, **32**, 59
55. Holborow, E. J. and Johnson, G. D. (1965). *Ann. N.Y. Acad. Sci.*, **124** part 2, 833
56. Fraser, K. B., Shirodaria, P. V. and Stanford, C. F. (1971). *Brit. Med. J.*, **3**, 707
57. Camargo, M. E., Leser, P. G. and Rocca, A. (1972). *Rev. Inst. Med. Trop. Sao Paulo.*, **14**, 310
58. Desmonts, G., Couvreur, J., Colin, J. and Peupion, J. (1972). *N. Presse Med.*, **1**, 339
59. Gispen, R., Nagel, J., Brand-Saathof, B. and de Graaf, S. (1975). *Clin. Exp. Immunol.*, **22**, 431
60. Hyde, B., Barnett, E. V. and Remington, J. S. (1975). *Proc. Soc. Exp. Biol. Med.*, **148**, 1184
61. Chantler, S. M., Devries, E., Allen, P. R. and Hurn, B. A. L. (1976). *J. Immunol. Methods*, **13**, 367
62. Handsher, R. and Fogel, A. (1977). *J. Clin. Microbiol.*, **5**, 588
63. Hannon, R., Haire, M., Wisdom, G. B. and Neill, D. W. (1975). *J. Immunol. Methods.*, **8**, 29
64. Gupta, J. D., Peterson, V., Stout, M. and Murphy, A. M. (1971). *J. Clin. Pathol.*, **24**, 547
65. Pattison, J. R. and Mace, J. E. (1973). *J. Clin. Pathol.*, **26**, 309
66. Bürgin-Wolff, A., Hernandez, R. and Just, M. (1971). *Lancet*, **2**, 1278
67. Pattison, J. R. and Mace, J. E. (1975). *J. Clin. Pathol.*, **28**, 670
68. Frisch-Niggemeyer, W. (1975). *J. Clin. Microbiol.*, **2**, 377
69. Remington, J. S. and Miller, M. J. (1966). *Proc. Soc. Exp. Biol. Med.*, **121**, 357
70. Desmyter, J., South, M. A. and Rawls, W. E. (1971). *J. Med. Microbiol.*, **4**, 107
71. Forghani, B., Schmidt, N. J. and Lennette, E. H. (1973). *Intervirology.*, **1**, 48
72. Remington, J. S. and Desmonts, G. (1973). *J. Pediatr.*, **83**, 27
73. Caul, E. O., Smyth, G. W. and Clarke, S. K. R. (1974). *J. Hyg.*, **73**, 329
74. Roggendorf, M., Schneweis, K. E. and Wolff, M. H. (1976). 261. *Zbl. Bakt. Hyg. I. Abt. Orig. A.*, **235**, 363
75. Newman, S., Horta-Barbosa, L. and Sever, J. L. (1969). *Lancet.*, **2**, 432
76. Schmitz, H. and Krainick-Riechert, C. M. (1974). *Intervirology*, **3**, 353
77. Forsgren, A. and Sjoquist, J. (1966). *J. Immunol.*, **97**, 822
78. Kronvall, G. and Williams, R. C. (1969). *J. Immunol.*, **103**, 828
79. Kronvall, G. and Frommel, D. (1970). *Immunochemistry.*, **1**, 124
80. Kronvall, G., Grey, H. M. and Williams, R. C. (1970). *J. Immunol.*, **105**, 1116
81. Ankerst, J., Christensen, P., Kjellen, L. and Kronvall, G. (1974). *J. Infect. Dis.*, **130**, 268
82. Janowski, M. A., Gut, W. L., Switalski, L., Imbs, D. and Kantoch, M. (1979). *Arch. Virol.*, **60**, 123
83. Mallison, H., Roberts, C. and Bruce White, G. B. (1976). *J. Clin. Pathol.*, **29**, 999

84. Skuag, K. and Gaarder, P. I. (1978). *Acta. Path. Microbiol. Scand. Sect. C.*, **86**, 33

85. Harbøe, M. and Følling, I. (1976). *Scan. J. Immunol.*, **3**, 471

86. Lind, I., Harboe, M. and Følling, I. (1975). *Scan. J. Immunol.*, **4**, 843

87. Schmitz, H., Shimizi, H., Kampe, D. and Doerr, H. W. (1975). *J. Clin. Microbiol.*, **1**, 132

88. Lehrich, J. R., Kassel, J. A. and Rossen, R. D. (1966). *J. Immunol.*, **97**, 654

89. Cooper, L. Z., Matters, B., Rosenblum, J. K. and Krugman, S. (1969). *J. Amer. Med. Assoc.*, **207**, 89

90. Remington, J. S., Miller, M. J. and Brownlee, I. (1968). *Paediatrics.*, **41**, 1082

91. Brenchley, P. (1975). Ph.D. Thesis University of Manchester

92. Jacoby, B. and Pepys, J. (1976). *J. Immunol. Methods.*, **11**, 37

93. Diment, J. A. and Pepys, J. (1978). In Hoffman-Ostelhof, O., Breitenbach, M., Koller, F., Kraft, D. and Scheiner, O., (eds.). *Affinity Chromatography.* p. 229. (Oxford: Pergamon Press)

94. Duermeyer, W. and van der Veen, J. (1978). *Lancet.*, **2**, 684

95. Duermeyer, W., Wielaard, F. and van der Veen, J. (1979). *J. Med. Virol.*, **4**, 25

96. Ertl, H. C. J., Gerlich, W. and Koszinowski, U. H. (1979). *J. Immunol. Methods.*, **28**, 163

97. Gerlich, W. H. and Luer, W. (1979). *J. Med. Virol.*, **4**, 227

98. Krech, U. and Wilhelm, J. A. (1979). *J. Gen. Virol.*, **44**, 281

99. Moller, A. M., and Mathiesen, L. R. (1979). *J. Clin. Microbiol.*, **10**, 628

100. Price, P. C. (1980). *J. Immunol. Methods.*, **32**, 261

29
Enzyme Immunoassays in Bacteriology

A. A. GLYNN and C. ISON

INTRODUCTION

In principle enzyme immunoassays (EIA) can be used to detect and measure any antigen or hapten as well as antibody and will distinguish the different immunoglobulin classes. They can be used to determine serum levels of antibiotics[1, 2] as well as antibodies in antibiotic-sensitive patients[3, 4]. With the attractions of relative simplicity, safety and general applicability why is it that such methods have not been used more widely in bacteriology? The deficit is mainly in diagnostic methods where the effort in virology and parasitology has been greater in volume and more concentrated in direction. The reasons become plain when one examines the diagnostic role of immunoassay or indeed of serology in general. In practice the most satisfactory method of establishing the presence of an infection is to demonstrate the causal agent. In bacteriology this means by culture or microscopy or both. Microscopy is more rapid, culture is more precise and also enables antibiotic sensitivities to be determined. In virology cultural methods are complex and slow and microscopy other than electronmicroscopy is of little help. Diagnosis from the presence of antibodies is, therefore, relatively important. Similarly culture of most parasites is not possible or practicable and diagnosis usually depends on visual demonstration of some stage of the life-cycle.

Diagnosis by antibody has its own problems of decision-making, as will be discussed below. Diagnosis by detection of antigen is more direct. Interpretation is simpler and does not really differ in principle from that of visual detection, though immunochemistry replaces microscopy.

USES

One would expect therefore that EIA would be tried first in conditions where the older techniques were least satisfactory. With some exceptions, this is true. It is no accident that in syphilis where serological tests are widely used, the causal bacterium cannot be grown *in vitro* and, except for the relatively few primary cases, microscopy is no help. So far EIA has been used relatively little in the diagnosis of syphilis, perhaps because the disease is less important than formerly and the tests already in use work reasonably well.

In leprosy EIA would conceivably be of value in investigating lepromatous compared with tuberculoid states but nothing has yet been published. There is a long history of attempts to use serology in tuberculosis. Nassau *et al.*[5] demonstrated a clear difference between tuberculous patients and controls by means of ELISA. However, in a complex disease like tuberculosis where so much depends on cell-mediated immunity, it remains unlikely that antibody measurements will ever be a useful guide to the state of infection. Since culture of *Mycobacterium tuberculosis*, though perfectly possible, is slow, microscopy is still a useful though less sensitive practice. To be detected in a strained film of sputum, tubercle bacilli need to present in a concentration of at least 50 000/ml. A rapid enzyme technique which could detect a smaller quantity of specific antigen would have a place. Draper (personal communication) has calculated from electronmicroscopic observations that a leprosy bacillus weighs about 0.1 pg. If one assumes that a tubercle bacillus is of the same order of size, 50 000 would weigh 5 ng. Since any one antigen would only be a small fraction of the whole, a system able to detect it in the picogram range would be needed, and this is getting to the limits of simple EIA. Ultrasensitive methods have been described but are complex[6].

Given the difficulties of culturing Rickettsiae, it is not surprising that attempts have been made to use EIA to detect antibody. A purified rickettsial antigen detected IgM and IgG antibodies more sensitively by ELISA than by established complement-fixation and microagglutination techniques in five patients with typhus[7]. ELISA has also been applied in the diagnosis of trench fever due to *Rochalimaea quintana*[8]. The new pathogen *Legionella pneumophila* can be cultured but expertise is still not general and antibody diagnosis is easier and for retrospective studies essential. So far microfluorescent techniques have been used but EIA is a possibility.

Enteric fever is best diagnosed by culture. The Widal reaction has a limited role and, for reasons which will become obvious, attempts to replace it by more sensitive haemagglutination tests or EIA[9] are unlikely to do any better.

Lipopolysaccharides are so widespread and so important in many Gram-negative infections that the use of EIA to detect both them and their antibodies is bound to develop further. Carlsson *et al.*[10] used a double-antibody method to look for *Escherichia coli* O antibody in the milk of Swedish and Pakistani mothers. They used similar methods to survey *E. coli* O antibodies in human milk, maternal serum and cord blood[11].

The appearance of IgG and IgM antibodies to the lipopolysaccharide of *Franciscella tularensis* in patients with tularaemia was followed by ELISA[12]. The lipopolysaccharide itself of *Yersinia entercolitica* was detected by Grippenberg *et al.*[13] but only if at least 0.5 μg was present. Antibodies to the lipopolysaccharide were also measured and often differed from those shown by haemagglutination.

Brucella, though cultivable, may be difficult to detect in chronic infections and antibody methods are widely used, particularly in veterinary medicine where the ability to detect carriers, especially by examination of serum or milk antibodies, is of importance in eradication programmes[14, 15].

An important line of advance is the potential increase in specificity offered by synthetic antigens. Thus Svenungsson and Lindberg[16] obtained high-titre antibody very specific for the salmonella O2 antigen by immunizing rabbits with the synthetic disaccharide paratose $\alpha1\rightarrow3$ mannose linked to bovine serum albumin.

Though not necessary for clinical diagnosis, EIA can be extremely useful in detecting soluble toxins where older methods are complex, insensitive, or inaccurate, or all three. Methods for detecting diphtheria, tetanus and botulinus toxin or antibodies to them have been described[17-19]. The exotoxin A of *Pseudomonas aeruginosa* was detected at a concentration of 30 pg/ml by Schultz *et al.*[20].

There are discrepancies between enteropathogenic strains of *E. coli* as defined by particular O serotypes and the ability of *E. coli* strains to produce toxin, so that a readily available method of toxin assay would be useful. The use of biological tests such as the effect on rabbit ileal loops or infant rabbit skin is clearly limited. So too is the use of cells in culture such as the Chinese hamster ovary cell or the Y-1 adrenal cell. The latter is extremely sensitive, detecting 0.1 pg/ml of toxin, but so is an ELISA described by Yolken *et al.*[21]. An interesting variation is the use of GM1 ganglioside, the cholera toxin receptor, instead of antitoxin to attach toxin to the plate. Since both cholera toxin and *E. coli* heat-labile enterotoxin bind to the same receptor, either could be measured, even in crude extracts[22, 23], using a ganglioside technique could detect 0.1 pg of *E. coli* toxin.

The proper diagnosis of acute meningitis is urgent and treatment cannot await the results of culture. Moreover early administration of antibiotics may have made culture impossible. At present counter immunoelectrophoresis is widely and successfully used to detect the antigens of the three commonest bacterial causes of meningitis[24]. The method is rapid, results being available within 2 h, but increased sensitivity would be welcome. Latex agglutination tests work well[25], though early attempts to detect *Haemophilus influenzae* antigen by haemagglutination techniques[26] never became common, presumably because of difficulty in standardizing and stabilizing reagents. Drow *et al.*[27], using EIA, could detect 1–5 ng of *H. influenzae* type b antigen in cerebrospinal fluid. In some patients as much as 5000 μg/ml antigen was

P

found. There were no cross-reactions with *E. coli* K100 which is antigenically similar.

In a rabbit model Harding *et al.*[28] could detect pneumococcal polysaccharide down to 1 ng/ml of cerebrospinal fluid compared with a lower limit of 25–50 times this amount with counter-immunoelectrophoresis. They had some trouble with variations in the commercial anti-pneumococcal serum but there were no cross-reactions with *H. influenzae* or *Neisseria meningitidis*. The method needs developing for man. It could be argued that since only a single qualitative yes or no result is needed, assay is not the right term to use. However, even the most evident qualitative test is based on underlying, often unacknowledged, quantitative adjustments, and only if antigens are properly assayed on a large scale will it be known whether the exercise is useful or not.

Antibodies to pneumococcal polysaccharides in immunized patients were measured by ELISA[29]. The results agreed badly with those of RIA probably because ELISA may not be good at picking up antibodies of low avidity[30].

The increasing frequency of serious infection of newborn infants by group B streptococci has led to investigations in which the phagocytic and protective function of antibodies have been measured in parallel with EIA[31]. Antibodies to the little-known type M proteins of group A streptococci have been investigated similarly[32].

Local antibodies to *Streptococcus mutans* are of considerable interest as possible factors protecting against dental caries. Salivary IgA antibodies were measured by ELISA by Bratthall *et al.*[33]. Differentiation of immunoglobulin classes among serum antibodies by means of ELISA was described by Ison and Glynn[34] in gonorrhoea. They also detected secretory antibody, mostly but not entirely IgA, present in circulating blood, presumably because of absorbence from sites of local production.

SOME STATISTICAL CONSTRAINTS

Though EIA has been applied to the detection of antigens of many different bacteria and their respective antibodies, it is clear that even in gonorrhoea, where there has perhaps been the most effort, no test yet forms part of current practice.

One knows intuitively that for a test to be useful it must be both sensitive and specific. It takes very little experience to learn that the two properties are inversely related. Raising thresholds or cut-off points increases specificity but reduces sensitivity. Lowering them does the opposite. Where the balance is struck depends on the circumstances and aims of the test. Subjective qualitative judgments can be made rigorously quantitative. How rigorously depends on one's inclination and aptitude for mathematics. Serological tests are only one example of decision-making in medicine and the application of simple information theory to such problems has been outlined by Vecchio[35] and by McNeil *et al.*[36].

The problem has been discussed in relation to gonorrhoeae[37,38] and chlamydial infection[39].

A new test is developed with the help of known positive sera to ensure that it is sufficiently sensitive and controlled with known negative sera to ensure that it is sufficiently specific (Table 29.1). It is then applied to a selected group of

Table 29.1 Some useful indices in the serological diagnosis of infection

$$\text{Sensitivity} = \frac{\text{No. of infected people with a positive test}}{\text{Total no. of infected people tested}}$$

$$\text{Specificity} = \frac{\text{No. of non-infected people with a negative test}}{\text{Total no. of non-infected people tested}}$$

$$\text{Predictive value of a positive result} = \frac{\text{No. of positive tests in infective people}}{\text{Total no. of positive tests}}$$

009n

$$\text{Predictive value of a negative result} = \frac{\text{No. of negative tests in uninfected people}}{\text{Total no of negative tests}}$$

patients with a large proportion suffering from the disease under investigation. If the preliminary work has been properly done, the results will be good or at least promising. A large number of more or less random sera from a wider population is then tested and it becomes obvious that something is not right. Cut-off points are manipulated, conditions modified and even reagents changed, but the chances are that the test will still not be entirely satisfactory. Why? The answer lies in calculations of predictive value (Table 29.1).

The predictive value of a positive test is the chance that it is a true rather than a false-positive. What is too often forgotten is that this depends not only on the sensitivity and specificity of the test but very much on the prevalence of the disease in the population tested (Figure 29.1). Thus if a disease has a prevalence of 2% in the normal population a test with 90% sensitivity and 90% specificity applied to 1000 people would give 116 positive results, of whom only 18 would be true positives; i.e. a predictive value of 15%. If the prevalence rises to 30% then the predictive value of a positive result is 79%.

Specificity has a greater effect than sensitivity (Figure 29.2). If the prevalence is 2% and sensitivity 95%, then even with a specificity of 98% the predictive value of a positive result is only just over 60%. At this point one wonders if any test is worth having. It depends on what the alternatives are and how important it is to make a diagnosis. Again the answer is given by current practice in serological tests for syphilis. Two tests are better than one. If two tests for the same infection detect independent chemically unrelated

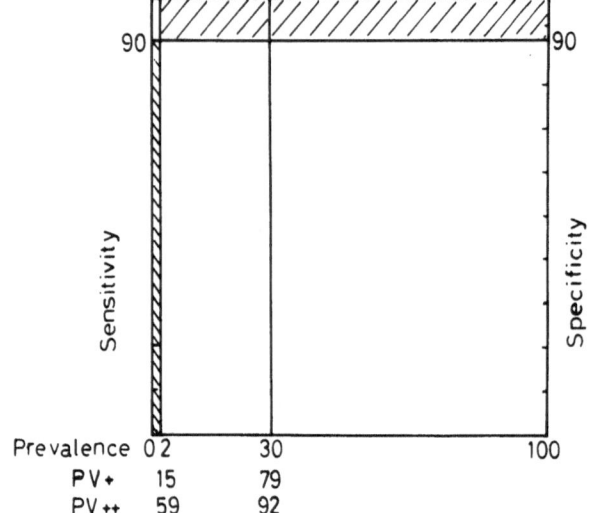

Figure 29.1   Effect of prevalence on predictive value given sensitivity and specificity both 90%. PV+, predictive value of a positive result in one test; PV + +, predictive value of a positive result in two sets for same infection using different antigens

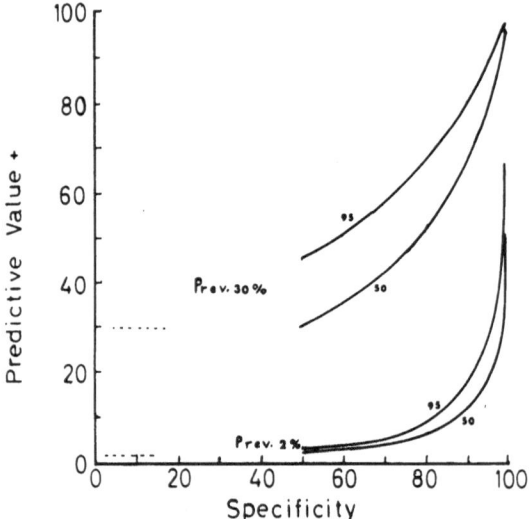

Figure 29.2   Relation between predictive value of a positive result (PV+) and specificity. Prev = prevalence (50 and 95 are percentage sensitivities)

antigens, then assuming for the sake of simplicity they each have sensitivities and specificities of 90%, then the predictive value of a positive result with each test singly in a population with a disease prevalence of 2% is, as before, 15%. However, in the infected 2% both tests will be positive in at worst 1.6%. In the rest of the population, however, if the antigens are sufficiently different, then the chances of cross-reactions are small and with the parameters chosen there is approximately a 1% chance of a double-positive in the unaffected group and the predictive value of a double-positive result rises to 59%. With a prevalence of 30%, the predictive value would be 92%.

Thus, although the highest possible specificity is desirable, it may well be easier to find two antigenic tests with specificities of 80-90% than one giving a specificity of over 98%. A traditional alternative is to look for rising antibody levels, but this involves delay.

SPECIFICITY

Antigenic specificity is the key to a good serological test. Bacterial antigens may define genera, species or strains. For diagnosis identification to species level is usually adequate though even this needs care since cross-reactions are common. Much difficulty has been encountered, for example, in serological tests for gonorrhoeae because of the widespread occurrence of antibodies to meningococci. Since *Neisseria meningitidis* and *N. gonorrhoeae* have some 80% of their DNA in common[40], this is not surprising. For epidemiological purposes differentiation between types or strains is often needed, e.g. in *Streptococcus pyogenes* or *Strept. pneumoniae*. It is history rather than science which decides that a change in a single oligosaccharide determinant distinguishes types of pneumococci while a difference of similar degree in the Salmonellae changes the species.

It has often been convenient and, under the right conditions, adequate to use whole bacteria as antigens. The increasingly precise requirements for specificity of EIA are making it necessary to use better-defined antigens. These are usually extracts of varying degrees of purity, e.g. the purified pilus protein of *N. gonorrhoeae*[41] or the partially purified mixture of outer membrane proteins of the same organism[42]. An indication of antibody to pili can, however, be gained with whole bacteria by comparing the reactions with pilated and non-pilated variants of the same strain of *N. gonorrhoeae* (Ison, Hadfield and Glynn, unpublished). Since most bacteria have a negative surface charge, they stick poorly to similarly charged polystyrene plates. The latter were, therefore, first coated with polylysine using an adaptation of the methods described for red cells[43] and lymphocytes[44].

The high degree of specificity obtained with synthetic oligosaccharide determinants[16] has been mentioned. Such an approach is not possible with proteins but genetic manipulation of bacterial strains to give high yields of specific antigens is technically feasible, and together with the production of highly specific monoclonal antibodies could revolutionize serology.

While much progress is being made in refining bacterial antigens, the increasing sensitivity of EIA and other assays has highlighted two phenomena which can cause much difficulty and, if unsuspected, major errors in interpretation. The ability of staphylococcal protein A to bind to many immunoglobulins is well known. Similar receptors for immunoglobulin occur among other bacteria, e.g. streptococci of groups A, C, and G. Christensen *et al.*[45] suggest that many of the experiments purporting to show cross-reactions between heart muscle and streptococci could be explained on the basis of this type of binding, so weakening the case for autoimmunity in rheumatic fever.

Serological tests can be disturbed even more seriously by the presence of antiglobulins[46]. While rheumatoid factor is the best known, antiglobulins may develop in chronic infections and it is likely that sensitive methods would also detect them in more acute infections. Although the rheumatoid factor commonly picked up by agglutination of IgG-coated latex particles or red cells is predominantly IgM, rheumatoid factors and anti-immunoglobulins of IgG and IgA types are well known. It is easy to see how in a sensitive EIA the unexpected binding of anti-immunoglobulin to the specific antigen–antibody complex could distort the results. Variations on EIA using labelled antigen or the use of Fab′ fragments[47] may overcome the problem.

Rheumatoid factors do not explain everything, however. In a survey of patients from an arthritis clinic an impossibly high proportion showed antibodies to gonococcal extracts (Ison, Seifert and Glynn, unpublished).

Such antibodies were more common in patients with rheumatoid factor. Nevertheless, when rheumatoid factor-positive sera were absorbed with IgG Sepharose particles until they became factor-negative, there was no significant change in antibody level.

References

1. Rubenstein, K. E. (1978). Homogeneous enzyme immunoassay. *Scand. J. Immunol.*, **8**, 57
2. Standefer, J. C. and Saunders, G. C. (1978). Enzyme immunoassay for gentamicin. *Clin. Chem.*, **24**, 1903
3. Haan, P. de, Bakker, W., Boorsma, D. M., Heidekamp, F. and Kalsbeek, G. L. (1978). Humoral aspects of penicillin sensitivity. *Dermatologica*, **156**, 303
4. Haan, P. de, Boorsma, D. M. and Kalsbeek, G. L. (1979). Penicillin hypersensitivity. *Allergy*, **34**, 111
5. Nassau, B., Parsons, E. R. and Johnson, G. D. (1976). The detection of antibodies to *Mycobacterium tuberculosis* by microplate enzyme-linked immunosorbent assay (ELISA). *Tubercle*, **57**, 67
6. Harris, C. C., Yolken, R. H., Krokan, H. and Hsu, I. C. (1979). Ultrasensitive enzymatic radioimmunoassay: application to detection of cholera toxin and rotavirus. *Proc. Natl. Acad. Sci. USA*, **76**, 5336
7. Halle, S., Dasch, G. A. and Weiss, E. (1977). Sensitive enzyme-linked immunosorbent assay for detection of antibodies against Typhus rickettsiae, *Rickettsia prowarekii* and *Rickettsia typhi*. *J. Clin. Microbiol.*, **6**, 101
8. Herrmann, J. E., Hollingdale, M. R., Collins, M. F. and Vinson, J. W. (1977). Enzyme immunoassay and radioimmunoprecipitation tests for the detection of antibodies to *Rochalimcea (Rickettsia) quintana*. *Proc. Soc. Exp. Biol. Med.*, **154**, 285
9. Carlsson, H. E., Lindberg, A. A. and Hammarström, S. (1972). Titration of antibodies to Salmonella O antigens by enzyme-linked immunosorbent assay. *Infect. Immun.*, **6**, 703

10. Carlsson, B., Ahlstedt, S., Hanson, L. A., Lidin-Janson, G., Lindblad, B. S. and Sultana, R. (1976). *Escherichia coli* O antibody content in milk from healthy Swedish mothers and mothers from a very low socio-economic group of a developing country. *Acta Paediatr. Scand.*, **65**, 417

11. Carlsson, B., Gothefors, L., Ahlstedt, S., Hanson, L. A. and Winberg, J. (1976). Studies of *Escherichia coli* O antigen specific antibodies in human milk, maternal serum and cord blood. *Acta Paediatr. Scand.*, **65**, 216

12. Carlsson, H. E., Lindberg, A. A., Lindberg, G., Hederstedt, B., Karlsson, K. A. and Agell, B. O. (1979). Enzyme-linked immunosorbent assay for immunological diagnosis of human tularaemia. *J. Clin. Microbiol.*, **10**, 615

13. Grippenberg, M., Nissinen, A., Väisänen, E. and Linder, E. (1979). Demonstration of antibodies against *Yersinia enterocolitica* lipopolysaccharide in human serum by enzyme-linked immunosorbent assay. *J. Clin. Microbiol.*, **10**, 279

14. Thoen, O., Piez, D. E., Armbrust, A. L. and Harrington, R. (1979). Enzyme immunoassay for detecting *Brucella abortus* antibodies in cow's milk. *J. Clin. Microbiol.*, **10**, 222

15. Byrd, J. W., Heck, F. C. and Hidalgo, R. J. (1979). Evaluation of the enzyme linked immunosorbent assay for detecting *Brucella abortus* antibodies. *Am. J. Vet. Res.*, **40**, 891

16. Svenungsson, B. and Lindberg, A. A. (1978). Synthetic disaccharide-protein antigen for production of specific O2 antiserum for immunofluorescence diagnosis of salmonella. *Acta Pathol. Microbiol. Scand., B*, **86**, 35

17. Svenson, S. B. and Larson, K. (1977). An enzyme linked immunosorbent assay (ELISA) for the determination of diphtheria toxin antibodies. *J. Immunol. Methods*, **17**, 249

18. Fruhwein, N. (1979). Tetanus antibodies in conventional gamma globulin preparations. *Fortschr. Med.*, **97**, 1063

19. Notermans, S., Dufrenne, J. and Schothorst, M. (1978). Enzyme-linked immunosorbent assay for detection of *Clostridium botulinum* toxin type A. *Jpn. J. Med. Sci. Biol.*, **31**, 81

20. Schultz, W. W., Phipps, T. J. and Pollack, M. (1979). Enzyme linked immunosorbent assay for *Pseudomonas aeruginosa* exotoxin A. *J. Clin. Microbiol.*, **9**, 705

21. Yolken, R. H., Greenberg, H. B., Merson, M. H., Sack, R. B. and Kapikian, A. Z. (1977). Enzyme-linked immunosorbent assay for detection of *Escherichia coli* heat-labile enterotoxin. *J. Clin. Microbiol.*, **6**, 439

22. Sack, D. A., Huda, S., Neogi, P. K. B., Daniel, R. R. and Spira, W. M. (1980). Microtiter ganglioside enzyme-linked immunosorbent assay for *Vibrio* and *Escherichia coli* heat-labile enterotoxins and antitoxin. *J. Clin. Microbiol.*, **11**, 35

23. Bach, E., Svennerholm, A. M., Holmgren, J. and Möllby, R. (1979). Evaluation of a ganglioside immunosorbent assay for detection of *Escherichia coli* heat labile enterotoxin. *J. Clin. Microbiol.*, **10**, 791

24. Greenwood, B. M., Whittle, H. C. and Dominic-RajKovic, O. (1971). Counter current immunoelectrophoresis in the diagnosis of meningococcal infections. *Lancet*, **2**, 519

25. Whittle, H. C., Tugwell, P., Egler, L. J. and Greenwood, B. M. (1974). Rapid bacteriological diagnosis of pyogenic meningitis by latex agglutination. *Lancet*, **2**, 619

26. Warburton, M. F., Keogh, E. V. and Williams, S. W. (1949). Haemagglutination test for diagnosis of influenzal meningitis. *Med. J. Aust.*, **1**, 135

27. Drow, D. L., Maki, D. G. and Manning, D. D. (1979). Indirect sandwich enzyme-linked immunosorbent assay for rapid detection of *Haemophilus influenzae* type b infection. *J. Clin. Microbiol.*, **10**, 442

28. Harding, S. A., Scheld, W. M., McGowan, M. D. and Sande, M. A. (1979). Enzyme-linked immunosorbent assay for detection of *Streptococcus pneumoniae* antigen. *J. Clin. Microbiol.*, **10**, 339

29. Callahan, L. T., Woodhour, A. F., Mecker, J. B. and Hilleman, M. R. (1979). Enzyme linked immunoassay for measurement of antibodies against pneumococcal polysaccharide antigens: comparison with radioimmunoassay. *J. Clin. Microbiol.*, **10**, 459

30 Butler, J. E., Feldbush, T. L., McGivern, P. L. and Stewart, N. (1978). The enzyme linked immunosorbent assay (ELISA): a measure of antibody concentration or affinity. *Immunochemistry*, **15**, 131

31. Rote, N. S., Taylor, N. L., Shigeoka, A. O., Scott, J. R. and Hill, H. R. (1980). Enzyme linked immunosorbent assay for Group B streptococcal antibodies. *Infect. Immun.*, **27**, 118

32. Russell, H., Facklam, R. R. and Edwards, L. R. (1976). Enzyme-linked immunosorbent assay for streptocococcal M protein antibodies. *J. Clin. Microbiol.*, **3**, 501

33. Bratthall, D., Gahnberg, L. and Krasse, B. (1978). Method for detecting IgA antibodies to *Streptococcus mutans* serotypes in parotid saliva. *Arch. Oral Biol.*, **23**, 843

34. Ison, C. A. and Glynn, A. A. (1979). Classes of antibodies in acute gonorrhoea. *Lancet*, **2**, 1165

35. Vecchio, T. J. (1966). Predictive value of a single diagnostic test in unselected populations. *N. Engl. J. Med.*, **274**, 1171

36. McNeil, B. J., Keeler, E. and Adelstein, S. J. (1975). Primer on certain elements of medical decision making. *N. Engl. J. Med.*, **293**, 212

37. Dans, P. E., Rothenberg, R. and Holmes, K. K. (1977). Gonococcal serology: how soon, how useful and how much? *J. Infect. Dis.*, **135**, 330

38. Holmes, K. K., Buchanan, T. M., Adam, J. L. and Eschenbach, D. A. (1978). Is serology useful in gonorrhoea? A critical analysis of factors influenzing serodiagnosis. In Brooks, G. F., Gotschlich, E. C., Holmes, K. K., Sawyer, W. D. and Young, F. E. (eds.) *Immunobiology of Neisseria Gonnorhoeae*, pp. 370–6. (Washington, DC: American Society for Immunobiology)

39. Schachter, J., Cles, L., Ray, R. and Hines, P. A. (1979). Failure of serology in diagnosing chlamydial infection of female genital tract. *J. Clin. Microbiol.*, **10**, 647

40. Kingsbury, D. T. (1967). Deoxyribonucleic acid homologies among species of the genus *Neisseria. J. Bacteriol.*, **94**, 870

41. Buchanan T. M. (1977). Surface antigens: pili. In Roberts, R. R. (ed.) *The Gonococcus*, pp. 255–72. (New York: Wiley)

42. Glynn, A. A. and Ison, C. A. (1978). Serological diagnosis of gonorrhoea by an enzyme-linked immunosorbent assay (ELISA). *Br. J. Vener. Dis.*, **54**, 97

43. Kennedy, J. C. and Axelrod, M. A. (1971). An improved assay for haemolytic plaque forming cells. *Immunology*, **20**, 253

44. Kedar, E., Landazuri, O. de and Bonavida, B. (1974). Cellular immunoadsorbents: a simplified technique for separation of lymphoid cell populations. *J. Immunol.*, **112**, 1231

45. Christensen, P., Schalen, C. and Holm, S. E. (1979). Reevaluation of experiments intended to demonstrate immunological cross-reactions between mammalian tissues and streptococci. *Progr. in Allergy*, **26**, 1

46. Yeni, P., Segond, P., Massias, P. and Pillot, J. (1978). False positive IgM anti-toxoplasma fluorescent test due to rheumatoid factor. *Lancet*, **1**, 219

47. Kato, K., Umeda, U., Suzuki, F., Hayashi, D. and Kosaka, A. (1979). Use of antibody Fab′ fragments to remove interference by rheumatoid factors with the enzyme-linked sandwich immunoassay. *FEBS Letters*, **102**, 253

30
Immunoassays in Mycology

D. W. R. MACKENZIE

In this chapter the values and limitations of immunoassays will be considered as they relate to the diagnosis and surveillance of diseases caused by fungi. No serious attempt will be made to present a comprehensive, or even a balanced, survey of this topic. Instead, specific areas or examples have been arbitrarily selected which have connection with the principal theme of immunoassays, and which may be of interest to workers largely unfamiliar with mycopathology.

It may be helpful at the outset to give brief indications of (1) what pathogenic fungi are, and (2) what diseases they cause in man. Firstly, fungi, apart from the unicellular yeasts, are micro-organisms with a branching filamentous habit. Lacking chlorophyll, they are committed to saprophytic or parasitic modes of life. An unusual feature, and one which has implications in the search for antigens suitable for use in immunoassays, is the gradient of age which exists along the length of an individual fungal hypha. Growth occurs only at the tip. Progressing proximally towards the point of origin involves a retracing of its entire lifespan, moving from the most recent and active region of cell wall synthesis through zones of increasing maturity and senescence. This age-gradient is accompanied by differences in metabolism along the hyphal length and in the associated cellular and extracellular products which are of potential interest as antigens.

Fungi cause disease in man by virtue of their allergenicity, toxigenicity or pathogenicity. Most immunoassays are used to detect products or host responses to *infection* and in this brief presentation consideration will be given only to this particular category of disease.

Infections are conveniently classified (Table 30.1) into four main groups:

(1) Superficial infections, such as ringworm, are confined to the outermost non-living layers of the epidermis and its appendages. Lesions are therefore usually obvious and readily diagnosed by a combination of

Table 30.1 Types of mycoses

Type	Example(s)
Superficial	ringworm
Implantation	mycetoma
Systemic	histoplasmosis
Opportunistic	candidosis aspergillosis

clinical appearance and history, and traditional laboratory procedures such as microscopy and culture. In this group, immunoassays are of very little value to the clinician.

(2) Mycoses of implantation (subcutaneous mycoses) occur when a pathogenic fungus is introduced into the subcutaneous tissues by traumatic implantation. Such infections are chronic and in some instances, e.g. mycetoma, can lead to extensive tissue destruction which may require amputation.

(3) Systemic mycoses such as histoplasmosis are acquired by inhalation of airborne fungal spores. The primary site of multiplication is therefore the lung. Exceptionally, there may be spread via the bloodstream and the development of disseminated or progressive disease, affecting almost any part of the body.

(4) Opportunistic mycoses such as candidosis or aspergillosis become established through localized or generalized predisposition of the host. Candidosis is unusual in being endogenous, originating from yeast cells which are already present in the body as commensals.

Table 30.2 shows the immunoassays used to measure antibodies and delayed hypersensitivity to the principal mycoses.

It is probably true to say that any immunoassay which has been developed has been or will be applied to the study of mycoses. Some tests are better than others in the sense that they correlate better with infection – or even disease. Largely through trial and error, a clearer understanding has been systematically gained on the limits of usefulness and applicability of individual immunoassays to individual mycoses.

There are several factors which have inhibited development of satisfactory immunoassays. The major problems are listed in Table 30.3.

Reference has already been made to the peculiar vegetative organization of filamentous fungi. A fungus grown in culture may be very different to the same organism growing in living tissues. This has not always been realized or taken into account in preparing antigens for use in immunoassays.

Fungal cells are packed with a wide range of enzymes and other proteins. Axelsen[1] used *Candida albicans* as the model for his elegant developmental studies with two-dimensional immunoelectrophoresis and enumerated 78

Table 30.2 Serological tests

	DD/CIE	CF	FA	Agglut. FC	IP	Skin test
Aspergillosis	+	(+)	(+)		+	+
Blastomycosis	(+)	+				+
Candidosis	+	(+)	+	(+)	(+)	+
Chromomycosis	(+)					
Coccidiomycosis	+	+	(+)		+	+
Cryptococcosis			(+)	(+)	+	
Histoplasmosis	+	+	(+)		+	+
Mycetoma	(+)					
Paracoccidioidomycosis	(+)	(+)				(+)
Phycomycosis	(+)					
Sporotrichosis	(+)	(+)	(+)			+

DD	= Double diffusion
CIE	= Counterimmunoelectrophoresis
CF	= Complement-fixation
+	= Test/reagent commercially available
(+)	= Test/reagent at special centres only
Agglut.	= Agglutination
FC	= Fungal cell
IP	= Inert particle
FA	= Fluorescent antibody

Table 30.3 Problems – immunoassays for detection of antibodies

(1) Antigens
   hyphal nature: dimorphism
   abundance of antigens
   biological function unknown
   cross-reacting antigens
   absence of reference reagents

(2) Antibodies
   cross-reactions with unrelated agents
   late or reduced production
   immunokinetics not fully understood

water-soluble antigens. In a recent paper presented at a meeting of the British Society for Mycopathology more than 700 proteins were demonstrated in yeast cells by two-dimensional separation using pH and molecular size gradients. Analysis of sera from patients with candidosis has not made it possible to discriminate between pathogenically significant and pathogenically irrelevant antigens. The mechanisms of fungal pathogenicity and virulence are poorly understood. How they invade living tissues remains conjectural and largely uninvestigated. Until and unless the biochemical events associated with tissue invasion are better known, however, selection of suitable serodiagnostic antigens must remain largely empirical. Only in

France have any sustained attempts been made to ascribe function to individual fungal antigens[2]. Cross-reacting antigens can be both common and troublesome. They are found in related and at times very dissimilar fungi. Their elimination by absorption procedures is practicable, but the increased specificity may be acquired at too high a price if the antibodies are directed principally against one or more of the cross-reacting antigens.

Reference reagents are sparse. Only one system has been subjected to a Collaborative Study by the WHO, *viz.* the histoplasmosis double-diffusion test developed at the CDC in Atlanta, Georgia. This test is effective, and its choice as a candidate system is justified on the basis of the long experience with both procedure and reagent and the good correlation which exists between a positive result and infection. Interest has recently been taken by the International Union of Immunological Societies in recognizing 'standard' *Candida* antigens, to be used for lymphocyte stimulation studies and for serological tests. These types of *Candida* antigen are presently lodged at the National Institute for Biological Standards and Control at Holly Hill. A Standing Committee of the International Society for Human and Animal Mycology is concerned with serodiagnostic reagents and procedures.

On the antibody side, there are problems caused by antibodies which react to non-specific antigens. In many instances, antibodies are formed too late to be of any real assistance with the diagnosis. This is particularly troublesome in acute life-threatening infections, and has led to the search for circulating antigens rather than antibodies.

The final problem listed is caused by the absence of precise information on the immunoglobulin classes involved in response to infection with different agents.

Antibodies to *Cryptococcus* are rarely found in the absence of infection. With *Candida*, however, the situation is different. Antibodies which react to *Candida albicans* are almost invariably demonstrable in human sera whether or not the subject has overt candidosis, and proliferation of *Candida* is very rapidly followed by an increase in antibody levels. In Figure 30.1 results are shown when sera drawn sequentially from a patient with *Candida* endocarditis were tested by counter-immunoelectrophoresis against cell wall polysac-charide (mannan) and cytoplasmic protein. At Day 3 a trace reaction against mannan is seen. Two days later the response is much stronger. Such tests are of real value in rather critically defined circumstances. Provided that the patient's antibody-forming mechanisms are fully functional (and in patients with *Candida* endocarditis they usually are) then serological studies can provide vital clues for the clinician on the state and progression of infection.

In Figure 30.2 precipitin titres to *C. albicans* are shown for a patient who had a successful aortic valve replacement (AVR). Similar profiles were obtained by agglutination and immunofluorescent procedures, and by RIA studies directed towards specific IgG and IgA immunoglobulins. In contrast, antibody titres to *C. parapsilosis* in another patient with endocarditis (Figure

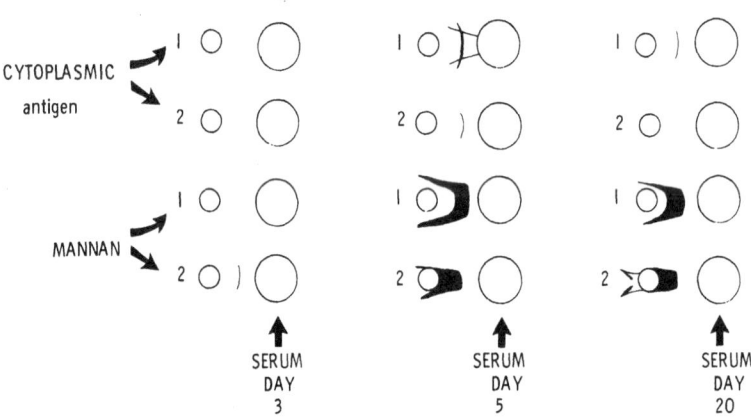

Figure 30.1 Antibody responses to *Candida albicans*

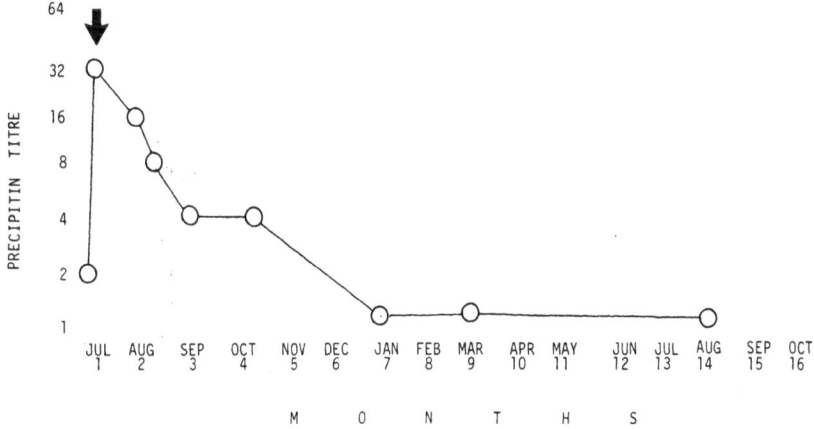

Figure 30.2 Precipitin titres to *Candida albicans*

30.3) show a different progression. In this case antibody levels remained high after completion of a course of antifungal therapy. Instead of diminishing, they subsequently rose to a very high level. An embolism was finally released from what was proven to be a recolonized valve and lodged in the patient's ankle. Histology and culture confirmed the cause of the embolism to be *C. parapsilosis*. Between the AVR and production of the embolism the patient was well. Only the high sustained precipitin titres hinted that the nidus of infection had not been eradicated and was becoming re-established.

Aspergillus infections are less amenable to diagnosis and surveillance by immunoassays since they usually occur in immunosuppressed patients. Attempts are being made to develop assay systems for detection of anti-genaemia, and these are badly needed, for early diagnosis of these opportun-

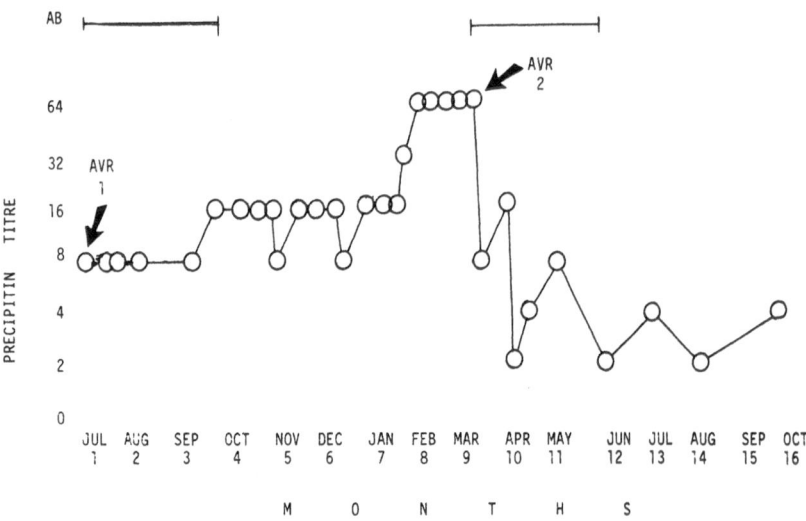

Figure 30.3 Precipitin titres to *Candida parapsilosis*

istic infections is essential, yet orthodox cultural and histological findings may not be helpful. Early results with ELISA[3, 4] have been encouraging, but much work needs to be done before immunoassays for antigen detection become accepted, reliable serological procedures in mycopathology. Several recent reviews describe in greater detail the use of immunoassays in mycology[5-8].

Rapid immunoassays have been used in situations where speed is a desirable or even necessary component of the immunoassay. The best known and most reliable of these is the latex agglutination test for capsular polysaccharide of *Cryptococcus neoformans*. This test, using latex particles coated with immunoglobulin from hyperimmunized rabbits, is both sensitive and specific. Antigen is readily detected in cerebrospinal fluid or serum of patients with cryptococcosis, and providing appropriate controls are used, 'false-positive' results can be eliminated. The test has prognostic, as well as diagnostic, value. Thus, the chances of survival of a patient are inversely proportional to the quantity of antigen detected, i.e. the LA titre.

Finally, an interesting and useful procedure that may be unfamiliar to many. It is a lineal descendant, perhaps, of the Elek test for recognition of toxigenic strains of *Corynebacterium diphtheriae*. This is the 'exo-antigen' system[9] for identification of the agents causing systemic mycoses. In this procedure, cultures are identified by flooding with merthiolate and concentrating the supernate × 25- or × 50-fold after overnight incubation. This is then used as antigen in double-diffusion against reference antisera to the major causes of systemic mycoses. The accuracy of the method is impressive. Cultures of these organisms can be slow-growing and they often fail to produce the diagnostic spores which make identification possible. Positive identification can take weeks or months, and in these circumstances management of a patient has to proceed according to presumptive evidence. It is not known how applicable this method is in other branches of microbiology for identification of genera or perhaps species.

The field of medical mycology presents both challenge and opportunity for the development and application of immunoassays as diagnostic and prognostic aids. Immunoassays have an important role in mycopathology and their potential is by no means fully realized. The future will certainly see both consolidation and extension of existing procedures, and the introduction of new methods and approaches for the study of antigens and antigen-associated responses.

References

1. Axelsen, N. (1973). Quantitative immunoelectrophoretic methods as tools of polyvalent approach to standardization in the immunochemistry of *Candida albicans*. *Infect. Immun.*, **7**, 949

2. Tran Van Ky, P., Uriel, J. and Rose, F. (1966). Caractérisation de types d'activités enzymatiques dans des extraits antigéniques d'*Aspergillus fumigatus* après électrophorese et immunoélectrophorèse en agarose. *Ann. Inst. Pasteur*, **111**, 161

3. Reiss, E. and Lehmann, P. (1979). Galactomannan antigenemia in invasive aspergillosis. *Infect. Immun.*, **25**, 357

4. Richardson, M. D., White, L. O. and Warren, R. C. (1979). Detection of circulating antigen of *Aspergillus fumigatus* in sera of mice and rabbits by enzyme-linked immunosorbent assay. *Mycopathology*, **67**, 83

5. Lehmann, P. (1980). Immunology of the fungi. In Lachmann, P. J. and Peters, D. K. (eds.) *Clinical Aspects of Immunology*, 4th Ed. (Oxford: Blackwell Scientific Publications. In preparation)

6. Mackenzie, D. W. R. (1979). Immune responses to fungal infections. In Dick, G. W. A. (ed.) *Immunological Aspects of Infectious Diseases*, pp. 21–75. (Lancaster: MTP Press Ltd)

7. Mackenzie, D. W. R., Proctor, A. G. J. and Philpot, C. M. (1980). *Basic Serodiagnostic Methods for Diseases Caused by Fungi and Actinomycetes*. PHLS Monograph Series 12, (London: HMSO)

8. Palmer, D. F., Kaufman, L., Kaplan, W. and Cavallaro, J. J. (1977). *Serodiagnosis of Mycotic Diseases*. (Springfield, Ill.: Charles C. Thomas.)

9. Kaufman, L. and Standard, P. (1978). Immuno-identification of cultures of fungi pathogenic to man. *Curr. Microbiol.*, **1**, 135

31
Some Applications of Immunoassays in Tropical Parasitic Infections

C. C. DRAPER and M. L. McLAREN

In parasitic infections the most certain method of diagnosis in the individual and in survey work is the demonstration of the infecting organism itself. This may often be difficult. The organism may be present in the blood, excreta or tissues at low densities, it may only be demonstrable intermittently or for a very limited period at the start of an infection, or the techniques needed may be sophisticated, time-consuming and expensive. However, most organisms elicit, sooner or later, an immune response; detection of this can be used as evidence of infection. This can be done by showing the presence of specific cell-mediated immunity, commonly by a skin test in which a reactive antigen from the organism is injected intradermally or, more frequently, by showing the presence in the blood of specific antibodies produced against the organism. The immunological response elicited by an organism may persist long after it has itself disappeared. Therefore, particularly in clinical work, an ideal test should differentiate between an active and a past cured infection. Unfortunately, in the field of tropical medicine, few such tests exist and it is usually necessary to make an inspired guess as to whether infection is still active or not by measuring the amounts of antibody present and, particularly, by looking for changes in the titre in serial specimens. The presence of specific IgM antibody may be indicative of recent infection and tests for this have been used in, for example, toxoplasma infections. The use of such tests needs to be explored further in other parasitic infections and it is to be hoped that new techniques will allow this. Notwithstanding difficulties in interpretation many of these immunodiagnostic tests are now established as useful aids in clinical practice, particularly for protozoal infections. Although they would be of great use, tests for helminthic infections have generally not been so valuable, chiefly because of difficulties in preparing specifically reactive antigens from these complex organisms.

In recent years increasing use has been made of immunodiagnostic tests in studying the epidemiology of several tropical infections. Skin tests (for example for leishmaniasis) have been used but because of frequent lack of specificity, serological tests have been more popular and this has given birth to the new discipline of seroepidemiology[1]. Blood is a convenient fluid to collect and test, and if a sample from a finger-prick, collected in capillary tubes or as drops on absorbent paper, can be used, a serological test may be easier and cheaper than searching for parasites in blood, excreta or tissue biopsies. Furthermore, the information obtained from a survey for specific antibodies, although it may not replace it entirely, will add greatly to that obtained from a parasite survey alone. The latter will indicate only the point prevalence of infections, detecting only those recently acquired, and will certainly miss some of these. Antibodies appear within days of infection and usually persist for months or years, depending on the intensity of the antigenic stimulus. Therefore, as well as more accurately detecting those recently infected an antibody survey will also indicate what has happened in the past, or in other words, the period prevalence of infection. From the proportions found with antibodies in different age-groups it is possible to assess the incidence rates of infection at different times using simple mathematical models[2]. Owing to the peculiar difficulties of isolating the infecting organisms such seroepidemiological surveys were first done on a large scale by virologists, for example for delineating the zones of yellow fever transmission. Tests are evolving which can be done on a large scale using small quantities of serum, and these are proving of use in tropical parasitic infections. They are likely to be of particular value at the lower levels of transmission, in situations where parasites may be present only in low densities or intermittently but where it is desirable to get accurate information on incidence and prevalence, and in surveying for infections where it is particularly difficult or tedious to isolate the organisms, as with Chagas' disease or *Schistosoma mansoni* infections.

A great variety of immunodiagnostic tests have been used for different tropical infections and their large number suggests that none is universally applicable. Table 31.1 shows the ideal criteria for a diagnostic test, particularly for one to be employed in developing countries. It is possible to discuss here only two of the more promising tests which meet some of these criteria.

Indirect fluorescent antibody (IFA) tests have been well evaluated over recent years and have been found to be of particular use for the diagnosis of protozoal infections both in individual clinical diagnosis and in survey work. Whole parasite antigens are usually employed which have advantages in simplicity of preparation and in reproducibility. The test has been less successful for diagnosis of helminth infections owing to problems with cross-reactions. The technique has also had wide applications in virology and bacteriology so that excellent equipment and reagents are available. Dis-

Table 31.1 Criteria of a diagnostic test

(1) High level of sensitivity

(2) High level of specificity

(3) Ease of sample collection
  (a) use of untrained personnel
  (b) socially acceptable method
  (c) cost effective

(4) Ease of test operation
  (a) use of untrained personnel
  (b) good test reproducibility
  (c) cost-effective

(5) Quantitative
  (a) able to differentiate active from past infection
  (b) responsive to intensity of infection
  (c) responsive to chemotherapeutic treatment

(6) Suitable for use in field laboratories

advantages are that the test is somewhat costly, time-consuming and the reading of the test is subjective. However, with modern microtechniques the time taken to test a set of sera for malaria antibodies, for example, is much less than that needed to examine an equal number of blood films.

The enzyme-linked immunosorbent assay (ELISA) has been adapted to several parasitic infections[3]. Because it uses only very small amounts of reagents it has the advantage that highly refined and specific antigens can be prepared, and it is also more objective in interpretation and can be carried out with less expensive apparatus than the IFA test; only one dilution of serum need be tested to obtain a quantitative result.

As has already been mentioned, it is particularly at the lower levels of transmission that immunodiagnosis is of practical epidemiological use. For example, towards the end of a successful malaria eradication scheme it is essential to detect any residual foci of transmission. Because malaria antibodies may persist for many years, particularly in those who have had much antigenic stimulation from repeated exposure in the past, it is necessary in such situations to look chiefly at the lower age-groups. An example of such a survey, in Mauritius, is shown in Figure 31.1. In this island a successful malaria control scheme was started in 1949 and it was thought that eradication of transmission had been achieved by 1971. However, in order to confirm this a serological survey was done in 1972. The district surveyed was the only one where some transmission might have lingered. Surveillance teams collected over 6000 samples of blood on absorbent paper, mostly from children. The absence of antibodies by the IFA test in those under 5 years old gave strong evidence, supporting parasite surveys, that little or no recent transmission had occurred. From the percentage prevalence of antibodies in different age-groups it was possible to calculate approximate inoculation rates

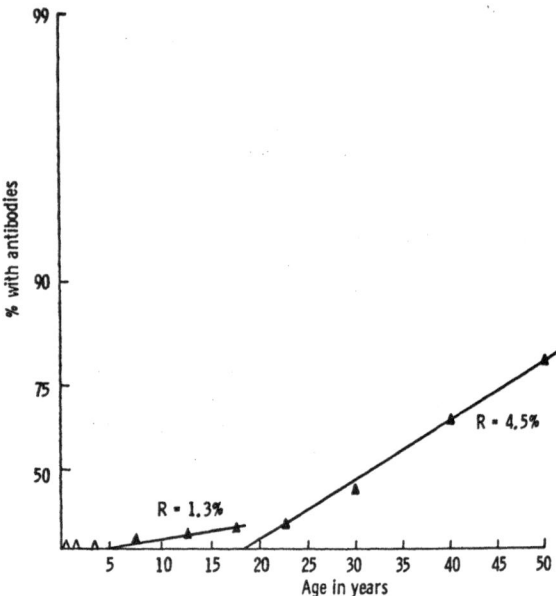

Figure 31.1 Mauritius Survey 1972. Total malaria antibodies by age-group. Black River district. Reverse log scale

(R) by a simple method[4], and to show that these had been decreasing over the years.

Conversely, serological surveys may be of value as sensitive indicators of the return of malaria into areas where eradication had previously been achieved. An interesting recent example of this was in the island of Grenada where there was a small outbreak of *Plasmodium malariae* malaria in 1978, probably arising from a recrudescence in an old case[5]. Because of the often low and fluctuating parasitaemia with this parasite serology was particularly useful in detecting cases. In order to exclude cross-reacting antibodies in older people, due to infections in the past with other malaria parasites, all positive sera were tested against all three malaria antigens. Only those with strong reactions against *P. malariae* which were greater than those with other antigens were considered as possibly being infected. The results of parasite and serological surveys are shown in Figure 31.2. Some 30 additional cases in a small community were detected by the latter.

An ELISA for malaria antibodies has been described but is not yet as sensitive or specific as the IFA test[6].

The third example (Figure 31.3) is taken from previously unpublished data from an area in Brazil where infection with *Trypanosoma cruzi* was endemic. Even more than in African trypanosomiasis, it is very difficult to demonstrate this organism except in the acute phase of the infection. The overall parasite rate in this community was well under 1%; however, the age-specific antibody

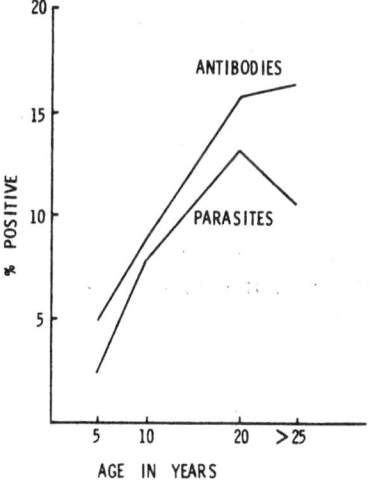

Figure 31.2 Grenada 1978. *P. malariae* parasite and antibody rates in 407 subjects

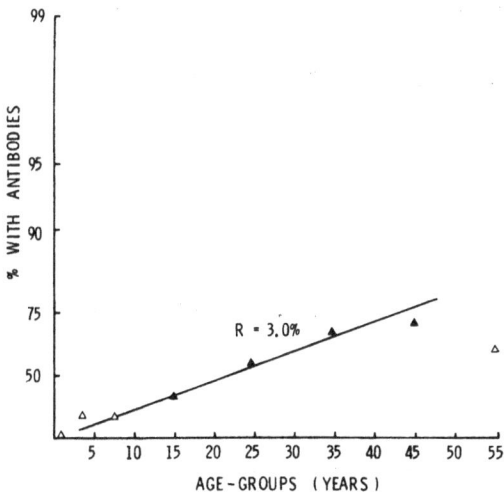

Figure 31.3 São Felipe, Bahia. *T. cruzi* antibodies by IFAT, by age-groups, 1971–2. Reverse log scale.

rates show that by the age of 35 years about 60% of the population had been exposed to infection, corresponding to an inoculation rate (R) of about 3% per year. The fall in the antibody rates in the older age-groups is probably due to the increased mortality of infected people. A reliable ELISA for *T. cruzi* antibodies, which can be performed more rapidly than the IFA test, has been described[3].

Infection with *Schistosoma mansoni* was endemic in the Caribbean island of St Lucia until an extensive and successful control scheme was started over 10 years ago, using chemotherapy, molluscicide, and provision of safe water supplies[7]. A problem has been how to monitor large numbers of children each year in order to detect any re-establishment of the infection. Stool examinations for ova of the parasite are expensive and time-consuming and only a limited number can be done. A trial was made in St Lucia of an ELISA[8,9] as an alternative to radioimmunoassay (RIA)[10] for antibody detection. Figure 31.4 shows a comparison of the different methods in an area where control had

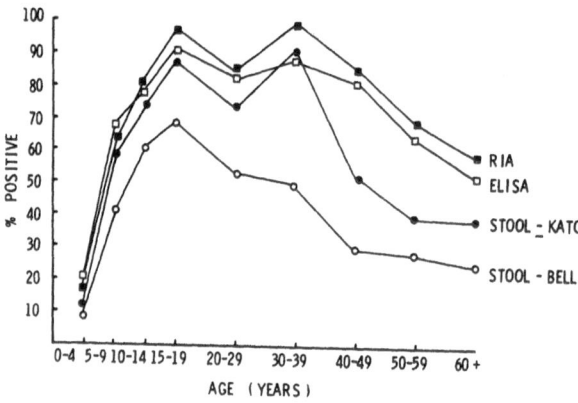

Figure 31.4   A. *S. mansoni* prevalence survey by stool and serology in an untreated community in St Lucia

not yet been started. In the younger age-groups both the ELISA and RIA show a higher level of infection, as judged by the presence of antibodies, than the standard Bell method of stool examination. This was confirmed when a more thorough stool examination was done by the Kato method by an experienced parasitologist. In the older age-groups there was some fall in the prevalence of antibodies and a lower proportion was accompanied by an active infection, probably due to a reduced exposure and possibly some acquired resistance. As a result of these studies the ELISA is being used for surveillance, in which 8000 capillary blood samples, collected on absorbent paper from children, are tested each year. Although equally sensitive and specific the RIA cannot be used routinely because of difficulties in obtaining regular supplies of labelled antigen and in maintaining sophisticated equipment. Some stool examinations are still done in a random sample to confirm the serological results, but the introduction of the ELISA for screening has greatly reduced both cost and time. One technician can process in a week from 500 to 1000 blood samples compared with 60 stool samples by the Bell technique.

Another approach to immunodiagnosis lies in the detection of parasites themselves, or of their circulating antigenic products. Several laboratories are engaged in attempts to identify relevant antigens and to prepare antisera to them which could be used in labelled antibody assays. Encouraging results have been obtained for schistosomiasis in experimental infections in animals and possibly in man[11], but less so with other parasitic infections. If successful, such techniques could provide sensitive methods for detecting active and, possibly, recent infections and, if applicable on a large scale, they could be useful tools. However, in most situations information is needed about period prevalence of an infection as well as about point prevalence. Therefore both types of survey would need to be done, and would complement each other.

Table 31.2 Advantages and disadvantages of parasitological and serological diagnostic tests

Advantages	Disadvantages
PARASITOLOGICAL TESTS	
Detects active infection	low sensitivity
Able to quantitate infection levels	not applicable to all infections
Specific	time-consuming
Often simple test procedure	expensive
Ease of technician training	sample collection can be socially unacceptable
SEROLOGICAL TESTS	
Very sensitive	variable specificity
Applicable to most infections	unable to distinguish active from past infection
Good test reproducibility	sophisticated techniques
Suitable for mass screening	often need highly trained personnel
Reflects period prevalence	
Cost-effective	

Table 31.2 summarizes some of the present relative advantages and disadvantages of parasitological and serological tests. Considerable advances are, however, being made in the latter and it can confidently be predicted that in the future they will provide useful tools both for the physician who is concerned with the diagnosis and treatment of tropical infections and for those who are concerned with the prevention of such infections at their source.

References

1. Lobel, H. O. and Kagan, I. G. (1978). Seroepidemiology of parasitic diseases. *Ann. Rev. Microbiol.*, **32**, 329
2. Draper, C. C., Voller, A. and Carpenter, R. G. (1972). The epidemiological interpretation of serologic data in malaria. *Am. J. Trop. Med. Hyg.*, **21**, 696
3. Voller, A., Bartlett, A. and Bidwell, D. E. (1976). Enzyme immunoassays for parasitic diseases. *Trans. R. Soc. Trop. Med. Hyg.*, **70**, 98

4. Bruce-Chwatt, L. J., Draper, C. C. and Konfortion, P. (1973). Seroepidemiological evidence of eradication of malaria from Mauritius. *Lancet*, **3**, 547

5. Tikasingh, E., Edwards, C. S., Hamilton, P. J. S., Commissiong, L. and Draper, C. C. (1980). An outbreak of malaria in Grenada due to *Plasmodium malariae*. *Am. J. Trop. Med. Hyg.* (In press)

6. Spencer, H. C., Collins, W. E. and Skinner, J. C. (1979). The enzyme linked immunosorbent assay (ELISA) for malaria. II. Comparison with the malaria indirect fluorescent antibody test (IFA). *Am. J. Trop. Med. Hyg.*, **28**, 933

7. Jordan, P. (1977). Schistosomiasis – research to control. *Am. J. Trop. Med. Hyg.*, **26**, 877

8. McLaren, M. L., Draper, C. C., Roberts, J. M., Minter-Goedbloed, E., Ligthart, G. S., Teesdale, C. H., Amin, M. A., Omer, A. H. S., Bartlett, A. and Voller, A. (1978). Studies on the ELISA test for *S. mansoni* infections. *Ann. Trop. Med. Parasitol.*, **72**, 243

9. McLaren, M. L., Long, E. G., Goodgame, R. W. and Lillywhite, J. E. (1979). Application of the ELISA for serodiagnosis of *S. mansoni* infection in St. Lucia. *Trans. R. Soc. Trop. Med. Hyg.*, **73**, 636

10. Pelley, R. P., Warren, R. S. and Jordan, P. (1977). Purified antigen radioimmunoassay in serological diagnosis of *S. mansoni*. *Lancet*, **2**, 781

11. Santoro, F., Vandemenlebrouha, B. and Capron, A. (1978). The use of the radioimmunoprecipitation–PEG assay (RIPEGA) to quantify circulating antigens in human and experimental schistosomiasis. *J. Immunol. Methods*, **24**, 229

32
Immunoassays in Veterinary Medicine

J. R. CROWTHER and E. M. E. ABU ELZEIN

INTRODUCTION

The advantages of high specificity and sensitivity gained by using immunological reactions in assay procedures have been illustrated by research in all fields of microbiology. The applications of immunoassay in veterinary science are wide-ranging and form the basis of most studies of infections in animals. Greatest emphasis is put on animal diseases where they may spread to man, or where the disease is economically devastating. Since animals are susceptible to a wide range of infectious agents, any reasonably brief discussion of immunoassays must concentrate on principles rather than describing many examples of their use.

The uses of immunoassays are two-fold. Firstly, to defect specific antigens in the diagnosis of disease, either directly from infected material or after attempting to grow the agent under suitable conditions, e.g. in tissue culture. Secondly, to measure specific antibodies from animal sera, for example, in epidemiogical surveys to assess the extent of disease, or the immune status of animals after vaccination.

The investigation of immunity in animals using *in vitro* methods is hampered by the lack of knowledge as to whether the antibodies detected have any relationship to protection. This knowledge can be increased where experiments comparing *in vivo* and *in vitro* tests can be conducted, although this is limited owing to the high costs involved in using economically important animals in statistically relevant numbers. Where this has been accomplished, good correlation between certain antibody levels and protection can be made; for example between serum neutralization (SN) test titres and cattle protection tests in foot and mouth disease (FMD) research.

Another handicap stems from the variable reactivities of different classes of immunoglobulins which may be stimulated by a particular pathogen. Most tests have evolved by extensive empirical research, whereby the 'best' tests to employ on particular situations with specific diseases have been discovered. The recent development of highly sensitive solid-phase assay techniques, making easy the detection and quantification of class-specific immunoglobulins from serum, for example IgA and IgE, may give valuable information which has hitherto been overlooked using routine tests.

It should be stressed that tests made *in vitro* on materials such as serum can be repeated on single or sequential samples, so that the chance of measuring protective antibody content is available. *In vitro* determinations of the activity of cell-mediated immune responses are not yet well developed, but may play an important future role in understanding protective mechanisms. When more knowledge of what immunoglobulins are responsible for protection and how cell-mediated immune processes work is available, it may become possible to correlate measurement of these factors with the degree of protection present. Here the veterinarian has a distinct advantage over the physician since he can assess the value of a vaccine or an antiserum in the same species of animal as that in which it is to be used. In man, such tests can only be done when evaluating innocuous pathogens.

Techniques used to detect antibody can be used, inversely, to detect and identify antigens. With the high specificity usually inherent in any antigen–antibody reaction, these tests not only provide a definitive method of identifying biological materials but also provide methods for qualitative comparison of antigens.

TYPES OF TESTS

Many methods are available for measuring the reactions between antibody and antigen. All of them depend on the properties of the complex which results. Table 32.1 illustrates several properties of the reactivity which are

Table 32.1 Properties of antigen–antibody reactions exploited in immunoassays

---

(1) Complexes are larger than individual reactants and can be separated by ultracentrifugation
(2) Complexes form lattice which is hydrophobic, yielding a visible precipitate
(3) Complexes have altered electrical charge and can be separated from individual components by electrophoretic methods
(4) Formation of complexes initiates activity of other factors, e.g. complement, phagocytosis
(5) Large particulate antigens may be 'tied' together to produce agglutination
(6) Reaction of antibody alters a property of antigen, e.g. haemagglutinating capacity reduced, infectivity reduced, toxicity reduced
(7) One of the reactants can be fixed to solid support and detected directly or indirectly with 'tagged' reagents, e.g. radioimmunoassay, enzyme-labelled assays

---

exploited in immunoassays. Tables 32.2a and 32.2b illustrate the types of immunoassays commonly used in veterinary research. The brief comments on each test, and examples of their applications, are intended only to illustrate the 'width' of the procedures employed. Two types of tests are shown. In the first, the combination of antibody with antigen is 'directly' observed. Tests of this type depend on precipitation or agglutination of the antigen. One of the reactants may be labelled with fluorescent or radioactive chemicals to aid localization of the complexes. The second group depend on the detection of secondary phenomena to show that a reaction has taken place. This may occur by a simple alteration to a test of the first type; e.g. antigens may be attached to larger particles which show agglutination in the presence of antibody instead of precipitation. The test can also be made more complex, as in the complement-fixation test, or in the neutralization of infectivity or toxicity. The development of immunoassays using tracers, and particularly the advent of enzyme-labelled assays (ELA) in the early 1970s, combined with the availability of solid-phase microtitre plate systems, has been a strong stimulus to veterinary researchers to use highly sensitive assays for the study of a wide variety of diseases. The ELA test, as is often quoted, combines the advantages of immunofluorescence and radioimmunoassay while overcoming the disadvantages of both.

It is useful to study an animal disease in detail and examine the development of immunoassays used in solving problems associated with the disease which are shared with most other animal/pathogen relationships.

Foot and mouth disease (FMD) occurs in most parts of the world and immunological studies are complicated by the existence of seven types of virus. Problems associated with the disease are outlined in Tables 32.3 and 32.4, which deal with those involving the virus as an antigen and antibodies produced against this antigen respectively.

IMMUNOASSAY AND FMD VIRUS

Diagnosis and serotyping of FMD virus

Seven serotypes of FMD virus can be distinguished which fail to produce cross-protective antibodies against infection with any other type. Thus, it is important not only to determine that a vesicular disease is caused by an FMD virus but also to identify the serotype so that relevant control measures may be taken; e.g. selection of the appropriate vaccine. The routine immunoassay at the Animal Virus Research Institute, Pirbright, which is the World Reference Laboratory for FMD, is the complement-fixation (CF) test. Field material is usually received in the form of epithelial tissue, which is ground into phosphate-buffered saline to release virus. Clarified suspensions are then titrated using the micro-CF test with standard typing sera produced after

Table 32.2 Immunoassays in veterinary research

Test	Comments	Applications
Neutralization	(1) Most relevant for study of immunity (2) 'Live' system needed after antigen–antibody reaction, e.g. tissue culture (3) Subject to high variation, laborious	Wide usage in measurement of antibodies to virus diseases Low levels of viruses needed Application to toxins
Haemagglutination inhibition	(1) *In vitro* 'neutralization' of activity of antigens which normally haemagglutinate various species of red blood cells	Many viruses haemagglutinate and can be used in their diagnosis, e.g. Newcastle disease virus, bovine para-influenza, influenza. Diagnosis of *Mycoplasma gallisepticum* infections in fowls Diagnosis of rinderpest using inhibition of measles haemagglutinin
Agglutination	(1) Simple test. Needs 'large' antigens (2) Slide agglutination tests (3) Qualitative agglutination utilizing secondary phenomena, antigens attached to solid support such as red blood cells, latex particles. Rapid tests	(1) Diagnosis of *Salmonella pullorum* and *Mycoplasma gallisepticum* virus. Diagnosis of contagious bovine pleuropneumonia (CBPP) caused by *M. mycoides* in cattle. (2) Salmonella serotyping. (3) Diagnosis of pregnancy in mares. Diagnosis of brucella, leptospira, salmonella, *Trichomonas foetus*, *Vibrio foetus*
Precipitation	(1) Simple – precipitates at interface of antigen–antibody (2) Double immunodiffusion. Wide usage for serum qualitative and quantitative assessments. Sensitivity increased by using radioactive labelled reagents	(1) Identification of species of animal from insect blood meals Identification of animal species in meat inspections Ascoli test for anthrax in carcases, hides, skins (2) Diagnosis of antibodies, e.g. swine vesicular disease, rinderpest, canine virus hepatitis, distemper, 'bluetongue' virus

(3) Immunoelectrophoresis. Useful in characterization of specific immunoglobulin reactions. Variations, e.g. rocket techniques

(3) Identification of non-specific reactive immunoglobulins from 'normal' sera against foot-and-mouth disease virus

(4) Immunoelectro-osmophoresis (IEOP). Rapid test where antigen and antibody are electrophoresed towards each other

(4) Diagnosis of African swine fever and swine fever viruses

(5) Immune electronmicroscopy

(5) Identification of many viruses, e.g. rotaviruses

Labelled reagents

Most recent development in immunoassays. Increased sensitivity due to high specific activities of incorporation of labels into antigens or antibodies

(1) Fluorescent dyes

(1) Wide applications as direct or indirect test on field or tissue culture material, e.g. diagnosis of rabies infection, identification of *Toxoplasma gondii* from stillborn lambs, rapid diagnosis of canine hepatitis, diagnosis of avian infectious bursitis, diagnosis of sarcocystis infections in sheep and swine. Can be used to identify antibodies, e.g. against *Babesia bigemina* in cattle sera, transmissible gastroenteritis in swine sera.

(2) Radioimmunoassay (RIA). Needs sophisticated equipment plus radioactive handling facilities. Versatile test which can be automated. Needs more exploitation in veterinary medicine.

(2) Wide use for detection and quantification of antibodies and antigens. Increasing use in veterinary research to measure hormones and drugs.

(3) Enzyme-labelled assays (ELA), enzyme-linked immunosorbent assays (ELISA)

(3) Large-scale diagnosis of Trichinella in infected pigs, indirect method used to detect Babesia infections and trypanosomiasis in cattle. Identification of Aujeszky's disease, African swine fever and many other virus diseases. Improved test for the measurement of Newcastle disease virus antibodies and diagnosis of rotavirus infections. Recent use to measure *Mycoplasma suipneumoniae* in pigs. Commercial kits now available, e.g. feline leukaemia virus

Table 32.3 Immunoassays used to study FMD virus antigen

Requirement	Problem	Test	Comments
Rapid diagnosis and serotyping.	Seven serotypes	(1) CF test routinely used. Results in 1–48 h	Cross-reactions between serotypes. Pro/anti-complementary factors. Passage of samples in tissue culture sometimes needed
		(2) Immunofluorescence	Laborious. Tissue culture needed
		(3) ELISA. Experimental so far. Indirect-sandwich tests best	10–100 times sensitivity of CF test. Low cross-reactions from crude samples. Needs long period of parallel testing with CF test to prove its worth
		(4) RIA. Similar techniques to above	Same results as with ELISA. Slightly more sensitive, cannot be read 'by eye'
Quantification of virus	Assay of whole virion in the presence of tissue culture, viral subunit and virus-induced proteins	(1) CF test. Modified test used attempting to make it more specific for whole virion by using adsorbed sera	Complicated results due to fixation of complement by unwanted antigen–antibody reactions
		(2) Single radial immunodiffusion (SRID)	Needs concentration of material – low sensitivity
		(3) Single radial haemolysis	Higher sensitivity than SRID. Little advantage over routine CF
		(4) ELISA. Sandwich tests used successfully	Can process large numbers of samples. High sensitivity and specificity achieved for whole virion antigen
		(5) RIA	May have advantage over ELISA for continuous measurement of virus during vaccine manufacture. More sensitive than ELISA
Qualitative tests	Comparison of virus isolates from the field to vaccine strains.	(1) CF. Routinely used for subtyping	Wide variation in results, with obscure relationships established owing to use of laboratory-prepared antisera
		(2) RIA. Double-antibody competition. Solid phase competition	Compares viruses using single pool of antiserum, strains related according to their relative avidity compared to homologous antigen–antibody reaction
		(3) ELISA. Solid-phase competition	Useful in comparing large number of field isolates when not purified. Relationships not correlated with field studies
		(4) Immunodiffusion (ID)	Insensitive. Improved by using radioactive

Table 32.4 Immunoassays used to study antibodies against FMD viruses

Requirement	Problem	Test	Comment
Antibody screening	Epidemiological studies	(1) SN test. Routinely used	Should be most relevant to field protection. Non-specific reactions from cattle in disease-free areas
		(2) Passive haemagglutination	Not fully exploited. Sensitive and versatile
		(3) ELISA. Indirect and sandwich. Competition assays	Non-specific reactions observed in SN test eliminated. Sensitive test. Results within 5 h
		(4) RIA. Double-antibody. Solid phase indirect	Rapid assay of total antibody. Same results
		(5) DID	Low sensitivity, can be used to establish which antibodies are non-specific
Quantification	Measurement after vaccine campaign	(1) SN test. Attempts to relate levels of antibody to protection	Complicated by non-specific reactions
		(2) ELISA. Indirect test	Correlation with SN titres good. Can be adapted to measure class antibodies, e.g. IgM, IgA, IgG_1, IgG_2
		(3) RIA	Similar results to ELISA, increased sensitivity

infecting guinea-pigs. This test is used successfully but can be influenced by three main difficulties. The first is that interfering reactions may produce pro- or anti-complementary activity so that typing is impossible. This activity cannot be predicted and the nature of the types of sample received, e.g. bacterial contamination, can be implicated in anticomplementary activity. The second difficulty is that samples may only contain low levels of virus so that typing on 'original' material is impossible and the level of virus has to be increased through growth in suitable tissue culture, producing a loss in time to achieve results. The third possible disadvantage is that the CF test detects varying degrees of cross-reactions between serotypes. These are probably due to the detection of cross-reactive subunit material and virus-induced antigens present in the samples by the hyperimmunized guinea-pig antisera. Methods to eliminate the cross-reactive antibodies from typing sera have been examined, for example by producing antisera against purified inactivated virus. Attempts to reduce the time of testing have met with some success since the specific homologous antiserum reactions are of higher avidity than those involving cross-reactions with the subunit material. However, the test becomes less sensitive and consequently the number of typings from original material is reduced. While the CF test remains the method of choice so far, it is interesting to compare the 'newer' techniques applied to this problem.

The double-sandwich enzyme-linked immunosorbent assay (ELISA), the principle of which is shown in Figure 32.1, has been used for serotyping with success[1]. This test was developed to be read 'by eye' so that it could be used

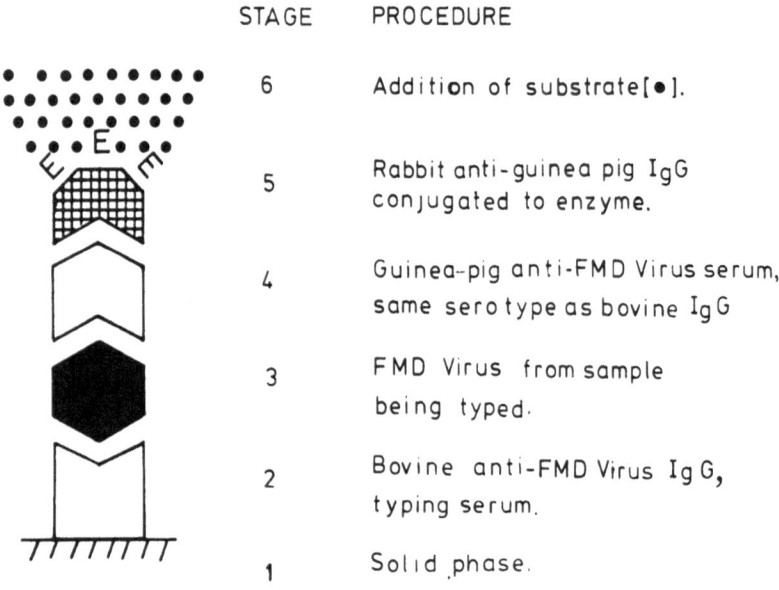

STAGE	PROCEDURE
6	Addition of substrate[●].
5	Rabbit anti-guinea pig IgG conjugated to enzyme.
4	Guinea-pig anti-FMD Virus serum, same serotype as bovine IgG
3	FMD Virus from sample being typed.
2	Bovine anti-FMD Virus IgG, typing serum.
1	Solid phase.

Figure 32.1 Principle of double-sandwich ELISA for identification of FMD virus types

more generally in laboratories where spectrophotometric equipment was not available. This emphasizes the need to evaluate the possible uses of any immunoassay before development. The ELISA test successfully typed all the FMD virus strains, using original epithelial tissue as shown in Table 32.5.

Table 32.5 Typing of FMD virus from bovine epithelium samples

Epithelium sample	ELISA* Original sample	CF Original sample	CF After passage in tissue culture
1	A	–	A
2	0	†	0
3	–	–	–
4	A	–	A
5	1	1	1
6	–	†	–
7	As 1	As 1	As 1
8	A	–	A
9	C	–	C
10	–	–	–
11	A	A	A
12	1	–	1
13	A	A	A
14	0	0	0
15	2	2	2
16	0	†	0
17	A	–	A
18	0	0	0
19	–	†	–
20	C	C	C
21	1	–	1
22	A	–	A
23	0	†	0

* Results obtained using neat, $\frac{1}{2}$ and $\frac{1}{4}$ of original sample.
† Anticomplementary
– No typing obtained

Results were obtained in 3 h using microplates already sensitized with the bovine typing serum and stored at $+4°C$. Only three dilutions of sample were needed to give specific typing and the higher sensitivity of this test over the CF test was demonstrated, since all 19 possible positive samples were identified from original material, whereas the CF test typed only eight samples and tissue culture passage was necessary before the rest could be typed. ELISA was unaffected by the anticomplementary nature of five of the samples.

Further studies have shown this type of ELISA to be a sensitive test for the unequivocal serotyping of FMD viruses. The use of sandwich techniques appears to reduce cross-reactions observed in the same samples when using CF tests. The ELISA test will probably be of most use in areas where typing resources are limited and tests on epithelial tissue are critical. Typing plates, sensitized with readily available type-specific bovine antibodies to FMD virus, can be produced in central laboratories, tested, and dispatched along with guinea-pig typing sera and enzyme-conjugated anti-guinea-pig antisera. Sensitized plates produced in these laboratories have remained usable for 18 months (so far). Collaborative studies to examine the use of such tests in the field are being made.

Subtyping of FMD viruses

FMD viruses isolated from the field can show antigenic variation within a serotype; enough sometimes to be able to break through low levels of protective antibody produced against antigenically different subtypes used in vaccines. Thus, field isolates are examined in a preliminary study before beginning vaccination campaigns to establish the relationship of these isolates to currently available vaccine strains. Virus isolates are also examined for subtype difference, where they occur in areas previously vaccinated against that serotype, to examine whether the breakdown in protection can be attributed to a large 'shift' in the antigenic nature of the new strain or is a result of vaccine failure. Routine subtyping of isolates sent from different countries with varying degrees of FMD virus control also gives an idea of the epidemiological significance of particular antigenic subtypes, both geographically and temporally.

The tests used mainly in these directions are the serum neutralization (SN) test and the micro-CF test. The former test attempts to examine the neutralizing ability of antisera raised against homologous virus (e.g. vaccine strains) or against heterologous viruses (e.g. field strains). Theoretically, this test should have the advantage of obtaining results which compare the properties of viruses relevant to cross-protective antibody production in animals. Even though the SN tests are laborious and not rapid, they offer the best approximation to what might occur under field conditions, in that they probably examine differences in the neutralizing antibody-inducing sites of the virus isolates.

The CF test is used to compare isolates by chequerboard titrations of dilutions of virus and antiserums. Homologous and heterologous systems are compared so that to obtain reasonable results, antisera against field isolates must be prepared. This entails at least 1 month's delay before results are available. Thus, this type of testing is of use only for taxonomic or broad epidemiological studies, and these are of retrospective value.

Immunoassays involving radioactive or enzyme tracers have been used to examine the epidemiological/taxonomic and vaccine problems posed by the existence of antigenic variants of FMD virus.

The direct double-antibody radioimmunoassay (RIA) was described by Crowther[2] and was used to examine relationships of several strains within FMD virus type SAT2. Briefly, the test involves the competitions of an unlabelled purified FMD virus dilution series for a pre-titrated reaction between radioactive [^{35}S]methionine-labelled purified virus and homologous antibody. A diagrammatic representation of a competition assay is shown in Figure 32.2. This type of test has the advantage that it can be used with any

Stage 1   Ab titration

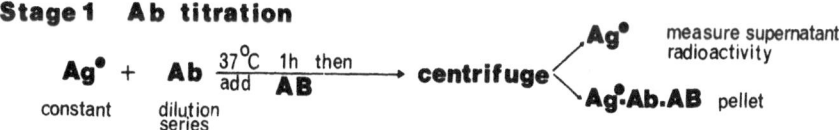

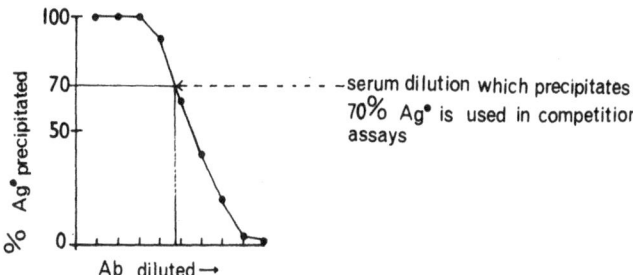

Stage 2   Competition Assay

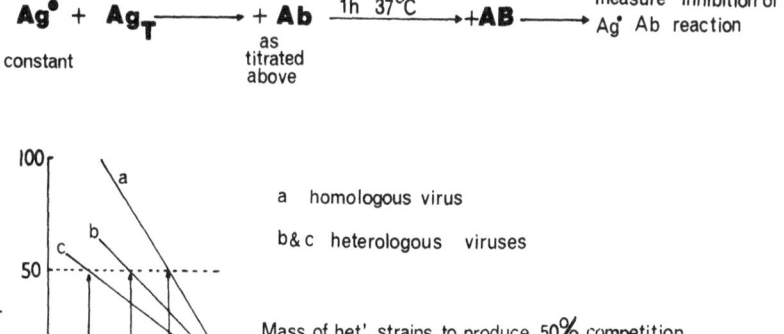

Figure 32.3 Outline of competition RIA. Ag●, [^{35}S]methionine-labelled 140S virus; Ab, homologous antibody; AB, anti-species antibody; Ag$_T$, dilution series of competing virus

species of serum, including bovine. This is not true of the CF test, which has to be modified for certain sera, so that CF inhibition tests, etc., have to be evolved where, for example, bovine serum does not fix complement. Some results of the RIA-competition test are shown in Figure 32.3. Several FMD type O viruses were compared using a homologous system of O$_1$, BFS 1860

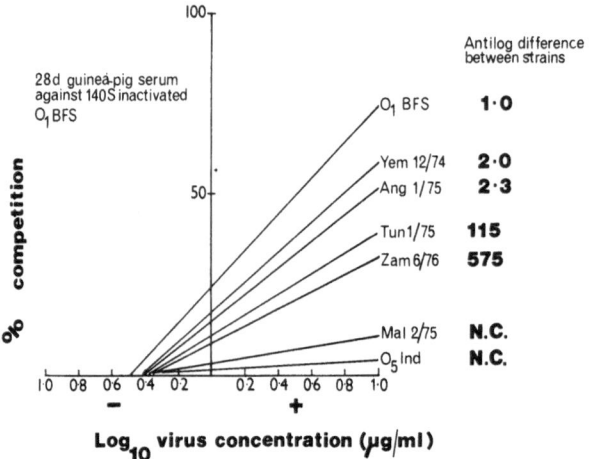

Figure 32.3   Comparison of type O FMD virus strains by competition RIA

radioactive virus with its respective guinea-pig antiserum. The values on the figure show the antilog values of the log difference in the competing ability of each strain compared (at 50% competition) with O_1, BFS 1860. The RIA results indicate that Yem 12/74 and Ang 1/75 are similar to O_1, BFS: Tun 1/75 and Zam 6/76 are intermediate in competition and Mal 2/75 and O_5 Ind do not compete under these conditions. Results of similar studies using other antisera are shown in Figure 32.4. Seven-day post-infection guinea-pig serum and hyperimmune (HI) guinea-pig serum obtained after infection and boosting of animal after 3 months are compared to cattle sera obtained 6 and 35 days after infection. Table 32.6 compares the relative differences in competition (antilog values at 50% competition) as determined from the graphs. The relative positions of most of the strains are similar for each serum; however, the scales of the masses of competing viruses are different. A salient point in this study is that early post-infection serum can be used to separate strains. It should be noted that Tun 1/75 does not react with the bovine antisera, indicating a different species response to an antigen, as discussed by Crumpton[3]. The change in discrimination by bovine serum from 6 to 35 days is interesting, since at 35 days the serum appears more specific for homologous virus as reflected by the reduction in competition for all the heterologous strains. HI guinea-pig serum, on the other hand, showed increased cross-reactivity with all strains, indicating an increased heterogeneity of antibodies to O_1, BFS 1860 with increased probability of cross-reactions with minor determinants shared by heterologous strains. It should be stressed, as in any immunoassay, that the particular antiserum used is the definitive factor in separation of strains. The competition patterns obtained are highly typical of the types of sera prepared as described, and have been obtained using several other homologous systems. The characterization of the reactivities of the different

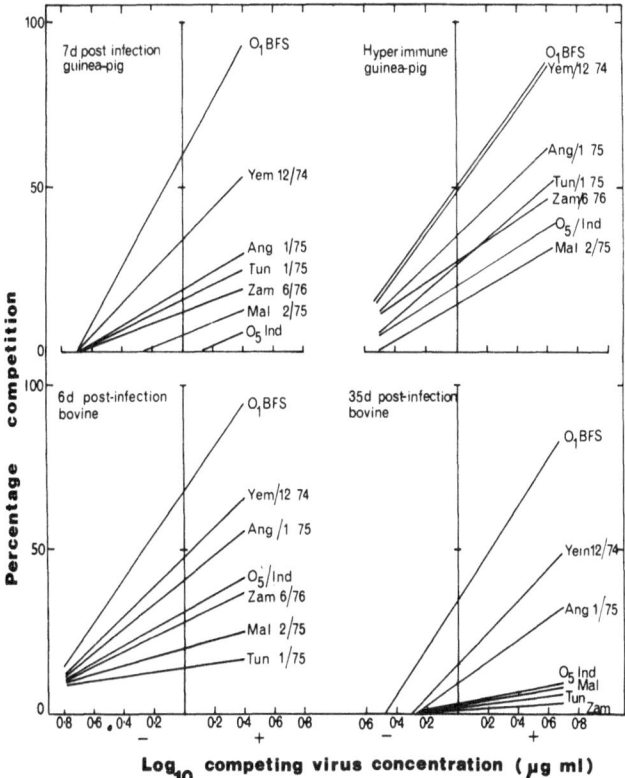

Figure 32.4 Comparison of type O FMD virus strains by RIA using different homologous antisera

Table 32.6 Relative mass of competing virus to inhibit 50% precipitation of radioactive O_1 BFS

Virus	Guinea-pig antisera			Bovine antisera	
	7d PI	28d-AEI virus	Hyperimmune	6d PI	35d PI
O_1 BFS	1	1	1	1	1
Yem 12/74	5	2	1	2	4
Ang 1/75	21	2	2	3	22
O_5 Ind	389	NC	10	9	NC
Zam 6/76	138	575	6	48	NC
Mal 2/75	200	NC	21	214	NC
Tun 1/75	29	115	4	NC	NC

NC, no competition

antisera has been dealt with at some length since it highlights the use of one immunoassay to define reagents which can then be exploited in other immunoassays, or gives valuable information by which other assay results can be interpreted. For example, the observation that the post-infection guinea-pig serum can distinguish between strains is of interest, since it has been established using radioimmunoprecipitation tests that this serum only reacts with antigenic determinants on the whole virion. Thus the competition RIA relationships using this antiserum are based on differences residing on the whole virion. Comparisons of SN test results relating the same strains show that there is good correlation between the differences obtained for both tests only when using early post-infected sera. Where IgG levels were increased there was less correlation between SN and RIA data. The use of natural early post-infectious serum – which cannot be used in CF tests and is usually of a low titre when used in neutralization testing, by the competition RIA – is probably most pertinent to field protection studies. Thus an immunoassay is available to compare the neutralizing antibody-inducing sites using naturally produced antiserum. This type of test has been used to examine differences between isolates which have been difficult to separate by other immu-nological tests, e.g. SN and CF. Using the competition RIA it has been established that SVD viruses do vary antigenically in the field, and new outbreaks can be characterized by definite changes in reactivity of the isolates with standardized reagents. In terms of diagnosis it has also been possible to rapidly distinguish between a recent English isolate appearing at a similar time to a Belgian isolate.

Solid-phase techniques

Solid-phase techniques using similar principles to those of competition assays described above, have simplified the comparison of strains. Both RIA and ELISA competition tests have been developed to solve various problems in comparing viral antigens and whole virions when purified and also a 'crude' preparation. An outline of two different methods for using solid-phase competition ELISA is shown in Figure 32.5. This methodology is also relevant to RIA, the tracer being radioactive instead of an enzyme.

This test has been evaluated in the comparison of FMD virus strains using ELISA. Viruses could be compared easily when produced in tissue culture with no need for purification. The solid-phase RIA test has been applied to the comparison of 'bluetongue' and other Orbiviruses where previous results have been ambiguous. This type of immunoassay is now being used to investigate the relationships of viruses, hitherto difficult to examine by 'conventional' immunoassays; in particular African swine fever, where it is hoped to relate the geographical differences of isolates with antigenic differences.

Measurement of immunizing antigens in vaccines

The likelihood of producing successful FMD virus vaccines is increased by

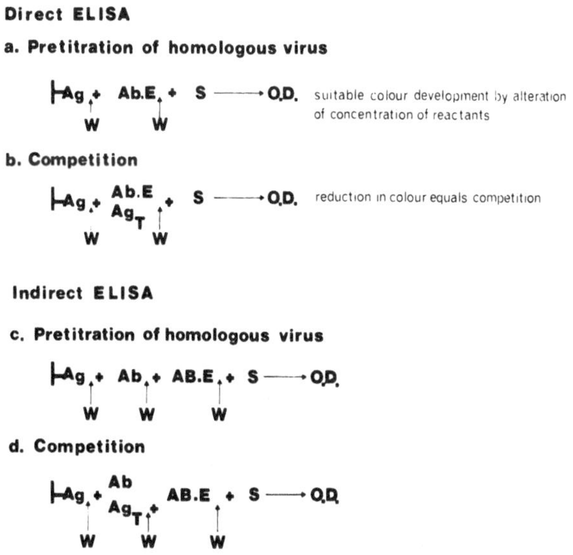

Direct ELISA

a. Pretitration of homologous virus

$$\vdash\!\!Ag_\downarrow + \ Ab.E_\downarrow + \ S \ \longrightarrow O.D. \quad \text{suitable colour development by alteration}$$
$$\ \ \ \ W \ \ \ \ \ W \qquad\qquad\qquad\qquad \text{of concentration of reactants}$$

b. Competition

$$\vdash\!\!Ag_\cdot + \ \begin{matrix} Ab.E \\ Ag_T \end{matrix}_\downarrow + \ S \ \longrightarrow O.D. \quad \text{reduction in colour equals competition}$$
$$\ \ \ \ W \ \ \ \ \ \ W$$

Indirect ELISA

c. Pretitration of homologous virus

$$\vdash\!\!Ag_\downarrow + \ Ab_\downarrow + \ AB.E_\downarrow + \ S \longrightarrow O.D.$$
$$\ \ \ \ W \ \ \ \ W \ \ \ \ \ \ W$$

d. Competition

$$\vdash\!\!Ag_\downarrow + \ \begin{matrix} Ab \\ Ag_T \end{matrix}_\downarrow + \ AB.E_\downarrow + \ S \longrightarrow O.D.$$
$$\ \ \ \ W \ \ \ \ \ W \ \ \ \ \ \ W$$

Figure 32.5 Outline of competition enzyme-labelled immunosorbent assay. ⊦, Solid-phase microtitre plate; Ag, FMD virus; Ag_T, dilution series of competing FMD virus; Ab, Antibody against Ag; AB, anti-species antiserum; .E, enzyme conjugated protein; S, substrate of enzyme; W, washing procedure to remove unreacted material

incorporating high levels of whole virions. Subunit material does not induce protection in animals, and so methods to determine the whole virion mass at different stages during manufacture are important. Garland et al.[4] reviewed the serological assays available at that time and compared them to the accurate though time-consuming physical method involving ultracentrifugation analysis on linear density gradients.

Quantitative CF tests are complicated since sera used to measure antigens have reacted with antigens on the whole virion and non-immunogenic subunit components present in cellular harvests. Fluorocarbon extraction has been used to remove subunit components present in cellular harvests, but this also removed variable amounts of whole virion.

Estimation of whole virion after sucrose density gradient centrifugation has been more reliable but this in itself can be used directly. It has proved difficult to establish a precise correlation between whole virion CF antigen activity and vaccine potency.

The single radial immunodiffusion (SRID) test has been used and detects 1.2 μg/ml of virus using convalescent guinea-pig antiserum containing IgM antibodies specific for the whole virion. To obtain good results the virus harvest had to be concentrated 30–50-fold, which is highly inconvenient.

Single radial haemolysis was applied with more success. Antibody to FMD virus was coupled to sheep erythrocytes using chromic chloride and the cell–antibody complex suspended in molten agar poured onto slides or plates.

Serial dilutions of FMD antigen were placed in wells cut into the gel and allowed to diffuse into the agar overnight at 4°C. Slides were then flooded with antiserum to FMD virus, together with guinea-pig serum as a complement source, and incubated at 37°C. Zones of lysis developed where virus reacted with antibody, the size of the zone being directly proportional to the concentration of virus in the sample. The test was reported to detect down to 1 μg of FMD virus antigen, a significant increase in sensitivity over straight immunodiffusion methods. However, the test proved unsuitable for measuring whole virion antigen from infected cells and attempts to make it more specific failed.

Recently the RIA and ELISA techniques have been used to measure FMD virus antigens. These show increased sensitivity and versatility providing convenient methods for processing large numbers of samples. The sandwich ELISA was used by Crowther and Abu Elzein[1] where plates were sensitized with γ-globulin from guinea-pig antiserum raised against a vaccine strain virus, and the same γ-globulin labelled with alkaline phosphate. This method provided a useful bonus in that it only detected whole virion antigen so that the assay was specific for whole particles. Standard curves relating colour development to purified virus of known mass (obtained by ultracentrifugation analysis) were constructed and test sample virus mass was 'read' from these (Figure 32.6). Virus titrations are easily made using infected tissue cultures, density gradient material and 'cocktails' of whole virion and subunit material. Thus ELISA offers two main advantages over previous immunoassays:

(1) Whole virion can be measured directly without the requirement of separation from subunit material. This has been necessary in the past with other tests.
(2) The high sensitivity of ELISA means that samples containing small amounts of virus (25 ng/ml and above) can be measured without need for concentration.

More routine applications of ELISA and RIA to detect and quantify other viruses have been made; e.g. African swine fever antigen[5], can be measured in 3 h with a sensitivity down to the equivalent of 50–500 HAD/50. Since the HA test takes up to 8 days to complete and involves tissue culture, the 'straightforward' sandwich techniques are of great value. Similar types of study on rinderpest and 'bluetongue' viruses confirm the success of the RIA in particular, in assessing low levels of antigen in tissue culture samples by tests taking much shorter times than tissue culture techniques.

EXAMINATION OF ANTIBODY

Detection of antibodies against FMD virus is important:

(1) to establish whether animals have been in contact with disease-free areas;

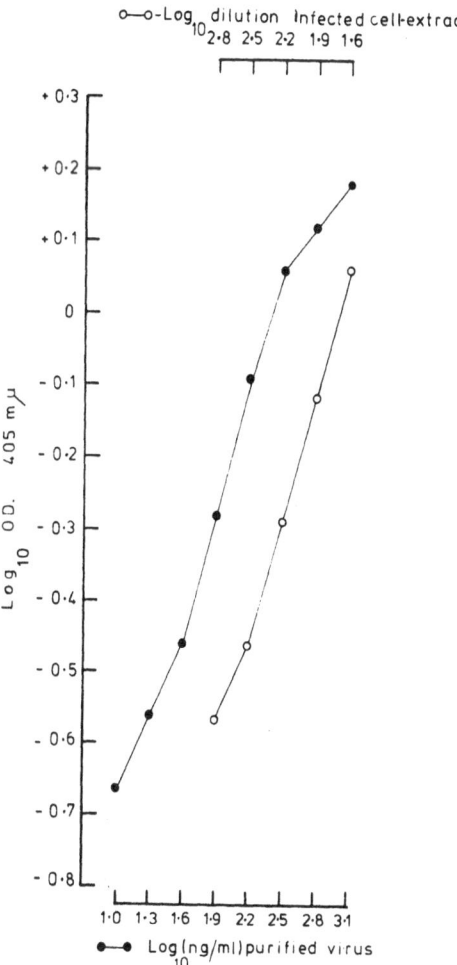

Figure 32.6 Titration of purified FMD virus and virus from infected cell extracts using sandwich ELISA

(2) as a means of establishing possible disease prevalence, and nature of type of FMD virus present in epidemiological studies before control measures can be formulated;

(3) to examine whether vaccination campaigns or laboratory-controlled vaccine schedules have induced an antibody response.

The likely protective quality of the antibody may also be examined in terms of its specific neutralizing ability or by the nature of the immunoglobulin where activity lies. As already indicated the 'protective' qualities of antisera should best be measured using SN tests. Thus, FMD virus screening is routinely made using SN tests in tissue culture using microtitre equipment. These do have some difficulties in that they are laborious and subject to variation.

Interpretation of SN test results is complicated since many cattle sera from disease-free countries produce low levels of antibody which react in the SN test (and may also be demonstrated by immunodiffusion and immunoelectrophoresis). Correlations relating SN test cattle antibody titres with protections to challenge can be made and defined ranges of close correlations are available where extensive studies on experimentally vaccinated animals have been made.

Recently ELISA has been used to detect and quantify antibodies against FMD viruses from cattle sera. Table 32.7 compares the results obtained by

Table 32.7   Examination of antibodies against FMD virus in cattle sera from Canada

Serotype examined	Total number cattle sera tested	Indirect ELISA	Double-sandwich ELISA	SN titres*			
				8	11	16	22
Anti-A	54	All < 5	All < 5	19	26	5	4
Anti-O	99	All < 5	All < 5	44	33	16	6
Anti-C	53	All < 5	All < 5	27	25	1	0

*Numbers of sera showing low-level cross-reactive titres

SNT and ELISA in a study of 206 cattle sera. Several advantages were noted for use of the indirect ELISA over the SNT and included:

(1) ELISA was sensitive; detecting specific antibodies for FMD virus at 3 days post-vaccination and infection of cattle under experimental conditions.
(2) ELISA was highly specific for the FMD serotype antibody detected and no false-positive reaction of the type found by the SMT test on the same samples was noted.
(3) ELISA was rapid (3 h) and large numbers of cattle sera could be handled using microtitre equipment. Results can be read very rapidly using modern multichannel spectrophotometers.

Studies to compare the SN test and ELISA are now being made to establish the possible routine use of the latter test in the AVRI.

A possible disadvantage of ELISA is that it measures total antibody reactive with the antigen attached to the plate. The specificity of the SN test renders a reaction with the neutralizing antibody-inducing site(s) on the virion. For this reason, the specificity of this test in ELISA might be defined by altering the antigen attached to the plates or, more easily, by measuring the classes of immunoglobulin where the antiviral activity lies. This is probably more important when assessing the effectiveness of vaccination campaigns and research is needed to establish the importance of particular levels of specific antibody to protection. This type of study has been made using ELISA. An increasingly popular technique in human medicine, where levels of antibodies specific for pathogenic agents give a useful idea of the state of disease, is to use the versatility of the solid-phase assay in RIA and ELISA. Thus, heavy chain-specific antibodies to the species of the test antiserum can be passively absorbed to microplates. Serum dilutions under test are then added and the subclass immunoglobulin reacts immunologically with the initial antibody. The specific antibody activity residing in the subclass fraction attached to the solid phase is then tested by addition of the relevant labelled antigen or antigen detection system. Such tests have been used to assess the levels of virus specific IgM, IgA, IgG$_1$ and IgG$_2$ from bovine sera after vaccination and infection. Results are shown in Figures 32.7 and 32.8 and are compared to SN test titres. The test is rapid; the intrinsic solid-phase separation of the subclass

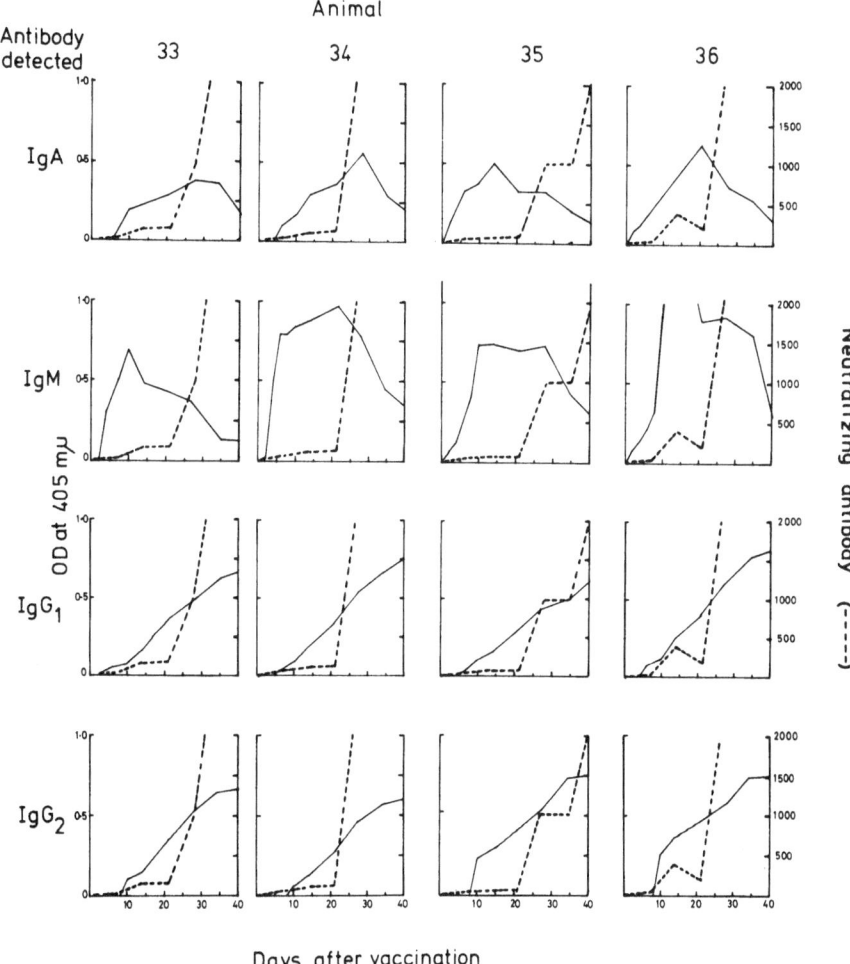

Figure 32.7 Examination of specific immunoglobulins in cattle sera after vaccination with type O$_1$, BFS 1860 FMD virus

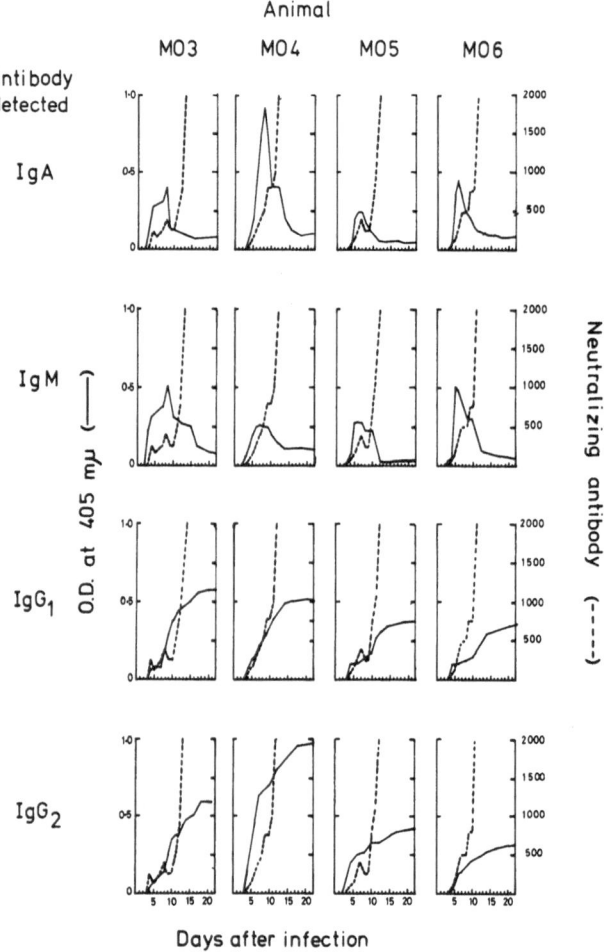

Figure 32.8 Examination of specific immunoglobulins in cattle sera after infection with type O_1 BFS 1800 FMD virus

immunoglobulin being the simplifying step. It should be mentioned that the relatively new immunoassays outlined above can run into difficulties when different systems are examined. The indirect test is the one of choice for detection of antibodies since it is relatively simple and needs a single anti-species tracer. Unwanted positive reactions occur in field sera obtained from animals in historically disease-free areas. Such reactions have been mentioned as being measured by SN test for FMD virus 'antibodies' in cattle sera. Here the ELISA did not detect those reactions under the test conditions employed.

Often, however, 'good' tests can be devised for antibody detection from animals experimentally vaccinated, or infected and preimmune sera can be used to obtain baseline 'zero' antibody titres. When these tests are used on field sera, results for so-called 'negative' animals can give variable and high backgrounds compared to the laboratory-produced zero antibody backgrounds. Limited studies on the reasons for this indicate that certain animal sera, notably from bovines, ovines and porcines, contain IgM antibodies which react indiscriminately with a range of different antigens. For this reason it may be necessary to increase the specificity of the detection system used with solid-phase techniques either by using positive antigens which can be shown not to react with 'normal' sera, e.g. by using purified antigen fractions of viruses or, more easily, by detecting specific antibodies using defined anti-immunoglobulin tracers, e.g. anti-heavy-chain IgG. This has proved successful in measuring ovine antibodies to 'bluetongue' virus.

The detection of antibodies to African swine fever (ASF) virus from porcine sera illustrates that the increased sensitivity of ELISA over other tests can cause problems in interpreting results in diagnosis. Wide variations in the levels of 'antibody' reacting with ASF from different pre-immune pigs, and day-to-day variations from individual pigs meant that a baseline 'negative' could not be obtained. Recently, a meeting held on behalf of the EEC agreed to prepare standard pools of antisera obtained from large numbers of uninfected pigs from disease-free areas. Participants also agreed to standardize the entire ELISA test chosen to diagnose ASF disease, including the conjugates. This type of cooperation is needed within animal disease research. Since the ELISA tests are relatively simple and large numbers of tests can be done rapidly, it should be possible to arrive quickly at valid conclusions as to its suitability as a world-wide test.

MONOCLONAL ANTIBODIES IN IMMUNOASSAY

Techniques are now available for producing monoclonal antibodies on a 'routine' basis. These are of interest to the diagnostician and research veterinary scientist since large quantities of antibody can be produced in tissue cultures or animal systems. Monoclonal antibodies have a single affinity for antigens and thus provide non-heterogeneous definitive reagents. Production and characterization of the reactivity of monoclonal antibodies may be made at central well-equipped laboratories, these can be distributed either as the final reagent or as tissue cultures. This means that standardized reagents might be available on a large scale, suitable for use with sensitive immunoassays such as ELISA and RIA. Problems may arise where highly specific reactions of the monoclonal antibodies arise, but 'panels' of mixtures of antibodies could be prepared to solve particular diagnostic and qualitative problems.

Research into the production of monoclonal antibodies in FMD virus is under way, with the aim of:

(1) producing large quantities of monospecific typing sera;

(2) producing sera reacting with whole virion components to measure these in relation to presence of other viral subunits;

(3) producing antibodies against the antigenic determinants of FMD virus so that they can be used to understand the structure/function relationships of the virion, as an aid to the production of better vaccines.

CELL-MEDIATED IMMUNITY

Assays involving measurement of cell-mediated immunity *in vitro* may have increasing importance in veterinary research. In general they have limited use in diagnosis and are used as an aid to understanding the basis of immunity in diseases. Such studies are undertaken where 'difficulties' arise in understanding classical disease processes, e.g. in ASF infections where no neutralizing antibody can be demonstrated.

IMMUNOASSAY IN THE 1980s

Immunoassays have generally developed as a direct response to disease problems coupled with advances in technology. Reliable methods established up to the 1970s are used to solve veterinary problems and will still be used where a country's veterinary facilities are limited – even in the face of demonstrably better immunoassay techniques such as ELISA and RIA. In this context, more exploitation of the 'established' methods might be made. For example, the very sensitive methods involving passive haemagglutination tests should be pursued, since these offer a directly visualized result and have a wide versatility.

Since the 1970s, the rapid growth of tracer techniques using solid-phase assays has revolutionized immunoassays, although we are still in a period of comparative testing. Commercial concerns are now committed to producing relatively cheap kits for the detection of antigens and antibodies of veterinary as well as medical interest. Rapid and relatively simple methodology means that semi- or fully automatic tests are feasible and several successful systems have been set up in individual laboratories for screening large numbers of samples. Solid-phase techniques can be used ingeniously for the continuous assessment of reactants throughout production runs in commercial operations. Increased 'turnover' of samples opens a new dimension in the study of diseases of animals and sensitive, highly specific assays, e.g. quantification of subclass immunoglobulins, can be made on large numbers of sera, where only limited numbers could be processed previously.

Services can also be provided by central laboratories similar to those in human medicine, e.g. for the measurement of hormone levels.

Immunoassays rely on the specific nature of the antigen–antibody reaction.

The ingenuity of the novel immunoassays sometimes obscures this fact and it is the 'duty' of research workers to maintain a basis of simplicity in this growing 'service' industry.

References

1. Crowther, J. R. and Abu Elzein, E. M. E. (1979). Application of the enzyme-linked immunosorbent assay to the detection and identification of foot-and-mouth disease viruses. *J. Hyg., Camb.*, **83**, 513

2. Crowther, J. R. (1977). Examination of differences between foot-and-mouth disease virus strains using a radioimmunoassay technique. International Symposium on Foot-and-Mouth Disease, Lyons 1976. *Developments in Biological Standardization*, Vol. 35, pp. 185–93. (Basel: Karger)

3. Crumpton, M. J. (1974). Protein antigens: The molecular bases of antigenicity and immunogenicity. In Sela, M. (ed.) *The Antigens*, Vol. 2, pp. 1–78. (New York: Academic Press)

4. Garland, A. J. M., Mowat, G. N. and Fletton, B. (1977). An evaluation of some methods of assay of foot-and-mouth disease antigen for vaccines. International Symposium on Foot-and-Mouth Disease, Lyons 1976. *Developments in Biological Standardization*, Vol. 35, pp. 323–32. (Basel: Karger)

5. Crowther, J. R., Wardley, R. C. and Wilkinson, P. J. (1979). Solid phase radioimmunoassay techniques for the detection of African swine fever antigen and antibody. *J. Hyg., Camb.*, **83**, 353

33
Immunoassays in Plant Virology

M. F. CLARK

INTRODUCTION

The specific antigenicity of a plant virus, tobacco mosaic virus, was first demonstrated more than 50 years ago[1]. Since then recognition of the combined advantages of speed and specificity has led to the use of serodiagnosis for a multitude of applications. These can be grouped into two major categories:

(1) as a means of pathogen identification or of determining the relationship of two or more serologically similar pathogens;
(2) as a qualitative probe or a quantitative assay for known pathogens.

Until recently the majority of applications were experimental and fell into the former category, while only sporadic attempts were made to exploit serology for the study of viruses in the field. This is perhaps surprising as the obvious advantages of serodiagnosis suggest that its potential should have been exploited more extensively. This paradox results from the inability of standard serological procedures to cope with difficulties arising from (a) the varied morphology of plant viruses, (b) the effect of inactivators and inhibitors in some plant extracts, (c) low virus concentrations in plants, and (d) the low proportion of infected plants in most plant populations. This chapter considers the current and future use of several immunoassay techniques for the serodiagnosis of viruses in field infections.

CHARACTERISTICS OF TRADITIONAL PROCEDURES

Precipitation-based procedures have been used for the majority of plant virus applications; in particular, immunodiffusion in agar and tube or micropreci-pitin tests. With partially purified virus preparations these procedures have been employed satisfactorily for characterizing viruses and for investigating serological interrelationships. For viruses in plant extracts, however, pre-cipitin tests are not generally suitable because the results are obscured by particulate components and by compounds in plants that either interfere with antigen–antibody interactions or cause non-specific precipitation. Immuno-diffusion procedures are less prone to these effects and have been used successfully both for disease diagnosis[2] and for comparing viruses when homologous and heterologous virus–antiserum combinations can be dis-tinguished by the formation of precipitation 'spurs'. The two major dis-advantages of immunodiffusion procedures are:

(1) their relative insensitivity; and
(2) their restriction to isometric viruses and those anisometric or fragmented viruses small enough to diffuse adequately through the gel matrix.

Although intact filamentous plant viruses cannot be assayed by gel immunodiffusion techniques it is possible to disrupt the capsid by physical or chemical means. For example, diffusible antigens have been produced by treating plant extracts containing virus with ethanolamine, pyridine, pyr-rolidine or sodium dodecyl sulphate[3, 4]. Practical immunoassays based on this approach have been used successfully for the large-scale diagnosis of potato viruses[3], citrus tristeza virus[5] and plum pox virus[6]. However, such treatment can significantly alter both antigenicity[7] and serological specificity[4] (Clark, unpublished results) so requiring the development of separate homologous antisera for intact and degraded virus particles.

A significant improvement in the sensitivity of virus detection was achieved by using flocculation procedures in which antibodies were passively adsorbed to tanned red cells, bentonite, or particles of polystyrene latex. Latex tests appeared to fulfil many of the requirements of an immunoassay for field use. The sensitized particles were easily prepared and used, they had a long shelf life, virus could be assayed in suitably diluted plant extracts, sub-microgram concentrations were detectable, and results were available within minutes. Accordingly, the test was employed to detect apple viruses[8], barley stripe mosaic virus[9], and several potato viruses[10]. However, despite its early promise practical problems were occasionally encountered and these, together with the inability of the test to provide truly quantitative results, have tended to discourage workers from applying it to more field disease situations.

Table 33.1 summarizes the relevant characteristics of precipitin, im-munodiffusion and latex flocculation tests for the serodiagnosis of plant virus diseases. This table also lists comparable characteristics of the two recently

Table 33.1 Characteristics of five immunoassay techniques for the detection of plant viruses

Technique	Sensitivity (ng/ml)	Viruses detected	Susceptibility to inhibitors	Batch testing	Quantitative potential	Technical requirements
Immunodiffusion	20 000	isometric disrupted filaments	low	no	low	low
Precipitin	2000	all	high	no	medium	low
Flocculation	200	all	medium	some	low	low
Immune electronmicroscopy	0.1–1.0	all	low	yes	high	high
Enzyme immunoassay	1.0–10.0	all	low	yes	high	medium

described techniques, immune electronmicroscopy and enzyme immunoassay. The considerable impact in plant pathology of the two latter techniques has been made the more significant by the limitations of traditional precipitation-based procedures which fail to fulfil all the requirements of a practical immunoassay.

IMMUNE ELECTRONMICROSCOPY

Although the quantitative potential of the electronmicroscope in virology has long been recognized, it has been regarded primarily as a specialist research instrument. Following the recent introduction of the techniques of immunosorbent electronmicroscopy and particle decoration[11, 12], however, the electronmicroscope has acquired a new importance as an everyday tool for virus detection and identification.

Immunosorbent electronmicroscopy (ISEM)

For ISEM studies microscope grids are coated with carbon, with or without a collodion or formvar supporting film[13]. Antiserum or γ-globulin, suitably diluted, is placed on the grid for some minutes, during which time the globulin adsorbs to the carbon surface. The grid is then washed and the test sample added and incubated for a further period to permit specific interaction between antigen and antibody. The grids are washed again, and contrasted by staining or shadowing.

The particular attraction of this technique is its extreme efficiency for trapping and detecting macromolecular antigens such as plant viruses and spiroplasmas[14], especially when these occur in low concentrations or when only small amounts of sample are available. Roberts and Harrison[15] used ISEM to determine the relative virus content of individuals of two aphid vector species of potato leafroll virus. Aphids of one species (*Myzus persicae* (Sulz.)) contained, on average, 25 times more virus particles than those of the other (*Macrosiphum euphorbiae* (Thos.)). Such a comparison was possible because of the approximate 1000-fold increase in sensitivity with ISEM compared with conventional electronmicroscopy.

Other uses of ISEM include seed testing[16] and indexing roses for viruses[17]. However, the relatively slow rate of processing (< 100 samples per day) limits the practical application of this method to small-scale surveys and specialist uses.

Particle decoration

In this method virus particles absorbed to the grid surface are exposed to specific antiserum so as to identify homologous antigens. The antibody halo

formed around homologous virus particles makes possible their recognition
and differentiation in a mixed population of morphologically similar particles

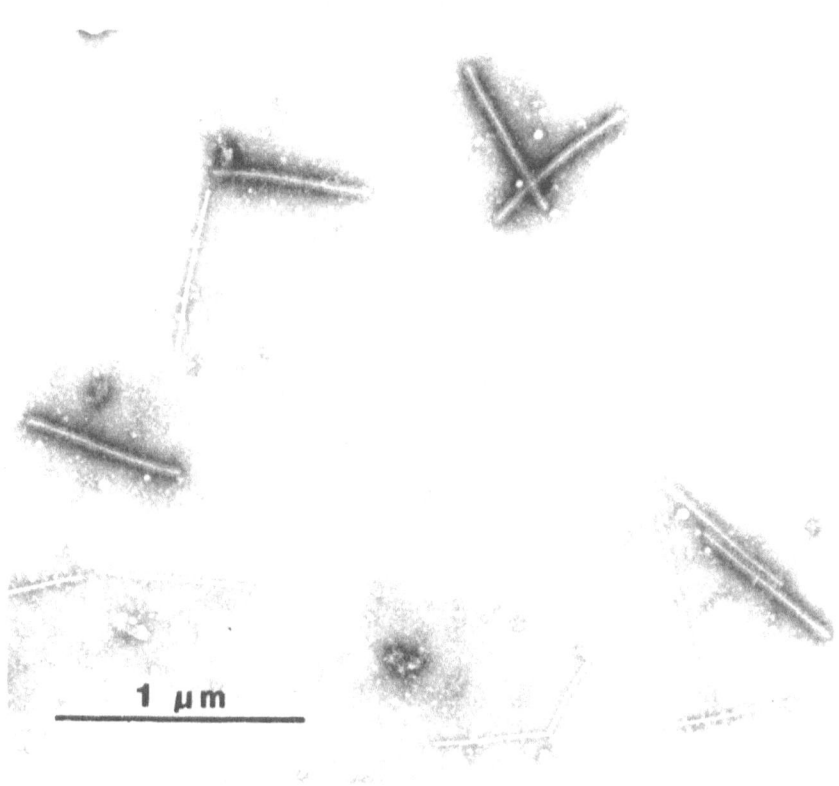

Figure 33.1 A mixture of hop mosaic and poplar mosaic virus particles treated according to the
decoration technique using anti-hop mosaic virus antiserum. Only the hop mosaic virus particles
have an antibody halo

(Figure 33.1). Such mixtures are frequently encountered in field infections.
For example, many established hop gardens are infected almost throughout
with the morphologically similar but otherwise distinct carlaviruses, hop
mosaic virus and hop latent virus. Serologically related viruses may also be
identified by this method by grading the degree of relatedness according to the
intensity of the antibody halo around the particles. This approach to
serological classification has been very useful for luteoviruses[18] which occur in
very low concentration in the plant.

ENZYME IMMUNOASSAY

Enzyme immunoassays were first introduced into plant pathology in 1976, following exploratory tests[19] by virologists at East Malling Research Station with collaborators at the Nuffield Laboratories of Comparative Medicine, London. In the ensuing 4 years the technique found ready international acceptance, particularly in plant virology. It is now firmly established as a powerful research technique and as an important practical diagnostic method for use by field officers and laboratories concerned with plant health.

Technique

For plant virus investigations a diagnostic technique is required which will directly detect the virus particles. Of the possible alternative procedures a heterogeneous assay based on the double-antibody sandwich method was selected as being most appropriate. The procedure involves four stages:

(1) specific antibody is passively absorbed to an inert solid phase;
(2) antigen in the sample is selectively trapped and immobilized by homologous antibody;
(3) immobilized antigen is reacted with enzyme-labelled specific antibody;
(4) substrate is added to reveal enzyme retained as a result of specific antigen present in the sample.

Various types of solid phase have been used but the microplate method[20] is most convenient. The characteristics of this procedure for use with plant viruses were originally described by Clark and Adams[21] and their protocol has been adopted essentially unchanged for the majority of research and field applications reported.

Reagents

The main objective in all developmental work has been to differentiate clearly between infected and healthy tissue. Such a distinction enables routine field assessments to be made on a visual $+/-$ basis, depending simply on the presence or absence of any colour in the final stage of the ELISA procedure. Thus, the prime reagent requirement has been for pathogen-specific, high-titre antisera, as the presence in the antiserum of antibodies to normal plant constituents results in non-specific and misleading production of colour. Some antisera prepared before the introduction of the ELISA procedure have been found unsuitable for this purpose although their use, appropriately diluted, in precipitin-based reactions has been quite satisfactory.

Clarity of result was also a dominant factor in the selection of alkaline phosphatase as the preferred enzyme. Despite the inefficiency of one-step glutaraldehyde conjugation[22], in which only about 4% of the enzyme may be coupled with γ-globulin (Clark, unpublished results), the complex conjugates so obtained are well suited to the detection of plant viruses and other macromolecular pathogens. Other enzymes and conjugation methods have been employed, especially in research and development, but for field use and general applications the combined advantages of ease of preparation, low background and linear reaction kinetics with substrate that are characteristic of alkaline phosphatase conjugates outweigh the principal disadvantage of their relatively high cost.

Antigens

A variety of antigens has been directly assayed by ELISA. In addition to plant viruses[23] these include viral components and ds-RNA (Clark and Barbara, unpublished results), bacterial[24, 25] spiroplasma[26] and fungal[27] pathogens.

The suitability of the microplate method of ELISA for pathogens with such diverse morphologies (Table 33.1) has enabled methodology to be standard-ized for nearly all these pathogens. A particularly important feature of the technique is its potential for assaying viruses in samples taken directly from untreated plant extracts as well as in partially purified virus preparations. This is possible because of the selective immobilization of virus on the solid phase. Thus, the detectability of plum pox virus was unaffected by diluting a partially purified preparation in buffer alone or with a plant extract (Figure 34.2). By contrast, many plants contain pectins, tannins, polyphenol oxidases or other components whose presence in the extract might interfere with virus detection although diluting the extract in buffers containing protective compounds has often overcome the effects of such inhibitors and inactivators[21,28].

Applications

The versatility of the ELISA procedure has enabled its use in many different areas of investigation, including those listed in Table 33.2. Its most significant practical impact, however, has been on methods of disease assessment and prevention. The success of ELISA in these areas results directly from its suitability for processing many samples rapidly, and with a high level of sensitivity for virus detection. The stimulus to utilize the procedure in practice arises from the limitations of the available alternative methods, especially for latent infections, some fruit tree and hop viruses, and for viruses that are difficult to transmit such as many of the aphid-borne circulative viruses of perennial and vegetatively-propagated crops. The following examples have been selected to illustrate the contribution that ELISA has already made in these two important areas of practical plant pathology.

Table 33.2   Applications of enzyme immunoassays in plant virology

Applied	Research
Disease assessment	virus purification
Disease prevention	serological classification
Seed testing	virus–host interactions
Epidemiology	virus replication and assembly
Plant breeding	

Disease assessment

Plum pox

The first field application of ELISA was for the serodiagnosis of plum pox disease[29]. This is caused by an aphid-borne filamentous virus that was first detected in this country in 1965[30]. It was probably introduced in infected planting material imported from mainland Europe where the disease was already widespread. Despite an immediate and sustained campaign to locate and destroy infected trees in orchards and nurseries, the number of infected sites continued to increase[31,32]. Among the many factors contributing to this increase was the practical difficulty of correctly identifying infected trees at a sufficiently early stage. Systemic movement of the virus from an infection site is slow and erratic, and the virus reaches only low concentrations in infected tissues. Any foliar symptoms are often faint, especially in some cultivars, and are easily missed or attributed to other causes. Prior to the introduction of ELISA, confirmation of the disease was by laborious and unreliable graft-inoculation of suspect material to indicator plants in glasshouse tests. Even when the graft test was successful symptoms could take up to 9 months to develop.

In early ELISA tests with partially purified preparations virus was detected at concentrations as low as 1 ng/ml[21] (Figure 33.2). Tests with experimentally infected herbaceous plants were equally encouraging and a joint investigation began with the Ministry of Agriculture to determine the suitability of the technique for monitoring natural infection. It rapidly became apparent that the uneven distribution of virus in trees made the results of any tests carried out with randomly collected samples of dubious value[31]. Consequently, in the UK there is continued heavy reliance on visual inspections and ELISA is used by the Ministry of Agriculture as a reliable confirmatory test for any trees suspected of being infected by the virus. Used in this way ELISA has successfully replaced the less reliable methods. The speed and precision with which it is now possible to diagnose plum pox has greatly improved prospects for containing the disease, although total eradication seems unlikely[32].

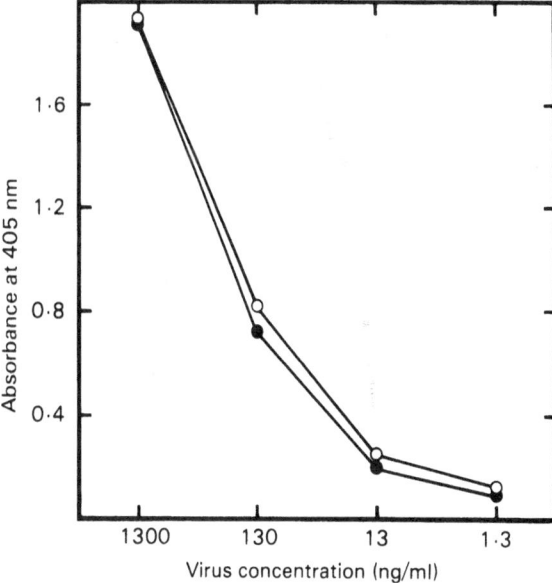

Figure 33.2 ELISA absorbence values for a purified preparation of plum pox virus diluted in buffer (O——O) and diluted in a 1 : 100 (w/v) extract of *Nicotiana clevelandii* in buffer (●——●) (from ref. 21)

Citrus tristeza

Citrus tristeza virus is a closterovirus transmitted semi-persistently by aphids. The particles are filamentous and are among the longest (about 2 μm) encountered in plant virology. The virus is confined to the phloem tissues where it occurs in low concentrations. Annually more than 300 000 trees are indexed in Israel and California, largely by batch graft-inoculating plants of the indicator 'Mexican' lime (*Citrus aurantifolia*) in glasshouses and screen-houses[23]. Conventional electronmicroscopy has also been used in attempts to improve and accelerate virus detection[33]. When an antiserum became available renewed attempts were made to modify existing serological indexing techniques. These led to experiments with fluorescent antibodies[34] and to an immunodiffusion method with sodium dodecyl sulphate-degraded virus[5]. Although the latter method showed serological detection to be practicable tests were limited to certain types of young tissue and were only reliable when the virus content of the trees was at its highest.

The introduction of the ELISA test for intact virus was immediately successful. Virus was readily detected in leaf and bark samples of all infected citrus species tested[35]. ELISA tests confirmed previous electronmicroscope observations that bark samples generally contained more virus than leaf samples, but that the best source of virus was fruit pedicels. Use of the latter type of tissue made possible tests with composite samples for field surveys and in 1978–9 more than 82 000 samples were indexed in Israel[23]. ELISA has now virtually replaced the lime test for routine indexing.

In contrast to the situation with plum pox virus detection of tristeza in symptomless trees is feasible. Thus, in a survey of 2811 citrus groves, testing five trees per grove, four new centres of symptomless infection were found[23]. Recently, a new approach was described for sampling trees to identify affected groves[36]. Tests were made with fruit pedicels subsampled from the fruit containers after delivery to the packing house. By sampling only five fruit taken at random from 350 kg containers it was possible to identify and discriminate between rates of infection of 0, 1.0 and 15%. The obvious success of ELISA in enabling the rapid and reliable diagnosis of citrus tristeza virus suggests that an enforced eradication programme will contain or virtually eliminate the disease from important fruit-growing areas.

Disease prevention

The need to assess the level of virus infection in 'seed' and ware potato crops has long been of major concern to certifying agencies. Routinely, crops for 'seed' production are grown outside the main potato-growing areas and are inspected in mid-season for symptoms of several viruses. Frequently, such inspections only measure infections introduced in tubers, and current-season spread is largely disregarded. However, during abnormal growing seasons, such as the hot summers of 1975–6, there may be significant spread of virus within the crop[37]. The implications of this for succeeding crops of ware potatoes can be serious, especially where growers have planted their own once-grown tubers instead of certified 'seed'. Interest in the possible use of ELISA to complement or replace current methods of indexing potato viruses is already international. Antisera against all but one of the most important viruses have been available for several years. Indeed, serological methods of detecting potato virus X (PVX) were first advocated in the UK over 30 years ago[38]. Potato leafroll virus (PLRV) is the one major virus for which no suitable antiserum was available until recently. However, laboratories in Japan, Europe and North America have now produced antisera to this virus of sufficiently high quality to be evaluated in ELISA tests.

A major problem encountered in devising a practical indexing procedure for more than one virus is the different distributions of the various viruses in the plant. The results of assays made separately with PLRV and potato virus Y (PVY) illustrate this problem. Both viruses occur in leaves and stems but PLRV is restricted to the vascular tissues, whereas PVY is more generally distributed and reaches somewhat higher concentrations. In primary infections PLRV is largely confined to the younger foliage while in secondary (that is tuber-borne) infections PLRV concentration is greatest in the middle and lower leaves[39] which are known to be most favoured by the principal aphid vector[40]. More important for indexing purposes is the difference in distribution of PLRV and PVY in tubers. ELISA tests are fairly reliable and show PLRV to occur in vascular tissue throughout the tuber, although its concentration drops with increasing distance from the heel end[41]. In contrast, the detection of PVY in freshly harvested tubers is erratic and less reliable. For this virus there is some evidence for an opposite concentration gradient. However, if young sprouts are indexed after breaking tuber dormancy the concentration gradients are less pronounced and both viruses are easily detected.

Practical programmes to use ELISA for virus indexing and certification purposes are currently being formulated in several countries. In the UK the main emphasis is directed toward determining the health status of once-grown potatoes to ascertain their suitability for replanting. This service has been available to commercial growers for several years at MAFF centres, and involves the 'growing on' of excised eyes under controlled conditions to observe foliar symptoms for PVX, PVY and PLRV. The potential of ELISA for this purpose is at present undergoing evaluation in a concurrent testing programme. Results now available indicate that the ELISA test is more accurate and reliable than the conventional 'growing on' method. In fact, because of its apparent suitability the test may be incorporated in a more comprehensive certification programme.

Such is the interest in the potential of ELISA in continental Europe that a full range of equipment has been designed specifically for indexing potatoes for the six most important viruses. Sets of this equipment have already been acquired by potato breeders and certification agencies in West Germany and Holland. If the initial promise of ELISA for potato virus indexing is fulfilled it seems likely that the global scale of operations will involve millions of tests per year.

FUTURE PROSPECTS

The full significance of the possibilities of using immune electronmicroscopy and enzyme immunoassays in plant virology is only now being recognized. The extent to which ELISA, in particular, is being incorporated into experimental and commercial applications reflects not only its suitability for such uses but also the inadequacy of alternative procedures. As sampling methods improve and techniques are refined to increase sensitivity so serodiagnosis will figure more prominently in all kinds of phytosanitary programmes.

Epidemiology is an area which is likely to benefit particularly from the prodigious amount of quantitative data that it is possible to generate by immunoassays. Already immunoassays have been used for monitoring virus spread into crops[42], in the search for vectors[43], for investigating virus–vector relationships[44], for identifying alternative natural plant hosts[45], and for discriminating among virus serotypes in separate and mixed infections[46,47]. With an increasing appreciation of the suitability of immunoassay procedures for collecting epidemiological data it should be possible to design and conduct investigations which will have a significant impact in all areas of applied virus research and should greatly increase our understanding of the complex interactions between plants and their pathogens.

Acknowledgments

I wish to thank B. D. Harrison, I. M. Roberts, P. Gugerli and M. Bar-Joseph for providing information and unpublished manuscripts.

References

1. Beale, H. P. (1928). Immunologic reactions with tobacco mosaic virus. *Proc. Soc. Exp. Biol., NY*, **25**, 702

2. Converse, R. H. (1976). Serological detection of viruses in *Rubus* sap. *Acta Hort.*, **66**, 53

3. Shepard, J. F. (1972). Gel diffusion methods for the serological detection of potato viruses X, S, and M. *Mont. Agric. Exp. Stn. Bull.* No. 662

4. Purcifull, D. E. and Batchelor, D. L. (1977). Immunodiffusion tests with sodium dodecyl sulphate (SDS)-treated plant viruses and plant viral inclusions. *Florida Agric. Exp. Stn. Bull.* No. 788

5. Garnsey, S. M., Gonsalves, O. and Purcifull, D. E. (1979). Rapid diagnosis of citrus tristeza virus by sodium dodecylsulfate-immunodiffusion procedures. *Phytopathology*, **69**, 88

6. Casper, R. (1975). Serodiagnosis of plum pox virus. *Acta Hort.*, **44**, 171

7. Hiebert, E. and McDonald, J. G. (1976). Capsid protein heterogeneity in turnip mosaic virus. *Virology*, **70**, 144

8. Sequeira, O. A. de and Lister, R. M. (1969). Applicability of latex flocculation serological testing to apple viruses. *Phytopathology*, **59**, 572

9. Lundsgaard, T. (1976). Routine seed health testing for barley stripe mosaic virus in barley seeds using the latex test. *Z. Pflanzenkr. Pflanzenschutz*, **83**, 278

10. Koenig, R. and Bode, O. (1978). Sensitive detection of Andean potato latent and Andean potato mottle viruses in potato tubers with the serological latex test. *Phytopathol. Z.*, **92**, 275

11. Derrick, K. S. (1973). Quantitative assay for plant viruses using serologically specific electron microscopy. *Virology*, **56**, 652

12. Yanagida, M. and Ahmad-Zadeh, C. (1970). Determination of gene-product positions in bacteriophage T4 by specific antibody association. *J. Mol. Biol.*, **51**, 411

13. Milne, R. G. and Luisoni, E. (1977). Rapid immune electron microscopy of virus preparations. In Maramorosch, K. and Koprowski, H. (eds.) *Methods in Virology*, Vol. VI, pp. 265–81

14. Derrick, K. S. and Brlansky, R. H. (1976). Assay for viruses and mycoplasmas using serologically specific electron microscopy. *Phytopathology*, **66**, 815

15. Roberts, I. M. and Harrison, B. D. (1979). Detection of potato leafroll and potato mop-top viruses by immunosorbent electron microscopy. *Ann. Appl. Biol.*, **93**, 289

16. Hamilton, R. I. and Nichols, C. (1978). Serological methods for detection of pea seed-borne mosaic virus in leaves and seeds of *Pisum sativum*. *Phytopathology*, **68**, 539

17. Thomas, B. J. (1980). The detection by serological methods of viruses infecting the rose. *Ann. Appl. Biol.*, **94**, 91

18. Roberts, I. M., Tamada, T. and Harrison, B. D. (1980). Relationship of potato leafroll virus

to luteoviruses: evidence from electron microscope serological tests. *J. Gen. Virol.*, **47**, 209

19. Voller, A., Bartlett, A., Bidwell, D. E., Clark, M. F. and Adams, A. N. (1976). The detection of viruses by enzyme-linked immunosorbent assay (ELISA). *J. Gen. Virol.*, **33**, 165

20. Voller, A., Bidwell, D., Huldt, G. and Engvall, E. (1974). A microplate method of enzyme-linked immunosorbent assay and its application to malaria. *Bull. WHO*, **51**, 209

21. Clark, M. F. and Adams, A. N. (1977). Characteristics of the microplate method of enzyme-linked immunosorbent assay for the detection of plant viruses. *J. Gen. Virol.*, **34**, 475

22. Avrameas, S. (1969). Coupling of enzymes to proteins with glutaraldehyde. Use of the conjugates for the detection of antigens and antibodies. *Immunochemistry*, **6**, 43

23. Bar-Joseph, M. and Garnsey, S. M. (1980). Enzyme-linked immunosorbent assay (ELISA): principles and applications for diagnosis of plant viruses. In Maramorosch, K. and Harris, K. F. (eds.) *Ecology of Plant Viruses* (New York and London: Academic Press Inc.) (In press)

24. Claflin, L. E. and Uyemoto, J. K. (1978). Serodiagnosis of *Corynebacterium sepedonicum* by enzyme-linked immunosorbent assay. *Phytopathol. News*, **12**, 156

25. Weaver, W. M. and Guthrie, J. W. (1978). Enzyme-linked immunospecific assay: application to the detection of seed borne bacteria. *Phytopathol. News*, **12**, 156

26. Clark, M. F., Flegg, C. L., Bar-Joseph, M. and Rottem, S. (1978). The detection of *Spiroplasma citri* by enzyme-linked immunosorbent assay (ELISA). *Phytopathol. Z.*, **92**, 332

27. Casper, R. and Mendgen, K. (1979). Quantitative serological estimation of a hyperparasite: detection of *Verticillium lecanii* in yellow rust infected wheat leaves by ELISA. *Phytopathol. Z.*, **94**, 89

28. McLaughlin, M. R. and Barnett, O. W. (1979). The influence of plant sap and antigen buffer additives on the enzyme-immunoassay of two plant viruses. *Phytopathology*, **69**, 1038 (abstr.)

29. Clark, M. F., Adams, A. N., Thresh, J. M. and Casper, R. (1976). The detection of plum pox and other viruses in woody hosts by enzyme-linked immunosorbent assay. *Acta Hort.*, **67**, 51

30. Cropley, R. (1968). The identification of plum pox (Sharka) virus in England. *Plant Pathol.*, **17**, 66

31. Adams, A. N. (1978). The incidence of plum pox virus in England and its control in orchards. In Scott, P. R. and Bainbridge, A. (eds.) *Plant Disease Epidemiology*, pp. 213–19. (Oxford: Blackwell Scientific Publications)

32. Pemberton, A. W. (1979). Campaigns against plant virus diseases in England and Wales. In Ebbels, D. L. and King, J. E. (eds.). *Plant Health*, pp. 239–46. (Oxford: Blackwell Scientific Publications)

33. Bar-Joseph, M., Loebenstein, G. and Oren, Y. (1974). Use of electron microscopy in eradication of tristeza sources recently found in Israel. In Weathers, L. G. and Cohen, M. (eds.) *Proceedings 6th Conf. Int. Organ. Citrus Virol.*, pp. 83–5. (Div. Agric. Sci., Univ. of California)

34. Tsuchizaki, T. A., Sasaki, A. and Saito, Y. (1978). Purification of citrus tristeza virus from diseased citrus fruits and the detection of the virus in citrus tissues by fluorescent antibody techniques. *Phytopathology*, **68**, 139

35. Bar-Joseph, M., Garnsey, S. M., Gonsalves, D., Moscovitz, M., Purcifull, D. E., Clark, M. F. and Loebenstein, G. (1979). The use of enzyme-linked immunosorbent assay for the detection of citrus tristeza virus. *Phytopathology*, **69**, 190

36. Bar-Joseph, M., Sacks, J. M. and Garnsey, S. M. (1978). Detection and estimation of citrus tristeza virus infection rates based on ELISA assays of packing house fruit samples. *Phytoparasitica*, **6**, 145

37. Hill, S. A. (1978). Current virus infection of seed potatoes in Britain. In Scott, P. R. and Bainbridge, A. (eds.) *Plant Disease Epidemiology*, pp. 229–34. (Oxford: Blackwell Scientific Publications)

38. Markham, R., Matthews, R. E. F. and Smith, K. M. (1948). Testing potato stocks for virus X. *Farming*, **2**, 41

39. Tamada, T. and Harrison, B. D. (1980). Factors affecting the detection of potato leafroll virus

in potato foliage by enzyme-linked immunosorbent assay. *Ann. Appl. Biol.*, **95**, 209

40. Taylor, C. E. (1955). Growth of the potato plant and aphid colonization. *Ann. Appl. Biol.*, **43**, 151

41. Gera, A., Loebenstein, G. and Raccah, B. (1979). Protein coats of two strains of cucumber mosaic virus affect transmission by *Aphis gossypii*. *Phytopathology*, **69**, 396

42. Bové, J. M., Moutous, G., Saillard, C., Fos, A., Bonfils, J., Vignault, J. C., Nhami, A., Abassi, M., Kabbage, K., Hafidi, B., Mouches, C. and Viennot-Bourgin, G. (1979). Mise en évidence de *Spiroplasma citri* l'agent causal de la maladie du 'stubborn' des agrumes dans 7 cicadelles du Maroc. *CR Acad. Sci.*, *Ser. D.*, **288**, 335

43. Thresh, J. M., Adams, A. N., Barbara, D. J. and Clark, M. F. (1977). The detection of three viruses of hop (*Humulus lupulus*) by enzyme-linked immunosorbent assay (ELISA). *Ann. Appl. Biol.*, **87**, 57

44. Gugerli, P. (1980). Potato leafroll virus concentration in the vascular region of potato tubers examined by enzyme-linked immunosorbent assay (ELISA). *Potato Res.*, 23. (In press)

45. Sweet, J. B. (1980). Hedgerow hawthorn (*Crataegus* spp.) and blackthorn (*Prunus spinosa*) as hosts of fruit tree viruses in Britain. *Ann. Appl. Biol.*, **94**, 83

46. Barbara, D. J., Clark, M. F., Thresh, J. M. and Casper, R. (1978). Rapid detection and serotyping of prunus necrotic ringspot virus in perennial crops by enzyme-linked immunosorbent assay. *Ann. Appl. Biol.*, **90**, 395

47. Rochow, W. F. and Carmichael, L. E. (1979). Specificity among barley yellow dwarf viruses in enzyme-immunosorbent assays. *Virology*, **95**, 415

Index